Surgery of the EYE

Volume I

Surgery of the EYE

Edited by

Stephen R. Waltman, M.D.
Professor, Department of Ophthalmology
Washington University School of Medicine
St. Louis, Missouri

Bartley R. Frueh, M.D.
Professor, Department of Ophthalmology
University of Michigan Medical School
Director, Eye Plastic and Orbital Surgery
Kellogg Eye Center
Ann Arbor, Michigan

Richard H. Keates, M.D.
Professor, Department of Ophthalmology
Ohio State University College of Medicine
Columbus, Ohio

Jonathan Herschler, M.D.
Director, Glaucoma Service
Oregon Lions Sight and Hearing Institute
Portland, Oregon

Creig S. Hoyt, M.D.
Professor of Ophthalmology and Pediatrics
University of California, San Francisco School of Medicine
San Francisco, California

Denis M. Carroll, M.D.
Assistant Clinical Professor, Department of Ophthalmology
University of Arizona College of Medicine
Tucson, Arizona

Illustrators

Diane Abeloff, M.A., A.M.I.
Craig A. Luce, M.S., A.M.I.
Sam Potthoff
Christine Gralap, M.A., A.M.I.
Betsy Palay, M.S., A.M.I.
Elizabeth Roselius, M.S., A.M.I.

Churchill Livingstone
New York, Edinburgh, London, Melbourne 1988

Library of Congress Cataloging in Publication Data

Surgery of the eye.

Includes bibliographies and index.
1. Eye—Surgery. I. Waltman, Stephen R. (Stephen Reeves), date. [DNLM: 1. Eye—surgery.
2. Surgery, Plastic—methods. WW 168 S9607]
RE80.S84 1988 617.7'1 87-18314
ISBN 0-443-08354-1

Distributed in the United Kingdom by Churchill Livingstone, Robert Stevenson House, 1-3 Baxter's Place, Leith Walk, Edinburgh EH1 3AF, and by associated companies, branches, and representatives throughout the world.

Accurate indications, adverse reactions, and dosage schedules for drugs are provided in this book, but it is possible that they may change. The reader is urged to review the package information data of the manufacturers of the medications mentioned.

Sponsoring Editor: *Linda Panzarella*
Copy Editor: *Ann Ruzycka*
Production Supervisor: *Sharon Tuder*

Printed in the United States of America

First published in 1988

Contributors

Thomas M. Aaberg, M.D.
Marjorie and Joseph F. Heil Professor of Ophthalmology, Department of Ophthalmology, Medical College of Wisconsin, Milwaukee, Wisconsin

Gary W. Abrams, M.D.
Professor, Department of Ophthalmology, Medical College of Wisconsin, Milwaukee, Wisconsin

Melvin G. Alper, M.D.
Clinical Professor of Ophthalmology and Neurological Surgery, Department of Ophthalmology, George Washington University School of Medicine and Health Sciences; Senior Attending Ophthalmologist and Chairman, Neuro-Ophthalmology Unit, Washington Hospital Center, Washington, D.C.

Hugh Beckman, M.D.
Clinical Associate Professor, Department of Ophthalmology, Kresge Eye Institute, Wayne State University School of Medicine; Chairman, Department of Ophthalmology, Sinai Hospital of Detroit, Detroit, Michigan

Frank A. Billson, M.D.
Professor, Department of Ophthalmology, The University of Sydney, Sydney Eye Hospital, Wooloomooloo, Australia

A. C. Bird, M.D., F.R.C.S.
Professor of Clinical Ophthalmology, Institute of Ophthalmology, University of London, London, England

George F. Buerger, Jr., M.D.
Clinical Associate Professor, Department of Ophthalmology, University of Pittsburgh School of Medicine; Medical Staff, Eye and Ear Hospital of Pittsburgh; Medical Staff, Department of Ophthalmology, Eye and Ear Institute of Pittsburgh, Pittsburgh, Pennsylvania

John A. Burns, M.D.
Clinical Professor, Department of Ophthalmology, Ohio State University College of Medicine; Grant Medical Center; Ophthalmic Surgeons and Consultants of Ohio, Incorporated, Columbus, Ohio

Kenneth V. Cahill, M.D.
Clinical Assistant Professor, Department of Ophthalmology, Ohio State University College of Medicine; Grant Medical Center; Ophthalmic Surgeons and Consultants of Ohio, Incorporated, Columbus, Ohio

N. Branson Call, M.D.
Chief, Division of Oculoplastics, Veterans Administration Hospital; Associate, Rocky Mountain Eye Center, Salt Lake City, Utah

Denis M. Carroll, M.D.
Assistant Clinical Professor, Department of Ophthalmology, University of Arizona College of Medicine, Tucson, Arizona

Steve Charles, M.D.
Chief, Vitreoretinal Service, Department of Ophthalmology, University of Tennessee Center for Health Sciences, Memphis, Tennessee

I. H. Chisholm, M.B., F.R.C.S.
Moorfields Eye Hospital, London, England; Consultant Ophthalmologist, Southampton Eye Hospital, Southampton, England

Frank H. Christensen, M.D.
Clinical Associate Professor, Department of Ophthalmology, University of North Carolina at Chapel Hill School of Medicine, Chapel Hill, North Carolina

Ian J. Constable, M.D.
Professor, Department of Ophthalmology, Royal Perth Hospital; Director, Lions Eye Institute, Perth, Australia

Joseph L. Dowling, Jr., M.D.
Associate Clinical Professor of Surgery/Ophthalmology, Brown University Program in Medicine, Providence, Rhode Island

Robert M. Dryden, M.D.
Adjunct Associate Professor, Department of Ophthalmology, University of Arizona College of Medicine, Tucson, Arizona

Michael K. Farley, M.D.
Jules Stein Eye Institute, University of California Center for Health Sciences, Los Angeles, California

Douglas P. Felt, M.D.
Private Practice, Odgen, Utah

Joseph C. Flanagan, M.D.
Professor, Department of Ophthalmology, Jefferson Medical College of Thomas Jefferson University; Director, Oculoplastic Surgery, Wills Eye Hospital; Associate in Ophthalmology, Lankenau Hospital, Philadelphia, Pennsylvania; Consultant in Oculoplastic Surgery, Mercy Catholic Medical Center of Southeast Pennsylvania, Darby, Pennsylvania

Bartley R. Frueh, M.D.
Professor, Department of Ophthalmology, University of Michigan Medical School; Director, Eye Plastic and Orbital Surgery, Kellogg Eye Center, Ann Arbor, Michigan

James L. Hargiss, M.D., M.Sc.(Med.)
Consultant in Oculoplastic Surgery, University of Washington School of Medicine, Seattle, Washington

Jonathan Herschler, M.D.
Director, Glaucoma Service, Oregon Lions Sight and Hearing Institute, Portland, Oregon

Tatsuo Hirose, M.D.
Associate Clinical Professor, Department of Ophthalmology, Harvard Medical School; Associate Surgeon, Massachusetts Eye and Ear Infirmary; Eye Research Institute of the Retina Foundation; Retina Associates, Boston, Massachusetts

H. Dunbar Hoskins, Jr., M.D.
Clinical Professor, Department of Ophthalmology, University of California, San Francisco, School of Medicine; Vice President, Foundation for Glaucoma Research, San Francisco, California

Creig S. Hoyt, M.D.
Professor of Ophthalmology and Pediatrics, University of California, San Francisco, School of Medicine, San Francisco, California

Leonard Joffe, M.D., F.C.S.(S.A.), F.R.C.S.Ed.
Clinical Assistant Professor, Department of Ophthalmology, University of Arizona College of Medicine, Tucson, Arizona

Stephen H. Johnson, M.D.
Assistant Clinical Professor, Department of Ophthalmology, University of California, Irvine, College of Medicine, Irvine, California

James F. Kapustiak, M.D.
Provisional Associate Staff, Christ Hospital and Medical Center, Oak Lawn, Illinois

Michael A. Kass, M.D.
Professor, Department of Ophthalmology, Washington University School of Medicine, St. Louis, Missouri

Herbert E. Kaufman, M.D.
Boyd Professor of Ophthalmology, and Pharmacology and Experimental Therapeutics, and Head, Department of Ophthalmology, Louisiana State University Medical Center School of Medicine, New Orleans; Director, LSU Eye Center, New Orleans, Louisiana

Richard H. Keates, M.D.
Professor, Department of Ophthalmology, Ohio State University College of Medicine, Columbus, Ohio

Stephen P. Kraft, M.D., F.R.C.S.C.
Assistant Professor, Department of Ophthalmology, University of Toronto Faculty of Medicine; Staff Ophthalmologist, The Hospital for Sick Children and Toronto General Hospital, Toronto, Ontario, Canada

Richard P. Kratz, M.D.
Clinical Professor, Department of Ophthalmology, University of California, Irvine, College of Medicine, Irvine, California; Clinical Professor of Ophthalmology, University of California, Los Angeles, UCLA School of Medicine, Los Angeles, California

Theodore Krupin, M.D.
Professor, Department of Ophthalmology, University of Pennsylvania School of Medicine; Scheie Eye Institute, Philadelphia, Pennsylvania

Dwight R. Kulwin, M.D.
Associate Professor, Department of Ophthalmology, Holmes Hospital, University of Cincinnati College of Medicine, Cincinnati, Ohio

Mark R. Levine, M.D.
Associate Clinical Professor, Department of Ophthalmology, Case Western Reserve University School of Medicine; Chief, Department of Ophthalmology, Mt. Sinai Medical Center; Director of Oculoplastic Service, University Hospitals of Cleveland, Cleveland, Ohio

Hunter L. Little, M.D.
Clinical Professor of Surgery/Ophthalmology, Stanford University School of Medicine; Stanford University Medical Center, Stanford, California

Richard L. McCammon, M.D.
Associate Professor, Department of Anesthesiology, Indiana University School of Medicine, Indianapolis, Indiana

Marguerite B. McDonald, M.D.
Associate Professor, Department of Ophthalmology, Louisiana State University Medical Center School of Medicine, New Orleans, LSU Eye Center, New Orleans, Louisiana

David J. McIntyre, M.D.
Consultant, Department of Ophthalmology, University of Washington School of Medicine, Seattle, Washington

Henry S. Metz, M.D.
Professor and Chairman, Department of Ophthalmology, University of Rochester School of Medicine and Dentistry, Rochester, New York

Donald S. Minckler, M.D.
Professor, Department of Ophthalmology, University of Southern California School of Medicine; Chief, Glaucoma Services, Estelle Doheny Eye Foundation, Los Angeles, California

William D. Myers, M.D.
Assistant Clinical Professor, Department of Ophthalmology, Michigan State University School of Human Medicine, East Lansing, Michigan; Director, Michigan Eye Institute, Southfield, Michigan

Thaddeus Nowinski, M.D.
Clinical Assistant Professor, Department of Ophthalmology, Jefferson Medical College of Thomas Jefferson University; Oculoplastics Department, Wills Eye Hospital, Philadelphia, Pennsylvania

Edward Okun, M.D.
Clinical Professor, Department of Ophthalmology, Washington University School of Medicine; Retina Consultants, Ltd., St. Louis, Missouri

J. Justin Older, M.D.
Associate Professor and Director, Oculoplastic Service, Department of Ophthalmology, University of South Florida College of Medicine, Tampa, Florida

Paul F. Olson, M.D.
Clinical Instructor, Department of Ophthalmology, University of California, Irvine, College of Medicine, Irvine, California

Frank M. Polack, M.D.
Adjunct Professor, Departments of Ophthalmology and Anatomy, University of Florida College of Medicine; Adjunct Clinical Professor, Department of Comparative Ophthalmology, University of Florida College of Veterinary Medicine; Attending Ophthalmologist, Alachua General Hospital and North Florida Regional Hospital, Gainesville, Florida; Medical Director, Medical Eye Bank of Orlando, Orlando, Florida

Allen M. Putterman, M.D.
Clinical Professor, Department of Ophthalmology, and Chief, Oculoplastic Service at the University of Illinois College of Medicine Eye and Ear Infirmary; Senior Attending Ophthalmologist and Director, Oculoplastic Surgery, Michael Reese Hospital and Medical Center, and the University of Chicago Hospitals, Chicago, Illinois

J. Earl Rathbun, M.D.
Associate Clinical Professor, Department of Ophthalmology, University of California, San Francisco, School of Medicine; Consultant, Ophthalmic Plastic and Reconstructive Surgery, Ft. Miley Veterans Administration Hospital, San Francisco, California

William E. Scott, M.D.
Professor, Department of Ophthalmology, University of Iowa College of Medicine; Director, Pediatric Ophthalmology and Strabismus, Department of Ophthalmology, University of Iowa Hospitals and Clinics, Iowa City, Iowa

Philip A. Shelton, M.D., J.D.
Assistant Clinical Professor of Surgery/Ophthalmology, University of Connecticut School of Medicine; Health Law Counsel, Tarlow, Levy, Mandell, and Kostin, P.C.,

Farmington, Connecticut; Senior Staff Attending Ophthalmologist, Hartford Hospital, Hartford, Connecticut; Eye Physician Associates of Hartford, West Hartford, Connecticut

Richard J. Simmons, M.D.
Associate Clinical Professor, Department of Ophthalmology, Harvard Medical School; Director, New England Glaucoma Research Foundation, Boston, Massachusetts

Omah S. Singh, M.D.
Incorporator and Chairwoman of the Institutional Review Board of the New England Glaucoma Research Foundation, Boston, Massachusetts

Alfred M. Solish, M.D.
Assistant Clinical Professor, Department of Ophthalmology, University of California, Los Angeles, UCLA School of Medicine; Director, Glaucoma Service, Wadsworth Veterans Administration Hospital, Los Angeles, California

George L. Spaeth, M.D.
Professor, Department of Ophthalmology, Jefferson Medical College of Thomas Jefferson University; Director, William and Anne Goldberg Glaucoma Service and Research Laboratories, Wills Eye Hospital, Philadelphia, Pennsylvania

Charles M. Stephenson, Sr., M.D.
Clinical Professor and Director, Ophthalmic Plastic Reconstructive and Orbital Surgery, Loma Linda University School of Medicine, Loma Linda, California; Associate Clinical Professor, Department of Ophthalmology, University of California, San Diego, School of Medicine, San Diego, California

William B. Stewart, M.D.
Director, Ophthalmic Plastic Reconstructive and Orbital Surgery, Department of Ophthalmology, Pacific-Presbyterian Medical Center, San Francisco, California

John H. Sullivan, M.D.
Associate Clinical Professor, Department of Ophthalmology, University of California, San Francisco, School of Medicine, San Francisco, California

Casimir A. Swinger, M.D.
Assistant Clinical Professor, Department of Ophthalmology, Mount Sinai School of Medicine of the City University of New York; Beth Israel Medical Center, New York, New York

Jerald L. Tennant, M.D.
Director, Dallas Eye Institute, Duncanville, Texas

William M. Townsend, M.D.
Associate Professor, Department of Ophthalmology, and Chief, Cornea Service, University of Puerto Rico School of Medicine, San Juan, Puerto Rico

Richard C. Troutman, M.D.
Professor Emeritus, Department of Ophthalmology, State University of New York Health Science Center at Brooklyn College of Medicine, Brooklyn, New York; Clinical Professor, Cornell University Medical College; Surgeon Director, Manhattan Eye, Ear and Throat Hospital, New York, New York

Stephen R. Waltman, M.D.
Professor, Department of Ophthalmology, Washington University School of Medicine, St. Louis, Missouri

Robert C. Watzke, M.D.
Professor, Department of Ophthalmology, and Chairman, Retina and Vitreous Services, Department of Ophthalmology, Oregon Health Sciences University School of Medicine, Portland, Oregon

Jacob Wilensky, M.D.
Clinical Professor, Department of Ophthalmology, University of Illinois College of Medicine; Director, Glaucoma Service, Eye and Ear Infirmary, Chicago, Illinois

John L. Wobig, M.D.
Associate Clinical Professor, Department of Ophthalmology, Oregon Health Sciences University School of Medicine, Portland, Oregon

Ted H. Wojno, M.D.
Assistant Professor, Department of Ophthalmology, Emory University School of Medicine; Head, Section of Oculoplastic and Orbital Surgery, The Emory Clinic, Atlanta, Georgia; Chief, Department of Ophthalmology, The Veterans Administration Medical Center, Decatur, Georgia

Allan E. Wulc, M.D.
Associate Professor, Department of Ophthalmology, Orbital Service, Scheie Eye Institute, University of Pennsylvania School Medicine, Philadelphia, Pennsylvania

Charles S. Zwerling, M.D., F.A.C.S., F.I.C.S.
Clinical Associate Professor, Department of Ophthalmology, University of North Carolina at Chapel Hill School of Medicine, Chapel Hill, North Carolina; Medical Director, Goldsboro Eye Clinic, Ltd., Goldsboro, North Carolina

Preface

Recent advances and refinements in ophthalmic surgical techniques now permit ophthalmic surgeons to greatly improve the quality of life of many patients with ocular disorders. The use of modern techniques of keratoplasty and cataract surgery results in rapid and dramatic improvements in visual acuity with low complication rates. Ophthalmic plastic and strabismus surgery usually provides functional and cosmetic improvement in most patients. Retinal and glaucoma surgery may restore or prolong useful vision in patients with severe ocular disorders. Recent advances in refractive surgery may allow patients to become less dependent on optical devices and therefore to function better in the tasks of daily life.

It is our purpose to provide a single text that elucidates the most commonly utilized ophthalmic surgical techniques and serves as an authoritative reference work for ophthalmic surgery. Within each section of the text, all of the various procedures likely to be performed by an ophthalmic surgeon are covered. There is no substitute for actual surgical experience, but the detail provided within each section is sufficient to allow a competent, well-trained ophthalmic surgeon to review and perform most common procedures. Sufficient information is provided so that he or she can undertake rarer procedures or be familiar with their details should referral to a subspecialist become necessary.

For each procedure the pertinent anatomy and techniques available for correction of the deformity are described. Each author, who is an expert within the field, then describes his or her preferred technique, and points out some of the common variations of it. Methods to avoid complications and to deal with intraoperative and postoperative deviations from expected results are described. Having each chapter written by an expert in the field with extensive experience allows the reader to share their experiences on a more personal basis. By so doing, we hope to raise the level of knowledge and understanding of each procedure and allow ophthalmic surgeons to be more comfortable and competent in undertaking them.

We express our appreciation to Linda Panzarella and Ann Ruzycka of Churchill Livingstone for their tireless assistance during all stages of this project.

Stephen R. Waltman, M.D.
Richard H. Keates, M.D.
Creig S. Hoyt, M.D.
Bartley R. Frueh, M.D.
Jonathan Herschler, M.D.
Denis M. Carroll, M.D.

Contents

Section I

GENERAL CONSIDERATIONS

Stephen R. Waltman

Section Editor

Ophthalmic Anesthesia

1

Richard L. McCammon

The primary goal of this chapter is to present an anesthesiologist's perspective of a number of common problems confronted by the ophthalmologist and anesthesiologist in caring for patients undergoing ophthalmic surgery. It is not the intention of this chapter to present a cookbook approach to ophthalmic anesthesia, nor is it meant to be a mere anecdotal report on how these cases are performed at my institution. Rarely is one anesthetic technique clearly right or wrong, nor is one anesthetic technique necessarily applicable to every patient.

Rather, this chapter discusses (1) the relative safety of local versus general anesthesia in patients undergoing ophthalmic surgery; (2) the preoperative evaluation of patients with particular emphasis on commonly encountered systemic illnesses in elderly patients and congenital anomalies and metabolic disorders in children; (3) the preoperative preparation of patients as regards choice of premedicants as well as what to do with their current systemic and ophthalmic medications; and (4) the choice of anesthesia. The advantages and disadvantages, complications, and side effects of local or regional versus general anesthesia are highlighted. Finally, problems unique to specific ophthalmic procedures are reviewed.

RISKS OF LOCAL VERSUS GENERAL ANESTHESIA IN PATIENTS UNDERGOING OPHTHALMIC SURGERY

The general requirements for ophthalmic anesthesia include (1) akinesia (immobility of the eye, including the extraocular and orbicularis muscles); (2) attainment of low to low-normal intraocular pressures (IOP), particularly prior to opening the globe; (3) avoidance of any intraoperative event that would result in loss of ocular contents once the globe is opened; (4) minimal bleeding; and (5) analgesia. In addition, anesthesiologists and their equipment must be positioned remotely from the patient's airway, the oculocardiac reflex must be anticipated at all times, and a smooth emergence from anesthesia must be an ever-sought-after ideal.

These requirements, along with the age, physical, and mental status of the patient, the type and length of the planned surgical procedure, the skills and temperaments of both the ophthalmologist and the anesthesiologist, and the desires of the patient, enter into the decision as to choice of anesthetic.

Ultimately, patient safety is the prime consideration. A central question is therefore: Is there a difference in morbidity and mortality rates or in incidences of ocular morbidity between local and general anesthesia in patients undergoing ophthalmic surgery? Mortality data in ophthalmology come from both retrospective questionnaire studies and anecdotal reporting of experience at various institutions. For example, Gartner and Billet in 1958 reported the results of a survey covering the years 1946 to 1956, in which 577 of 922 ophthalmologists polled responded.[1] Although a mortality rate could not be gleaned from this report, certain conclusions could be drawn. For example, most deaths occurred in children. This reflects, however, an era in which the methods, equipment, and personnel involved with delivery of anesthesia made anesthesia an all too risky affair for this age group. Likewise, the low numbers of deaths in adults in this report reflect a period in which extensive procedures on the vitreous or retina were not performed and a time when practically all adult operations were done under local anesthesia.

Duncalf et al.[2] subsequently surveyed all members of the American Society of Ophthalmology regarding cases done in 1967. Forty-nine percent of those surveyed responded (197,000 cases), and the noted mortality rate was approximately equal between local (0.62 per 1,000) and general (0.65 per 1,000) anesthesia. Again, most deaths occurred in children.

The earliest of the anecdotal reports were from Quigley,[3] Petruscak et al.,[4] and Kaplan and Reba.[5] For example, Quigley reported 49 deaths in 47,001 ophthalmic cases believed to be related to the events of surgery and anesthesia over the period 1952 to 1972 (0.10 percent mortality rate). The leading causes of death in order of frequency were pulmonary embolism, myocardial infarction, cerebrovascular accident (CVA), and anesthesia-related. Although mortality rates for local and general anesthesia were the same, Quigley correctly concludes that this should not be taken to prove necessarily that both are equally safe. In this study, as in most, the comparability of the two groups—those given local versus those given general anesthesia—is dubious at best.

Petruscak and co-workers[4] analyzed the period 1962 to 1971 and reported 19 deaths in 32,322 ophthalmic procedures. The overall mortality ratio in this study was 0.35 per 1,000 for general anesthesia and 0.69 per 1,000 for local anesthesia. The most common cause of death in this study was a perioperative myocardial infarction; the most important factor contributing to death was the preexisting medical condition of the patient.

Kaplan and Reba[5] reported a mortality rate of 0.14 percent (30 deaths in 21,400 cases) at their institution between 1958 and 1970. These investigators were able to have autopsied 19 of the 30 patients, nine of whom were noted to have sustained a pulmonary embolus (only two of these had been suspected clinically). This study as well as Quigley's serve as a reminder of this ever-present complication.

A more recent report comes from Backer et al.,[6] who reported two deaths in 10,278 cases between 1962 and 1977 (0.05 percent mortality rate).[6] Almost all these operations were done using local or retrobulbar blocks, or both. Of special consideration is the fact that 195 of these patients, who underwent 288 separate operations, had previously suffered a documented myocardial infarction. Not a single reinfarction or death occurred in this group. Two hundred fifty-five other patients with known coronary artery disease, but without a history or evidence of a previous infarction, underwent 373 separate procedures. Two of these patients suffered a postoperative infarction, although neither died. Two other patients died suddenly 4 and 7 days postoperatively, but an autopsy was not performed. It should also be noted that 21 patients with a prior infarction underwent 26 separate procedures under general anesthesia during this same period. No reinfarction occurred in this group either. Because of the small size of the group who underwent general anesthesia, Backer and colleagues correctly concluded they could not categorically state that local is safer than general anesthesia in these patients. They do correctly note, however, that their reported reinfarction rate (0 percent) in patients undergoing ophthalmic surgery under local anesthesia is much lower than in similar patients undergoing nonophthalmic surgery of similar duration.[7]

Lang et al.[8] recently reported on 14,889 procedures done at the Massachusettes Eye and Ear Infirmary between 1977 and 1979. The distribution between local and general anesthesia was about even. These investigators reported only two deaths. One patient died of septicemia following drainage of an advanced lacrimal gland infection, and a diabetic with severe complications died suddenly 20 hours postoperatively of unknown causes. The most common complications included urinary retention and nonfatal cardiac complications, including myocardial infarction and arrhythmias. At variance with previous studies was the low incidence of pulmonary embolism. This was attributed to the use of elastic stockings and early ambulation.

Interestingly, available data comparing local and general anesthesia have not demonstrated a significant difference in rates of ocular morbidity (vitreous loss, iris or lens prolapse, or wound dehiscence) between the two techniques.[9,10] I personally find this intriguing in light of the fact that most studies indicate a higher incidence of nausea and vomiting following general anesthesia—events likely to increase the chance of a poor result.

What, if any, conclusions can be drawn from this array of data? First, it becomes evident that no definitive answer exists. None of the existing studies permits direct comparison of local versus general anesthesia. There simply are too many variables involved. Nevertheless, it is clear that mortality rates in ophthalmic patients should be very low. It therefore behooves each institution to compare its own data with the findings noted in the series cited. If their own mortality rate is much higher than that noted, a search for the cause(s) is in order.

Second, local anesthesia has proved very safe. There is an interesting side question to this issue: Is standby necessary? This question was examined recently by Meyers et al.[11] In their study, although the incidence of complications intraoperatively was similar in patients undergoing intraocular surgery without or with standby; the complications with standby were not as severe and were more quickly controlled. Although my opinion on this matter is biased, I believe that standby enables surgeons to concentrate on the surgery and not try to divide their attention between the procedure and the patient.

Finally, as newer anesthetic agents and techniques have appeared, better monitoring techniques have developed and, probably most importantly, as more well-trained personnel involved in delivery of anesthesia have emerged, general anesthesia is now much safer. Certainly, the high incidence of deaths in pediatric patients reported in some of the earlier series has been corrected. In elderly patients, the severity of their coexisting systemic diseases still most closely correlates with their risk of general anesthesia.

THE PREOPERATIVE EVALUATION OF SEVERAL COMMON DISEASE STATES FOUND AMONG ADULT OPHTHALMIC PATIENTS

Coronary Artery Disease

Coronary artery disease is one of the most commonly encountered systemic diseases in adult patients presenting for ophthalmic surgery. Patients are often known to have coronary artery disease, since they manifest symptoms of angina pectoris or have a history of a prior myocardial infarction, congestive heart failure, or a coronary artery bypass graft (CABG) procedure. It should be appreciated, however, that "silent" coronary artery disease is very common in elderly patients and must be suspected in any patient with several of the known risk factors for the development of coronary artery disease. In addition to advancing age, these include increased serum cholesterol and glucose concentrations, elevated arterial blood pressure, male sex, cigarette smoking, and a positive family history.

The presence of coronary artery disease in patients undergoing noncardiac surgery is associated with increased morbidity and mortality.[7,12] For example, a history of a prior myocardial infarction dramatically increases the likelihood of perioperative complications. Specifically, the incidence of a perioperative reinfarction does not stabilize until 6 months after the prior infarction. Even then, the incidence approaches 5 to 6 percent, as compared with 0.13 percent in patients without known coronary artery disease. This incidence forms the basis for the recommendation that elective surgery be postponed for at least 6 months following a myocardial infarction.

Nevertheless, these figures paint an overly dismal picture. Most ophthalmic operations are of reasonably short duration and are not as stressful as major surgeries in which body cavities are invaded. As noted in Backer's study,[6] ophthalmic procedures performed on patients with known or suspected coronary artery disease are associated with a relatively low incidence of perioperative infarction. Still, a myocardial infarction remains one of the most common causes of perioperative mortality in ophthalmic patients.

Those factors that are of most concern to an anesthesiologist in evaluating a patient with known or suspected coronary artery disease are as follows[13]: (1) Is there any evidence of congestive heart failure? (2) Has there been any change in the character of the patient's angina pectoris? (3) Is there any coexisting noncardiac disease present? (4) What medications is the patient currently taking?

Indeed, congestive heart failure has been shown to be the single most important determinant contributing to postoperative cardiac morbidity.[14] Thus, no patient with symptoms or signs suggestive of congestive heart failure should undergo elective surgery. Likewise, anginal pain produced with less activity than usual or lasting for more prolonged periods than usual is considered characteristic of unstable angina pectoris and may signal an impending myocardial infarction. In addition, patients with coronary artery disease are likely to have several coexisting noncardiac diseases, including severe peripheral vascular disease, chronic obstructive lung disease (COLD), renal dysfunction, and diabetes mellitus. These diseases must also be adequately evaluated along with the impact they have on the conduct of anesthesia appreciated.

The drugs most likely encountered in patients with coronary artery disease are the nitrates, β-adrenoceptor antagonists, and calcium-channel blocking agents. In addition, these patients may be receiving antihypertensives, diuretics, and digitalis. Most anesthesiologists prefer to maintain these drugs during the perioperative period. In fact, in view of the short half-life of many of these medications, the usual morning doses of these medications should be administered with the premedicants. Not only is the overwhelming evidence in the literature that this practice is safe in light of better anesthetic drugs and monitoring techniques,[15–17] but abrupt withdrawal of drugs such as the β-adrenoceptor antagonists or calcium-channel blockers may be associated with myocardial infarction, arrhythmias, and sudden death as well.[18] Evidence of adverse or side effects of β-adrenoceptor antagonists such as high-grade atrioventricular (AV) block, congestive heart failure, and bronchospasm should, however, be sought preoperatively.

Likewise, digitalis should be maintained if the patient is receiving it for recent or recurrent bouts of congestive heart failure or for control of the ventricular response to atrial tachydysrhythmias. Here again, evidence of digitalis toxicity must be sought preoperatively. Gastrointestinal symptoms such as anorexia and nausea are common. Similarly, numerous arrhythmias may occur in association with digitalis toxicity.[19]

Hypertension

Hypertension is also a very common coexisting medical problem confronted in ophthalmic patients. Of primary concern to the anesthesiologist are the degree of blood pressure control achieved and the presence and extent of deleterious effects the hypertension has produced on the brain, heart, and kidneys. Regarding the latter, the anesthesiologist is primarily concerned if there is any evidence of congestive heart failure, coronary or carotid arterial disease, and the degree of renal dysfunction. This should be ascertained from the history, physical, and appropriate laboratory testing.

Commonly used antihypertensive medications are listed in Table 1-1. The key question that has been discussed extensively in the literature is whether these drugs should be discontinued preoperatively.[20–23] On the basis of available information, most anesthesiologists believe that antihypertensive drug therapy (excepting monamine oxidase inhibitors) should be continued up to and including the morning of surgery and restarted as soon as possible postoperatively. In fact, sudden withdrawal of β-adrenoceptor antagonists (i.e., propranolol) or clonidine has been associated with severe rebound hypertension and significant adverse sequelae.[18,24]

An often confronted question is how well controlled the patient's blood pressure must be before

Table 1-1. Chronic Oral Antihypertensive Therapy

Site of Action[a]	Total Daily Dose	Frequency of Dose
Central sympatholytic drugs		
Reserpine (Serpasil)	0.1–0.25 mg	Daily
Methyldopa (Aldomet)	0.5–2 g	2–4/day
Clonidine (Catapres)	0.2–0.8 mg	2–3/day
Peripheral sympatholytic drug		
Guanethidine (Ismelin)	25–100 mg	Daily
β-Adrenergic blocking drugs		
Propranolol (Inderal)	120–360 mg	2–3/day
Metoprolol (Lopressor)	100–400 mg	2/day
Nadolol (Corgard)	40–320 mg	Daily
Atenolol (Tenormin)	50–100 mg	Daily
α-Adrenergic blocking drugs		
Prazosin (Minipress)	3–20 mg	3/day
Dilators of vascular smooth muscle		
Hydralazine (Apresoline)	40–200 mg	4/day
Minoxidil (Loniten)	10– 40 mg	1–3/day

[a] Generic name is followed by proprietary name (in parentheses).

allowing elective surgery. Ideally, all patients with essential hypertension should be rendered normotensive prior to performance of an elective operation. As a general statement, most anesthesiologists would agree that the incidence of perioperative hypotension, hypertension, and myocardial ischemia is greater in hypertensive than in normotensive patients. However, there is no evidence that the incidence of cardiac complications is increased when hypertensive patients undergo elective surgery as long as the preoperative diastolic blood pressure does not exceed 110 mmHg and *if* appropriate therapeutic interventions are made perioperatively.[25] It should be appreciated, however, that the better the control preoperatively, the less the incidence of hemodynamic events requiring treatment (both hypotensive and hypertensive episodes) intraoperatively and postoperatively.

Pulmonary Disease

The salient features in the preoperative evaluation of the patient with chronic obstructive lung disease (emphysema or chronic bronchitis) are to determine the severity of the disease and to elucidate any reversible components such as infection or bronchospasm.[26] It is firmly established that preoperative recognition and treatment of these reversible components will lessen the incidence of postoperative pulmonary complications.[27] It is also important to inquire regarding the patient's ability to lie supine and the severity of any accompanying cough as regards decision-making processes of local versus general anesthesia. Certainly if the patient is receiving bronchodilating medications for a reversible bronchospastic component of chronic lung disease or for asthma, these medications should be maintained during the perioperative period.

Diabetes Mellitus

Diabetes mellitus is the most common endocrine disease encountered in patients presenting for ophthalmic surgery. Several factors are of concern to the anesthesiologist in the preoperative evaluation: (1) type of diabetes (juvenile-onset versus maturity onset); (2) type of medications the patient is receiving (oral hypoglycemics or an insulin preparation); (3) degree of control of the diabetes; and (4) presence and significance of complications of diabetes mellitus.[28]

Juvenile-onset diabetics usually require insulin to prevent ketoacidosis, whereas maturity-onset diabetics, although they may require exogenous insulin, are not susceptible to ketosis. Clearly, no diabetic patient should be allowed to undergo elective surgery in the presence of marked hyperglycemia (i.e., >400 mg %) or ketosis.

There are two basic goals in the management of anesthesia for the patient with diabetes. First, hypoglycemia must be prevented. This is generally ensured by providing an adequate supply of exogenous glucose. Second, ketoacidosis, with asso-

Table 1-2. Commercially Available Preparations of Insulin

Preparation	Onset (hr)	Peak Effect (hr)	Duration (hr)
Short acting			
Crystalline	1	2–4	6–8
Semilente	1.5	5–7	12–18
Intermediate acting			
NPH	1–2	10–20	20–24
Lente	1–2	14–18	20–24
Prolonged			
Protamine	6–8	16–24	24–36
Ultralente	6–8	22–26	24–36

ciated hyperglycemia, dehydration, and electrolyte abnormalities, must be avoided. This may require the administration of exogenous insulin. Many successful routines have been reported in the literature for accomplishing these goals.[29,30] It behooves the ophthalmologist to ensure that a physician is assigned to take charge and follow through on a perioperative plan—the ophthalmologist, the anesthesiologist, or the patient's internist.

The key to any of the described techniques is to appreciate the pharmacology of the oral hypoglycemics and insulin preparations (Table 1-2), monitor the blood glucose concentration periodically, respond to abnormalities with either more glucose or more insulin, and continue to manage the patient during the postoperative period until the patient resumes a normal caloric intake and prior medications.

Myasthenia Gravis

Patients with myasthenia gravis often present for ophthalmic surgery. Myasthenia gravis is a chronic disease involving the neuromuscular junction.[31] The hallmark of the disease is weakness and rapid fatigability of voluntary muscles with repetitive use, followed by partial recovery with rest.

Myasthenia gravis may be classified on the basis of the muscles involved and the severity of symptoms. There are milder forms in which involvement is limited to the extraocular muscles. By contrast, other more severe types progress to involve basically all muscle groups, including the muscles involved with respiration as well as pharyngeal and laryngeal muscles. Patients in the latter group are thus susceptible to respiratory insufficiency and are at risk of aspiration.

The primary drugs used in therapy of this condition are the anticholinesterases and corticosteroids. Neostigmine and pyridostigmine are the anticholinesterase drugs most often selected to treat myasthenia. These drugs are effective because they inhibit the enzyme responsible for the hydrolysis of acetylcholine (ACh). This serves to increase the amount of neurotransmitter available at the neuromuscular junction and thus improve muscle strength.

Excessive anticholinesterase effect may result in drug-induced weakness, known as a cholinergic crisis. The presence of muscarinic side effects (salivation, miosis, bradycardia) plus accentuated muscle weakness confirms this diagnosis. Likewise, many of these patients are on the corticosteroid prednisone. Presumably, corticosteroids interfere with production of antibodies responsible for degradation of cholinergic receptors. Corticosteroids must also be maintained perioperatively.

The pertinent considerations preoperatively are as follows: (1) the effectiveness of drug therapy (how often and severe are either the myasthenic or cholinergic crises); (2) the potential potentiation in response to muscle relaxants given during general anesthesia; and (3) the appreciation of the potential need for ventilator support. In this regard, preoperative medicants should be used with caution, if at all. This also applies to the use of sedatives and tranquilizers given intraoperatively for sedation during local procedures.

THE PREOPERATIVE EVALUATION OF PEDIATRIC PATIENTS

Most children, regardless of the diagnostic or operative procedure necessitated by their ocular pathology, require general anesthesia. Not infrequently, these children have coexisting congenital syndromes or metabolic disorders. A detailed discussion of the medical and anesthetic considerations for each of these various syndromes is beyond the intended scope of this chapter. For those involved in the care of pediatric ophthalmic problems, several excellent reviews are offered.[32–33]

It is axiomatic that the presence of one anomaly should prompt the physician to search for others. Rather than discuss a few of these syndromes individually, the following discussion addresses some of the general problems common to a number of these syndromes. For example, many of these syndromes are associated with various craniofacial anomalies, such as cleft lip or palate, a high arched palate, a large tongue, and prognathism. The anesthesiologist should be forewarned so that appropriate evaluation of the airway can be performed preoperatively. This allows a plan of attack to be formulated. Such abnormalities also increase the patient's aspiration risk, so that drugs that decrease gastric volume and acidity should be included in the preoperative regimen.

A number of other skeletal malformations are associated with these conditions. These include odontoid hypoplasia, cervical spine fusion, scoliosis, kyphosis, and lumbar lordosis. Such abnormalities further complicate airway management, and the ability to position the patient can be associated with coexisting pulmonary infections and potentially are associated with increased likelihood of postoperative pulmonary insufficiency and infections.

The entire gamut of cyanotic and acyanotic congenital heart lesions may be found in these patients. It is vital to understand that the management of anesthesia for patients with congenital heart disease requires a thorough knowledge of the pathophysiology of each cardiac defect.

Finally, a partial listing of other associated problems includes (1) autonomic nervous system dysfunction (loss of temperature and respiratory control, postural hypotension), (2) various endocrine abnormalities (diabetes mellitus, thyroid dysfunction); (3) CNS disorders (mental retardation, cerebral palsy, patients with seizure histories), (4) renal dysfunction, (5) sickle cell anemia, and (6) a variety of muscular dystrophies. Once again, each of these problems deserves a thorough workup preoperatively and should be evaluated by the anesthesiologist.

PREMEDICATION

It must be emphasized that psychological preparation of patients prior to surgery is as at least as important as pharmacologic premedication. This too begins in the surgeon's office. Interestingly, the incidence and extent of anxiety in patients who are visited preoperatively are reduced as compared with patients receiving only a pharmacologic premedication.[34] A preoperative visit permits evaluation of the patient's overall condition and a thorough description of the planned anesthetic and events to anticipate in the perioperative period.

Nevertheless, patients generally receive some type of pharmacologic premedication. The goals of pharmacologic premedication in ophthalmic patients are multiple and must be individualized to meet each patient's unique requirements. Probably in no other area of anesthesia is there as much variance in the means to accomplish these goals, however. The best drug or drug combination is not known and is most often influenced by the individual physician's previous experience. Other factors affecting premedicant choice include the patient's age, weight, coexisting medical problems, and the planned anesthetic approach.

Commonly accepted goals of pharmacologic premedication include relief of anxiety, sedation, analgesia, and amnesia. In selected instances, an antisialagogue effect (decreased oral and airway secretions) may be desirable. Likewise, in patients who are to undergo general anesthesia, many anesthesiologists prefer to administer with the premedicants, drugs that either elevate gastric fluid pH and/or reduce gastric fluid volume. Similarly, many anesthesiologists believe that pharmacologic premedication facilitates induction of general anesthesia as well as decreases intraoperative anesthetic requirements. In addition, premedicants are given by some in an effort to provide analgesia and prevent nausea and emesis postoperatively. It is this author's opinion, shared by many others, that these latter goals are better achieved with an intravenous injection near the end of anesthesia. Finally, the potential undesirable effects of the drugs

Table 1-3. Drugs and Doses Used for Pharmacologic Premedication

Classification	Drug	Typical Adult Dose	Route of Administration
Barbiturates	Secobarbital	50–150 mg	Oral, IM
	Pentobarbital	50–150 mg	Oral, IM
Narcotics	Morphine	5–15 mg	IM
	Meperidine	50–100 mg	IM
Benzodiazepines	Diazepam	5–10 mg	Oral
	Lorazepam	2–4 mg	Oral, IM
Butyrophenones	Droperidol	2.5–5 mg	IM
Antihistamines	Diphenhydramine	25–75 mg	Oral, IM
	Promethazine	25–50 mg	IM
	Hydroxyzine	50 mg	IM
Anticholinergics	Atropine	0.3–0.6 mg	IM
	Scopolamine	0.3–0.6 mg	IM
	Glycopyrrolate	0.2–0.3 mg	IM
H_2-antagonists	Cimetidine	300 mg	Oral, IM, IV
	Ranitidine	150 mg	Oral
Antacids	Particulate	15–30 ml	Oral
	Nonparticulate	15–30 ml	Oral
Stimulants of gastric motility	Metoclopramide	5–10 mg	Oral, IM, IV

available must always be appreciated and weighed against their desirable effects.

Table 1-3 lists the commonly used premedicants, their typical dosages, and the routes of administration. The following discussion highlights the relative advantages and disadvantages of these various classes of drugs, with particular emphasis on points relating to ophthalmic patients. Although choice of premedicants usually falls within the realm of the anesthesiologist's responsibility in patients scheduled for general anesthesia or local standby, it behooves the ophthalmologist to understand the relative merits of the various drug classes.

Barbiturates

Advantages of barbiturates as used for pharmacologic premedication include sedation, minimal ventilatory depression as evidenced by an unchanged response to carbon dioxide,[35] minimal circulatory depression, rarity of nausea and vomiting, and effectiveness when administered orally. Disadvantages in the use of barbiturates for premedication in ophthalmic surgery include a lack of analgesia (in fact, disorientation and an anti-analgesic effect in the presence of pain have been reported), a variable sedative effect, little anxiolysis, and absence of a specific antagonist. Prolonged sedation and confusion, combined with the absence of an antagonist, may be particularly troublesome in an elderly ophthalmic patient.

Narcotics

The use of narcotics as part of the premedicant regimen in ophthalmic patients is highly controversial. Although most ophthalmic operations are not associated with tremendous pain, the analgesic effect of narcotics may prove beneficial in a patient who has eye pain preoperatively or in whom a painful regional block is planned. Similarly, if a narcotic–nitrous oxide general anesthetic technique (balanced anesthesia) is planned, a narcotic premedicant may be a reasonable choice. In addition, many patients experience a euphoric effect after receiving a narcotic. The latter may prove extremely beneficial in the highly anxious patient scheduled under local anesthesia.

By contrast other anesthesiologists and ophthalmologists believe that the potential for nausea and vomiting that may follow administration of any narcotic relatively contraindicate their use in patients undergoing ophthalmic sugery. This can be a real problem for which there is no ready treatment other than oxygen, reassurance, and time. Perhaps a middle-of-the-road approach would be that when the advantages of a narcotic premedicant are thought to be great, an antiemetic drug such as phenergan should be included in the premedicant regimen.

Finally, it must be appreciated that certainly other adverse effects are associated with narcotics that the ophthalmologist should be aware of. The most significant of these are depression of the medullary respiratory center as evidenced by hypoventilation and carbon dioxide retention and orthostatic hypotension secondary to venodilatation. In addition, the euphoric effect of narcotics may be dysphoria in occasional patients. Finally, narcotic-induced smooth muscle constriction may cause choledochoduodenal sphincter spasm manifesting as right upper quadrant abdominal pain similar to an attack of acute cholecystitis.[36] This effect, as well as the respiratory depression, can be reversed by naloxone.

Benzodiazepines

Diazepam and lorazepam are widely used sedative-hypnotics that also produce selective antianxiety effects at doses that generally do not produce excessive sedation or cardiopulmonary depression. These drugs, and particularly lorazepam, also produce a suppression of recall of events that occur during the period following their administration. As with the barbiturates, the primary disadvantage of benzodiazepines as used for premedication is the occasional production of excessive or prolonged sedation for which there is no reliable antagonist. There is no good evidence in human that doses of benzodiazepines as used for premedication reduce the likelihood of local anesthetic toxicity.[37]

In the case of diazepam, the drug is better absorbed orally, achieving higher blood levels than when given intramuscularly.[38] Intravenously administered diazepam may be associated with pain on injection and often causes phlebitis. By contrast, lorazepam is equally well absorbed after intramuscular or oral administration. Furthermore, lorazepam metabolites are inactive in contrast to the significant pharmacologic activity of the major metabolite of diazepam, *n*-desmethyl diazepam.

Butyrophenones

The use of the butyrophenone droperidol for premedication is limited because of the occasional production of dysphoria following its administration.[39] Other potential disadvantages include its production of dopaminergic receptor block, which may produce extrapyramidal symptoms, and the mild α-adrenoceptor blockade, which may lead to hypotension. Advocates of its use cite its potential antiemetic effect as a strong indication for its inclusion in the premedicant regimen.

Antihistamines

Certainly nausea and vomiting in the perioperative period of ophthalmic surgery are undesirable. Much has been written regarding the effectiveness of various antiemetics. Some authorities believe that a long-acting antiemetic should always be included in the premedicant regimen. They cite good results with the phenothiazine, promethazine, or the antihistamine, hydroxyzine. These drugs also have the quality of producing an additive sedative effect when combined with narcotics without producing an increase in the ventilatory depression.[40] Others, the author being one, believe that these drugs are more effective if given intravenously 20 to 30 minutes prior to the anticipated termination of anesthesia.[41] Droperidol has proved particularly useful in this regard.

Anticholinergics

The most frequent reasons cited for administering an anticholinergic drug are (1) the production of an antisialagogue effect (drying of oral secretions) prior to general anethesia, (2) production of sedative and amnestic effects (scopolamine), and (3) prevention of reflex bradycardia. All three available drugs—atropine, scopolamine, and glycopyrrolate—are effective as antisialagogues, but only scopolamine provides significant sedation and amnesia.[42] Anticholinergics have not proved efficacious in attenuating bradycardia associated with the oculocardiac reflex when given intramuscularly as part of premedicant regimen (see the section on the oculocardiac reflex).

The need for including an anticholinergic drug in the premedicant to produce an antisialagogue effect has been questioned with the newer inhaled anesthetics. Nevertheless, when a difficult intubation is anticipated, more satisfactory conditions exist if an anticholinergic has been administered. Anticholinergics are unnecessary when local anesthesia is planned.

In addition, a number of potentially undesirable

effects are associated with anticholinergics. Central nervous system (CNS) toxicity manifests as delerium or prolonged somnolence. This is most likely with scopolamine. Physostigmine is effective in reversing this effect. All three anticholinergics may produce mydriasis and cycloplegia such that patients may experience visual impairment postoperatively. Scopolamine has a greater mydriatic effect than does atropine or glycopyrrolate.[43] Conceivably, this could interfere with drainage of aqueous humor. There is, however, no convincing evidence that inclusion of an anticholinergic drug in the commonly employed doses is contraindicated in the patient with glaucoma.[44,45] Nevertheless, miotic eyedrops should be continued throughout the perioperative period in those patients with glaucoma.

Other potential drawbacks to anticholinergic administration include the production of tachycardia or increased ventricular response in patients with supraventricular tachyarrhythmias (unlikely in clinically used doses), relaxation of the lower esophageal sphincter (unlikely with intramuscular administration), elevation of body temperature (contraindicated in patients with a temperature), and excessive drying of airway secretions (may cause atelectasis in the bronchitic patient with a chronic productive cough).

H_2-Histamine Receptor Antagonist-Antacids

Although the incidence of clinically significant aspiration of gastric contents in patients subjected to general anesthesia is relatively low, it remains an ever-present danger during the perioperative period. Likewise, the patient undergoing ophthalmic surgery under local anesthesia is not immune from this danger either. Their premedicants, drugs administered in the room for supplementation, local anesthetics, and anxiety with its associated increase in gastric acid production, all combine to increase the risk of nausea and emesis.

From animal experiments it is known that the severity of pneumonitis following aspiration of gastric contents is related to the gastric fluid pH (acidity) and the volume and character of the aspirate (tonicity, presence of food particles).[46,47] Data in the literature have clearly indicated that either H_2-histamine receptor antagonists or antacids are capable of increasing gastric fluid pH and in some cases lowering gastric volume.[48,49] Although this should not be interpreted as evidence that the actual incidence of aspiration will be lowered, it does imply that the severity (thus morbidity and possible mortality) of the subsequent pneumonitis should be less. Many anesthesiologists therefore prefer to include these drugs with the premedicants when general anesthesia is planned. Their inclusion in the premedicant regimen in patients scheduled for local anesthesia is not altogether unreasonable, particularly if the patient has trouble with reflux esophagitis or a hypersecretory gastric acid state.

Although on the whole these drugs as used for premedicants have proved quite safe, one reported drawback associated with H_2-histamine receptor blocking agents is their potential to inhibit the mixed function oxidase system (P_{450}) in the liver and decrease liver blood flow.[50] This can result in higher blood levels and prolonged effects of any drug that relies on the liver for its termination of effect. Ranitidine is purportedly superior to cimetidine in this regard, although the clinical experience with ranitidine is much more limited than that of cimetidine.[51]

Conclusion

There are some patient subsets in which a "heavy" premedication is very desirable. The patient with coronary artery disease and good left ventricular function presenting for ophthalmic surgery is far less likely to manifest tachycardia, hypertension, and possible ischemic symptoms if he or she is well premedicated. Keeping in mind, however, that most ophthalmic patients are elderly, most should not receive excessive premedication. It is far better to underestimate their requirements and then titrate supplemental medications intravenously in the operating room while monitoring the patient than to overmedicate the patient on the ward. Finally, emphasis is again placed on maintaining those medications being taken for coexisting medical problems.

SYSTEMIC EFFECTS OF OPHTHALMIC DRUGS

Ophthalmologists must be constantly cognizant of the fact that medications they administer topically are absorbed and can result in systemic effects. Indeed, systemic absorption of these medications can have a dramatic effect on the conduct of anesthesia. The most commonly involved drugs in this regard are timolol, echothiophate, phenylephrine, epinephrine, and cocaine. Likewise, the systemic effects of the carbonic anhydrase inhibitor, acetazolamide, and the osmotic diuretics must be appreciated.

Timolol (Timoptic)

Timolol is a nonspecific β-adrenoceptor blocking agent that may produce systemic toxicity. Cardiovascular dysfunction as manifested by signs of β-blockade, including sinus bradycardia, heart block, syncope, and congestive heart failure, have all been reported.[52] Similarly, exacerbation of asthma (bronchospasm) and of myasthenia gravis have been reported.[53,54] Nonspecific signs of systemic β-blockade, such as lightheadedness, fatigue, and general depression of the CNS, have also been noted. Timolol should therefore be used with caution if at all in patients with known contraindications to the systemic use of this class of drugs. Patients presenting for ophthalmic surgery taking this drug must be carefully evaluated for the above side effects.

Echothiophate Iodide

Echothiophate is a long-acting antiacetylcholinesterase used to treat glaucoma. It also inhibits the enzyme pseudocholinesterase, which is responsible for the inactivation of the commonly used muscle relaxant, succinylcholine, and the amino-ester-type local anesthetics (procaine, chloroprocaine, tetracaine). Pseudocholinesterase activity purportedly begins to decrease after several days of topical ophthalmic application.[55] It may take 3 to 6 weeks for return of normal activity after the drug is discontinued. When dealing with a patient who has been taking echothiophate iodide within the previous 4 weeks, drugs that are metabolized by pseudocholinesterase (succinylcholine, procaine, chloroprocaine, tetracaine) should be reduced in dosage or avoided altogether when acceptable alternatives are available.

Phenylephrine

Phenylephrine is used to produce capillary decongestion and pupillary dilation. Although systemic effects following topical application of phenylephrine are infrequent, case reports of arrhythmias, severe hypertension, and subarachnoid hemorrhage are attributed to its use.[56] These reactions usually occurred within 1 to 20 minutes after topical application and have generally only occurred after the application of the 10 percent solution which contains 5 mg of the drug per single drop. Statements made in the literature indicate that there is little increase in the mydriatic effect in a solution more concentrated than 5 percent.[57] Phenylephrine is also marketed as a 2.5 percent solution, and to date I am aware of no reported adverse reactions with this concentration.

It is therefore recommended that the 2.5 percent solution be used in children to avoid relative overdosage. Similarly, it should be limited to one drop in patients who would be at increased risk of adverse sequelae should significant absorption be encountered. This would include patients with hypertension, coronary artery disease, left ventricular dysfunction, and cerebrovascular disease.

Epinephrine

Epinephrine is also used in the management of glaucoma. Again, although relatively safe, occasionally hypertension, dysrhythmias, tachycardia, and angina can occur.[58] It also raises one potential intraoperative drug interaction. That is, the inhalation agents, and in particular halothane, sensitize the heart to catecholamines.[59]

Cocaine

Cocaine is unique in that it is the only local anesthetic that inherently causes vasoconstriction and shrinkage of mucous membranes. As such, it is often employed as a nasal spray or in a nasal pack during dacryocystorhinostomies. It is important to appreciate that not only does significant absorption of cocaine from mucosal surfaces occur but also, once absorbed, it inhibits catecholamine uptake and has a sympathetic potentiating effect.

Meyers,[60] for example, reported two cases of cocaine toxicity during dacryocystorhinostomies. Similarly, Chung et al.[61] recommended that drugs such as halothane that sensitize the myocardium to catecholamines are theoretically best avoided with cocaine. One must also question the concomitant use of sympathomimetics such as epinephrine. The recommended maximum dose in clinical practice is 3 mg/kg, up to a total dose of 200 mg.

Acetazolamide

The carbonic anhydrase inhibitor, acetazolamide, is commonly used and is often ordered preoperatively or intraoperatively to lower IOP. It interferes with the sodium pump mechanism responsible for the production of aqueous humor. Acetazolamide, 500 mg IV, acts within 5 minutes and reaches its maximum intraocular hypotensive effect within 20 to 30 minutes.[62] It must be appreciated that chronic acetazolamide therapy may be associated with potassium depletion and relative hypovolemia. Both of these may profoundly affect the conduct of anesthesia and may require correction prior to anesthesia.

Osmotic Agents

Osmotic agents increase plasma oncotic pressure relative to that of aqueous and vitreous. The resulting dehydration of the vitreous humor produces a drop in IOP.[63] Agents clinically useful in this regard include urea, mannitol, and glycerol. Urea has been largely supplanted by mannitol because of the potential for significant tissue damage in the event of extravasation of urea. Mannitol (1 g/kg), given as a 20 percent solution, results in a reduction in IOP within 30 to 45 minutes, with a return to baseline level in 5 to 6 hours. Mannitol infusion results in a brisk osmotic diuresis with a loss of potassium. To prevent overdistention of the bladder with resulting pain and potentially reflex bradycardia, catheterization of the bladder must be considered, particularly during a general anesthetic. Similarly, the transient increase in plasma volume may precipitate acute left ventricular dysfunction. Likewise, the resulting diuresis may result in volume depletion and hypotension as well as electrolyte abnormalities. Thus, caution must be exercised in using a rapid mannitol infusion in patients with a history of congestive heart failure, hypertension, or chronic hypokalemia. Although glycerol is effective orally, it may cause trapping of water in the stomach. Many strongly believe that this effect relatively contraindicates its use, as this most likely increases the chance of aspiration.

LOCAL ANESTHESIA

The two basic requirements for ophthalmic surgery—akinesia and analgesia—can both be fulfilled with a combination of a facial nerve block and retrobulbar block anesthesia. Ophthalmologists have surely developed their own techniques of performing these blocks. Likewise, several excellent reviews of the various techniques exist in the literature.[64,65] This brief discussion will therefore focus on the pharmacology of the available local anesthetics as well as the potential complications relating to these drugs that may occur intraoperatively.

The safe use of local anesthetics requires a sound understanding of their clinical pharmacology.[66] Certainly, there are now a number of drugs to choose from (Table 1-4). For example, it has become clear that certain drugs can preferentially affect either motor, sensory, or autonomic fibers. Similarly, agents vary in their period of latency, that is, their speed of onset of blockade. Although the duration of action of a given drug varies with the dose, concentration, and whether or not epinephrine is added; there is also an intrinsic difference in the duration of action of drugs given in equiblocking concentrations. Likewise, these drugs vary in their toxic potential.

In ophthalmic anesthesia, however, usually only low dosages are required and thus a toxic reaction is relatively rare. Nevertheless, all possible precautions need to be taken beforehand. This includes

Table 1-4. Local Anesthetics

Generic Drug	Tradename	Relative Potency	Relative Onset	Relative Duration	Dose Producing CNS Toxicity in Humans (mg/kg)
Procaine	Novocain	1	Slow	Short	19.2
Chloroprocaine	Nesacaine	1	Fast	Short	22.8
Tetracaine	Pontocaine	8	Slow	Long	2.5
Lidocaine	Xylocaine	2	Fast	Medium	6.4
Mepivacaine	Carbocaine	2	Fast	Medium	9.8
Bupivacaine	Marcaine	8	Medium	Long	1.6
Etidocaine	Duranest	6	Fast	Long	3.4

beginning an intravenous infusion preblock as well as ongoing monitoring of the ECG and blood pressure. Appropriate resuscitative equipment and drugs must be at hand and ready to use. Finally, someone must be in immediate attendance who knows how to recognize the manifestations of the various reactions or side effects that can occur following local anesthesia. That individual must be equally skilled at treating these problems.

The two major groups of local anesthetics are the amino amides and the amino esters. The amides are primarily broken down by enzymes in the liver while the esters are rapidly hydrolyzed in the plasma.

The Amides

Lidocaine (Xylocaine)

Lidocaine is an ideal agent for most block procedures requiring rapid onset. Effective infiltrative blockade can be produced with 0.5, 1, and 2 percent solutions either with or without epinephrine. The 0.5 percent solution alone provides a duration of analgesia of approximately 75 minutes (30- to 90-minute range) lasting up to 200 minutes (60 to 300 minutes) when 1 : 200,000 epinephrine is added. The 1 percent solution has a duration of 120 minutes (90 to 140 minutes) lasting up to 400 minutes (360 to 410 minutes) with epinephrine. Similarly, for peripheral nerve blocks both the 0.5, 1, and 2 percent solutions with or without epinephrine may be used. Onset of anesthesia here requires 5 to 10 minutes. Similarly, the higher concentrations should be used if motor blockade is desired. Duration of anesthesia is approximately 60 minutes without epinephrine and 120 minutes with epinephrine. The published safe dosage is 400 mg without epinephrine and 500 mg with epinephrine. Lidocaine is primarily detoxified in the liver. States in which there is a known decrease in the integrity of hepatic cells or any state known to be associated with decreased liver blood flow (congestive heart failure) should necessitate a reduction in lidocaine dosage.

Mepivacaine (Carbocaine)

Effective concentrations for infiltrative or peripheral nerve block anesthesia are the same as for lidocaine. In general it results in a slower onset of anesthesia than with lidocaine. Its duration of action is slightly longer than equal doses of lidocaine, and blood levels are not as sensitive to inclusion of epinephrine. Its duration of action is reported to be in the range of 90 to 180 minutes. The reported maximum dose is 400 mg alone or 500 mg with epinephrine.

Bupivacaine (Marcaine)

For infiltrative anesthesia, 0.25 to 0.5 percent, is generally effective. Onset of effect following infiltration is rapid. Its duration of effect is approximately 200 minutes if used alone and 400 minutes if combined with epinephrine. For peripheral nerve block most clinicians prefer to use 0.5 to 0.75 percent solution. Onset of action is slower (10 to 20 minutes) than with lidocaine. Duration of action is approximately 400 minutes, and the addition of epinephrine has only a minimal effect in increasing duration. The reported dose limits are 150 to 175 mg when used alone and 225 mg when used with epinephrine.

Etidocaine (Duranest)

For infiltrative anesthesia, effective blockade is provided by a 0.5 percent solution without epinephrine. Onset is extremely rapid, and duration is similar to that of bupivacaine. For peripheral nerve blocks, solutions of 0.5 percent with or without epinephrine are effective. When used this way its onset of action is more rapid than that of bupivacaine. The safe dose without epinephrine is 300 mg and with epinephrine it is 400 mg. Again, the duration of anesthesia is similar to that of bupivacaine. It does differ from most local anesthetics in that it relatively provides a greater degree of motor blockade. Etidocaine undergoes extensive hepatic clearance as well as tissue binding, thus enhancing its safety as compared to bupivacaine.

The Esters

Procaine (Novacaine)

For infiltrative or peripheral nerve anesthesia, effective concentrations are similar to those of lidocaine. Procaine has a slower onset (5 to 15 minutes) as compared with lidocaine and a shorter duration of action (45 to 90 minutes). It is however less toxic than lidocaine with a recommended safe dose of 500 mg when used alone and 750 mg with epinephrine. The drug is hydrolyzed by plasma (pseudo) cholinesterase to paraaminobenzoic acid and diethylaminoethanol.

Chloroprocaine (Nesacaine)

Because of its more rapid hydrolysis via plasma cholinesterase, its toxicity is very low. For infiltrative anesthesia, a 1 percent solution has a rapid onset and a duration of 45 to 60 minutes, which is prolonged to 70 to 80 minutes with epinephrine. Similarly, a 1 percent solution is effective for peripheral nerve block. It has a rapid onset of effect but a duration of action limited to about 45 minutes when used alone or to 70 minutes with epinephrine. The recommended dosage limits are 600 mg plain and 800 mg with epinephrine. Both procaine and chloroprocaine appear to be safe for regional block in a patient with a history of malignant hyperthermia.

Tetracaine (Pontocaine)

Tetracaine is not extensively used for infiltration or peripheral nerve blocks. Nevertheless, when used in a concentration of 0.1 to 0.15 percent, it has been shown to be a useful alternative for the administration of many blocks. Epinephrine should be added to all solutions of tetracaine because of the slow plasma hydrolysis of tetracaine. Onset of blockade is slow and may take as long as 30 minutes. Duration of anesthesia ranges from 4 to 6 hours. The recommended safe dose is 100 mg when used alone or 150 mg with epinephrine.

Role of Epinephrine

Vasoconstrictors are used to permit more prolonged exposure or application of the local anesthetic to the nerve fiber and to slow drug absorption (thus reduce systemic toxicity). Likewise when an infiltrative injection is made into a relatively vascular area (lid), a great deal of bloody oozing is prevented. A 1 : 200,000 concentration seems to produce the desired vasoconstriction. The principle side effects are the possibility of hypertension, tachycardia, palpitations, arrhythmias, nervousness, and apprehension. Such reactions are of course most likely if the local anesthetic solution is given intravascularly. Donlon et al demonstrated that when the amount of exogenous epinephrine added to eyelid and retrobulbar local anesthetic injection is limited to 0.06 mg (12 ml vol with 1 : 200,000 epinephrine), systemic uptake was minimal and should not be sufficient to produce untoward effects.[67] Nevertheless caution should be exercised in the use of epinephrine containing solutions in patients with coronary artery disease. Likewise the anesthesiologist should be informed, as halothane particularly sensitizes the heart to catecholamines.

Hyaluronidase

This mucolytic enzyme renders tissues more permeable to injected fluids by depolymerizing hyaluronic acid. It traditionally was used to aid the spread of local anesthetic solutions although most present-day local anesthetics have excellent spreading powers in their own right. Nevertheless, in ophthalmology, hyaluronidase may increase the effective area of an injected anesthetic as well as shorten the time of onset of anesthesia significantly.[68]

Local Anesthetic Effects and Reactions

Toxic reactions from local anesthetics can result from high blood levels secondary to direct intravascular injection or systemic absorption from their site of administration. High blood concentrations result primarily in a gamut of CNS and cardiovascular effects. Central nervous system effects are by far the most common side effects of local anesthetic drugs. There are a number of premonitory symptoms, which vary from subject to subject. Initially a number of excitatory symptoms become manifest. These include lightheadedness, numbness of the tongue and circumoral tissues, tinnitus, a constellation of visual disturbances, disorientation, and occasional drowsiness. Slurred speech, shivering, muscle twitching, and tremors, initially involving facial muscles, may progress to a generalized convulsion. If blood levels continue to rise, there is subsequent CNS depression leading to coma and respiratory depression or arrest. Numerous studies have shown that hypercarbia, hypoxemia, and acidosis markedly potentiate the CNS toxicity of local anesthetics.[69]

Classically, it has been accepted that local anesthetic drugs cause a dose-dependent depression of the myocardium and a direct vasodilatory effect on the peripheral vasculature and prolong conduction time and depress excitability of the heart. However, these effects in general occur at higher blood levels than cause the CNS effects unless hypoxemia or hypercarbia from the respiratory depression are allowed to occur.

An intravascular injection of a local anesthetic results in a toxic reaction of almost immediate onset. In fact, a convulsion may be its first manifestation, as blood levels increase so rapidly that many of the premonitory signs simply do not have time to become manifest. Certainly, this possibility can be minimized by aspiration before and intermittently during injection of a local anesthetic solution. Occasionally, even aspiration will not reveal the misplacement of the needle if the vein is small or if excessive negative pressure results in collapse of a thin venous wall. This emphasizes the need to be prepared to treat a toxic reaction immediately when local anesthetics are used.

Reactions due to systemic absorption are due to a relative imbalance between absorption and concomitant distribution of the local anesthetic throughout the tissues of the body as well as ongoing biotransformation or renal elimination from the body. Absorption is influenced by the specific local anesthetic employed, the dosage, whether a vasopressor was employed, and the site and speed of injection. It should be appreciated that the concentration of a particular anesthetic solution in clinically used ranges has little if any influence on attained blood levels. Thus a higher concentration of a particular local anesthetic results in the same blood levels as a lower concentration if the same total dose of local anesthetic is administered. Similarly, body weight has been shown to correlate poorly with attained blood concentrations. Thus, a heavier patient does not require or cannot tolerate a higher dose of local anesthetic than can a thin patient. Finally, patients with cardiovascular disease states associated with decreased liver blood flow are predisposed to attain higher blood concentrations of anesthetics than are normal patients. Systemic toxic reactions resulting from absorption usually occur from 5 to 25 minutes postinjection. The more vascular the site of injection, the greater is the likelihood of the toxic reaction. Because blood levels progressively increase, the previously described premonitory symptoms and signs are almost always present.

An occasional toxic reaction is unavoidable. It therefore becomes mandatory to be prepared and know how to treat a toxic reaction. If the early premonitory signs of increasing blood levels of local anesthetics appear, treatment should consist of constant verbal contact with the patient, administration of supplemental oxygen, encouragement of the patient to maintain a normal rate and depth of respiration, and continuance of minute-to-minute cardiovascular monitoring.

The primary treatment should a convulsion occur is directed at attenuating the rapidly developing hypercarbia, hypoxemia, and acidosis.[70] Thus the key is to establish and maintain an adequate airway while providing supplemental oxygen via assisted or controlled ventilation. Frequently convulsions are self-limiting. If convulsions persist, the most commonly employed medications used to control them are the ultra-short-acting barbiturates or the benzodiazepines. Intravenous barbiturates are very effective in treating convulsions and are commonly the first choice of anesthesiologists because of their availability and familiarity. Their dosage should, however, be reduced (1 to 2 mg/kg thiopental) because of the potential to exaggerate the cardiopulmonary depression of the local anesthetic.

The benzodiazepines (diazepam, 0.1 to 0.2 mg/kg IV) are also extremely useful in terminating seizures. They are of slightly slower onset than are the barbiturates, but they are also associated with less cardiovascular depression. Another drawback associated with benzodiazepines is respiratory depression, an effect that can persist longer than the barbiturates because of their longer elimination half-life.

If cardiovascular depression ensues, elevation of the legs, head-down positioning, and an increase in the rate of fluid administration may suffice. Otherwise, the administration of vasoactive drugs, preferably those with both α- and β-receptor agonist effects, would be appropriate.

Certainly, equally if not more common problems associated with injections of local anesthetics are related to the effects of additives. For example, epinephrine absorption may manifest as sweating, tachycardia and palpitations, hypertension, apprehension, and headache. Often awareness of the problem and thus reassurance of the patient and the administration of supplemental oxygen are all that are required. Obviously, if these symptoms or signs become manifest before the injection has been completed, it should be terminated.

Similarly, vasovagal reactions are commonly encountered in practice. These manifest most commonly after a painful stimulus such as the beginning of an IV line or the injection of the local anesthetics. These reactions manifest as bradycardia, hypotension, pallor, faintness, and CNS aberrations. Such reactions usually respond to head-down positioning and supplemental oxygen. Occasionally, intravenous atropine may be required.

Finally, local anesthetic allergies are extremely rare. Most documented cases are associated with the amino-ester type of local anesthetics and are believed to be associated with the paraaminobenzoic acid moeity. By contrast, allergic reactions to the amino amide local anesthetics are very rare. In fact the preservative methylparaben used is some of the amide local anesthetics may be the offending agent. Skin testing has not proved particularly reliable in testing for possible allergy. When these reactions do occur, they may manifest with generalized erythema, edema, hypotension, tachycardia, and wheezing. As in the case of systemic toxic reactions, all necessary equipment and medications must be available to treat anaphylactic reactions whenever local anesthetics are administered.

FACTORS INFLUENCING INTRAOCULAR PRESSURE

Numerous studies have looked at the impact of various drugs and techniques on IOP. Among these studies, however, there are many differences in premedication, in the dosage and timing of administration of the drugs themselves, in the timing and methods of measurement of IOP, and in concomitantly administered drugs. This makes direct comparison of these studies difficult. The material that follows gives some of the specifics for individual drugs or techniques that highlight clinical points. A discussion of general anesthetic techniques for intraocular surgery follows that attempts to bring this hodge-podge of data together in a meaningful format.

The greatest increases in IOP are usually secondary to increases in venous pressure.[71] This increase results from the impedance of aqueous humor outflow from the canal of Schlemm secondary to backpressure that develops in the venous system draining the eye and from direct compression of the globe by dilated episcleral veins. Numerous perioperative events can lead to increases in venous pressure. For example, vomiting during the perioperative period secondary to narcotics, general anesthetics, or anxiety often occurs. Any straining, bucking, breathholding, or airway obstruction during the course of anesthesia will also increase venous pressure dramatically. Coughing in an awake patient (chronic bronchitic) under local anesthesia or postoperatively in patients with lung disease following general anesthesia can prove equally deleterious. Although many of these events cannot be absolutely avoided, their incidence and severity can be minimized. In a related matter, advantage should be taken of slightly (10 to 15 degrees) head-up positioning to promote venous drainage during surgery.

Also relating to this topic is the IOP response to laryngoscopy and intubation of the trachea during induction of general anesthesia. A stormy induction with the patient bucking at the time of laryngoscopy can prove disastrous if the eye is open. Indeed, laryngoscopy and tracheal intubation results in an increase in IOP in the closed globe even in the absence of any apparent reaction to intubation.[72] This response can, however, be attenuated in the presence of "deep" anesthesia as may be provided by a large dose of one of the ultrashort acting barbiturates (i.e., thiopental) or with inhalation agents. Thus the importance of a smooth induction of anesthesia in patients undergoing ophthalmic surgery, particularly in the situation of an open eye injury.

Increases in systemic blood pressure in general have much less effect on IOP.[73] A sudden increase in blood pressure intraoperatively may cause a transient acute rise in IOP in the closed globe until the aqueous flow dynamics can accommodate. This rise in IOP is not, however, of nearly the same magnitude as IOP increases following venous congestion. Moderate decreases in arterial pressure also have little effect on IOP, but at values of systolic pressure less than 85 to 90 mmHg marked reductions in IOP begin to occur.[74]

Hypoventilation, with resulting hypercarbia, results in increased IOP and must be avoided.[75,76] This may arise secondary to drugs given as supplements during local anesthesia or to agents used in the induction and maintenance of general anesthesia. Thus adequacy of ventilation must be ensured. Hypoxemia may also contribute to increased IOP through vasodilation of choroidal vessels. By contrast, hyperventilation tends to lower IOP.

Many of the drugs used during general anesthesia affect IOP. Inhalation agents (halothane, enflurane, isoflurane) are alleged to cause dose-related decreases in IOP.[77-80] The mechanism(s) suggested to be responsible for these decreases include a reduction of aqueous humor production, depression of a CNS control center, a facilitatory effect on aqueous humor outflow, and a decrease in extraocular muscle or orbicularis muscle tension. The concept of dose-related decreases in IOP has been challenged recently by a group of investigators who believe that if preoperative sedation is adequate before control measurements are made, inhalational agents will produce no significant change in IOP.[80]

Most central nervous system depressants, such as barbiturates, narcotics, neuroleptics, and tranquilizers, tend to lower IOP.[81] Drugs used for induction of anesthesia, namely ultra-short-acting barbiturates and etomidate, cause a lowering of IOP. For example, Litwiller et al.[82] showed that intravenous thiopental, 3 to 4 mg/kg, will cause a 25 percent decrease in IOP lasting 3 to 5 minutes. Etomidate is a recently introduced intravenous anesthetic induction agent. Purported advantages of this drug over the ultra-short-acting barbiturates include greater rapidity of recovery, less cumulation of effect on repeated doses, and greater cardiovascular stability. Oji and co-workers[83] demonstrated that a typical induction dose of etomidate, 0.3 mg/kg IV, resulted in a fall in IOP that was apparent at 30 seconds and this persisted in some patients for as long as 20 minutes.

Narcotics such as morphine, meperidine (Demerol), or one of the newer synthetic compounds such as fentanyl or sufentanyl, may be administered as part of a balanced general anesthetic technique.[84] Provided that hypercarbia secondary to the resulting respiratory depression is avoided, narcotics in general have been noted to decrease IOP slightly.

Ketamine, given intravenously or intramuscularly, was originally reported to increase IOP.[85] More recent studies, however, have shown no significant change in IOP after ketamine administration.[86] Ketamine may be considered inadvisable in ophthalmic anesthesia for other reasons however in that it can cause blepharospasm and nystagmus.

Succinylcholine (SCh) has been shown to increase IOP. As early as 1955, Lincoff et al.[71] reported vitreous humor loss following SCh administration in the presence of an open eye. An increase in IOP occurs within the first minute after SCh administration, with an average peak increase of 6 to 8 torr between 1 and 4 minutes and a return to control measurements by 5 to 7 minutes[87] (Fig. 1-1). This occurs whether SCh is given as a single intravenous injection, intramuscularly, or by continuous infusion.[88] Prolonged tonic contraction of the extraocular muscles produced by SCh is the most likely mechanism for this increased IOP. Patients with glaucoma do not appear to have unusually exaggerated or prolonged IOP responses following SCh administration.[89]

Several techniques have been advocated to prevent or minimize the IOP increase following SCh. Carballo claims that the preoperative administration of a carbonic anhydrase inhibitor (acetazolamide) abolishes this response.[90] Establishment of a deep level of anesthesia prior to SCh administration has also been claimed to attenuate the increase in pressure.[88] There is still controversy regarding the efficacy of pretreatment with nondepolarizing muscle relaxants. For example, Miller and coworkers[91] found that pretreatment with *d*-tubocurarine or gallamine inhibited the pressure increase. By contrast, Meyers et al.[92] found that similar pretreatment doses could not reliably block this response. Since SCh-induced increases of IOP cannot always be prevented, many anesthesiologists advocate avoidance of SCh during induction of anesthesia in a patient with an open eye injury.

In contrast to succinylcholine, small (pretreatment) doses of the nondepolarizing muscle relaxants produces no significant change in IOP. Fully paralyzing doses in general have been shown to reduce IOP.[82] Presumably their predominant effect is secondary to their actions on the extraocular muscles. Reversal of neuromuscular blockade with commonly utilized dosages of the anticholinesterase, neostigmine, and the anticholinergic, atropine, has been shown not to affect IOP adversely either.[93,94]

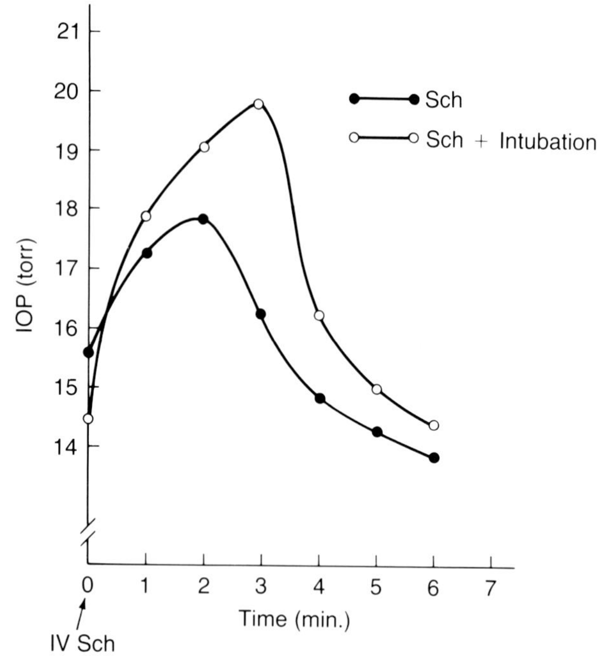

Fig. 1-1. Effect of succinylcholine (SCh) and intubation on intraocular pressure. (•—•) SCh; (O—O) SCh and intubation. (Data from Pandey K, Badola R, Kumar S: Time course of intraocular hypertension produced by suxamethonium. Br J Anaesth 44:191, 1972.)

ANESTHETIC MANAGEMENT OF PATIENTS UNDERGOING INTRAOCULAR PROCEDURES

Intraocular pressure should be reasonably low prior to opening the globe. High pressures at this time can result in loss of the iris, lens, or vitreous through the incision site or in shearing stresses on ocular vessels with a resultant expulsive hemorrhage. Once the globe is opened, IOP functionally becomes zero (i.e., atmospheric). At this time, concern should be focused on avoiding events that either extrinsically compress the globe or increase the relative volume of the vitreous or choroid. The former may occur secondary to fixation sutures or improper placement of an eyelid speculum, to a retrobulbar hematoma, or to squeezing of the orbicularis or extraocular muscles (secondary to "light" anesthesia or succinylcholine). Increases in choroidal volume may occur secondary to elevations of arterial carbon dioxide tension, acute increases in systemic blood pressure, or increases in central venous pressure. The vitreous volume can increase if overzealous hydration of the patient is carried out. In any event, any of these factors can result in loss of ocular contents through the incision site and must be avoided.

Ideally, the induction of general anesthesia should be as smooth and as safe as possible. The actual choice of drugs for induction of general anesthesia is primarily dependent on the physiologic makeup of the patient, the expected duration of the procedure, and the familiarity of the anesthesiologist with each particular technique, and not with the particular eye pathology present.

Thus, in all likelihood it is the smoothness of induction that is vital. IOP will remain at acceptable values if straining or bucking at the time of laryngoscopy and intubation are avoided or at least attenuated. This may be accomplished by ensuring an unobstructed airway during mask ventilation, performing a rapid laryngoscopy, and providing an adequate depth of anesthesia. Adequate depth can be attained using large doses of the ultra-short-acting barbiturates or etomidate. The hemodynamic response to laryngoscopy and intubation can be attenuated with lidocaine (topical or intravenous).[95]

Again, the drugs chosen for maintenance of anesthesia are most influenced by the anticipated duration of surgery and the physiologic makeup of the patient.[41] An inhalation or volatile agent such as halothane, enflurane, or isoflurane is often a good choice. All these agents in a dose-related manner seem to lower IOP. As compared with narcotic-based techniques (balanced anesthetic), volatile agents provide easier control of depth of anesthesia and are associated with a slightly lower incidence of nausea and vomiting. They permit more rapid adjustment of depth of anesthesia than narcotic-based techniques and provide some muscle relaxing properties in their own right. Likewise, volatile agents are more commonly able to control intraoperative tachycardia and hypertension than balanced techniques.

The alternative approach of using a balanced anesthetic of narcotic-nitrous oxide often requires the supplemental use of a volatile agent to control hypertension and muscle relaxants to ensure no patient movement. In principle, not all patients need to be paralyzed during the procedure. It is mandatory, however, that sufficient depth of anesthesia be provided to ensure lack of patient movement. Many times, in elderly patients, use of muscle relaxants are required however.

During surgical repair of retinal detachments, intravitreal injection of sulfur hexafluoride gas (SF_6) or air may be employed. It must be appreciated that if nitrous oxide is used as part of the general anesthetic technique, it will diffuse into the gaseous bubble.[96,97] This can be of such magnitude as to compromise retinal blood flow. Likewise, when nitrous oxide is discontinued, a dramatic fall in IOP can occur as the nitrous oxide is reabsorbed. The easiest way to handle this problem is to avoid using nitrous oxide in these cases.

Extubation of the trachea and emergence from anesthesia should likewise be as smooth as possible. If not already performed, gastric air and fluid should be emptied via an orogastric tube before the patient awakens. Similarly, the pharynx should be suctioned while the patient is still reasonably deeply anesthetized. Many anesthesiologists are advocates of the prophylactic use of a potent antiemetic such as droperidol (1.25 to 2.5 mg IV) 20 to 30 minutes prior to emergence. It becomes a matter of clinical judgement and experience as to when to extubate a patient. Some have advocated intravenous lidocaine as an adjunct to allow the patient to tolerate the endotracheal tube longer and cough less following extubation.[98] Once extubated, the patient should be placed on their nonoperated side down, the head slightly raised, and supplemental oxygen administered unless the nature of the surgery dictates that a specific position be maintained.

Oculocardiac Reflex

The oculocardiac reflex is an ever present danger during ophthalmic surgery.[99] Originally described in 1908, its afferent impulses originate in the long and short ciliary nerves and subsequently traverse the ciliary ganglion, the ophthalmic division of the trigeminal nerve, and the gasserion ganglion, to terminate in the main sensory nucleus of the trigeminal nerve near the fourth ventricle of the brain. The efferent impulses travel via the vagus nerve.

The most common manifestation of this trigeminal-vagal reflex is a decrease of 10 to 50 percent in heart rate, although other arrhythmias, including junctional rhythm, atrioventricular block, ventricular bigeminy, and cardiac standstill have been reported.The reported incidence of cardiac rhythm changes during eye muscle surgery varies widely. This wide range is primarily accounted for by the variation in defining how much slowing of heart rate constitutes the occurrence of the reflex.[100,101] Traction of the extraocular muscles, particularly the medial or lateral rectus muscles, is most likely to elicit this reflex. Other causes include pressure on the globe during surgical manipulation, occlusive dressings, pinching of the conjunctiva, or pressure applied while performing or following a retrobulbar block. Hypercarbia or hypoxemia and increased vagal tone as in children or secondary to drugs most likely increase the incidence and severity of this reflex.

Various techniques have been recommended to abolish and/or decrease the incidence and severity of this reflex. None has proved entirely effective, and each introduces some risk. Studies indicate that neither atropine nor any of the other anticholinergics given intramuscularly in clinically used dosages are of value in preventing this reflex.[102] By contrast, the decrease in incidence by intravenously administered anticholinergics depends on both dosage and timing of administration.[103–106] For example, Meyers and co-workers[103] have shown that both atropine and glycopyrrolate given just prior to induction of anesthesia are very effective in preventing the oculocardiac reflex in pediatric patients. Reed and McCaughey[64] also have reported excellent success with intravenous atropine in preventing cardiac rhythm changes during pediatric ophthalmic surgery. Atropine is, however, associated with a greater degree of tachycardia and a higher likelihood of central anticholinergic syndrome than is glycopyrrolate.[105,106] Similarly, others have noted that frequently other more severe arrhythmias may occur when atropine has been administered.[107] Likewise, the routine use of intravenously administered atropine for adults has not consistently been found to decrease the incidence of this reflex.[108] In fact, the resulting increase in heart rate following anticholinergics may be harmful in adult patients with cardiac disease.

The protective effect of retrobulbar block is controversial. In fact, the risk associated with retrobulbar block may exceed the risk of the reflex itself. These include (1) stimulation of the reflex arc itself, (2) retrobulbar hemorrhage, and (3) optic nerve injury.

In the final analysis, the most important aspect of care is anticipation of the reflex. All patients undergoing ophthalmic surgery should therefore be monitored with an ECG regardless of the procedure or the type of anesthetic. Additionally, ready access of a patent IV line and ready availability of an anticholinergic must be ensured. Should a dysrhythmia occur, initial management consists of stopping surgical manipulation while concomitantly reassessing the patient's oxygenation and ventilatory status. Most often, heart rate returns spontaneously to initial levels. The surgeon can usually then proceed safely, as this reflex often fatigues.[109] If the initial presentation is severe (profound bradycardia, sinus arrest, severe hypotension), most anesthesiologists would consider the use of intravenous atropine. If the reflex recurs repeatedly deepening of the anesthetic, ensurance of adequacy of ventilation, and local infiltration of the recti muscle with a local anesthetic in addition to anticholinertgic administration, may prove beneficial.

Monitoring during Ophthalmic Surgery

The requirements for monitoring patients undergoing ophthalmic surgery ideally should be the same regardless of the type of anesthetic employed. As previously alluded to, ECG monitoring is essential because of the ever-present danger of the oculocardiac reflex. Whether performed under local or general anesthesia, ophthalmic patients are covered with the surgical drapes, their face and upper chest hidden from view. It is therefore imperative that someone be assigned to monitor the patient. Thus, in addition to ECG monitoring, the blood pressure must periodically be monitored (auscultory, Doppler, automated), and an IV line must be patent and readily accessible (preferably on the side of the person monitoring the patient), a precordial stethoscope for monitoring both breath sounds and heart tones must be used, and access to one of the patient's hands to assess color, capillary filling, and the radial pulse is mandatory. Although having someone in attendance does increase the cost of the overall procedure, it can prove invaluable. High-flow oxygen should be delivered around the face to ensure adequate carbon dioxide dilution and removal.

The most common intraoperative complications under local anesthesia are due to oversedation and hypoventilation causing hypoxemia and hypercarbia.[11] These may result in arrhythmias and ischemia. Likewise, an undersedated patient may experience anxiety and stress and subsequently manifest tachycardia, hypertension, and angina pectoris.

Attention must be paid to proper patient positioning particularly when long procedures are performed under general anesthesia. This includes padding of any potential pressure points or exposed peripheral nerves and a pillow under the knees. The nonoperated eye must be protected from a corneal abrasion. Cross and Krupin[110] showed that both basal and reflex tear production are decreased under general anesthesia (Fig. 1-2). Thus, the nonoperated eye must be protected with an eye lubricant and should be closed mechanically. The importance of monitoring temperature in pediatric patients is stressed in the section on pediatric ophthalmic anesthesia.

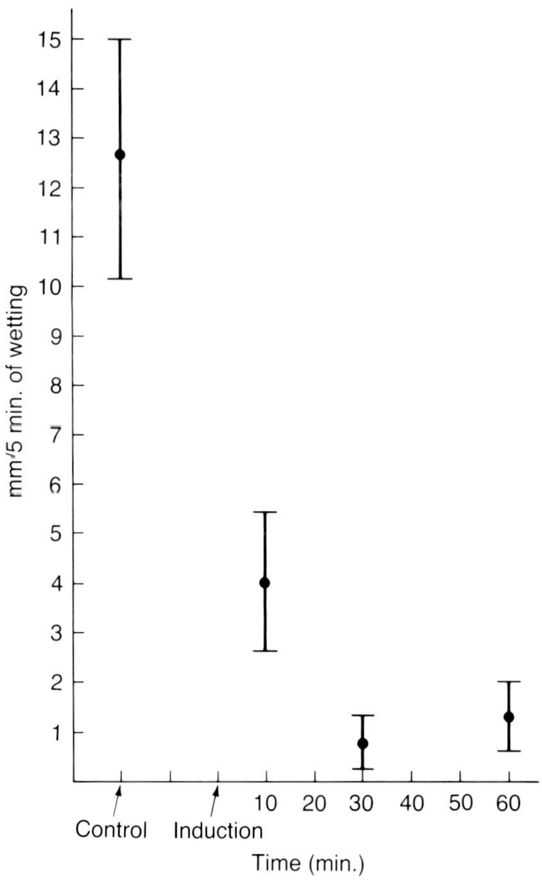

Fig. 1-2. Effect of general anesthesia on basal tear production. (Redrawn from Cross D, Krupin T: Implications of the effects of general anesthesia on basal tear production. Anesth Analg 56:35, 1977.)

OPEN EYE INJURY

The patient with a penetrating eye injury presents one of the most challenging problems faced by the ophthalmologist and anesthesiologist. As with any emergency, these patients must be assumed to have a stomach full of partially digested food. The patient is therefore at increased risk for aspiration and subsequent pneumonitis. The anesthesiologist must thus weigh the effects of various maneuvers and drugs used to protect the patient from aspiration against the effect those same techniques or drugs have on the likelihood of causing an increase in the volume of intraocular contents or extrinsic pressure on the globe. Either of the latter events results in an increased likelihood of loss of intraocular contents through the open wound. Thus the anesthesiologist is caught in the dilemma of the potential loss of vision in an eye versus the potential loss of life. A realistic appraisal of the likelihood that the eye is salvagable is sometimes known by the ophthalmologist; this likelihood should be shared with the anesthesiologist. Any well-trained anesthesiologist should be willing to try everything possible to save the eye, yet to place a patient at increased risk for aspiration when an eye is in all likelihood unsalvagable is worse. In addition, associated injuries must be evaluated, as they may affect anesthetic decisions dramatically. Finally, it should be appreciated that the patient who has undergone recent intraocular surgery should be treated with the same precautions afforded the patient with an open eye injury.

Preanesthetic medication in the adult must be individualized; it may include a sedative-hypnotic, an antisialagogue, an antacid or H_2-receptor blocking agent, and an antiemetic. Many anesthesiologists would argue that narcotics are contraindicated in these patients because of their potential emetic effect. The preoperative administration of acetazolamide or osmotic agents are of minimal value in protecting the patient from loss of intraocular contents in this situation. Attempted emptying of the stomach via placement of an nasogastric tube is contraindicated in light of the likelihood of vomiting.

The induction of anesthesia is the most critical period. Important general considerations in this regard include (1) avoidance of external pressure on the globe (i.e., mask, anesthesiologist's hands, or instruments), (2) minimization of any increase in venous pressure (i.e., vomiting, coughing, straining), and (3) adherence to basic full stomach precautions (i.e., preoxygenation, head-up positioning, rapid-sequence intravenous induction, cricoid pressure).

Anecdotal reporting has indicated a number of different induction techniques to be efficacious. Perhaps more importantly, it should be appreciated that a few techniques have definitely proved unsatisfactory. For example, succinylcholine should never be used alone, not as part of an induction sequence nor once the eye is opened in response to patient movement. Numerous reports attest to the subsequent loss of intraocular contents following administration of succinylcholine in these situations. Likewise, the choice of a local anesthetic utilizing a retrobulbar block is relatively contraindicated, as the block itself may result in loss of intraocular contents. Similarly, awake intubation techniques are relatively contraindicated in view of the inability to reliably prevent the patient from coughing during the transtracheal block or intubation itself.

Previously, the most commonly used technique for induction of anesthesia and subsequent intubation was pretreatment with a nondepolarizing muscle relaxant–thiopental–succinylcholine technique. Controversy continues, however, regarding the effectiveness of pretreatment in preventing the increase in IOP associated with succinylcholine administration.[91,92] It must be stated, however, that this author is unaware of any reports in the literature of loss of intraocular contents when this technique is used.

Because of the concerns regarding the effectiveness of pretreatment in attenuating the rise in IOP following succinylcholine, techniques employing thiopental and one of the nondepolarizing muscle relaxants have been used. These techniques are associated with minimal to no change in IOP in closed globe models and have also been used successfully in many cases.[82,111] Some very real drawbacks are associated with their usage, however. For example, conditions acceptable for intubation take longer to attain (i.e., slower onset of block) than with pretreatment-succinylcholine. This problem can be overcome somewhat by using larger doses of the nondepolarizing muscle relaxants, yet this results in prolonged neuromuscular blockade. In fact, with pancuronium (0.15 to 0.2 mg/kg), the duration of neuromuscular blockade could be 2 to 4 hours. Two recently introduced nondepolarizing muscle relaxants, atracurium (0.5 to 0.6 mg/kg) and vecuronium (0.1 to 0.15 mg/kg), offset this latter drawback, however, since their duration of action in this dose range is significantly shorter (range: 60 minutes). Nevertheless, the patient and his family should be informed of the possibility of intubation in the postoperative period if the surgical procedure is short and a thiopental-nondepolarizing muscle relaxant technique has been chosen. Likewise these techiques are relatively contraindicated when the ability to intubate the patient easily is questioned.

It probably makes little difference whether inhalation agents or narcotic-muscle relaxants are chosen for maintenance of anesthesia. It is imperative that the anesthesiologist ensure adequate depth of anesthesia during the procedure, and in fact many anesthesiologists consider both controlled ventilation and neuromuscular blockade desirable. Consideration should also be given to emptying the stomach with a gastric tube intraoperatively as well as use of an antiemetic near the end of the procedure.

Finally, pharyngeal suctioning should be performed while the patient is still anesthetized relatively deeply. The importance of extubation while deep is not as critical today as in the past in view of improved surgical closure although it remains a desirable goal.

PEDIATRIC OPHTHALMIC ANESTHESIA

By far the most commonly performed procedure in pediatric ophthalmology is strabismus surgery. The most common intraoperative problem associated with strabismus surgery is the occurrence of the oculocardiac reflex (see section on oculocardiac reflex). Other issues of concern include the impact of succinylcholine on the forced duction test and the propensity of these patients to malignant hyperthermia.

It is well accepted that succinylcholine causes a sustained tonic contraction of the Felderstruktur fibers of the extraocular muscles. Smith[112] reported that this effect makes interpretation of the forced duction test unreliable for 15 to 20 minutes postadministration of succinylcholine, while pancuronium did not seem to influence the forced duction test. Others have not considered this a significant clinical problem.

Malignant hyperthermia (MH) has an incidence of 1 : 15,000 in anesthetized children. Several cases of MH reported in the literature have however been found in patients having strabismus surgery. Tammisto et al.[113] speculate that strabismus may be a sign of a latent muscle system disturbance. These workers reported that succinylcholine caused a fourfold increase in the incidence of myoglobinuria and a threefold greater frequency of increased CPK levels in patients with strabismus compared to general surgical patients. It thus behooves the ophthalmologist to know something about MH.

The susceptible patient possesses a genetic predisposition for development of this disease, which is usually not manifested until exposure to a triggering agent such as a drug or stressful environmental factor occurs. It is currently believed that the mode of transmission is polygenic and that the inheritance pattern can be recessive or dominant. Most patients have a positive family history for the disease. Thus the question must be raised in the properative evaluation of any patient for eye muscle surgery. A family history of hyperthermia or unexplained death following administration of an anesthetic is highly suggestive. Two thirds of susceptible patients manifest this syndrome during their first anesthetic induction (locals and general anesthetics). It must be emphasized, however, that patients can undergo anesthesia uneventfully and yet have an MH episode triggered with subsequent exposures.

From an overall viewpoint, the priorities are these.[114] First, anyone with a positive history should be identified. Susceptible patients can be treated prophylactically preoperatively with oral dantrolene. Although no one anesthetic technique has proved entirely safe, some drugs have been more highly incriminated as triggering agents than others. Second, all those involved with the patient's care must be familiar with the presenting signs, and all preparations for the treatment of MH must be made prior to the induction of anesthesia.

Malignant hyperthermia is characterized by signs and symptoms of hypermetabolism. One of the earliest signs of MH is tachycardia that cannot be attributed to other causes. This hypermetabolic state also results in hypoxemia, hypercarbia, and a metabolic acidosis. The tachycardia and tachypnea are manifestations of these changes. Cardiac arrhythmias, hyperkalemia, and hypotension may ensue. Temperature elevation is often a late manifestation of MH. Indeed, the diagnosis of MH should not depend on a rise in body temperature. Nevertheless, an increase in body temperature may be precipitous, increasing at a rate of 0.5°C every 15 minutes, and reaching levels as high as 46°C.

Successful management of MH depends on early recognition of the syndrome and institution of a preplanned therapeutic regimen. Treatment of MH can be divided into an etiologic and symptomatic approach. Etiologic treatment is directed at correction of the underlying causative mechanism. Symptomatic therapy is directed toward maintenance of renal function and correction of hyperthermia, acidosis, and arterial hypoxemia.

Dantrolene, administered intravenously, is the

only drug that is reliably effective for the etiologic treatment of MH. Symptomatic treatment for MH includes immediate termination of the administration of inhaled anesthetics and the surgical procedure. The lungs of the patient should be aggressively hyperventilated with 100 percent oxygen and active cooling initiated. Other symptomatic therapy includes intravenous infusion of sodium bicarbonate to correct metabolic acidosis, hydration with normal saline, maintenance of urine output at 1 to 2 ml/kg/hr with osmotic and/or tubular diuretics, and administration of glucose.

REFERENCES

1. Gartner S, Billet E: A study on mortality rates during general anesthesia for ophthalmic surgery. Am J Ophthal 45:847, 1958
2. Duncalf D, Gartner S, Carol B: Mortality in association with ophthalmic surgery. Am J Ophthalmol 69:610, 1970
3. Quigley H: Mortality associated with ophthalmic surgery. Am J Ophthalmol 77:518, 1974
4. Petruscak J, Smith R, Breslin P: Mortality related to ophthalmological surgery. Arch Ophthalmol 89:106, 1973
5. Kaplan M, Reba R: Pulmonary embolism as the leading cause of ophthalmic surgical mortality. Amer J Ophthalmol 73:159, 1972
6. Backer C, Tinker J, Robertson D, Vlietstra R: Myocardial reinfarction following local anesthesia for ophthalmic surgery. Anesth Analg 59:257, 1980
7. Steen P, Tinker J, Tarhan S: Myocardial reinfarction after anesthesia and surgery. JAMA 239:2566, 1978
8. Lang D: Morbidity and mortality in ophthalmology. p. 195. In Bruce R, McGoldrick K, Oppenheimer P (eds): Anesthesia for Ophthalmology. Aesculapius, Birmingham, 1982
9. Snow J, Sensel S: Review of cataract extraction under local and general anesthesia at MEEI. Anesth Analg 45:742, 1966
10. Lynch S, Wolf G, Berlin I: 2200 cases of cataract surgery under general anesthesia. Anesth Analg 53:909, 1974
11. Meyers E: Problems during eye surgery under local anesthesia—Is standby necessary? Anesthesiol Rev 6:23, 1979
12. Tarhan S, Moffitt E, Taylor W, Guiliani E: Myocardial infarction after general anesthesia. JAMA 220:145, 1972
13. McCammon R: Coronary artery disease. p. 1. In Stoelting R, Dierdorf S (eds): Anesthesia and Co-Existing Disease. Churchill Livingstone, New York, 1983
14. Goldman L, Caldera D, Nussbaum S, et al: Multifactorial index of cardiac risk in noncardiac surgical procedures. N Engl J Med 297:845, 1977
15. Koprivac C, Brown A, Pappas G: Hemodynamics during general anesthesia in patients receiving propranolol. Anesthesiology 48:28, 1978
16. Slogoff S, Keats A, Ott E: Preoperative propranolol therapy and aorto-coronary bypass operation. JAMA 240:1487, 1978
17. Kates R: Calcium antagonists. Drugs 25:113, 1983
18. Nattel S, Rango R, VanLoon G: Mechanism of propranolol withdrawal phenomenon. Circulation 59:1158, 1979
19. Chung D: Anaesthetic problems associated with the treatment of cardiovascular disease—Digitalis toxicity. Can Anaesth Soc J 28:6, 1981
20. Crandell D: The anethestic hazards in patients on antihypertensive therapy. JAMA 179:495, 1962
21. Katz R, Weintraub H, Papper E: Anesthesia, surgery and rauwolfia. Anesthesiology 25:142, 1964
22. Prys-Roberts C, Meloche R, Foex P: Studies of anesthesia in relation to hypertension. Br J Anaesth 43:122, 1971
23. Dingle H: Antihypertensive drugs and anesthesia. Anaesthesia 21:151, 1966
24. Bruce D, Croley T, Lee J: Preoperative clonidine withdrawal syndrome. Anesthesiology 51:90, 1979
25. Goldman L, Caldera D: Risks of general anesthesia and elective operation in the hypertensive patient. Anesthesiology 50:285, 1979
26. LoSasso A, Gibbs P, Moorthy S: Obstructive lung disease. p. 171. In Stoelting R, Dierdorf S (eds): Anesthesia and Co-Existing Disease. Churchill Livingstone, New York, 1983
27. Stein M, Cassara E: Preoperative pulmonary evaluation and therapy for surgery patients. JAMA 211:787, 1970
28. Moorthy S: Metabolism and nutrition. p. 485. In Stoelting R, Dierdorf S (eds): Anesthesia and Co-Existing Disease. Churchill Livingstone, New York, 1983
29. Walts L, Miller J, Davidson M, Brown J: Perioperative management of diabetes mellitus. Anesthesiology 55: 104, 1981
30. Taitelman U, Reece E, Bessman A: Insulin in the

management of the diabetic surgical patient. JAMA 237:658, 1977
31. Drachman D: Myesthenia gravis. N Engl J Med 298:136, 1978
32. Stewart R: Craniofacial malformations—Clinical and genetic considerations. Pediatr Clin North Am 25:485, 1978
33. McGoldrick K: Anesthetic implications of congenital and metabolic diseases with ocular pathology. p. 139. In Bruce R, McGoldrick K, Oppenheimer P (eds): Anesthesia for Ophthalmology. Aescucapius, Birmingham, AL, 1982
34. Egbert L, Battit G, Turndorf H, et al: The value of the preoperative visit by an anesthetist. JAMA 185:553, 1963
35. Smith T, Stephen G, Zeiger L, et al: Effects of premedication drugs on respiration and gas exchange in man. Anesthesiology 28:883, 1967
36. Chessick K, Black S, Haye S: Spasm and operative cholangiography. Arch Surg. 110:53, 1975
37. Moore D, Balfour R, Fitzgibbons D: Convulsive arterial plasma Levels of bupivacaine and the response to diazepam therapy. Anesthesiology 50:454, 1979
38. Hillestad L, Hansen T, Melsom H, et al: Diazepam metabolism in normal man. Clin Pharm Ther 16:479, 1974
39. Lee C, Yeakel A: Patient refusal of surgery following innovar premedication. Anesth Analg 54:224, 1975
40. Keats A, Telford J, Jurousu Y: "Protentiation" of meperidine by promethazine. Anesthesiology 22:34, 1961
41. Donlon J: Anesthesia for eye, ear, nose, and throat surgery. p. 1265. In Miller R (ed): Anesthesia. Churchill Livingstone, New York, 1981
42. Frumin M, Herekar V, Jarvik M: Amnesic actions of diazepam and scopolamine in man. Anesthesiology 45:406, 1976
43. Garde J, Aston R, Endler G, et al: Racial mydriatic responses to belladona premedication. Anesth Analg 57:572, 1978
44. Schwartz H, deRoeth A, Papper E: Preanesthetic use of atropine in patients with glaucoma. JAMA 165:144, 1957
45. CoZanitis D, Dundee J, Buchanan T, Archer D: Atropine versus glycopyrrolate. Anaesthesia 34:236, 1979
46. Teabeaut J: Aspiration of gastric contents. Am J Pathol 28:51, 1952
47. Roberts R, Shirley M: Reducing the risk of acid aspiration during cesarean section. Anesth Analg 53:859, 1974
48. Manchikanti L, Kraus J, Edds S: Cimetidine and related drugs in anesthesia. Anesth Analg 61:595, 1982
49. Gibbs C, Spohr L, Schmidt D: The effectiveness of sodium citrate as an antacid. Anesthesiology 51:380, 1979
50. Klotz U, Reimann I: Delayed clearance of diazepam due to cimetidine. N Engl J Med 302:1012, 1980
51. Woodings E, Dixon G, Harrison C, et al: Ranitidine — A new H_2-receptor antagonist. Gut 21:187, 1980
52. McMahon C, Schaffer R, Hoskins H, et al: Adverse effects experienced by patients taking timolol. Am J Ophthalmol 88:736, 1979
53. Jones F, Eckberg N: Exacerbation of asthma by timolol. N Engl J Med 301:270, 1979
54. Shavitz S: Timolol and myasthenia gravis. JAMA 242:1612, 1979
55. deRoeth A, Dettbarn W, Rosenberg P: Effect of phospholine iodide on blood cholinesterace levels. Am J Ophthalmol 59:586, 1965
56. Fraunfelder F, Scafidi A: Possible adverse effects from topical ocular 10% phenylephrine. Am J Ophthalmol 85:447, 1978
57. Haddad N, Moyer N, Riley F: Mydriatic effect of phenylephrine hydrochloride. Am J Ophthalmol 70:729, 1970
58. Lansche R: Systemic reactions to topical epinephrine and phenylephrine. Am J Ophthalmol 49:95, 1966
59. Johnston R, Eger E, Wilson C: A comparative interaction of epinephrine with enflurane, isoflurane, and halothane in man. Anesth Analg 55:709, 1976
60. Myers E: Cocaine toxicity during dacryocystorhin ostomy. Arch Ophthal 98:842, 1980
61. Chung B, Naraghi M, Adriani J: Sympathomimetic effects of cocaine and their influence on halothane and enflurane anesthesia. Anesth Rev 5:16, 1978
62. Havener W: Secretory inhibitors. p. 575. In Havener W (ed): Ocular Pharmacology. CV Mosby, St. Louis, 1983
63. Havener W. Osmotic agents. p. 539. In Havener W (ed): Ocular Pharmacology CV Mosby, St. Louis, 1983
64. Eriksson E: Illustrated Handbook in Local Anaesthesia. 2nd Ed. WB Saunders, Philadelphia, 1980
65. Havener W: Anesthesia. p. 72. In Havener W (ed): Ocular Pharmacology. CV Mosby, St. Louis, 1983
66. Scott D, Cousins M: Clinical pharmacology of local anesthetic agents. p. 86. In Cousins M, Briden-

baugh P (eds): Neural Blockade. JB Lippincott, Philadelphia, 1980
67. Donlon J, Moss J: Plasma catecholamine levels during local anesthesia for cataract operations. Anesthesiology 51:471, 1979
68. Mindel J: Value of hyaluronidase in ocular surgical akinesia. Am J Ophthalmol 85:643, 1978
69. Covino B, Vassallo H: Local Anesthetics. Grune & Stratton, New York, 1976
70. Moore, D, Crawford R, Scurlock J: Severe hypoxia and acidosis following local anesthetic-induced convulsions. Anesthesiology 53:259, 1980
71. Lincoff H, Ellis C, DeVoe A, et al: The effect of succinylcholine on intraocular pressure. Am J Ophthalmol 40:501, 1955
72. Joshi C, Bruce D: Thiopental and succinylcholine: Action on intraocular pressure. Anesth Analg 54:471, 1975
73. Bain W, Maurice D: Physiologic variations in intraocular pressure. Trans Ophthalmol Soc UK 72:249, 1959
74. Schroeder M, Linssen G. Intraocular pressure and anaesthesia. Anaesthesia 27:165, 1972
75. Duncalf D, Weitzner S: Ventilation and hypercapnia on intraocular pressure during anesthesia. Anesth Analg 43:232, 1963
76. Samuel J, Beaugie A: Effect of carbon dioxide on the intraocular pressure in man during general anaesthesia. Br J Ophthalmol 58:62, 1974
77. Kornbleuth W, Aledjenoof L, Magora F: Influence of general anesthesia on intraocular pressure in man. Arch Ophthalmol 61:84, 1959
78. Magora F, Collins V: The influence of general anesthetic agents on intraocular pressure in man. Arch Ophthalmol 66:806, 1962
79. Ausinsch B, Graves S: Intraocular pressure in children during isoflurane and halothane anesthesia. Anesthesiology 42:167, 1975
81. Duncalf D, Foldes F: Effect of anesthetic drugs and muscle relaxants on intraocular pressure. Int Ophthalmol Clin 13:21, 1973
82. Litwiller R, Difazio C, Rushia E: Pancuronium and intraocular pressure. Anesthesiology 42:750, 1975
83. Oji E, Holdcroft E: The ocular effects of etomidate. Anaesthesia 34:245, 1979
84. Ivankovich A, Lowe H: The influence of methoxyflurane and neuroleptanalgesia on intraocular pressure in man. Anesth Analg 48:933, 1969
85. Yoshikawa K, Murai Y: The effect of ketamine on intraocular pressure in children. Anesth Analg 50:199, 1971
86. Ausinsch B, Rayburn R, Munson E, et al: Ketamine and intraocular pressure in children. Anesth Analg 55:773, 1976
87. Pandey K, Badola R, Kumar S: Time course of intraocular hypertension produced by suxamethonium. Br J Anaesth 44:191, 1972
88. Craythorne N, Rottenstein H, Dripps R: The effect of succinylcholine on intraocular pressure during general anesthesia. Anesthesiology 21:59, 1960
89. Taylor T, Mulcahy M, Nightengale D: Suxamethonium chloride in intraocular surgery. Br J Anaesth 40:113, 1968
90. Carballo A: Succinylcholine and acetazolamide in anesthesia for ocular surgery. Can Anaesth Soc J 12:486, 1965
91. Miller R, Way W, Hickey F: Inhibition of succinylcholine-induced intraocular pressure by nondepolarizing muscle relaxants. Anesthesiology 29:123, 1968
92. Meyers E, Krupin T, Johnson M, et al: Failure of nondepolarizing neuromuscular blockers to inhibit succinylcholine-induced increased intraocular pressure. Anesthesiology 48:149, 1978
93. Schwartz H, Apt L: Mydriatic effect of anticholinergic drugs used during reversal of nondepolarizing muscle relaxants. Am J Ophthalmol 88:608, 1979
94. Balamoutsos N, Drossou F, Alevizou F, Tjovairi E, Papastephanou C, et al: Pupil size during reversal of muscle relaxants. Anesth Analg 59:615, 1980
95. Stoelting R: Blood pressure and heart rate changes during laryngoscopy for intubation. Anesth Analg 57:197, 1978
96. Fineberg E, Machemer R, Sullivan P, et al: Sulfur hexafluoride in owl monkey vitreous cavity. Am J Ophthalmol 79:67, 1975
97. Stinson T, Donlon J: Interaction of SF_6 and air with nitrous oxide. Anesthesiology 51:S16, 1979
98. Bidwai A, Rogers C, Stanley T: Prevention of postextubation laryngospasm after tonsillectomy. Anesthesiology 51:S50, 1979
99. Snow J: Anesthesia in Otolaryngocology and Ophthalmocology. 2nd Ed. Appleton-Century-Crofts, E. Norwalk, CT, 1982
100. Bosomworth P, Ziegler C, Jacoby J: The oculocardiac reflex in eye muscle surgery. Anesthesiology 19:7, 1958
101. Apt L, Isenberg B, Gaffney W: The oculocardiac reflex in strabismus surgery. Am J. Ophthalmol 76:533, 1973
102. Alexander J: Reflex disturbances of cardiac rhythm

during ophthalmic surgery. Br J Ophthalmol 59:518, 1975

103. Meyers E, Tomeldan S: Glycopyrrolate compared with atropine in prevention of the oculocardiac reflex during eye muscle surgery. Anesthesiology 51:350, 1979
104. Reed H, McCaughey T: Cardiac slowing during strabismus surgery. Br J Ophthalmol 46:112, 1962
105. Mirakhur R, Jones C, Dundee J, Archer D: IM or IV atropine or glycopyrrolate for the prevention of oculocardiac reflex in children undergoing squint surgery. Br J Anaesth 54:1059, 1982
106. Hunsley J, Jones C: A study of glycopyrrolate and atropine in the suppression of the oculocardiac reflex during strabismus surgery in children. Br J Anaesth 54:459, 1982
107. Katz R, Bigger T: Cardiac arrhythmias during anesthesia. Anesthesiology 33:193, 1970
108. Meyers E, Charles P: Glycopyrrolate compared with atropine in patients undergoing intraocular operations with local anesthesia. Anesthesiology 49:370, 1978
109. Moonie G, Rees D, Eton D: The oculocardiac reflex during strabismus surgery. Can Anaesth Soc J 11:621, 1964
110. Cross D, Krupin T: Implications of the effects of general anesthesia on basal tear production. Anesth Analg 56:35, 1977
111. Fabian L: The experts opine. Surv Anesthesiol 23:134, 1979
112. Smith R: Succinylcholine and the forced duction test. Ophthalmol Surg 5:53, 1974
113. Tammisto T, Brander P, Airaksinen M: Strabismus as a possible sign of latent muscular disease predisposing to succinylcholine induced muscle injury. Ann Clin Res 2:126, 1970
114. Krisha G, Haselby K, Rao C, et al: The pediatric patient. p. 741. In Stoelting R, Dierdorf S (eds): Anesthesia and Co-Existing Disease. Churchill Livingstone, New York, 1983

The Surgical Microscope

2

Richard C. Troutman
Casimir A. Swinger

Twenty years ago, in 1966, a small internationally based group of surgeons met at the behest of Professor Heinrich Harms, Dr. Gunter Mackensen, and myself to discuss, with several interested manufacturers and each other, how we might encourage the use of the surgical microscope in ophthalmology. Several of us had been using surgical microscopes for 10 years or longer. Convinced that the improved visualization would reduce surgical trauma and improve technique, we approached the next most important group of individuals necessary to implement such a program: the manufacturing community. For the first time, and for most, the last time, the manufacturers cooperated to design a better instrument or instruments. During this brief commercial armistice many new ideas were proposed both by the profession and by manufacturers in our common meeting. Those manufacturers, convinced by our enthusiasm, went back to their various factories and began to produce microscopes designed specifically for ophthalmology. Although there were some false starts, out of this group have come the major microscopes in use by the profession today. This was not only true for microscopes, but also for instruments, needles, suture materials, and other instrumentation complimenting or reinforcing microsurgical techniques.

For this chapter it was my proposal that, rather than discuss a single microscope from a single manufacturer, I would use the format of the meeting in Tubingen and discuss the microscope from the standpoint of its systems. Each manufacturer has incorporated some or all of the system components to be described in their microscope as manufactured today. The ophthalmic microsurgeon, in choosing and learning to operate a surgical microscope, should be cognizant of the various systems and their component functions not only to acquire the best instrument for the specific task but also to make the most efficient use of the instrument selected. It should be the surgeon who orders the instrument with the necessary systems and system components and controls. If it is the manufacturer who dictates the systems to the surgeon, there may be unnecessary functions, or there may be necessary functions that have been omitted. From this description the surgeon should gain a better knowledge of his or her microscope by looking at it much as we were taught to look at the human body, from the standpoint of its systems and system function.

POSITIONING SYSTEM

Every major microscope requires the use of a positioning system, not only for positioning the microscope but also for positioning the surgeon and the patient.

The microscope is suspended above the patient either from a floor mount or from a ceiling mount (Fig. 2-1). The surgeon sits on a surgical chair that has armrests that position the arms and hands within the surgical field. Armrests can be mounted on the chair (Fig. 2-1A), reducing the possibility of the movement of the patient's head, or on the table top, supporting a handrest (Fig. 2-1B), or both.

The floor mount should be designed to be positioned in relation to the operating table without interfering with assistants or with the surgeon. When in position it should be able to be locked in such a way that vibrations or small movements are prevented. This is best accomplished by retracting

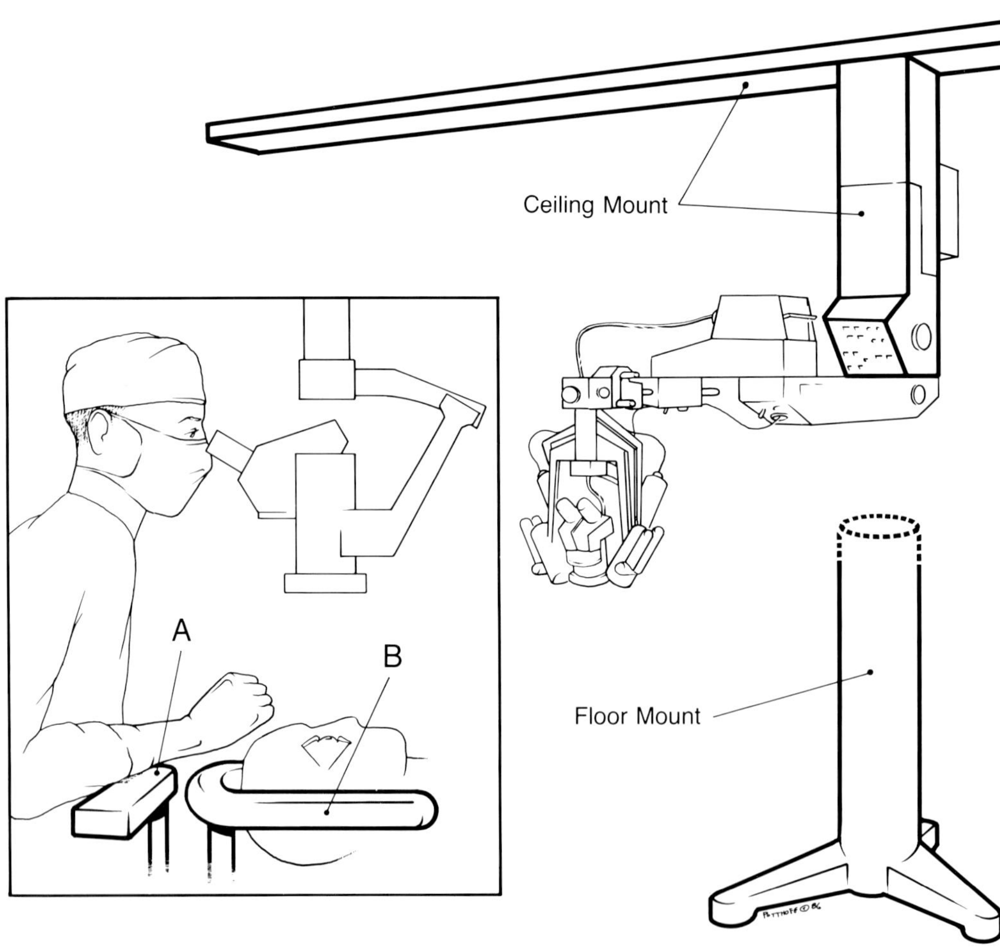

Fig. 2-1. Ceiling mount, floor mount. The ceiling mount suspends the microscope from a column containing basic microscope controls. These are duplicated on a wall switch plate (not illustrated). The floor mount is, in effect, an inverted ceiling mount that supports the microscope suspension arms and controls. It sets firmly on the floor when its casters are retracted. **(A)** Surgeon's armrest, which is attached to the chair. **(B)** Tabletop armrest (alternative).

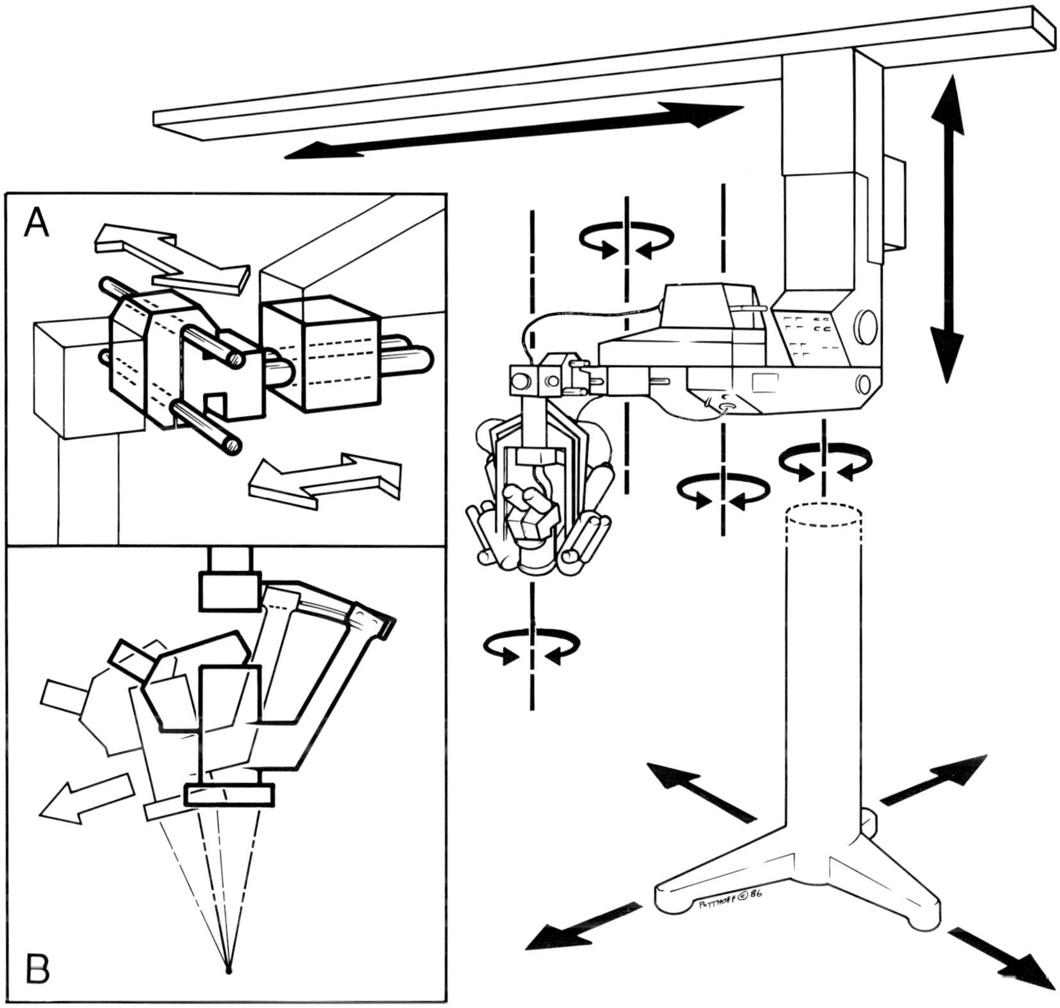

Fig. 2-2. Right. Top: Ceiling track supporting vertical ceiling support column above floor mount (alternate). Middle: Microscope shoulder, elbow, and wrist joints controlling position of the support arms of the microscope over the surgical field. Microscope on coaxial pivot. All joints are locked firmly by tension knobs when the microscope is in position. **(A)** X – Y positioning device, motor controlled, incorporating automatic centering device and speed control. **(B)** Planetary tilt mechanism allowing tilting of the microscope from the vertical position toward the surgeon without loss of focus or field.

positioning wheels into a heavy base, which then rests firmly on the floor (Figs. 2-1, 2-2).

The ceiling mount has the advantage of being fixed firmly overhead. When purchasing a ceiling mount the surgeon should investigate the stability of the ceiling upon which the microscope is to be mounted. There should be written assurance from the building contractor and the manufacturer that the ceiling structure is rigid enough to prevent vibration of the microscope. It may not be possible in some buildings to mount a ceiling track that will be completely stable. Structural modifications, sometimes expensive, will prevent disturbing movements. The ceiling track must be located in such a way that when in position the microscope and operating table are fully accessible to assistants, anesthesiologist, and nursing personnel and that ancillary equipment can be positioned as closely to the patient as possible.

A ceiling mount (Fig. 2-2, top left), motor driven to its surgical position, is more convenient to operating personnel than a manually positioned system. A motor-driven vertical column (Fig. 2-2, right) facilitates final positioning of the microscope to the surgical level more readily than does a manual lowering and retracting system. The microscope in turn should be supported on two equal-length arms extending from the vertical ceiling column (Fig. 2-2, center). The arm should be able to be moved in plane and fixed when positioned at the shoulder, elbow, and wrist. The shoulder portion is suspended from the top of the floor mount or base of the ceiling mount. The elbow, together with the wrist, which supports the microscope, provides full mobility of the arm in plane for X–Y positioning.

The microscope positioning unit is made up of an X–Y positioning system (Fig. 2-2A), a vertical coaxial support, which allows the microscope to be rotated around a 360 degree axis without changing the field position (Fig. 2-2, left center), and a tilting position, which ideally should be planetary, to permit the microscope to be changed from vertical to oblique again without losing focus or field position (Fig. 2-2B). All microscopes, except that from one manufacturer, however, use a tilting mechanism, which, of necessity, changes focus and field. This inconvenience is occasioned, according to the manufacturers, to make it possible for their microscope to be used by other disciplines that may require more tilting than available from the planetary tilt systems.

All of the positioning systems come into play during the rough and final positionings of the microscope for surgery. The floor or ceiling mount (Fig. 2-2, top, bottom) moves the microscope into position approximately over the surgical field. When the knobs locking the support arms are loosened the microscope can be moved in a rough X–Y direction to an approximate position over the eye. All friction knobs are locked in the final position so that the microscope is squared in relation to the X–Y. The X–Y mechanism, which should have a speed control and automatic centering device, moved to the neutral position, accomplishes the final positioning of the microscope over the surgical field.

ILLUMINATION SYSTEM

Of all of the microscope systems, the illumination system is probably the least understood and most inappropriately used. All modern surgical microscopes have a coaxial illumination system (Fig. 2-3A). The coaxial system was the first illumination system developed for surgical microscopes. The initial use of surgical microscopes was for otology and culposcopy to allow visualization of deep structures through small apertures. The ophthalmic use of a coaxial illumination system began with the introduction of extracapsular cataract extraction by phacoemulsification. The oblique illumination system (Fig. 2-3B,C) was an intermediate development. Before phacoemulsification made it necessary to view a red reflex, obliquely directed focal illuminators, one usually incorporating a slit lamp (Fig. 2-3C), were the only illumination systems used.

Oblique illumination causes less glare and enhances depth perception better than coaxially directed light. For some years ophthalmic microscopes were not equipped with coaxial systems because they were detrimental to viewing and performance of then common procedures. With modern surgical techniques both systems should be used, the coaxial system for viewing at the level of the iris and deeper, the oblique illumination system for viewing anterior to the iris. Coaxial illumination systems are also useful in extraocular muscle surgery or for some plastic procedures, for example, surgery of the lacrimal apparatus. During the extracapsular cataract operation, the coaxial system is used for the surgery of the lens. It should be shielded or shut off during all anterior segment surgery and surgery of the cornea.

There is abundant evidence that prolonged exposure of the retina to coaxial illumination during surgery may induce irreversible changes in retinal structures. Inadequate heat shielding of both coaxial and focal illuminators can produce dehydration and has resulted in corneal, conjunctival, and lid burns. Modern illumination systems are protected by ultraviolet and heat absorbing filters to minimize these problems. Nevertheless, when working with the coaxial illumination system the surgeon

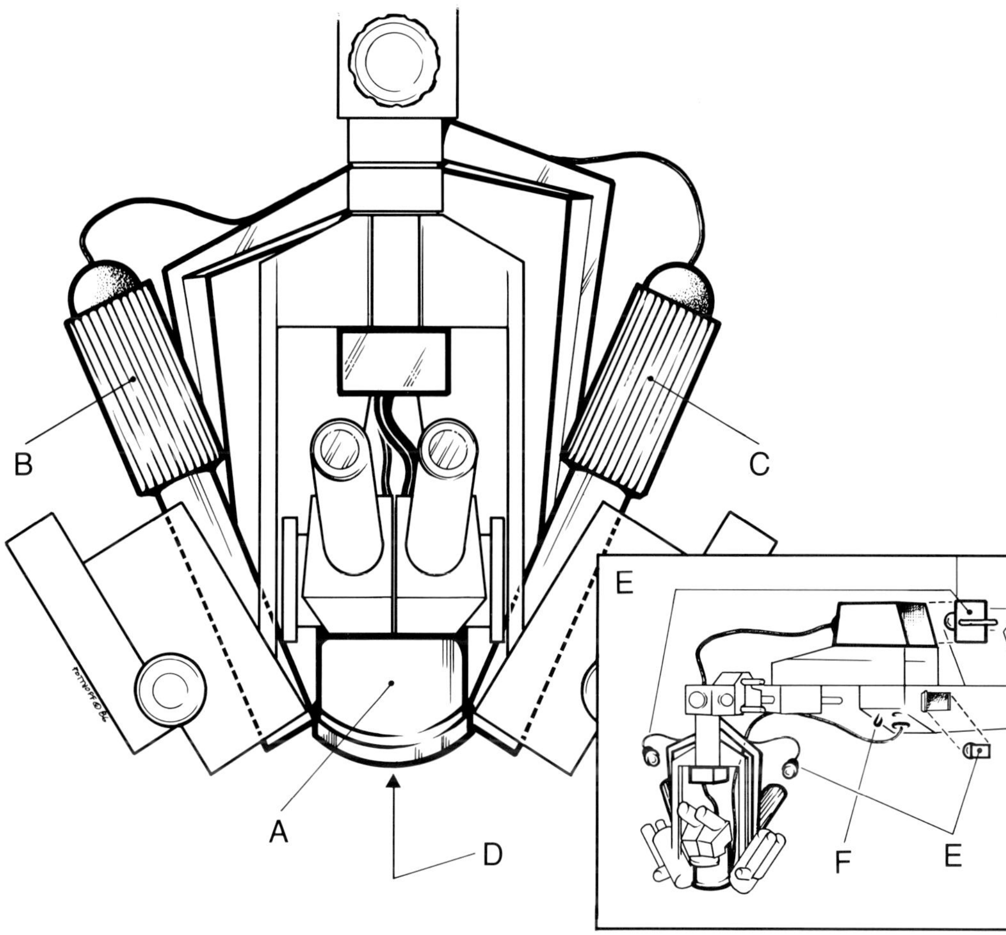

Fig. 2-3. Illumination systems. **(A)** Microscope body containing coaxial illumination system and LED centration light. Coaxial system illuminated through fiberoptic bundle seen centered above binoculars. **(B,C)** Focal illuminators left, focal only, right, focal incorporating slit lamp. **(D)** Surgical keratometer. **(E)** Quick change bulb installations for unit change of bulbs to focal illuminators, coaxial illuminator and keratometer. **(F)** Toggle switch for LED fixation light.

must prevent intense direct light from impinging on the macular region. The best way to accomplish this is to shut off the coaxial illumination system, using only the oblique system except when working specifically where the coaxial system must be used. Central occluders have been introduced into the coaxial optical system that induce a blackout of the central portion of the beam. Many surgeons, however, find this roving black spot disturbing.

All illuminator bulbs should be able to be changed readily during surgical procedures (Fig. 2-3E, inset). The change should be made using a bulb carrier so as to avoid touching the bulb during the change. Touching an incandescent or halogen bulb can cause early failure. Skin oil or deposited foreign bodies on the bulb can cause it to burn out prematurely. Figure 2-3E,F shows a method employed to change bulbs using carrier units that can be removed and replaced in a few seconds.

An auxiliary illumination system that is experiencing increasing use is the surgical keratometer (Figs. 2-3D, 2-5A,B) attached to the microscope body, which also contains the fiberoptic illuminated front surface mirror directing the light coaxially into the eye (Fig. 2-3A). The keratometer illustrated, that of the author, has 12 lights displayed in a circle centered around the objective of the microscope. Between the binocular microscope objectives is a centered fixation light (Fig. 2-5A). When activated (Fig. 2-3F) the light is fixated by the patient and the surgeon can mark the approximate optical center of the cornea. This fixation light when centered in the light ring also serves to verify the verticality of the microscope. When marking one must view the patient fixation light binocularly to determine the exact centration. In order to mark accurately the optical center of the cornea, the patient's visual axis, the surgeon should observe the parallax induced by shutting one eye and then the other alternately. A marking instrument is placed at an intermediate position between the observed parallax-deviated fixation light.

MICROSCOPE OPTICAL SYSTEM

The microscope optical system employs a conventional dissecting microscope especially modified for microsurgical use (Fig. 2-4A,B). The surgeon's microscope has its binocular (Fig. 2-4A) inclined at 40 to 45 degrees to the vertical so that he or she may view an object through the vertical objective without having to flex the neck. The body (Fig. 2-4B) incorporates, in addition to the binoculars, the zoom magnification system, the right and left beam splitters, and the objectives (Fig. 2-5A). The beam splitters allow the use of two optical devices, such as cameras or television, for recording a surgical procedure. The zoom system gives the surgeon a continuous magnification of between 6 and 24× depending upon the manufacturer. The working distance to the field from the microscope objective varies, depending upon the manufacturer, from 150 to 200 mm. The longer the working distance the less the magnification and the larger the field. For practical purposes, all current surgical microscopes have approximately the same field size when corrected for the working distance. As a general rule, the shorter the distance between the objective and the field, the more comfortable the working position of the surgeon.

The surgical microscope incorporates the pre-

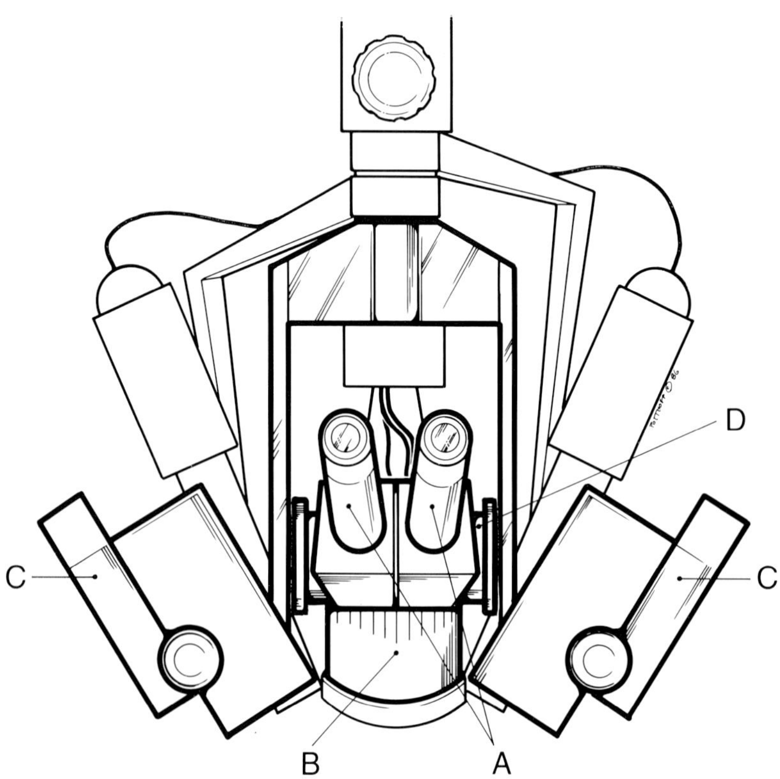

Fig. 2-4. Optical systems. **(A)** Binoculars. **(B)** Zoom magnification system. **(C)** Assistant's microscope left and right. **(D)** Beam splitters.

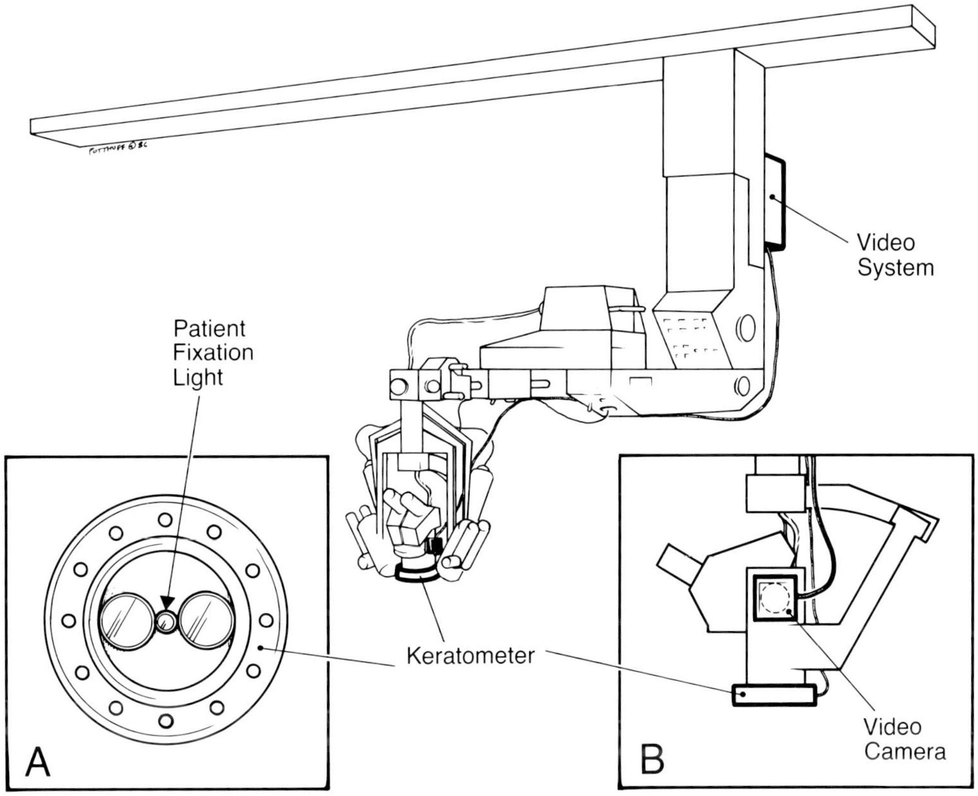

Fig. 2-5. Top. Video system control box leading to video camera attached to beam splitter right of microscope body. **(A,B)** Keratometer as integrated to microscope from lateral and inferior view. **(A)** Patient fixation light. **(B)** Video camera attached to beam splitter.

viously described surgical keratometer and LED patient fixation light (Figs. 2-5, 2-5A,B). When a television camera is attached to the beam splitter (Fig. 2-5B), the control system is mounted on the vertical ceiling column or floor mount (Fig. 2-1). Beam splitters are placed in such a way so as not to interfere with other optical or viewing systems (Figs. 2-4D, 2-5B). To the surgeon's microscope are attached the right and left surgical assistant microscopes (Fig. 2-4C). These microscopes view obliquely to the field and have separate galilean or zoom focusing systems incorporated so the assistant can maintain the magnification at the level of the surgeon or alter it. It is often important that the assistant have less magnification than the surgeon so that he or she may monitor the field outside the surgeon's area of attention. An assistant's microscope can be attached to the beam splitter.

When an assistant's microscope is coupled to the beam splitter, the assistant observes through only one of the surgeon's microscope objectives. This reduces illumination 50 percent and eliminates binocularity, making it difficult for the assistant to function accurately. His or her functioning is impeded also by the fact that the assistant's microscope must work at the same magnification as the surgeon's microscope. This does not permit the assistant to use a reduced magnification for better overall viewing of the field.

One manufacturer has an assistant's microscope capable of binocular, almost coaxial, viewing. This is accomplished by the flat prism table, which centers and verticalizes the objective of the tilted assistant's microscope. Since it has the disadvantage of interfering with the illumination by the surgical keratometer it is most useful in procedures in the posterior segment, where the surgical keratometer is not used.

MICROSCOPE FUNCTION CONTROLS

Microscope functions are controlled either by a foot switch panel (Fig. 2-6, right) or by a hand-operated panel mounted to the right or left of the surgical microscope. Ophthalmic surgeons seem almost universally to prefer a foot-operated panel incorporating all of the functions necessary to position the microscope and focus it. In addition, the foot panel incorporates a switch for alternately selecting illumination (Fig. 2-6C) and switch for activation (Fig. 2-6D) of ancillary equipment such as a camera. The foot switch illustrated (Fig. 2-6) shows two rocker panels, one of which controls the focusing of the microscope (E), and the other the zoom (F). A joy stick (A) controls the X–Y unit, moving the microscope right, left, forward, backward, or obliquely. The switches (B) on the sides of the unit forward tilt the microscope in or out. The three-position switch (C) on the left side of the unit turns the coaxial system on, the oblique illumination system on, or all three on. The right switch (D) controls the camera or other auxiliary equipment at the election of the surgeon.

Other functions of the microscope, such as gross vertical movement of the column for initial positioning of the microscope and change of intensity of illumination, are controlled by means of rheostats from a column or wall-mounted auxiliary switching panel (Fig. 2-1). Keratometer illumination, also controlled at the auxiliary control panel (Fig. 2-1), is left on throughout the procedure. The LED fixation light (Fig. 2-5A) again, since it does not interfere with the surgical viewing, can also be left on during the procedure and is controlled from a separate switch (Fig. 2-3F) mounted to one of the support arms. X–Y centration and speed control (Fig. 2-2A) are mounted on that unit and activated only between procedures.

Recently, several manufacturers have introduced voice-controlled systems that directly control microscope functions by the surgeon speaking a command such as "focus up" or "focus down" to a computer that has been trained to recognize his or

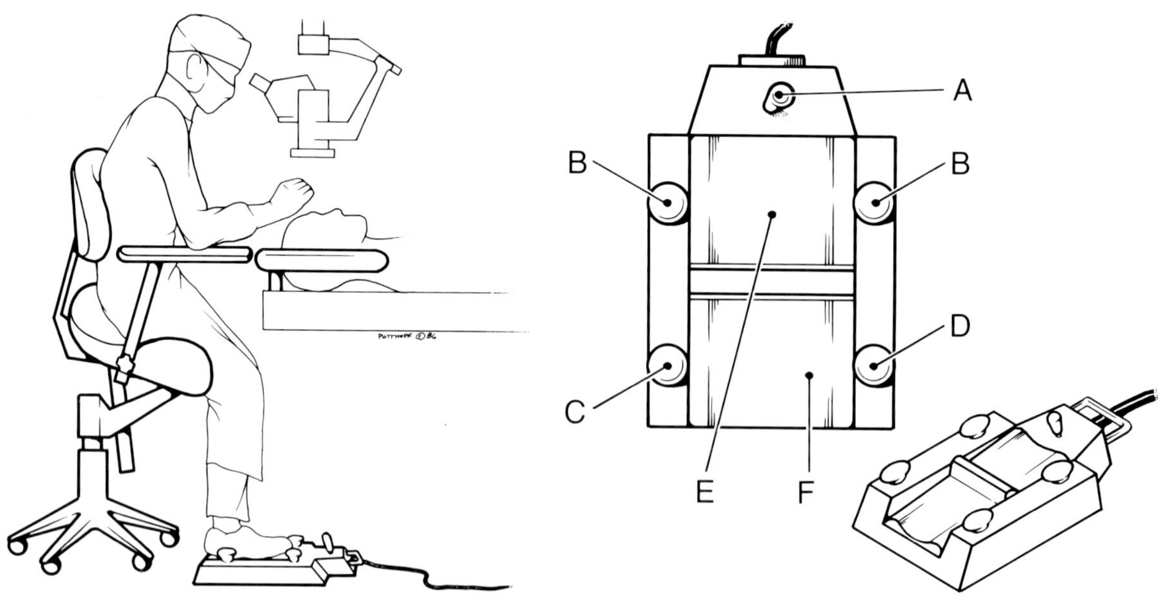

Fig. 2-6. Left: Ergonomically designed chair (Pos chair™). A neutral-posture chair incorporating adjustments for tilt, back support and elevation, and depression that allows the surgeon to work in a neutral-posture position, significantly decreasing fatigue during surgery. Right: **(A)** Joy stick for X–Y positioning. **(B,** right, left) Tilt controls. **(C)** Light on–off switch. **(D)** Auxilliary switch. **(E)** Foot switch operating focus. **(F)** Zoom.

her voice, or, indirectly by the surgeon speaking a function such as "focus," which activates a foot control for movement of focus up or down as desired. A proximity switch mounted above and between the surgeon's binoculars allows the surgeon to activate or inactivate the unit merely by moving a millimeter or two toward or away from the proximity switch.

PATIENT AND SURGEON POSITIONING

The patient is positioned under the microscope on an operating platform or table. At the present time such tables are adapted from existing general surgical equipment. This has been necessitated by the occasional need for rapid repositioning of the patient in the event of anesthetic emergency. Improvement in these patient support systems has been primarily in the method to move the patient to and from the table. In some instances the table top can be transferred directly from a gurney to a permanent floor-mounted pedestal. In others the entire operating table moves in and out of the room and doubles as a recovery stretcher.

The surgeon's chair has received even less attention and it is only recently that an ergonomically designed chair has been introduced that offers improved seating for the surgeon. One has only to visit an operating room and observe surgeons at work or moving painfully between cases to see the extent to which current surgical chairs fail to give him or her the sort of comfort required for long sessions of microsurgery. The position of the surgeon during microsurgery is such that back support with presently used stools and chairs is virtually unattainable. Pressure on the posterior thigh area is universal. The new chair illustrated in Figure 2-6 incorporates a tilting seat on which the back also tilts to give the surgeon firm back support when leaning into the microscope. The surgeon is maintained in this forward-leaning position by the shape of the chair bottom. This chair bottom incorporates a pommel to prevent the surgeon from sliding forward on the tilted pan with a waterfall front to either side so that the backs of the thighs will not be compressed by the edge of the chair bottom. Compared to the vertical right-angle-only seat position of most chairs this chair has three positioning systems controlling elevation, back support, and tilt. The surgeon is not only more comfortable but better ergonomic support has been shown to significantly increase surgical efficiency and performance.

SUMMARY

The primary tool of ophthalmic microsurgery is the surgical microscope. Understanding of the various systems that make up the surgical microscope will increase the facility of its use by the individual surgeon. The initial positioning of the microscope from its retracted position is the responsibility of the surgeon. Understanding the support mechanism enables this to be done quickly, efficiently, and accurately. Understanding the illumination system in its various functions enables the surgeon to illuminate the surgical field in the most efficient manner for the particular procedure being performed. This not only provides the best visualization but also the greatest protection for the eye. Measuring systems, such as the surgical keratometer and the centering LED, and recording systems, such as the television camera and still cameras, must be understood, as they, too, are important to the better performance of the procedure and its adequate record. The foot control should be so familiar to the surgeon that it can be operated without needing to see it at any time during the procedure. It should contain all the necessary functions to control both positioning and illumination for the greatest facility of surgery and the best protection of the patient.

Finally, both the patient and the surgeon must be firmly and comfortably positioned so that, particularly under local anesthesia, the patient will not suffer skeletal or muscular discomfort, and the surgeon will not be tired by his or her poor positioning on an adequate surgical chair. Stabilization of the seated surgeon and of his or her arms and hands in an ergonomically comfortable position for the duration of the procedure is essential to the best surgical performance. Within limits, the higher the magnification the surgeon can use comfortably to perform the procedure, the less trauma he or she will inflict and the less morbidity will result from the operation. A firm stable microscope support, appropriate illumination, facile function control, and an ergonomically comfortable position of both patient and surgeon combine to allow the use of the highest magnification possible and effective for a given surgical technique improving both the quality and performance of a given microsurgical procedure.

Lasers

3

Richard H. Keates

Ophthalmology has been one of the pioneer surgical specialties using therapeutic lasers in medicine. Eventually, the whole electromagnetic spectrum may conceivably have therapeutic applications. The two mechanisms of action of laser light that have particular value for the ophthalmologist are based on either thermal effects or photodisruptive effects.

The laser light may have a "hot" or a "cold" effect. The mechanism of action of the "hot" thermal effect is that light is absorbed by the target and converted into heat. The heat causes the tissue temperature to rise, thus causing a thermal damage. Argon, krypton, ruby, and CO_2 lasers cause lesions by photocoagulation.

The "cold" laser effect is via photodisruption. The Nd:YAG laser is an example of this type of mechanism. The power is delivered over an extremely short (10^{-12}-second) time period, causing rapid ionization of the target. The ionized tissue with sheered-off electrons is called a plasma state. Tissue damage results from an acoustic and mechanical shock wave produced at the plasma formation. The temperature in the center of the plasma is in excess of 15,000°C. The area of the temperature elevation is extremely small (less than 0.1 mm). Although a thermal effect is generated, the area is so small that photocoagulation per se does not occur.

Several important differences must be discussed before the clinical applications can be reviewed. As the energy is increased

$$E = P \times t$$

where E is energy, P is power, and t is time, the photocoagulation effect increases linearly. The energy can be increased by either raising the power of the laser or lengthening the duration of the laser burn, or both.

The photodisrupting laser is nonlinear and an all-or-none phenomenon. Below the threshold, optical breakdown does not occur. Since the duration of laser pulse is held constant, the energy is increased by increasing the power. Some models may also increase the energy be increasing the number of bursts per pulse. The spot size is held constant for a photodisrupting laser, whereas the photocoagulating laser spot size may be changed from 50 to 1,000 μm.

From this point on, for ease of discussion and understanding, the clinical application of the photocoagulating and photodisrupting lasers is discussed separately.

PHOTOCOAGULATION

Laser Delivery

In general, a laser system is composed of a laser cavity that emits light of a particular wavelength. This is delivered through the laser's own optical system to the target. The surgeon views the aiming beam and the target through the optical system of the slit lamp (Fig. 3-1).

Aiming Beam

The aiming beam is an attenuated laser treatment beam. The energy of the aiming beam is low enough so as not to cause tissue damage. When the laser is fired the aiming beam increases to the desired setting and becomes the treatment beam. The same optical path is used, and the spot size of the treatment beam will be the same as that of the aiming beam.

Laser Wavelength

Table 3-1 shows the available lasers and their characteristics. Each laser's usefulness is dictated by its wavelength. Table 3-1 shows which wavelengths are absorbed by the pigmented ocular structures. The Nd:YAG laser is absorbed by all tissues and is dependent on its point of focus. The CO_2 laser is largely absorbed by water. It is therefore most effective in procedures limited to the surface of the eye. The surgeon may choose a wavelength that will allow for the best treatment of specific disease entities.

Table 3-1. Comparison of Lasers and Their Respective Wavelengths

Laser	Color	Wavelength
Excimer ArF	Ultraviolet	193
Argon	Blue	488
Argon	Green	514
Krypton	Yellow	568
Helium-neon	Red	632
Krypton	Red	647
Ruby	Red	694
Nd:YAG	Infrared	1,064
Erbium YLF	Infrared	1,228
Carbon dioxide	Infrared	10,600

Focusing

Focusing the optical system of the laser delivery apparatus and the slit lamp is critical. If the surgeon and the laser are not parfocal, the spot size will be incorrect. This is extremely important when the 50- and 100-μm spot size is used. Although this is not as important for the 500-μm spot size, proceeding without focusing would be poor technique.

For most lasers, the focal point for the 50- and 100-μm spot size will be parfocal with the focal point of the slit lamp. The laser delivery system achieves a 200- to 1,000-μm spot size by defocusing the 100-μm spot size. Therefore, for the same laser power, the smaller spot size has the same power but increased power density. To focus the laser, the following steps should be followed.

1. Set the spot size to 100 μm and project the aiming beam onto the target rod.
2. With one eye open, adjust the slit lamp with the joy stick to achieve the smallest-diameter aiming beam. If the target rod is not in focus simultaneously, turn the reticle to adjust the power of the oculars until the target rod is in focus.
3. Focus the other eye monocularly until the tar-

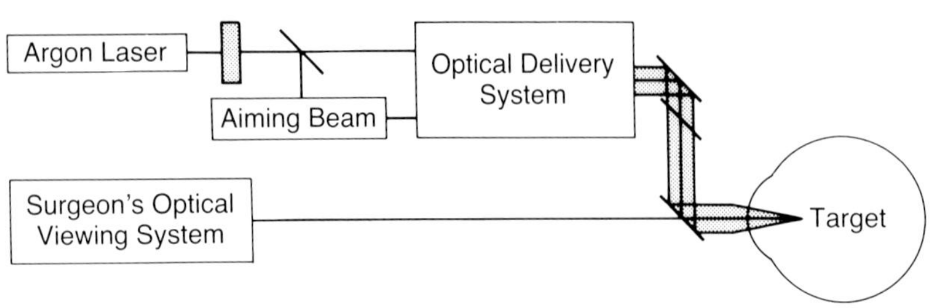

Fig. 3-1. Argon laser delivery system.

get rod is in focus. Now, with both eyes open, the target rod should be in clear focus while the aiming beam maintains the smallest diameter. The system will now be in focus. This procedure should be done by all surgeons prior to using the laser.

Hints before Proceeding

Laser treatments are easier to perform in a cooperative patient. Patient education regarding what to expect will usually relax the patient during the procedure. Both the surgeon and the patient should be situated at the laser in a comfortable position. Finally, if a gonioprism will be used, the surgeon should be able to rest an arm comfortably to facilitate manipulation of the gonioprism.

TREATMENT AREAS

Eyelids

Treatment of hemangioma of the eyelid that has a potential to cause amblyopia in children has been recommended. Xenon, argon, and CO_2 lasers have been used.

Cornea

Pterygia

Pterygia have been treated with argon lasers. The goal is to halt the advancing pterygium. Although the laser may close off blood vessels within the pterygia, it may also stimulate granulation tissue. The cornea is treated with topical anesthesia prior to treatment. The 50- or 100-μm spot size is focused directly onto blood vessels within the ptergium. With a duration of 0.2 seconds, it should be started at 300 mW and the power increased as necessary. Spot sizes larger than 100 μm should not be used. It should be remembered that a 500-μm spot size is really a defocused 100-μm spot size. If the larger spot sizes are used, the laser will actually be focused deep into the pterygium. This may cause an unwanted anterior chamber burn.

Sutures

Sutures may be divided with the argon laser in patients who present a difficulty with standard techniques. Settings of 50 μm, 0.2 seconds, and 500 to 700 mW should be used. The globe may be immobilized with an Abraham lens to facilitate suture division.

Iris

The techniques for argon laser iridectomy and iridoplasty are taken from a manual by Ritch.[1]

Iridectomy

The patient is pretreated with 650 mg aspirin orally 1 hour prior to treatment. The aspirin helps prevent inflammation by inhibiting prostaglandins. The pupil should be constricted with 2 to 4 percent pilocarpine if maximal miosis is not already obtained. If the pupil is not miotic, the iris will be thicker and will require more energy to produce a peripheral iridectomy. The patient should continue with all glaucoma medications.

Topical anesthesia is applied followed by the Abrahams lens. This lens increases the cone angle and thus decreases the spot size (Fig. 3-2). By de-

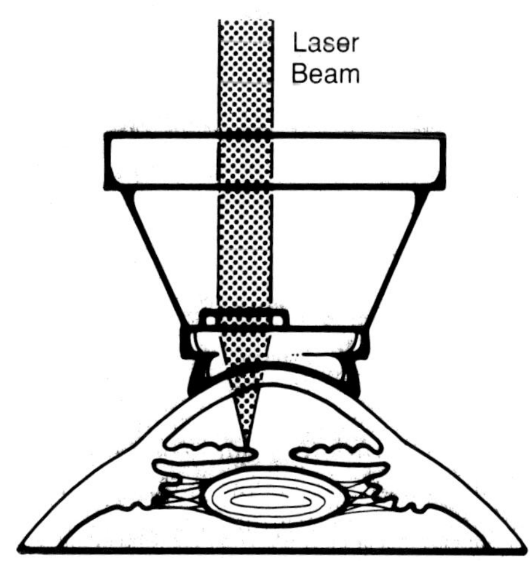

Fig. 3-2. Using an Abraham lens will increase the cone angle and thereby decrease the spot size; that is, power density is increased.

Table 3-2. Various Types of Laser Burn Techniques Used in Argon Laser Iridectomies

	Spot Size (μm)	Duration (sec)	Power (mW)
Contraction	500	0.5	200
Punch	50	0.02	1,200–1,500
Penetration	50	0.05 or 0.1	1,000 or 500
Cleanup	50	0.1–0.2	300

(Modified from Ritch R: Techniques of argon laser iridectomy and iridoplasty. Coherent Medical, Palo Alto, CA, 1983.)

creasing the spot size, the power density is increased. The settings are dependent on the pigmentation of the iris. In all irides, the superior nasal quadrant should be used when possible to avoid retinal complications and be covered by the upper lid. The types of application to be used would be a contraction burn to shrink the iris stroma, a punch-and-penetration burn to create a hole in the iris, and a cleanup burn to enlarge the opening (Table 3-2).

Dark Brown Irides

This author recommends finding a crypt in the superior nasal area and beginning with punch burns. The shorter-duration, high-power beams will prevent a pigmented crust from forming over the iridectomy site. The pigment crust is more common in heavily pigmented irides when longer duration burns are applied. The pigment crust will absorb the laser and prevent the progression through the iris. The number of applications is variable. Using the punch technique may require 300 to 400 applications. Signs that the posterior chamber has been entered are reflection of the aiming beam off the lens capsule and a puff of pigment into the anterior chamber as fluid passes from the posterior to anterior chamber through the iridectomy.

Light Brown Irides

These are probably the easiest irides to penetrate. This author has found penetration burns to be most useful. Again, a crypt should be identified for the site of treatment. Penetration burns are placed until a full-thickness iridectomy has been formed.

Blue or Gray Irides

With these irides a contraction burn must be used. This will usually cause some pigmentation of the iris. Actually, the iris stroma is being compacted; thus the pigment is also being concentrated. Punch burns are then used to perform an iridectomy in the center of the contraction burn. Care should be taken to focus carefully on the superficial layers. If the pigment epithelium is removed before the anterior stroma is penetrated, the remainder of the procedure will be almost impossible. Once a full-thickness iridectomy is completed, the opening can be enlarged with cleanup burns.

Postoperative Care

Topical steroid three times daily is recommended, with intraocular pressure checks made at 2 and 24 hours postlaser treatment. Pressure elevation should be treated appropriately. The patient should return on the first postoperative day for evaluation of the patency of the peripheral iridectomy and the status of the intraocular pressure.

Iridoplasty

Pretreatment consists of aspirin therapy and miotic therapy similar to that used in laser iridectomy. The laser settings are set to that of a contraction burn. Figure 3-3 shows the location of the laser applications. Light irides may require more power than do dark irides. One should start low and gradually increase the power until the desired effect is obtained.

Use of the argon laser permits manipulation of the iris for specific disease entities. If the iris is obstructing the angle structures, iridoplasty may be useful for pulling the iris out of the angle. Iridoplasty would therefore be very useful for angle closure glaucoma not controlled by medications in which an iridectomy has been unsuccessful. Plateau iris, nanophthalmis, and ciliary block glaucoma also respond well. Finally, iridoplasty should be performed prior to laser trabeculoplasty in patients with both a chronic open-angle glaucoma and a narrow-angle component. The iridoplasty will remove the iris from the angle and therefore

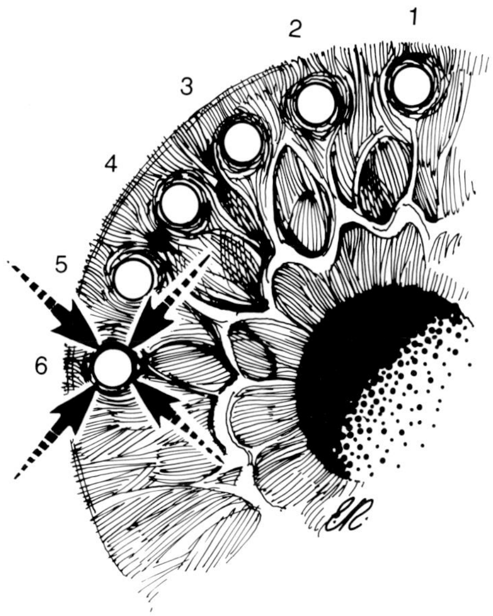

Fig. 3-3. The contraction burn pulls tissue toward the center of the burn, thus pulling iris tissue away from the angle structures.

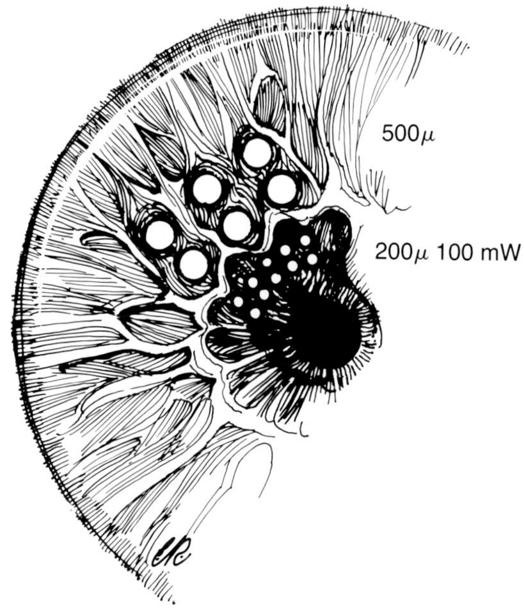

Fig. 3-4. Pupiloplasty with small contraction burns near the pupil and large burns in the mid-periphery of the iris.

enable the surgeon to complete the laser trabeculoplasty.

Postoperative care consists of topical steroids every 2 hours for 24 hours, followed by three times daily for 72 hours. Intraocular pressure elevation should be monitored and treated appropriately.

Pupiloplasty

The argon laser can also be used for eccentric pupils and chronic miosis. The patient is pretreated with 650 mg aspirin 1 hour prior to the laser treatment. A miotic pupil may be enlarged by placing contraction burns just outside the pupillary border of the iris (Fig. 3-4). In this case, this author recommends using a 200-μm spot and starting at 100 mW power. Contraction burns can be placed elsewhere on the iris to increase the effect. Burns farther away from the pupil should be 500 μm in size.

Postoperative care consists of topical steroids every 2 hours for the first 24 hours, and then three times daily for the next 3 days. Intraocular pressure must be followed postoperatively at 2 hours and 24 hours. Increases in intraocular pressure are treated appropriately.

For an updrawn pupil with the inferior portion of the iris obstructing the visual axis, the contraction burn should also be used. Contraction burns placed on the inferior iris will pull the iris inferiorly.

Trabecular Meshwork

The technique for argon laser trabeculoplasty is largely taken from Mandall and Terry.[2] Argon laser trabeculoplasty for treatment of chronic open-angle glaucoma not responsive to maximal tolerated medical therapy has become very popular since the original article by Wise.[2a] It has proved a useful technique for lowering intraocular pressure. Studies are currently being completed to determine the value of its use prior to maximally tolerated medically therapy. Contraindications include not being able to visualize the trabecular meshwork.

Preoperative Care

The patient should be maintained on medical therapy. If the patient is on a carbonic anhydrase inhibitor, an additional dose should be given 2

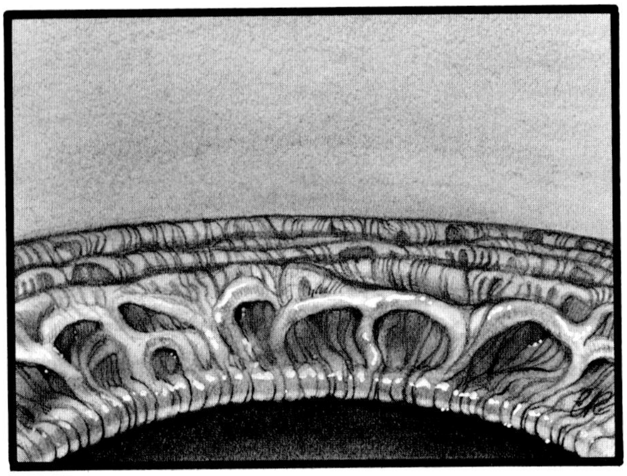

Fig. 3-5. Poor visualization of angle structures.

hours preoperatively. Aspirin 650 mg PO is given 2 hours preoperatively.

Explaining the procedure to the patient is crucial. An informed patient will be more cooperative. Slit-lamp examination is also extremely important. The angle structures should be identified 360 degrees prior to the treatment. Having a good mental image of Schwalbe's line, the trabecular meshwork, and the scleral spur will facilitate the laser treatment. The surgeon must also be certain that the treatment is placed correctly. Pigment anterior to Schwalbe's line (Sampaolasi line) may cause the treatment to be placed on the corneal endothelium rather than the trabecular meshwork (Figs. 3-5 and 3-6). Incorrect location of treatment can cause increasing glaucoma rather than lowering the intraocular pressure.

Treatment consists of placing a total of 100 burns of 50-μm spot size and 0.1-second duration. The power setting is started at 500 mW and is increased until the desired effect is reached. The surgeon is looking for a tiny bubble to form or a slight blanching of the tissue. The site of treatment is at the junction of nonpigmented and pigmented trabecular meshwork (Fig. 3-6).

In patients with advanced glaucoma, the surgeon may consider two separate 180-degree treatments in an attempt to keep the postoperative pressure rise down.

Postoperative care consists of topical steroids every hour while awake followed by three times daily for 1 week. The intraocular pressure must be checked 1 hour and 24 hours postoperatively. Again, unacceptable pressure increases should be treated appropriately.

Rubeosis

Treatment of early rubeosis in the angle may be of benefit if performed prior to the formation of fibrosis. Unfortunately, most patients do not

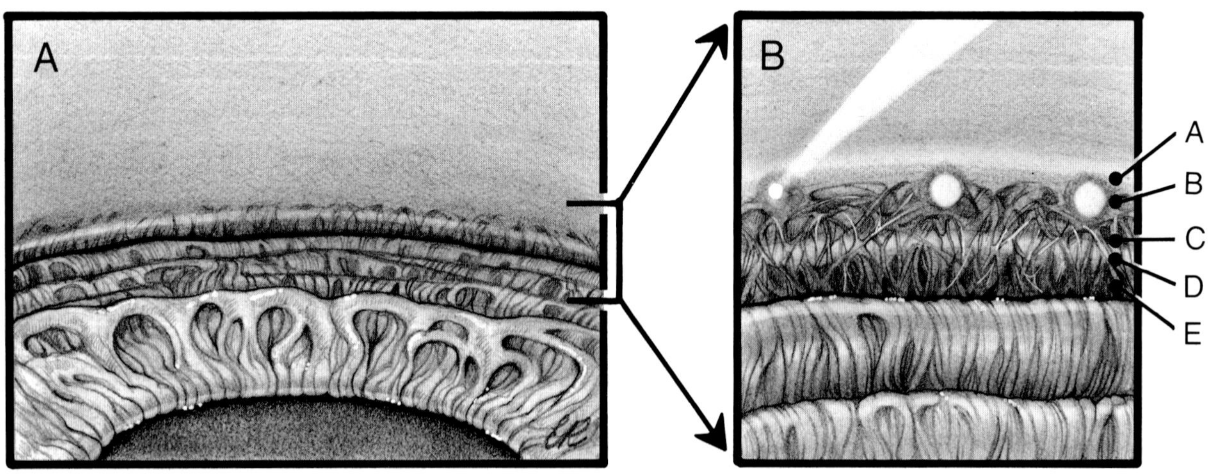

Fig. 3-6. Good visualization of angle structures. **(A)** Schwalbe's line. **(B)** Nonpigmented trabecular network. **(C)** Pigmented trabecular meshwork. **(D)** Scleral spur. **(E)** Ciliary band. The site of treatment with the argon laser is at the junction of nonpigmented and pigmented trabecular meshwork.

present at this early stage. The vessels can be occluded by using a gonio lens with the laser set to a 50-μm spot size for 0.1 seconds and a power of 500 mW. Postoperative care consists of treating the underlying cause of the rubeosis and short-term topical steroid therapy.

Choroid and Retina

Diabetic Retinopathy

Argon laser treatment has been shown to prevent the loss of vision in patients with diabetic retinopathy. Between 5 and 10 percent of diabetics will develop visual loss from diabetic retinopathy. Proliferative diabetic retinopathy occurs with retinal ischemia from capillary nonperfusion. A postulated vasoproliferative substance is released to induce neovascularization.

Diabetic retinopathy is divided into background and proliferative forms. Both forms may have macular edema. Patients with background retinopathy are not treated with laser therapy. A study is under way to determine the potential benefits of early treatment. Currently, persistent macular edema is the only indication for treatment in background retinopathy.

Macular edema may be produced by leaking vessels around the fovea. If foveal leaks can be identified on the fluoroscein angiogram, they should be specifically treated. Applications of 200-μm spots of 0.1-second duration is recommended. Excessive treatment should be avoided. The prognosis for improved vision is good when the leakage is focal. In patients with diffuse macular leakage the prognosis is poor. With diffuse leakage, a scatter pattern of 200-μm spots may be applied. The area of capillary nonperfusion must be avoided.

Treatment of the macula should be done with a fundus lens. The fluoroscein angiogram should be projected on a screen at the same time in order to locate the focal treatment sites. Areas of retinal hemorrhage and hard exudate should be avoided. The adjacent area may be treated instead (Fig. 3-7). The surgeon may prefer a retrobulbar injection to prevent the patient from looking directly into the aiming beam.

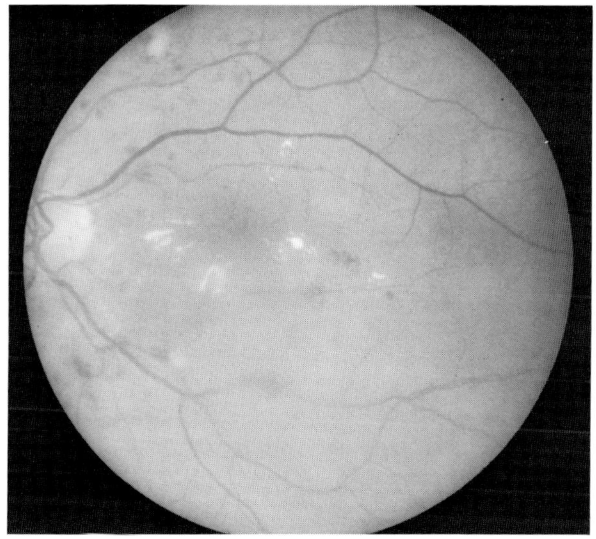

Fig. 3-7. Macular edema treatment by Argon laser.

Proliferative Diabetic Retinopathy

Peripherial retinal ablation has been shown to be effective in preventing loss of vision. There are four risk factors to consider before initiating treatment. The patient usually has two or more risk factors to qualify for therapy: (1) neovascularization elsewhere, (2) neovascularization of the disc, (3) neovascularization larger than one disc diameter, and (4) vitreous hemorrhage.

Once the surgeon has decided to treat, the eye should be maximally dilated and topical anesthesia applied. This author prefers to first outline the treatment areas. This approach gives an additional safety factor when using the mirrored peripheral retinal lenses.

First, a row of lesions are placed just outside the arcade (Fig. 3-8). A 500-μm spot size should be used for 0.1 to 0.2 seconds with the indirect type retinal lens. Next the fovea is located and spots are placed two disc diameters temporal to the fovea. The nasal retina is then treated. Lesions are placed one disc diameter away from the disc. If disc neovascularization is present, this area is avoided. The goal is to ablate retina and not treat neovascularization focally. Direct treatment can be used in selected cases but may cause hemorrhage, which will make photocoagulation more difficult.

Now that the area of nontreatment has been out-

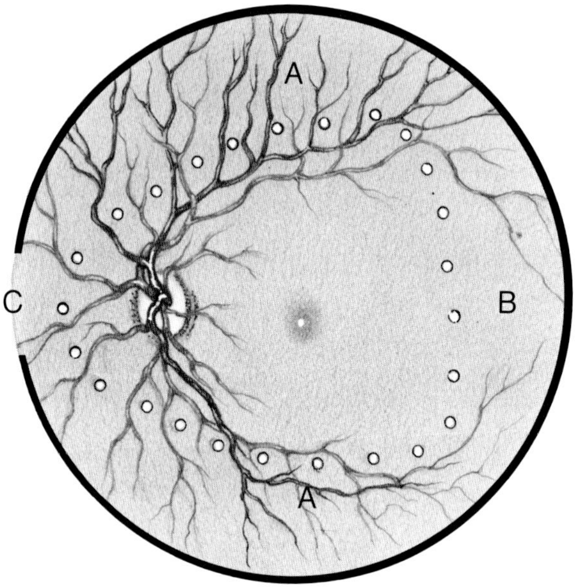

Fig. 3-8. Initial placement of Argon laser application for proliferative diabetic retinopathy.

lined, the peripheral retina can be treated. If the posterior portion of the peripheral retina is treated first, this will decrease the risk of macular edema when the peripheral retina is treated. The panfunduscopic retinal lens is an excellent lens with which to treat the central periphery. The surgeon must remember that this lens gives the same view as indirect ophthalmoscopy. No more than one half the central periphery can be treated at the first session. This will decrease the possibility of posttreatment choroidal effusion. A 500-μm spot size, 0.1 to 0.2 seconds in duration, is used. The power setting is gradually increased until a slight blanching of the pigment epithelium is obtained. Lesions are placed a distance of approximately one half spot size apart.

Although some patients may experience some discomfort with the laser treatment, most will not require retrobulbar injection for anesthesia. On subsequent visits, the more peripheral retina should be treated. The mirrored retinal lens must be utilized. Fifty percent of the remaining area should be treated.

Areas of tractional retinal detachment should be outlined during the first treatment session. This area may be treated more safely after 4 weeks, when a firm chorioretinal adhesion has formed. The laser can cause a retinal hole in the area of tractional retinal detachment.

Vascular Occlusion

Central retinal vein occlusion and branch vein occlusion may cause either macular edema or neovascularization secondary to retinal ischemia, or both. Patients with neovascularization should be treated with retinal photocoagulation in areas of fluoroscein angiography-proven nonperfusion. This treatment is similar to that of proliferative diabetic retinopathy. Macular edema from vascular occlusion may also improve with a scatter pattern around the fovea and to the area of capillary nonperfusion.

MACULAR SUBRETINAL NEOVASCULARIZATION

The laser has opened exciting vistas for the retinal surgeon. Previously, one could only watch helplessly as a subretinal neovascular membrane extended into the macula leading to subretinal hemorrhage and fibrinosis. Now, in selected cases, the retinal surgeon can ablate subretinal neovascular membranes. Currently, the argon and krypton red lasers have clinical applications in treating subretinal membranes.

The argon laser emits light in the blue (488.0-nm) and green (514.5-nm) wavelength and was originally developed to produce vascular closure. The blue-green spectrum is absorbed by the three pigmented layers in the fundus: (1) xanthophyll in the macula, (2) hemoglobin within the vessels, and (3) melanin in the retinal pigment epithelium. This allows for an efficient generation of thermal energy in the spot vicinity without excessively heating the ocular media. The disadvantage of the blue wavelength is that it is well absorbed by the yellow macular xanthophyll pigment, which leads to inner retinal and nerve fiber layer damage. Argon laser-emitting green light only significantly decreases this effect and permits juxtafoveal treatment of subretinal nets.[3,4]

The histopathology of argon retinal burns

usually shows some necrosis. The thermal damage to the vessel presumably accounts for vessel leakage seen on fluorescein angiography. The adjacent nerve fiber layer and ganglion cell layer will display coagulation necrosis. This is especially important around the optic nerve and around the macula, where the capillary network is the densest. It is in these regions in which extensive destruction of the nerve fiber layer may be produced by even weak argon burns. For this reason, attention has been directed to the krypton laser for treating macular and perimacular subretinal membranes.

The krypton laser can produce several wavelengths, but the red (647.1-nm) wavelength has been investigated most because of its clinical characteristics. The krypton red wavelength passes easily through cataracts, vitreous hemorrhage, xanthophyll pigment, and retina. The krypton red wavelength is strongly absorbed by the choroid and retinal pigment epithelium. This wavelength has the theoretical advantage of sparing normal retina while efficiently transferring energy to subretinal pathology.

The efficacy of argon laser treatment of extrafoveal choroidal neovascularization (CNV) in aging macular degeneration, presumed ocular histoplasmosis syndrome, and idiopathic choroidal neovascularization has recently been proved by the macular photocoagulation study.[4–6] Extrafoveal choroidal neovascularization in aging macular degeneration, presumed ocular histoplasmosis syndrome, and idiopathic choroidal neovascularization have proved responsive to argon laser treatment in selected cases.

In treating subretinal neovascularization, the first step is to determine its relationship to the fovea. Macular photocoagulation has not been found effective for lesions closer than 200 μm to the center of the foveal avascular zone, in patients with poorly defined subretinal neovascularization, or if blood is obscuring the limits of the neovascularization. Subfoveal neovascularization falls within this category, since treatment of the lesion would destroy most, if not all, of the macula. Juxtafoveal neovascularization extends from the limits of the foveal avascular zone toward the center of the fovea while extrafoveal neovascularization never enters the foveal avascular zone. Generally, the affected area is outlined with nonoverlaying 100-μm, 0.2-second burns that extend 100 μm beyond the margins of the neovascularization. The spot size then is increased to 200 μm of 0.5-second duration and of sufficient intensity to produce an intense white burn (Fig. 3.9). The patient is followed with serial fluorescein angiograms at appropriate intervals and treated as indicated.

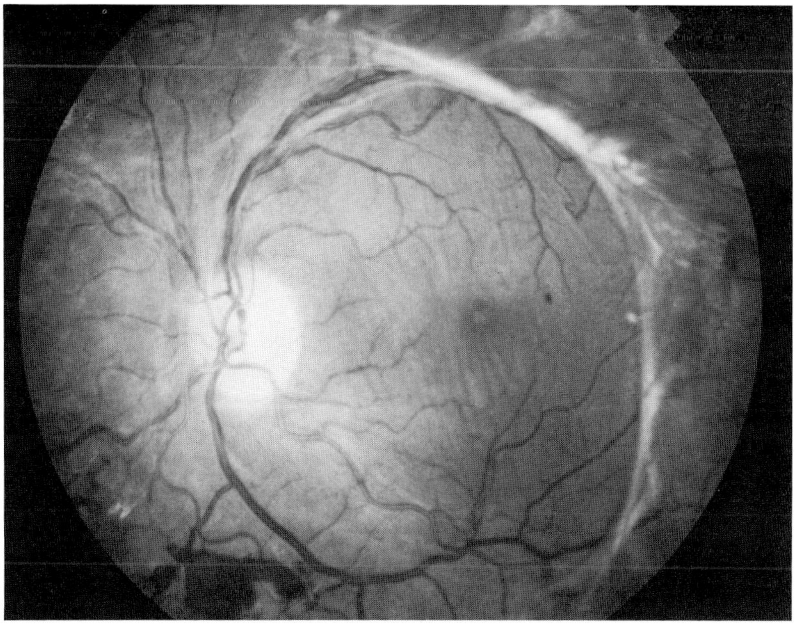

Fig. 3-9. Macular neovascularization after treatment.

The krypton red laser is currently being evaluated by the macular photocoagulation study and may play a role in treating subretinal neovascularization.

ARGON LASER COMPLICATIONS

Corneal Burns

These are frequently seen as small white opacities in the corneal epithelium or superficial stroma. They are particularly likely to happen in the periphery when treating angle structures. The major difficulty is that the opacity produced may impair the treatment. The burn will readily clear without therapy and is not considered significant.

Transient Increase in Intraocular Pressure

The energy delivered to the anterior segment may cause elevations of intraocular pressure within 1 to 2 hours. The mechanism of the pressure rise remains obscure. Rarely, a marked rise in pressure may lead to further damage in a compromised eye with advanced glaucoma. Generally, the use of carbonic anhydrase inhibitors and β-blockers will control undesirable pressure elevations.

Hyphema

This complication is generally not seen for routine argon iridotomy or trabeculoplasty but may be seen when treating rubeosis. Mild pressure applied to the eye will elevate the pressure and stop the bleeding.

Cataracts

Lens damage during iridotomy may cause nonprogressive, small, white subcapsular opacities that have not advanced to significant cataract.

Damage to the Fovea

Inadvertent movement by the patient when the laser is fired could result in the laser focusing on the macula. This is not very likely with anterior segment treatment but may occur with posterior segment work. Special care must be taken when using the indirect panfundoscopic retinal lens to check orientation repeatedly with regard to the fovea.

Nd:YAG LASER APPLICATIONS IN THE ANTERIOR SEGMENT

The Nd:YAG laser light passes through optically clear tissue without damaging it and produces photodisruption at the point of focus. This property was initially exploited to lyse opacified posterior capsules but now this laser is used in a variety of intraocular surgeries (Fig. 3-10).[7-9]

Peripheral Iridotomy

The Nd:YAG laser is ideally suited to perform peripheral iridotomies at the slit lamp. The primary advantage is that the laser effect is independent of the iris pigmentation, frequently requiring less applications than the argon laser. The technique is very similar to argon peripheral iridotomy. The laser power setting is set to 5 mJ and focused at a superior, peripheral portion of the iris. As always, the focus must be critical to ensure that iris stroma and not corneal endothelium is being destroyed. As a pit is being formed, the surgeon must remember to focus into the bottom of the pit; otherwise the power delivered will be ineffective. Similarly, a shower of pigment particles into the anterior chamber signifies a successful opening (Fig. 3-11). Great care must be exercised to prevent injury to the underlying lens capsule. Generally, 8 to 15 applications or less will provide an adequate opening.

Finally, this author uses an Abraham YAG laser contact lens to perform iridotomies. This lens provides globe immobility and a very high-energy

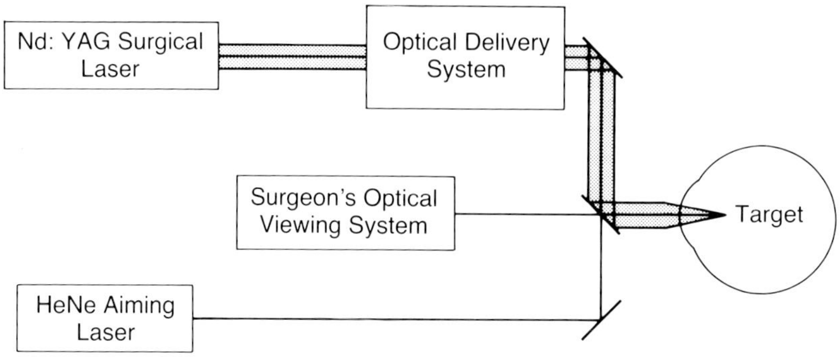

Fig. 3-10. Nd: YAG laser delivery system.

density at the focal point, thereby maximizing the chances of success.

Lysis of Vitreous Strands

Prior to the Nd: YAG laser, the lysis of vitreous strands entailed intraocular surgery. This procedure can now be done at the slit lamp aided by the use of a goniolens. In a patient with cystoid macular edema and vitreous strands distorting the pupil, Nd: YAG laser lysis is a logical step. It has been the author's experience that these strands are best cut within a short distance from the wound with a power setting of 3 to 5 mJ (Fig. 3-12). It is very difficult to cut tags and strands that are not under

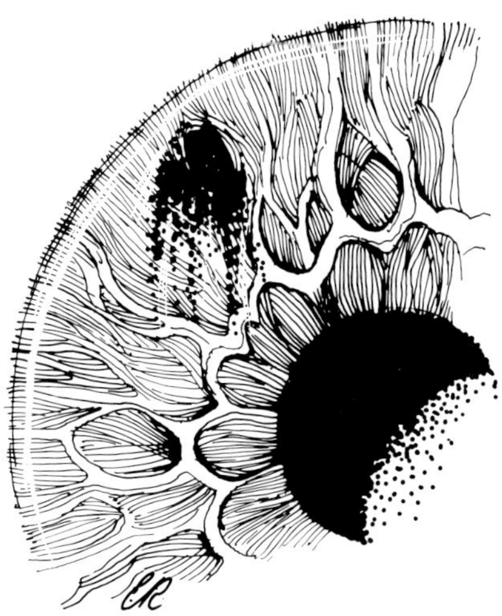

Fig. 3-11. Nd: YAG iridotomy. A shower of pigment into the anterior chamber indicates a successful opening.

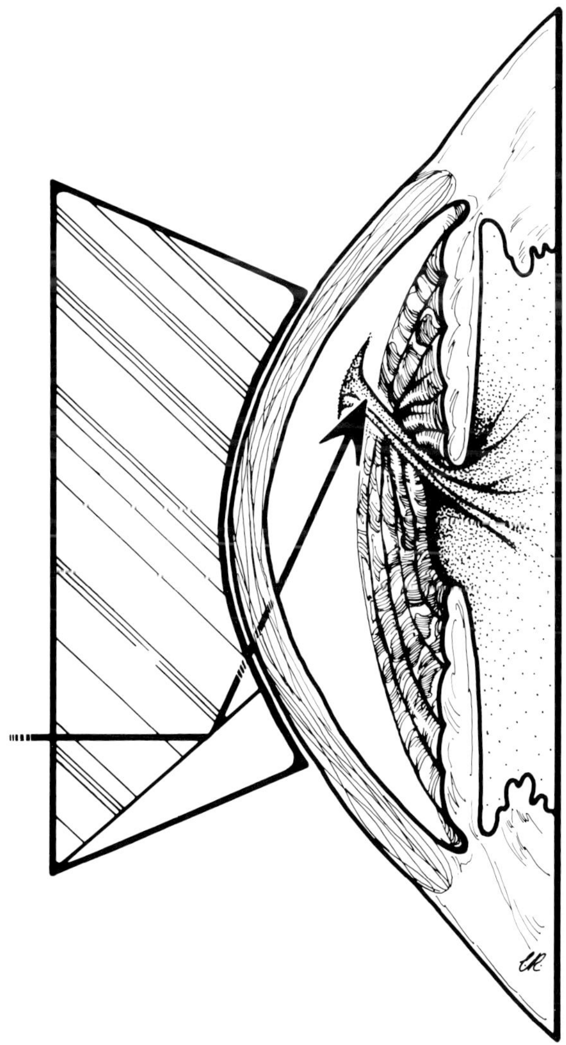

Fig. 3-12. Cutting of vitreous strand with Nd: YAG laser.

tension. Constricting the pupil places the strands under tension. As always, the focus must be precise and far enough away from the endothelium to limit any damage to this area.

Anterior Capsulotomy

Anterior capsulotomy may be used prior to cataract extraction to minimize traction on the zonules and capsule at surgery. The most effective approach has been the creation of a postage-stamp type of series of defects just beneath the capsule. These lesions cause minute perforations without widely opening the capsule. This permits fluid imbibition by the nucleus and allows the surgeon to readily strip away the capsule in the operating room. Phacolytic glaucoma may result from released lens protein.

Softening of the Nucleus

This is a new procedure with little clinical experience reported. It involves setting the laser at approximately 3 to 5 mJ, focusing deep into the nucleus, and placing from 70 to 150 shots. This apparently causes lamellar clefts in the harder portions of the nucleus. The technique involves placing the deeper shots first, followed by the middle portions and then the anterior portion. The nucleus may cause marked aberration of the laser beam. Great care must be used to prevent posterior capsule rupture using this technique. Advocates of this procedure believe that using the Nd : YAG laser in this way will permit a reduction in phacoemulsification time.

Posterior Capsulotomy

The most widespread use of the Nd: YAG laser has been the posterior capsulotomy. Thousands of capsulotomies have been performed in this manner, which appears to be safe and efficacious. The usual technique is to focus the laser just behind an intraocular lens or on the capsule. The power level should be set at 1 to 2 mJ. The surgeon must be careful not to hit the implant, as small marks may occur. Although no reduction in acuity or damage from chemicals released by the intraocular lens has been proved, the long-term effects have yet to be demonstrated. The capsule can be opened to a 1- to 3-mm area (Fig. 3-13).

This author prefers to start above at the 12 o'clock position coming down vertically toward six o'clock. Once this vertical rent has been formed, it is extended to the right and left to end up with a six-sided opening, as shown in the accompanying schematic (Fig. 3-14). In aphakic patients, it is recommended to begin anteriorly and work posteriorly so as to decrease the chance of rupturing the vitreous face. A smaller opening is also made in aphakes because the intraocular lens is not present to support the vitreous. Although dilation is not necessary, this author prefers it, since one is able to

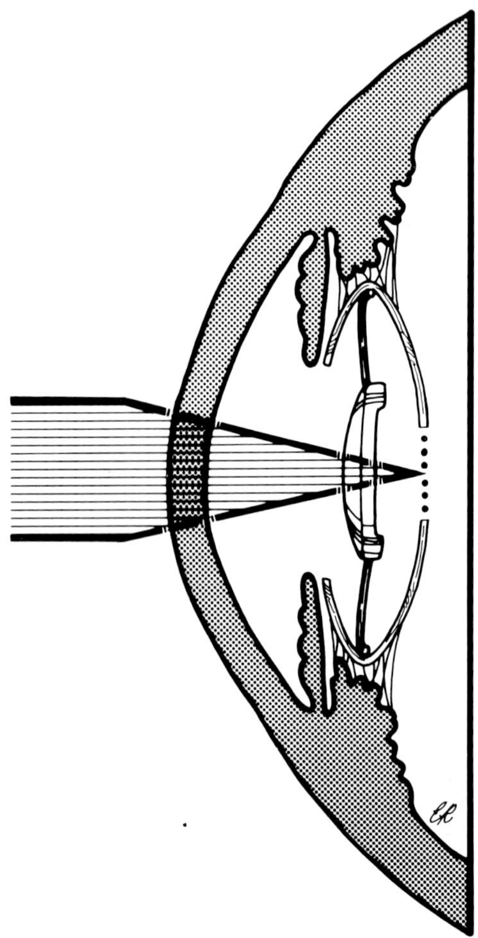

Fig. 3-13. Focus on partially opened capsule.

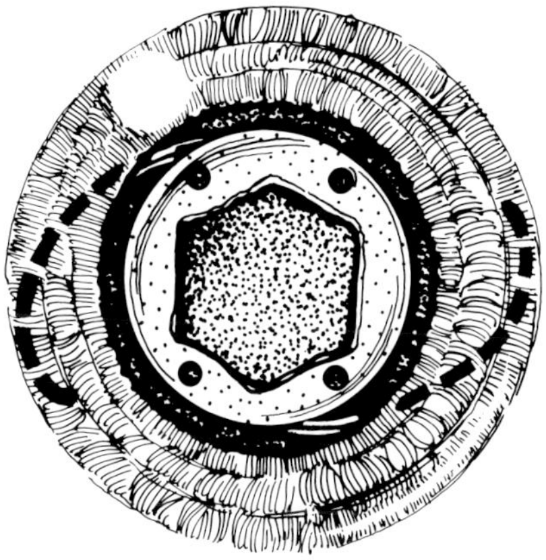

Fig. 3-14. Placement of applications during a Nd:YAG capsulotomy.

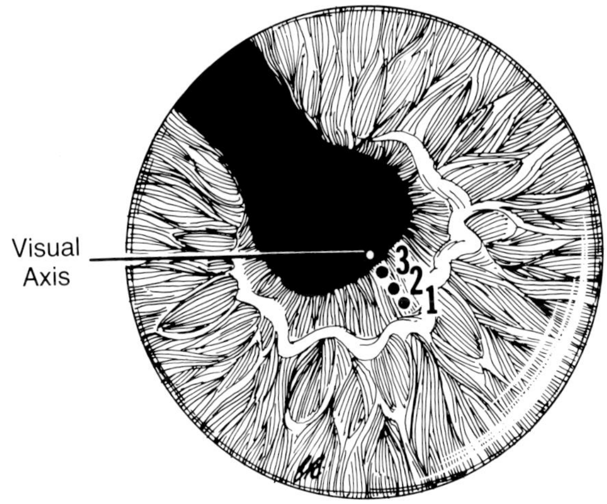

Fig. 3-15. Placement of Nd:YAG laser applications during a sphincterotomy.

perceive what is happening to the capsular flaps. The higher the power setting, the more likely one will mark the lens. It is important to keep the beam perpendicular to the target.

Sphincterotomy

The Nd:YAG laser will readily cut the iris and is an excellent tool for performing a sphincterotomy. If bleeding occurs, it will usually arise from the pupillary edge. By starting in the midpheriphery and moving towards the pupillary edge the bleeding can be kept to a minimum (Fig. 3-15). Slight pressure against the globe with the contact lens will elevate the intraocular pressure and control the bleeding. This author finds that using an Abraham lens with a power of 3 to 5 mJ will allow for the least amount of shots.

Sutures

Sutures may be cut with the Nd:YAG laser, although the efficiency is not as great as with an argon laser. Taught sutures are more easily cut than are loose sutures.

Membranes

Membranes may be lysed behind artificial corneas, such as Cardona nut-and-bolt devices by focusing through the telescope. These membranes may be cleared away without having to use a knife. This is a very specialized technique. The key to success is to have the beam perpendicular to the telescope in order to not fire within the telescope. This should not be performed by a novice Nd:YAG surgeon. Membranes elsewhere in the anterior chamber would be treated similarly to posterior capsule membranes.

Lysis of Vitreous Face in Malignant Glaucoma

In some patients with malignant glaucoma, it was found that vitreous was plugging the iridotomy and pupil. The Nd:YAG can be used at the 3- to 5-mJ level to rupture the vitreous face and break the pupillary block. There is a striking effect produced by the Nd:YAG, and no other laser actually does this as well.

Tabeculectomy

The Nd:YAG laser has been used after a nonpenetrating trabeculectomy where a sclera flap is cut almost into the anterior chamber. The flap is then closed and the internally trabeculectomy completed with the Nd:YAG laser through a gonioprism (Fig. 3-16). The power setting is 8 to 10 mJ and may take 30 to 40 shots. One can create a tra-

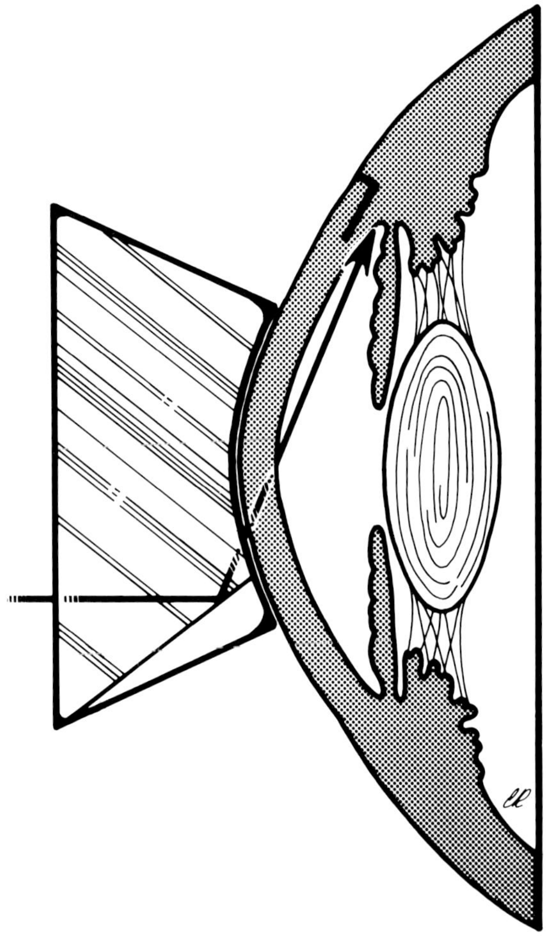

Fig. 3-16. Internal trabeculectomy by Nd:YAG laser following nonpenetrating trabeculectomy.

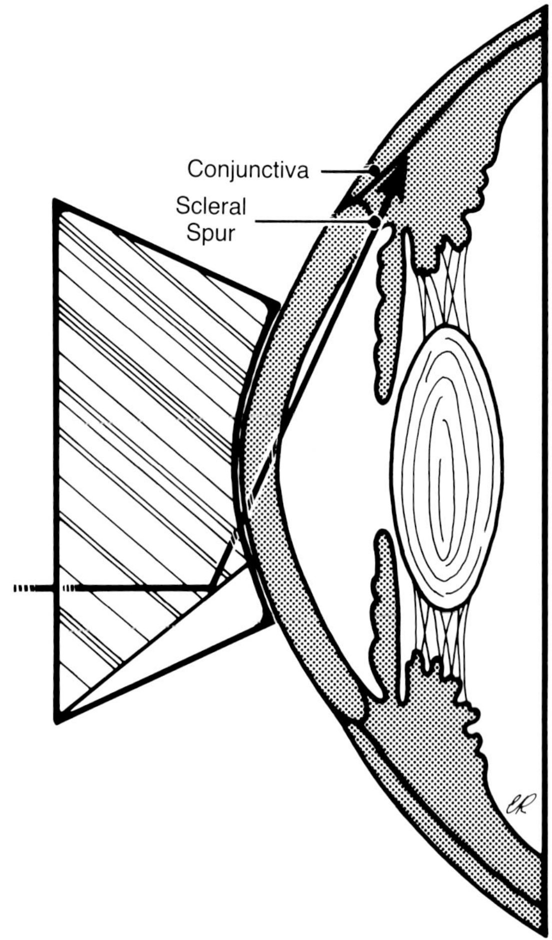

Fig. 3-17. Internal trabeculectomy by Nd:YAG laser without a previous nonpenetrating trabeculectomy flap.

beculectomy without loss of the anterior chamber and without the bleeding sometimes seen with the usual trabeculectomy. In addition, there have been preliminary reports of successful internal trabeculectomy using only the Nd:YAG laser, that is, without the need for a previous nonpenetrating trabeculectomy flap (Fig. 3-17). If this should prove effective in the long term, it will become a very significant advance, especially for failed trabeculectomy flaps plugged by vitreous or fibrosis. These tracts may be opened as long as there is not extensive fibrosis of the subconjunctival tissue. High-power settings in the 8- to 10-mJ level; repeated shots are necessary for this to be effective.

COMPLICATIONS OF ANTERIOR SEGMENT Nd:YAG LASER

Corneal Disruption

One can cause vacoules and burns in the cornea, but they are extremely transient. It is possible that if the successive bursts are near enough to the cornea to destroy endothelial cells, decompensation could occur. Generally, as long as the burst is farther than 1 mm from the cornea, this should not be a problem.

Glaucoma

The most common complication of Nd: YAG anterior laser in the anterior segment has been transient elevation of intraocular pressure. This occurs most frequently in those patients whose preoperative pressures are over 20 mmHg, or who have a history of glaucoma.[10] A significant number of patients' pressures will be elevated, but only a small number will rise over 30 mmHg. The pressure may go to 50 or 60 mmHg in rare cases and these patients should be treated appropriately with carbonic anhydrase inhibitors and β-blockers. The pressure is usually transient and subsides within 24 to 48 hours. Patients may occasionally show prolonged elevations of pressure but it is suspected that these patients are borderline glaucoma patients prior to treatment, and the laser may have ended up as a provocative test.

Hyphema

It is possible to have iris bleeding when performing iridotomy or pupiloplasty. The hyphemas are usually extremely small and can be readily stopped by pressure on the eye and have not proved of any significance.

Damage to the Lens or Cataract Formation

As of this writing, there have been no reported cases of cataract formation following the use of the Nd: YAG laser.

Damage to the Intraocular Lens

The melting point of most of the plastics used in intraocular lenses requires an energy level of somewhere between 1 and 2 mJ. To minimize the chance of marking an intraocular lens, it is important to focus behind the lens and keep the energy level low. Clinically, it would take a great number of hits to cause a large-opacity reducing visual acuity. The most significant factor in damage to an intraocular lens may be with a glass lens. A number of cases have been reported in which the glass optic was cracked by a Nd: YAG laser shot. The Nd: YAG laser should be used with great caution when the implant is glass intraocular lenses.

Nd: YAG APPLICATIONS IN THE POSTERIOR CHAMBER

Nd:YAG laser applications in the posterior chamber involve lysing vitreous strands, cyclitic membranes, and preretinal membranes. These generally require special lenses for focusing in the vitreous and higher energy levels (5 to 10 mJ). The tighter the band the easier it is to cut. The problem is that the closer one gets to the retina (certainly within 2 mm), the greater the possibility of causing retinal hemorrhage or a retinal hole. In the future, the Nd: YAG may be useful in lysing vitreous bands and retinal membranes allowing the retina to settle prior to detachment surgery. The use of the optical micrometer allows the precise focusing that would be required.

Few prospective studies have been conducted at this time. Improvements in the focusing of these lasers will result in greater applications to retinal surgery.

REFERENCES

1. Ritch R: Techniques of argon laser iridectomy and iridoplasty. Coherent Medical, Palto Alto, CA, 1983
2. Mandell AI, Terry SA: Manual of argon laser trabeculoplasty. Coherent Medical, 1982

2a. Wise JB, Witter SL: Argon laser therapy for open angle glaucoma: A pilot study. Arch Ophthalmol 97:319, 1979

3. Macular Photocoagulation Study Group: Argon laser photocoagulation for senile macular degeneration; results of a randomized clinical trial. Arch Ophthalmol 100:912, 1982

4. Macular Photocoagulation Study Group: Argon laser photocoagulation for ocular histoplasmosis; results of a randomized clinical trial. Arch Ophthalmol 101:1347, 1983
5. Macular Photocoagulation Study Group: Argon laser photocoagulation for idiopathic neovascularization; results of a randomized clinical trial. Arch Ophthalmol 101:1358, 1983
6. Singerman LJ: Important points in management of patients with choroidal neovascularization. Ophthalmology 92: 610, 1985
7. Constable IJ, Ming Arthur LS: Laser, Its Clinical Uses in Eye Diseases. Churchill Livingstone, New York, 1981
8. Buratto L: Nd:YAG Laser Applications. Sifi, Catania, Italy, 1985
9. Steinert RF, Puliafito CA: The Nd:YAG Laser in Ophthalmology. Principles and Clinical Applications of Photodisruption. WB Saunders, Philadelphia, 1985
10. Keates RH, Steiner RF, Puliafito CA, Maxwell SC: Long term follow-up of Nd:YAG laser posterior capsulotomy. Am Intraocul Implant Soc J 10, 1984

Viscoelastic Materials

4

Richard H. Keates

Since the advent of ophthalmic microsurgery, it has become readily apparent that surgical results depend considerably on meticulous technique. During the mid-1970s, investigators demonstrated that collapse of the anterior chamber with an intraocular lens in place could produce disastrous results. Contact between the intraocular lens and the corneal endothelium led to destruction of these cells.[1-3] Corneal edema was also a late manifestation of apparently uncomplicated intraocular lens implantation. As ophthalmologists became aware of these facts, intense efforts were made to develop new surgical techniques to limit endothelial damage. Air bubbles, autologous serum, polyvinyl pyrrolidione, and several viscoelastic materials were employed in various types of ocular surgery. Of the viscoelastic materials tried, sodium hyaluronate proved the most successful.[4,5] A testimony to the efficacy of sodium hyaluronate (and the related compound chondroitin sulfate) has been its widespread use in diverse forms of intraocular surgery.

The major clinical properties of sodium hyaluronate are its ability to coat tissue surfaces and maintain space and a high degree of water solubility.[6]

Once ocular tissue is coated with sodium hyaluronate, a dense lubricating film is formed that resists contact between the coated tissue and other structures or offending agents. In addition, this film provides an excellent lubricating surface that prevents damage to the coated tissue. The high viscosity of sodium hyaluronate permits the surgeon to inject the material into a space or cavity and maintain its shape. This is particularly useful when the surgeon wishes to maintain delicate intraocular tissues with a minimum of trauma. Finally, sodium hyaluronate is miscible; that is, it will gradually dissolve in aqueous and slowly percolate out of the eye through the anterior chamber angle.

CLINICAL APPLICATIONS

Phacoemulsification and Extracapsular Cataract Extraction

During extracapsular cataract extraction (ECCE) with or without phacoemulsification (PEM), sodium hyaluronate should be used to assist during the anterior capsulotomy and in intraocular lens implantation. After the surgeon has entered the anterior chamber, sodium hyaluronate is injected to maintain the space between the corneal endothelium and the anterior capsule (Fig. 4-1). This

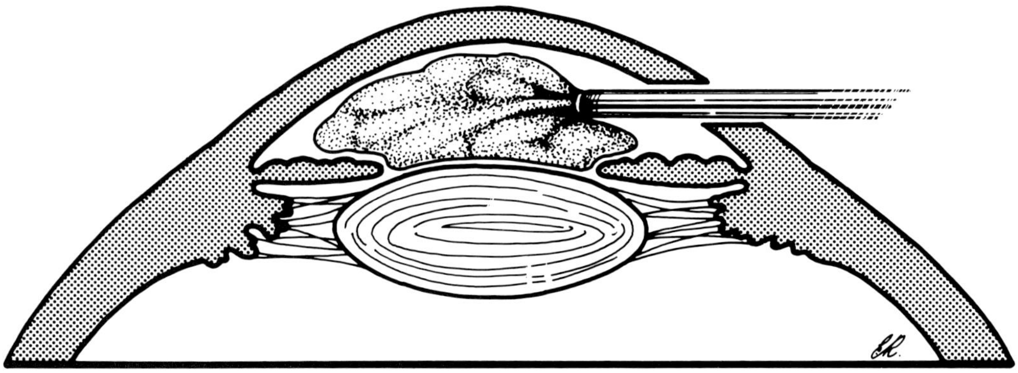

Fig. 4-1. Injection of sodium hyaluronate into the anterior chamber to maintain space between the corneal endothelium and the anterior capsule.

obviates the need for a capsulotomy under air or irrigation. Visualization of the capsule is far superior under sodium hyaluronate than the latter two techniques; it protects the endothelium if contacted. If the entry wound is excessive (greater than 2 mm), sodium hyaluronate may leak out of the anterior chamber and cause it to become shallow.

This author prefers to start the capsulotomy at the 12 o'clock position and to extend first clock-

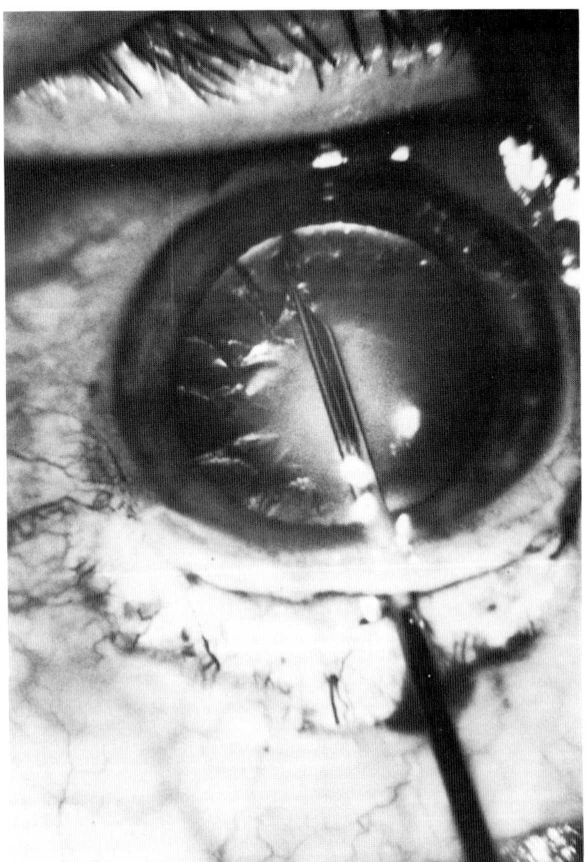

Fig. 4-2. Anterior capsulotomy performed under sodium hyaluronate.

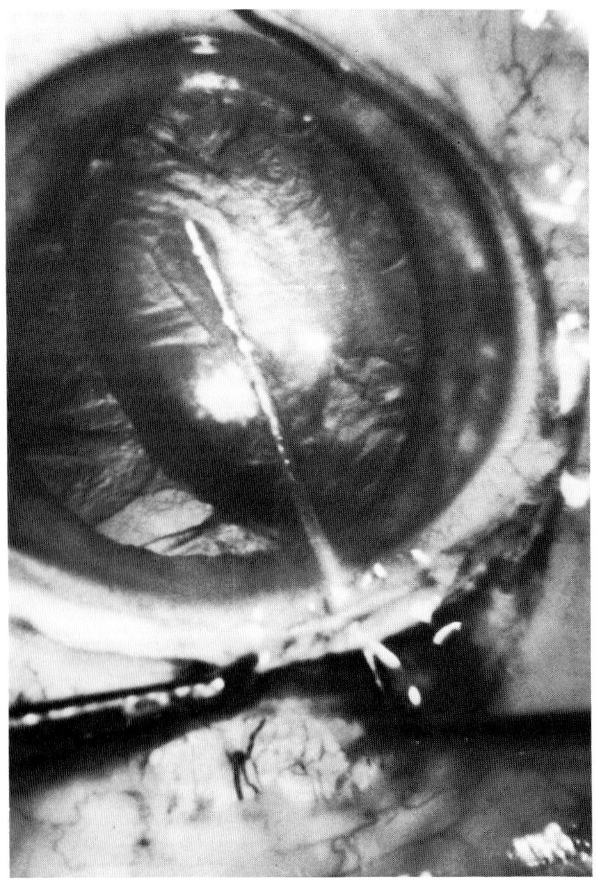

Fig. 4-3. Initial lateral motion of nucleus prior to dislocation into anterior chamber.

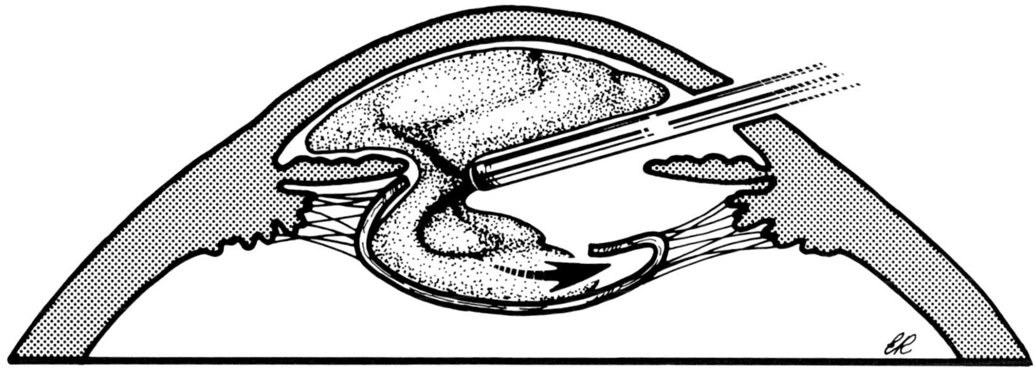

Fig. 4-4. "Inflation" of capsular bag with sodium hyaluronate to facilitate placement of intraocular lens.

wise, then counterclockwise to meet at 6 o'clock (Fig. 4-2). The cystotome is withdrawn once the capsulotomy is complete and a 0.25-mm-diameter cyclodialysis spatula is used to enter the cataract nucleus just to the right of the center. The nucleus is then dislocated into the anterior chamber with first a lateral motion followed by an upward and contralateral motion (Fig. 4-3). The cyclodialysis spatula is then removed; the surgeon may proceed with an ECCE or phacoemulsification. This author believes that this technique is safer in preventing inadvertent posterior capsular rupture.

Once the lens has been delivered, the wound closed, and the residual lens cortex aspirated, the anterior and posterior chamber may again be formed with sodium hyaluronate. The surgeon inserts the cannula tip between the anterior capsule flap and the posterior capsule and inflates the capsular bag with sodium hyaluronate to facilitate placing the intraocular lens in the bag (Fig. 4-4). Once the lens has been positioned (Fig. 4-5), the surgeon should remove the bulk of the sodium hyaluronate with the irrigation/aspiration tip. This maneuver has two objectives: (1) it allows Miochol or Miostat to produce miosis more rapidly, and (2) it reduces the volume of material presented to the trabecular meshwork. The intent is to reduce the peak and duration of the postoperative pressure rise associated with viscoelastic materials.[7–9]

In the process of performing an ECCE, the posterior capsule may be ruptured. If the tear in the capsule is small enough and there is minimal vitreous prolapse, the surgeon may still safely proceed with implanting the posterior chamber lens. This may be achieved by layering a sufficiently thick coat of viscoelastic material over the tear to prevent vitreous prolapse without extending the tear (Fig. 4-6). By contrast, if there is a large tear with extensive vitreous prolapse, the surgeon should first perform a vitrectomy with automated vitrectomy equipment. A large air bubble should be

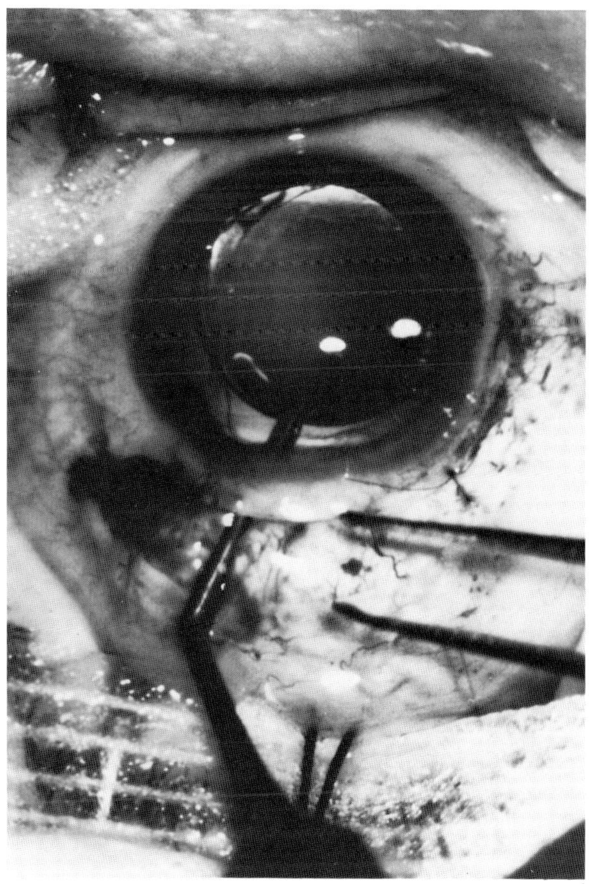

Fig. 4-5. Positioning of intraocular lens.

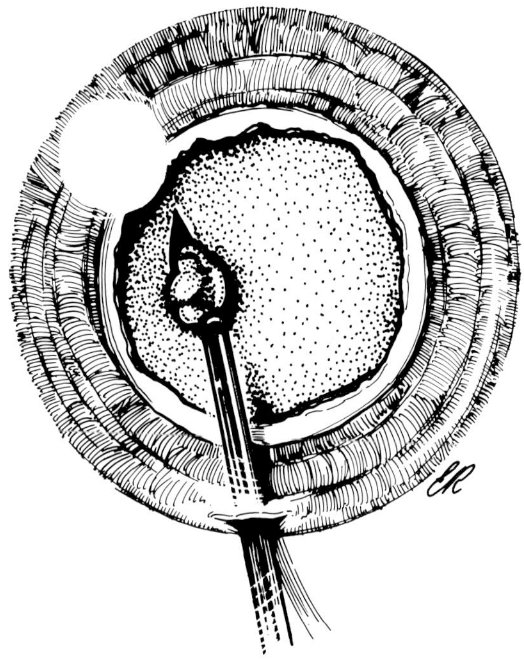

Fig. 4-6. Pushing vitreous back with sodium hyaluronate.

placed into the anterior chamber, which will help demonstrate vitreous strands at the wound and pupillary margin. After the surgeon is satisfied that the anterior chamber has been completely cleared of vitreous, it should be reformed with sodium hyaluronate. This author perfers to insert a small-gauge cannula tip and to slowly advance it. Once the anterior chamber has been formed with sodium hyaluronate and the vitreous has been tamponaded, the surgeon may proceed with an anterior chamber implant (Fig. 4-5).

Some surgeons prefer to use sodium hyaluronate only to coat the intraocular lens immediately before inserting it into the anterior chamber. This author strongly believes that sodium hyaluronate should be used throughout the procedure to provide as much protection to the corneal endothelium as possible.

The surgeon must verify that the cannula tip has entered the anterior chamber before injecting any substance. It is quite possible to strip Descemet's membrane when using sodium hyaluronate. In addition, one should not overinflate the eye, since it is possible to rupture the posterior capsule and theoretically possible to collapse the central retinal artery.

INTRACAPSULAR CATARACT EXTRACTION

For those surgeons who find the rare need to perform an intracapsular cataract extraction, sodium hyaluronate is definitely indicated. Sodium hyaluronte should be used to form the anterior chamber prior to extending the limbal incision. It may be wiped from the lens surface with a cellulose sponge just prior to placing the cryoprobe. In this way, the degree of injury to the endothelium is reduced. If an anterior chamber lens is to be placed, it should also be performed under sodium hyaluronate.

PENETRATING KERATOPLASTY

In phakic penetrating keratoplasty, once the recipient bed has been prepared, the surgeon must thinly coat the iris, lens, and wound edge (Fig. 4-7). It is not desirable to fill the recipient bed completely, since this author advises against irrigating sodium hyaluronate out of the anterior chamber once the donor button has been sutured into position. Most importantly, the donor endothelium may be lightly coated just before placing the cornea into the recipient bed (Fig. 4-8), thus protecting the endothelium during suturing.[10,11]

When faced with an aphakic penetrating keratoplasty, the surgeon must protect the donor endothelium and control vitreous. If vitreous is adherent to the previous wound, it should be divided and trimmed back to the plane of the iris with a vitreous-suction cutter instrument. If there are no iridectomies the surgeon should perform at least one. After covering the peripheral iridectomy and pupil with sodium hyaluronate, the chamber is then slightly filled with sodium hyaluronate (Fig. 4-9). By covering the peripheral iridectomy and pupil, the surgeon has created a barrier to further vitreous prolapse (Fig. 4-10). One should then proceed as for a phakic penetrating keratoplasty. The surgeon must never carelessly inject sodium hyaluro-

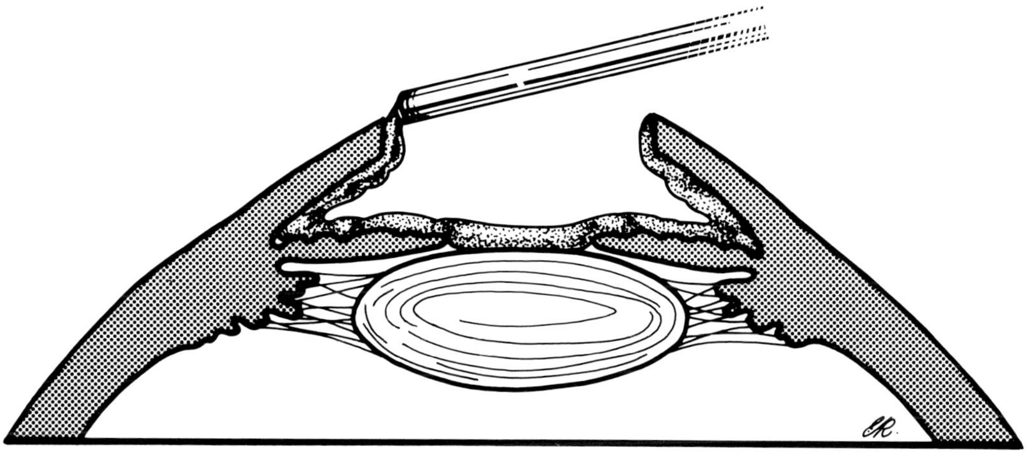

Fig. 4-7. Coating of iris, lens, and wound edge with sodium hyaluronate during penetrating keratoplasty.

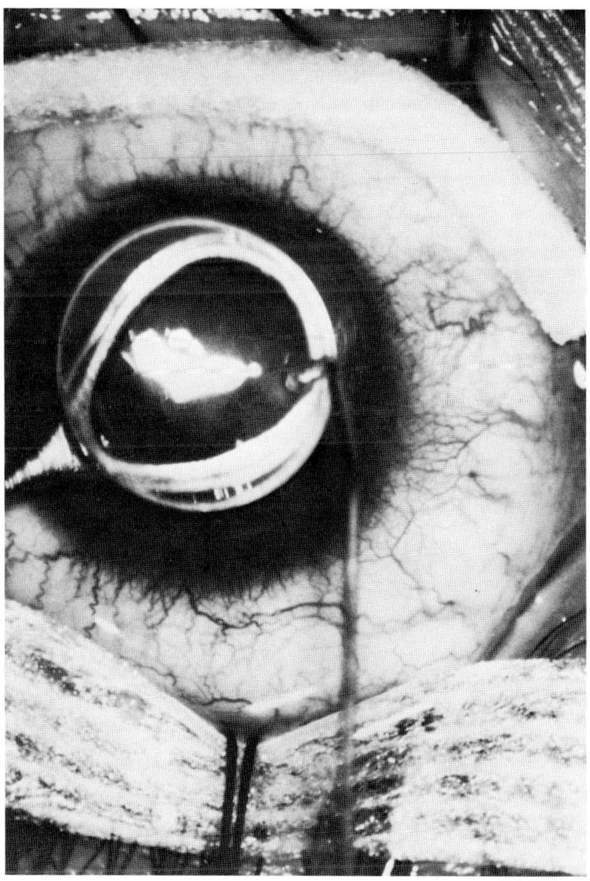

Fig. 4-8. Coating donor button to protect endothelium during suturing.

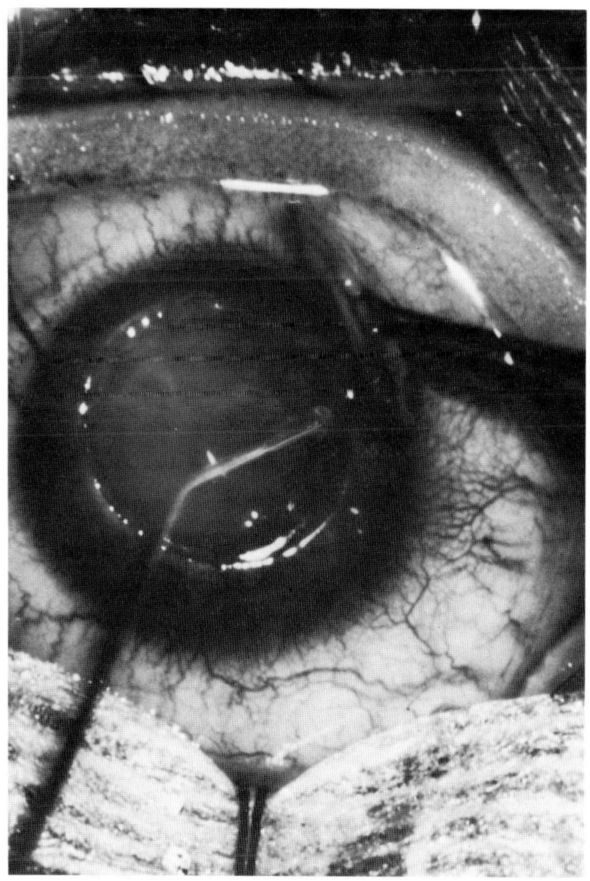

Fig. 4-9. Filling of chamber with sodium hyaluronate.

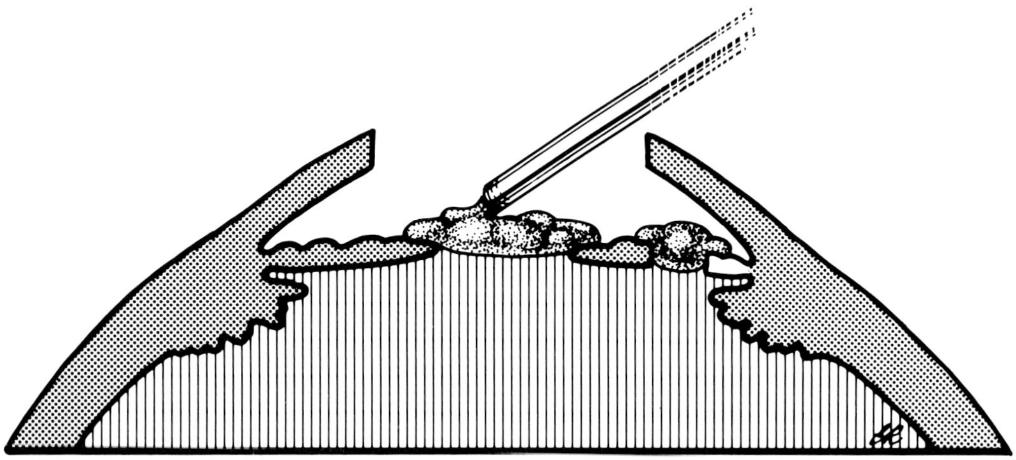

Fig. 4-10. Covering of peripheral iridectomy and pupil with sodium hyaluronate to prevent further vitreous prolapse.

nate into the vitreous. The sodium hyaluronate may track posteriorly and force vitreous into the anterior chamber.

When an intraocular lens is left in the anterior or posterior chamber in conjunction with a penetrating keratoplasty, it is imperative that the lens be coated prior to placing the donor button.

SECONDARY INTRAOCULAR LENS IMPLANTATION

As long as vitreous is not adherent to the pupil, iridectomies, or prior wound, the procedure is straightforward. All vitreous adhesions should be removed prior to secondary lens implantation. After filling the anterior chamber with air the surgeon should gently fill the chambr with HA by first covering the pupil and iridectomy(ies). This will hold vitreous back, while the anterior chamber is filled with HA (Figs. 4-11 and 4-12). Next, grasp the wound margin and lift just enough to insert the intraocular lens. Viscoelastic material is superior to air in maintaining the anterior chamber especially if an anterior corneal incision is used. After the lens

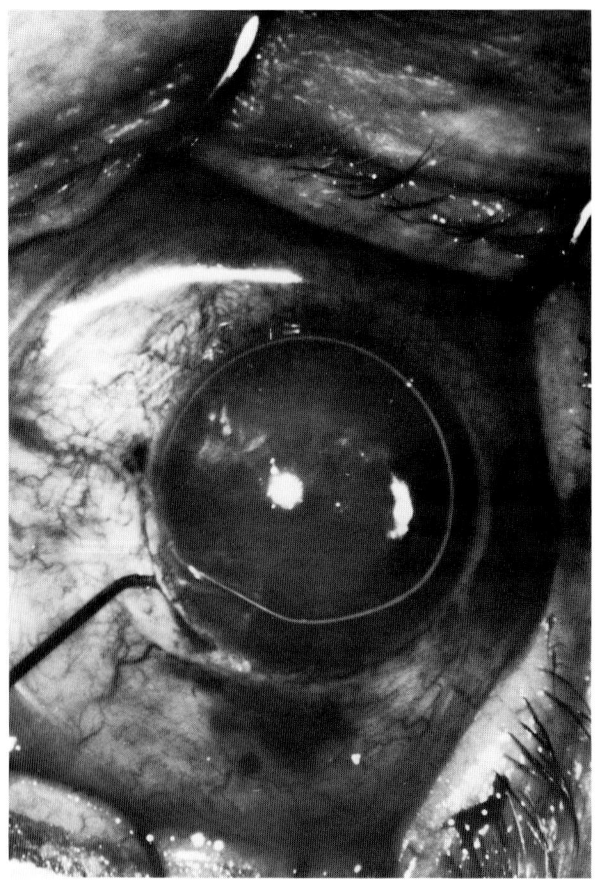

Fig. 4-11. Placement of sodium hyaluronate following air injection.

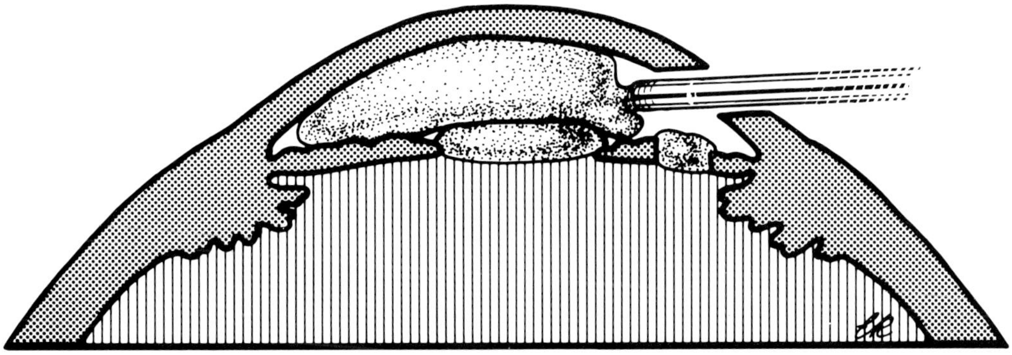

Fig. 4-12. Placement of sodium hyaluronate during secondary intraocular lens implantation.

has been positioned, the residual sodium hyaluronate should be removed with an irrigating/aspirating device.

If vitreous is present in the previous wound or extensively prolapsed into the anterior chamber, it must be controlled. This author finds that injecting an air bubble in the anterior chamber will often allow the vitreous to recede into the posterior chamber. In those cases in which the air leaks out through the wound, a light bead of sodium hyaluronate along the inner wound margin will tamponade the wound and prevent further air leaks. If vitreous is firmly adherent to the wound or an adhesion is suspected, this author finds that an air bubble is indispensible. By placing an air bubble in the anterior chamber the vitreous strands are placed on tension and they will reveal themselves by distorting the pupil (Fig. 4-13). It is a simple maneuver to sweep them from the wound and pupil with a cyclodialysis spatula. Alternatively, a vitreous suction cutter may be used. The irrigation inflow should be minimal, and great care must be taken to avoid injury to the iris.

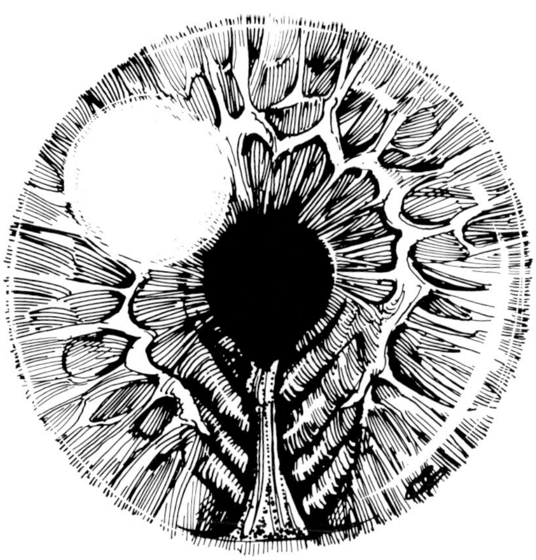

Fig. 4-13. Vitreous strands are placed under tension by placing air into the anterior chamber.

If the vitreous is not incarcerated in the wound but refuses to regress into the posterior chamber when an air bubble is placed, the anterior chamber may be filled with viscoelastic material, forcing the vitreous back and a lens glide may be placed over the vitreous. Once the lens is in position and the glide removed, the surgeon must inspect the iris for strands distorting the pupil margin. The cyclodialysis spatula can be used to sweep the vitreous and free the pupil.

Throughout these maneuvers, it is possible to differentiate between sodium hyaluronate or vitreous at the wound margin with a dry cellulose sponge. Sodium hyaluronate will adhere to the sponge but allows it to be withdrawn without distorting the pupillary margin or peripheral iridectomy. On the otherhand, vitreous will not part easily from the sponge and will produce strands that transmit tension to the iris and distorts its configuration (Fig. 4-14).

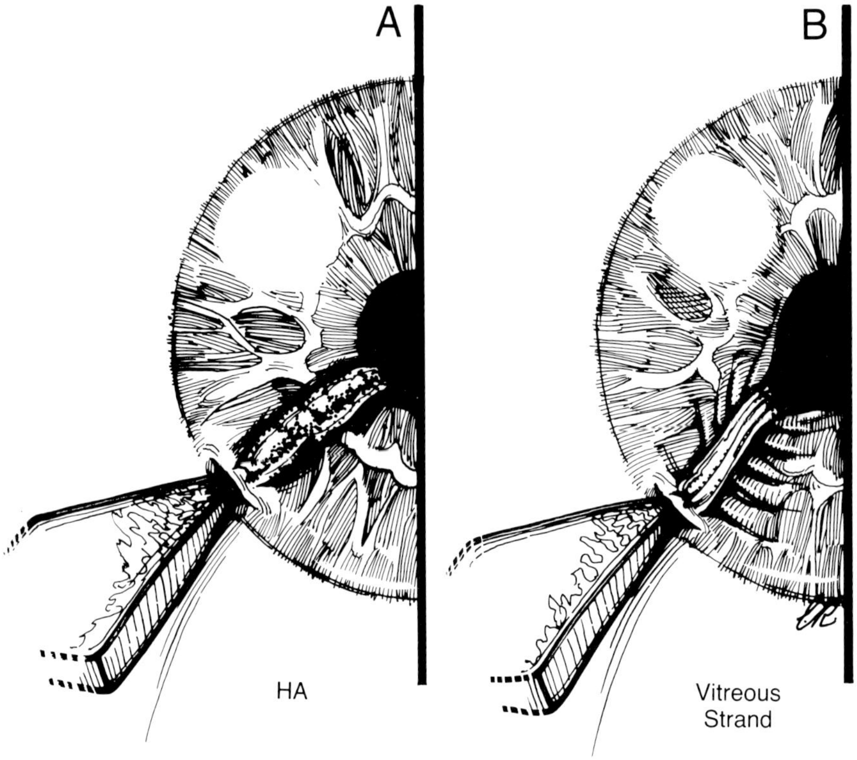

Fig. 4-14. Maneuvers to differentiate between sodium hyaluronate and vitreous.

GLAUCOMA

Sodium hyaluronate can be used to maintain the anterior chamber in filtering procedures. This author prefers to perform a temporal paracentesis and partially fill the anterior chamber with sodium hyaluronate in the area where the trabeculectomy will be performed (Fig. 4-15). Once the trabecular block has been excised, there is less tendency for the anterior chamber to collapse completely and for blood to enter the eye. Although it is theoretically appealing to inject viscoelastic material under the conjunctival flap to prevent early bleb failure, this author is not aware of any controlled studies that have proved this to be true.

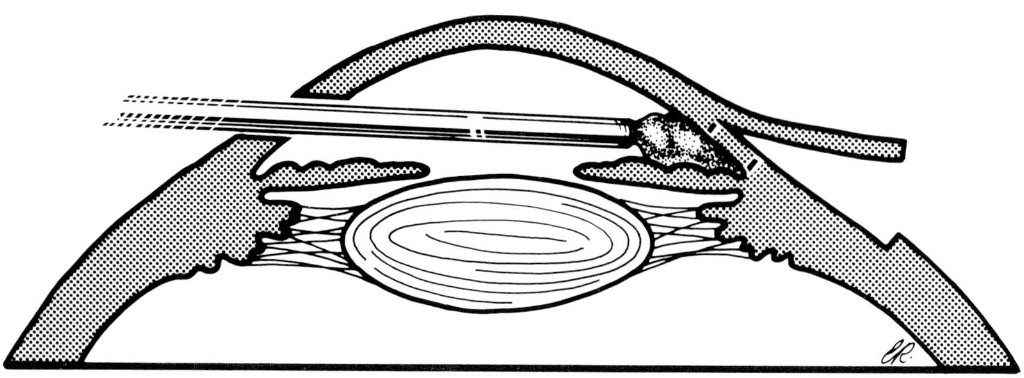

Fig. 4-15. Sodium hyaluronate maintaining the anterior chamber during filtering procedures.

TRAUMA

Sodium hyaluronate can be an extremely useful tool in reconstructive surgery. It can be used as a soft spatula to manipulate iris tissue and temporarily incarcerate a small foreign body or a bleeding vessel. Often, the anterior chamber can be reformed allowing correct tissue apposition even with extensive lacerations. Sodium hyaluronate can be extremely valuable in tamponading a persistent bleeding site and allowing adequate inspection of the damaged area. This will often aid the surgeon in reestablishing the globe integrity and applying sutures or cautery.

COMPLICATIONS FROM USING SODIUM HYALURONATE

The major disadvantage of viscoelastic materials is the transient intraocular pressure rise seen for 24 to 48 hours after surgery in many patients. The presumed mechanism is mechanical plugging of trabecular meshwork. The pressure elevation is usually mild, generally less than 30 mmHg. However, there can be dramatic pressure elevations requiring full medical treatment.[12] These unnerving elevations in intraocular pressure tend to occur in eyes with severely compromised trabecular meshwork or when a large amount of material is left in the anterior chamber.[7,8] For these reasons, this author routinely removes residual sodium hyaluronate from all procedures except penetrating keratoplasty. The small amounts used and the risk of further endothelial damage are thought to outweigh the risk of an elevation in intraocular pressure. Unless contraindicated, Timolol 0.5 percent and carbonic anhydrase inhibitors are prescribed and the intraocular pressure checked in 24 hours. A subtle sign of elevated intraocular pressure may be in those patients who complain of nausea for the first 24 hours yet who do not have their intraocular pressure checked until 48 hours or later.

A minor complication of sodium hyluronate use results from the fact that it may incarcerate blood and slow its resorption for 3 to 4 days. This has not proved significant.

THE FUTURE OF VISCOELASTIC MATERIALS

There are several exciting areas involving the experimental use of sodium hyaluronate and related compounds in ophthalmology. Investigators are using it in applications such as tear film stabilizers and vehicles for topical and intraocular drug delivery.[13] Certainly these intriguing developments may result in improved quality of care and the advancement of ophthalmology. Sodium hyaluronate has clearly changed the way in which ophthalmologists perform surgery and has improved their results.

REFERENCES

1. Kaufman HE, Katz JI: Endothelial damage from intraocular lens insertion. Invest Ophthalmol 15:996, 1976
2. Miller D, O'Connor P, Williams J: Use of Na-hyaluronate during intraocular lens implantation in rabbits. Ophthalmic Surg 11:19, 1980
3. Miller D, Stegman R: Use of Na-hyaluronate in anterior segment eye surgery. Am Intraocular Implant Soc J 6:13, 1980
4. Grave EL, Polack FM, Balazs EA: The protective effect of Na-hyaluronate to corneal endothelium. Exp Eye Res 31:119, 1980
5. Pape LG, Balazs EA: The use of Na-hyaluronate (Healon®) in human anterior segment surgery. Ophthalmology 87:699, 1980
6. Balazs EA, Miller D, Stegmann R: Viscosurgery and the use of Na-hyaluronate in intraocular lens implantation. Paper presented at the International Congress and First Film Festival on Intraocular Lens Implantation, Cannes, France, 1979
7. Schuber H, Denliner JL, Balazs EA: Na-hyaluronate injected into the anterior chamber of the owl mon-

key: Effect on IOP and rate of disappearance. Invest Ophthalmol Vis Sci 20(suppl):118, 1981
8. Genstler DE, Keates RH: Amvisc® in extracapsular cataract extraction. Am intraocular Implant Soc J 9:317, 1983
9. Galin MA, Long-Kuang L, Osterbaum SA: Cataract extraction and intraocular pressure. Trans Ophthalmol Soc UK 98:124, 1978
10. Miller D, Stegmann R: Use of Na-hyaluronate in corneal transplantation. J Ocul Ther Surg 1:28, 1981
11. Bourne WM: Reduction of endothelial cell loss during phakic penetrating keratoplasty. Am J Ophthalmol 89:787, 1980
12. Binkhorst CD: Inflammation and intraocular pressure after the use of Healon® in intraocular lens surgery. Am Intraocular Implant Soc J 6:340, 1980
13. Polack FM, Balazs EA, McNiece M: The use of sodium hyaluronate (Healon®) in the treatment of keratitis sicca. Scientific Poster. American Academy of Ophthalmology, Atlanta, Ga, Nov. 1981

Endophthalmitis

5

Leonard Joffe

Endophthalmitis is the term applied to inflammation of the intraocular contents. This inflammation may be sterile or infectious, endogenous or exogenous, and the term can be applied to a broad range of clinical conditions.

This chapter, presents discussion of the clinical picture and management of endophthalmitis occurring in the postoperative period. Whether immediate or delayed, postoperative infectious endophthalmitis is always a potentially catastrophic event, and the ophthalmologist must be alert for the earliest clinical symptoms and signs to improve the prognosis for treatment.

HISTORIC PERSPECTIVE OF POSTOPERATIVE ENDOPHTHALMITIS

The management of postoperative endophthalmitis presents one of the most challenging problems in ophthalmology and has undergone many changes in recent years, with a definite trend toward improved visual results and salvaged eyes. The current approaches are aggressive. Reviews of endophthalmitis in the English-language literature between 1944 and 1966 reported 103 cases. Results were dismal, with 73 percent retaining no useful vision, whereas only 27 percent demonstrated visual acuities allowing finger counting or better.[1] Maylath and Leopold demonstrated in rabbits that it was possible for the anterior chamber (AC) aspiration to be culture negative while the vitreous aspiration was culture positive.[2] Allansmith et al. recovered 5 positive AC cultures in 14 patients with postoperative endophthalmitis, three of whom had prophylactic systemic antibiotics prior to surgery.[3] Prophylactic use of systemic antibiotics is not effective in preventing endophthalmitis routinely, nor do systemic antibiotics control the condition in all cases once an infection is established. Furthermore, anterior chamber cultures are not uniformly satisfactory to confirm the clinical impression of intraocular infection.[4]

With this rather poor record in management and results of treatment, new avenues of investigation were necessary. In the mid 1940s, Von Sallman and colleagues[5–7] and Leopold[8] investigated the intravitreal use of antibiotics. The extraocular route of antibiotic therapy has, however, persisted until recently. Peyman and his colleagues[9–16] have provided much new information on the use of the more recently discovered and more effective antibiotics.

Several authors have explored the use of vitrectomy as an adjunct to the management of infectious endophthalmitis.[17-19] There is little doubt that vitrectomy has become part of the armamentarium of the therapy of infectious endophthalmitis in at least some cases.

CLINICAL PICTURE

The clinical presentation of postoperative endophthalmitis varies greatly. It is most important to have a high index of suspicion in any patient with an unexpected inflammation in the postoperative period. The severity of symptoms and signs is most directly related to the virulence of the organism.

Postoperative endophthalmitis generally presents early in the postoperative period, usually after 48 to 72 hours, but may present at any time from 24 hours to 6 weeks or more after surgery. I regard those patients presenting in the first 10 postoperative days as being surgical infections, innoculation occurring at the time of the surgery, whereas those patients presenting after 2 weeks are considered to have either less virulent intraoperative infections or secondary infections through the incompletely healed incision. In my experience, those eyes with endophthalmitis after 4 weeks frequently have a gap in the wound, suggesting that an incompletely sealed incision may have allowed the entry of the organism into the eye. In the late (6 weeks or more) postoperative presentation, one should consider fungal infection even though these infections are very rare.

The most common symptoms of bacterial endophthalmitis are pain and loss of vision, but again, these features vary. Visual loss is often rapid, due presumably to the effect of toxic breakdown products on the retina, and is out of proportion to the clinical signs in the early stages. An eye with poor vision and anterior chamber and vitreous cells alerts one to suspect early endophthalmitis. Observation over a short period frequently shows increased cells, fibrin formation, hypopyon, synechiae, pupillary membrane, and vitreous opacification. A hypopyon is a strong indication of bacterial infection, but it can often be very small and may even be missed.

Ciliary injection, periorbital edema, photophobia, corneal edema, and secondary glaucoma are very frequent clinical signs (Figs. 5-1 – 5-3). Pain is usually prominent, starting early in the development of infection and increasing rapidly and severely to a point where strong analgesics may be indicated. It is, however, vital to recognize that pain is not invariable and can be mild. Many patients with endophthalmitis relate only a very brief episode of pain often relieved by cycloplegics, and the absence of this symptom should not bring one a false sense of security.

In those patients presenting in the relatively early stages, biomicroscopy of the vitreous is very helpful. Vitreous debris, seen as aggregations of cells and opacification of the vitreous fibrils, are common findings in infectious cases. In the most severe cases, the vitreous becomes an infected abscess, a cavity filled with pus. Acuity can be reduced to bare light perception in these cases. Considerable recovery of vision is possible, even in those eyes with bare light perception, if treatment is successful.

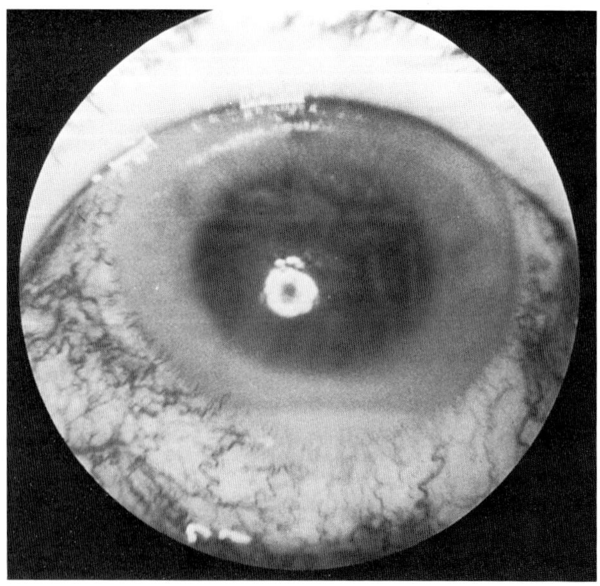

Fig. 5-1. *Staphylococcus epidermidis* endophthalmitis 6 days after cataract surgery. Note ciliary injection, corneal edema, and small hypopyon.

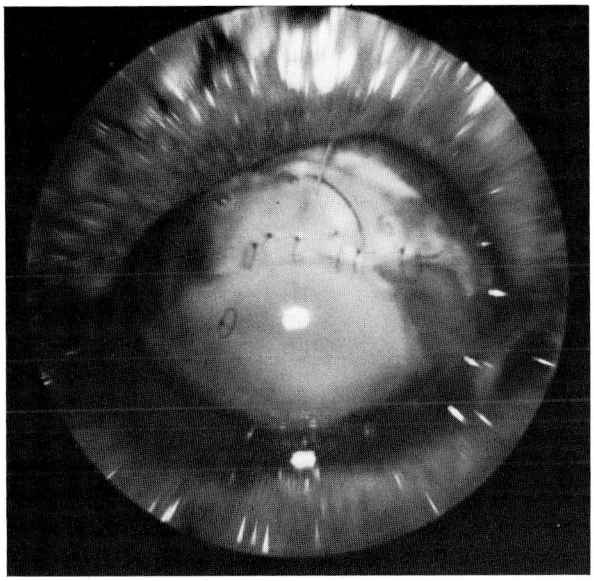

Fig. 5-2. Fulminating staphylococcal endophthalmitis 12 days after cataract extraction. Note wound disruption, purulent discharge, and abscess of eye, which was later enucleated.

Discharge from the affected eye is usually watery but can occasionally be purulent. Culture of the purulent discharge, when positive, usually reveals the same organism as that identified from the aspirate of intraocular contents.

Systemic features are also variable. Many patients show the typical features of infection, with pain, fever, vomiting, and prostration, whereas some are only minimally disturbed and appear relatively well, especially after analgesia or sedation.

Whereas the diagnosis is easily made in severe and advanced cases, it is in the milder or early case where the diagnosis is often missed or delayed. There is frequently a subconscious denial by the ophthalmologist, who feels that he is simply witnessing an inordinately severe sterile inflammatory reaction. This complacency is hazardous, as the delay in diagnosis is dangerous and may have disastrous consequences for the eye. It is preferable to have a high index of suspicion and to be overcautious in management. Postoperative patients complaining of pain and/or loss of vision should receive immediate attention. If one elects not to treat the eye as an infectious endophthalmitis, then the ophthalmologist should be very cautious, perhaps seeing the patient just a few hours later. At least if the infection is of a virulent nature, the change will become obvious very rapidly. In milder, lower-grade infections, the changes and progression may be much slower.

The trend toward the use of lens implants in cataract surgery over the past 10 years or more, and to extracapsular surgery with posterior chamber lens

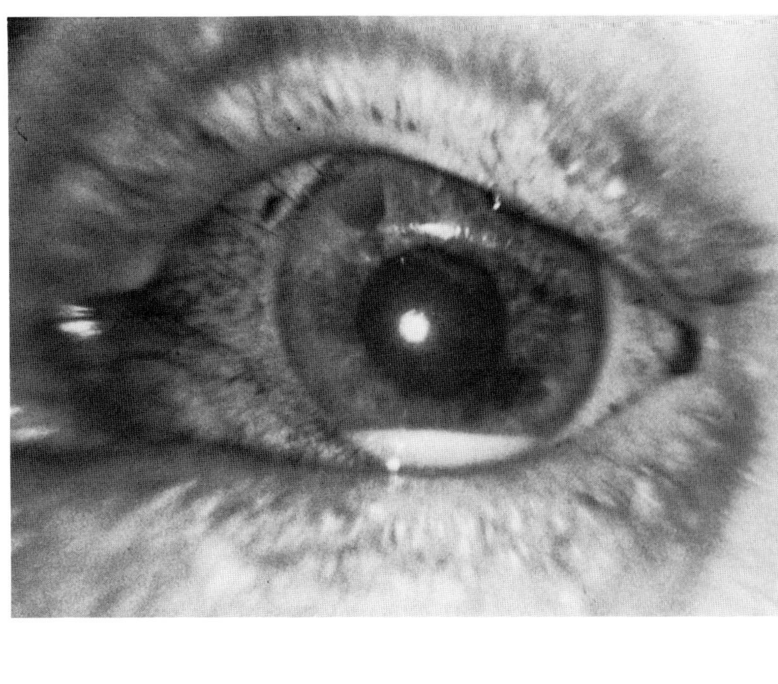

Fig. 5-3. Hypopyon in exogenous staphylococcal endophthalmitis 1 week after cataract surgery.

implants, has added a new dimension to the diagnosis and management. Although there have not been any major studies of the influence of the newer surgical techniques on the incidence of postoperative endophthalmitis, it is my impression and that of many of my colleagues who manage endophthalmitis that there was a dramatic increase in the incidence. If true, one suspects that the increase was due to the learning of new techniques of surgery, the multiplicity of new instruments being introduced into the anterior chamber, and perhaps a lengthening of the time taken for the surgical procedure in the learning period. It is my recent observation that the frequency of occurrence of endophthalmitis is diminishing, perhaps in association with the learning process and new surgical expertise and prowess.

The physical presence of a lens implant somewhat alters the clinical presentation of postoperative endophthalmitis. Anterior chamber reaction and hypopyon, vitreous exudation, and opacification are all similar. Synechiae occur early, and a prominent finding is the formation of a fibrinous membrane across the lens implant surface in the pupillary space. In the presence of these inflammatory changes, one must assume that bacterial infection has occurred and act accordingly. In the earlier implantation years, many hypopyon eyes were often regarded as sterile, but there is little doubt that infection is the most common cause of these clinical features, and it is much safer to err on the side of overdiagnosis than to delay by underdiagnosis.

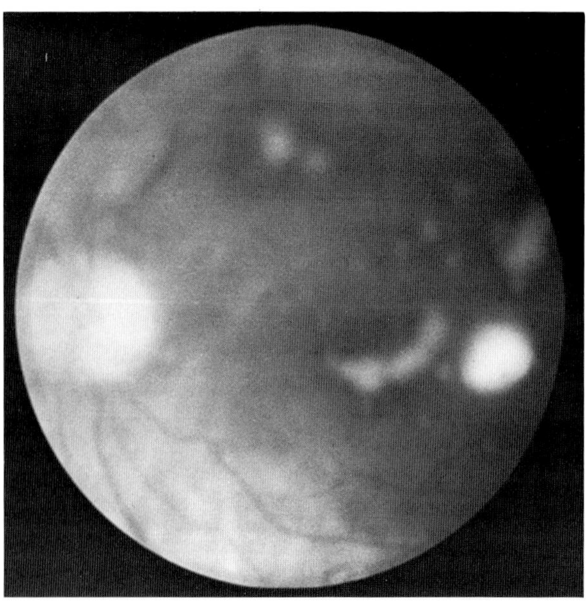

Fig. 5-4. Endogenous candida endophthalmitis. Note hazy media, "puff-ball" lesions on retina and in vitreous.

"Bleb" Endophthalmitis

This is a group of infections often occurring very late after filtration surgery or when other intraocular surgery leaves an intentional or inadvertent bleb or fistula. The organism enters the eye through the often thin conjunctiva and elicits an inflammatory response not dissimilar from other forms of exogenous endophthalmitis. Many of these patients are phakic, and the severity of these cases and resultant loss of vision and eyes cannot be overstressed.

Posttraumatic Endophthalmitis

The clinical presentation of posttraumatic endophthalmitis is often clouded by the damage done by the initial trauma, by the variable degree of ocular disorganization, and by the periorbital edema and pain arising out of the primary injury. Perforating trauma is, of course, much more likely to cause infection than is blunt trauma, and the perforating agent, if contaminated, is the usual source of the organism. Wood and other plant matter are frequently infected, often by unusual organisms, and even by various rare fungi.

A good general principle is that one should again have a high index of suspicion in perforating injury and that any deviation from the expected course of progress, such as increasing pain and swelling or decreasing vision, should lead one to suspect such a possibility and re-evaluate the eye with infection in mind. Blood in the eye easily masks the inflammatory reaction and complicates the diagnosis.

Fungal Endophthalmitis

Fungal endophthalmitis is very rare as a postoperative infection unless introduced by contamination of instruments, implants, or intraocular fluid infusion.

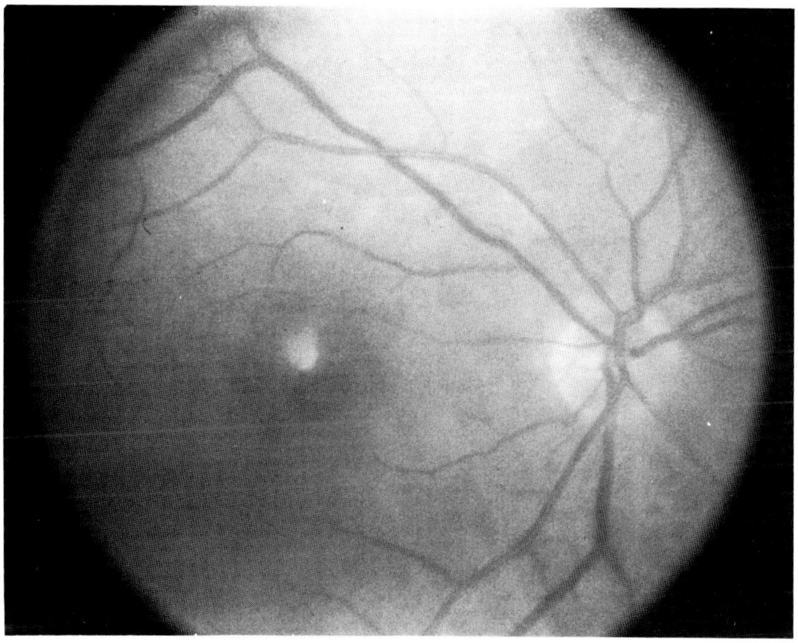

Fig. 5-5. Endogenous candida endophthalmitis with foveal fungal lesion.

The features of fungal infection are somewhat different from those of other types of endophthalmitis. In general, inflammatory reaction is of a much lower grade, with mild anterior chamber reaction. The appearance of the vitreous is also somewhat different, often demonstrating large clumps of vitreous debris in the posterior pole and inferior periphery, described as "puff balls" (Figs. 5-4–5-6). Visual loss is generally mild, and pain mild to even nonexistent. These infections are rarely fulminating. Peripheral uveitis occasionally mimics fungal infection with similar vitreous lesions (Fig. 5-7).

Time of onset is very important in the classical presentation of fungal infection. Generally the onset of symptoms and clinical suspicion occur much later than with bacterial infections, often 6 weeks to 3 months later. It is important to recognize findings suggestive of fungal infection, as they do then have bearing on the subsequent management.

Endogenous Endophthalmitis

Endogenous endophthalmitis is often missed, and therefore often diagnosed late, because almost invariably the patient is ill due to some primary serious illness. Most patients who develop endogenous intraocular infection are in the throws of a septicemia such as bacterial endocarditis or, in the case of fungal endogenous infection, they have had longstanding intravascular channels for hyperalimentation or indwelling catheters for bladder dis-

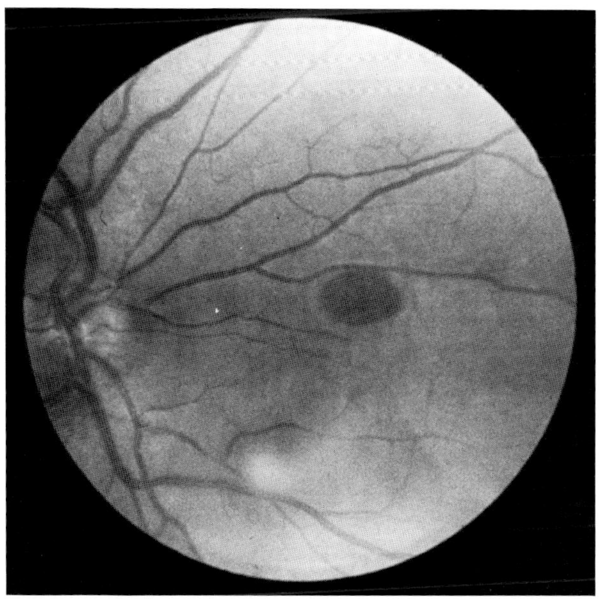

Fig. 5-6. Hole in nasal posterior retina 2 years after candida endophthalmitis, cured by systemic antifungal therapy. Note free operculum.

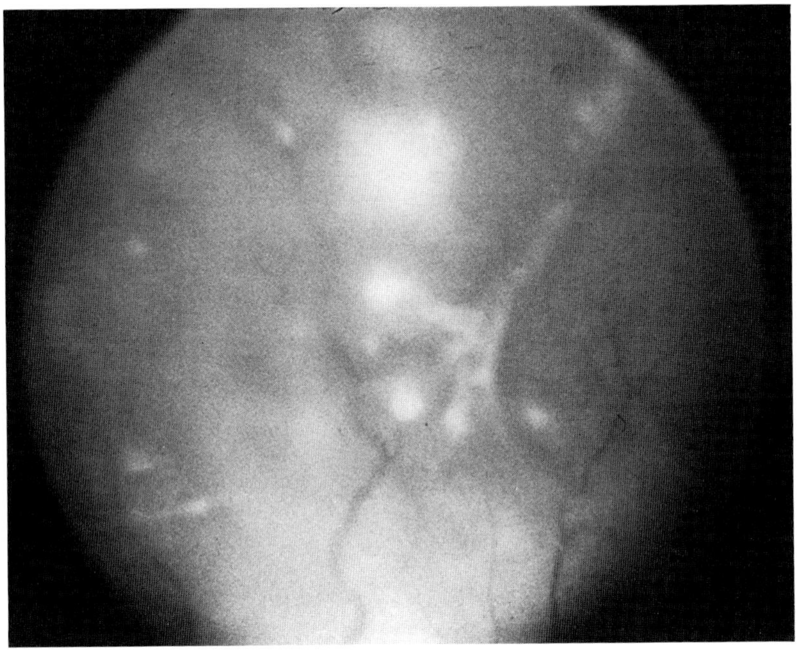

Fig. 5-7. Multiple "puff-balls" and strands in mid periphery of patient with peripheral uveitis, simulating Candida infection.

ease. Intravenous drug abusers are also at risk. By far, the most common fungal infection is Candidiasis.

The clinical course of endogenous endophthalmitis is generally determined by the nature of the responsible organism, and it may vary from fulminating, as in systemic and intraocular streptococcal infection, to mild, low-grade inflammation, as in systemic and intraocular Candidiasis. Endogenous endophthalmitis can be bilateral, though not necessarily symmetrical.

Affliction of the visual system can be the first presentation in endogenous infection, especially when a fungal organism is responsible. However, in seriously ill septicemic patients, intraocular extension of infection may not be noted by the patient nor his physician until much later when the patient is well enough to report visual symptoms such as blurring, floaters, or pain.

MICROBIOLOGY OF ENDOPHTHALMITIS

It is not my intention to provide a full and intense bacteriological guide and text in this chapter, but to emphasize those organisms most commonly encountered in endophthalmitis, especially in postoperative cases.

Gram-Positive Organisms

Staphylococcus epidermidis

Staphylococcus epidermidis is by far the most frequent etiologic organism, occurring in over 40 percent of my series of over 70 cases (unpublished data). As in many other nonophthalmological postsurgical infections, this organism was considered a contaminant at one time, but is now recognized as a pathogenic organism. While sometimes causing only mild, low-grade infection, it is frequently virulent and highly destructive in its pathogenic effects. Its discovery should not lull the physician into complacency, and aggressive management should continue. This organism is usually penicillin resistant, but very sensitive to methicillin and cefazolin.

Alpha-hemolytic Streptococcus

Alpha-hemolytic streptococcus is a very virulent organism, usually causing fulminating infections. Severe visual loss, pain, and hypopyon are common and rapid in onset. In the few cases I have seen, the visual outcome has been extremely poor even though the infection was controlled, presumably

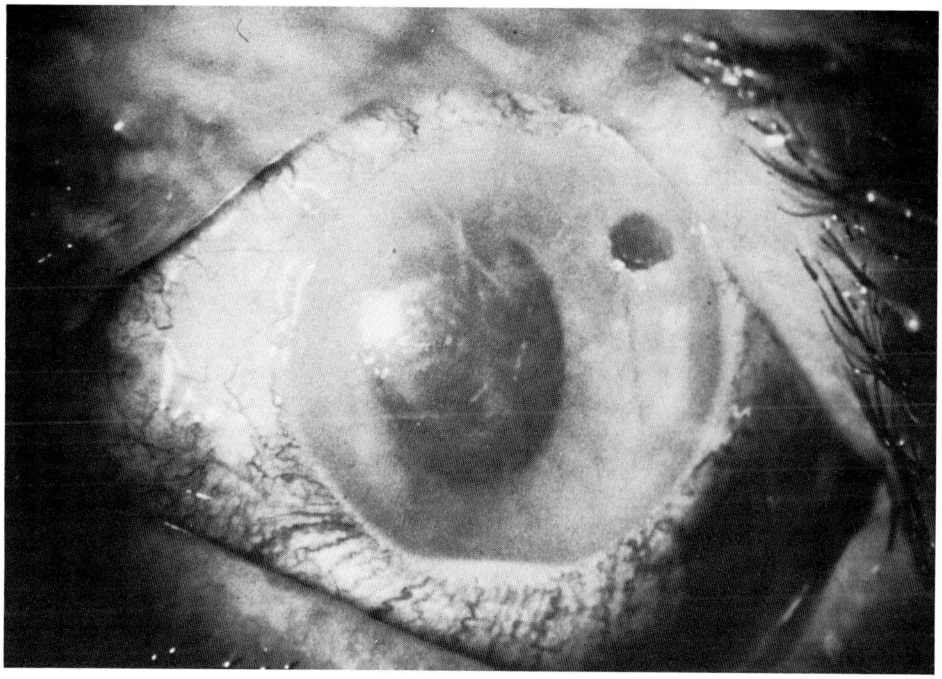

Fig. 5-8. Aspergillus fungal endophthalmitis 5 weeks following cataract surgery. Note fibrin and fungus in pupil and hypopyon.

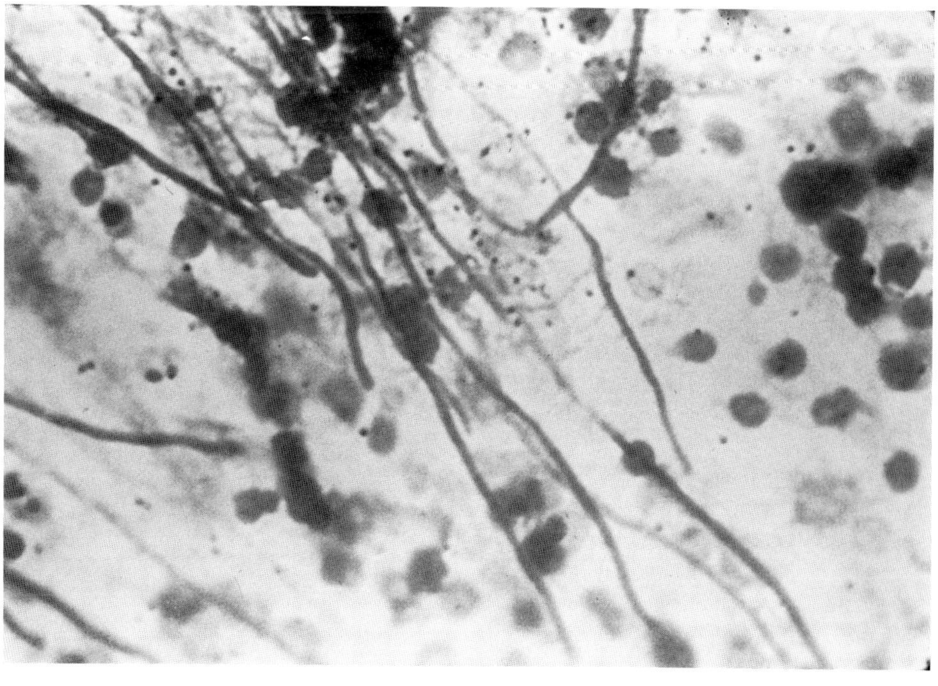

Fig. 5-9. Fungal elements of aspergillus in vitreous specimen. (Gram stain ×400)

due to severe toxic effects on the retina. Penicillin is the drug of choice for this organism unless the patient is allergic to penicillin, when cefazolin may be used.

Gram-Negative Organisms

Pseudomonas aeruginosa

Justifiably feared for its highly destructive effects in the eye, this organism is not uncommon as a cause of endophthalmitis. As with Streptococcus, the visual prognosis is poor even with appropriate treatment. In one of my patients the infection recurred within days of cessation of a full 10-day course of treatment, the only recurrence I have ever seen. Antibiotic of choice is piperacillin, with gentamicin or tobramycin somewhat effective for this generally resistant organism.

Proteus species

This group of organisms, now subdivided into *Proteus* sp. and *Morganella* sp., is generally highly virulent and relatively resistant to antibiotics. This group is a not-infrequent cause of endophthalmitis. Treatment is directed by sensitivity results, but gentamicin or tobramycin are often effective.

Fungi

Candida species

Of the rare fungal occurrences, Candida is the most common. This is especially the case in *endogenous* fungal endophthalmitis. The infections are generally low grade, with "puff balls" in the vitreous (Figs. 5-4 – 5-6). Prognosis with antifungal therapy (amphotericin B, miconazole), often supported by surgical vitrectomy, is reasonably favorable.

Aspergillus species

Much more devastating, this fungus is fortunately a rare cause of endophthalmitis (Figs. 5-8, 5-9). Management consists of surgical vitrectomy, sometimes repeated, and appropriate antifungal agents.

MANAGEMENT OF POSTOPERATIVE ENDOPHTHALMITIS

The problem often faced by the ophthalmologist in managing a case of postoperative inflammation is twofold:

1. Is the case one of *infectious* endophthalmitis?
2. Who should manage the case?

It is probably safest to assume that the case is indeed infected, to direct one's management toward confirming or excluding the diagnosis, and to begin treatment while waiting for the result. Occasionally, the inflammatory reaction is so mild that one does not have enough evidence to even begin the somewhat invasive investigation nor to treat it. Some physicians simply begin with topical therapy and periocular antibiotic injections, but the disadvantage of this approach is that a firm diagnosis is not established and that the resultant therapy is generally inadequate to properly manage a true virulent infection. I prefer to observe a suspected case very closely if definitive therapy is not instituted, and to re-examine the patient in a few hours, during which time I direct therapy at symptoms such as pain and at relieving synechiae with mydriatics and perhaps reducing inflammatory reaction with topical steroids. The short-term use of topical steroids is unlikely to mask a developing case to a point where the diagnosis is missed or delayed.

The decision as to who will manage the case is critical. Fortunately, most ophthalmologists see only two or three cases in their careers, whereas some of the larger institutions or retinovitreal groups tend to see significant numbers on referral. Naturally, a certain degree of expertise and experience is developed that is beneficial to the overall management. Furthermore, the laboratory facilities, availability of infectious disease experts, and familiarity with often toxic drug therapies in their hands is a positive step toward better and safer therapy. Referral to a subspecialist or center competent to manage the case is often a wise decision, if geographically possible, and relieves the primary ophthalmologist of the pressures and responsibilities. If the primary ophthalmologist elects to treat the patient, he should be familiar with all the techniques and have available the facilities for investigation and treatment of the problem.

Once a clinical diagnosis is made, therapy can be delayed only a very short time so as to allow for the proper specific cultures to be taken. By doing so, the responsible organism is easier to identify without the influence of prior antibiotic therapy. If the delay is expected to be more than an hour or if the referral specialist or center are at some distance away, then therapy should be begun immediately with topical mydriatics, steroids and antibiotics, and even systemic agents. In cases where I have begun treatment several hours before getting a vitreous culture, I have still generally been able to identify the responsible organism.

In general, any patient with endophthalmitis, suspected or proven, should be admitted to hospital for investigation and treatment. Management as an outpatient cannot be intensive enough for obvious logistic reasons.

The traditional therapy has been to institute topical, periocular, and systemic antibiotic treatment, and there is little doubt that such treatment can be effective in less virulent infections. This treatment is by nature "hit and miss," using combinations of often toxic antibiotics for an unidentified organism for fairly long periods of time. Furthermore, if it turns out that the organism is virulent, requiring more aggressive therapy, then valuable time has been lost in directing specific definitive therapy at the organism and in allowing the conditions to deteriorate further before instituting such measures. The value of identifying the organism and then directing specific therapy at it cannot be overstressed and often avoids the unnecessary use of the more toxic antibiotics in mostly elderly patients.

Three recent advances in the management of endophthalmitis are:

1. Recognition that the vitreous is the most likely site for identification of the specifically responsible organism.
2. Confirmation of the safety of techniques for intraocular injection of antibiotic solutions and advances in the effectivity of the newer antibiotics in general.
3. The use of vitrectomy, at least as an adjunct, in the therapy of endophthalmitis.

The first two advances mentioned are generally accepted by most authorities, whereas the third, vitrectomy, has not yet gained wide acceptance.

Vitreous Biopsy

Traditionally, cultures were taken from the conjunctival sac, but this site is subject to many variables and cannot be efficiently relied upon. Anterior chamber tap is very helpful if an organism can be identified, but false-negative results are common. Vitreous biopsy is most likely to provide a reliable culture result and should be undertaken if at all possible. Combination of conjunctival culture, AC tap, and vitreous biopsy are theoretically likely to give the highest yield. The technique of vitreous biopsy will depend on the nature of the case. I prefer not to go through the limbus or wound with a needle, as a permanent anterior vitreous adhesion is almost inevitable and certainly undesirable. Extracapsular techniques and posterior chamber lens implants make such an entry even less desirable. My preference would be to enter through the pars plana, 3 to 4 mm behind the limbus, with a 25G or 23G needle and then to aspirate a small amount of vitreous, even 0.1 ml being adequate. This aspiration technique requires effective topical anesthesia, and probably at least retrobulbar anesthesia, as the eye is often painful and tender. It may be difficult and dangerous to perform this technique in a congested eye with thick material, and it is not without risk. The recent surgical incision can be distorted and a dehiscence may result from the required pressure on the eye. The aspiration of vitreous through a needle is usually combined with the subsequent injection of intravitreal antibiotics with or without steroids. The procedure is best performed in the operating room.

Intravitreal Antibiotics

Thanks to the work of Peyman and colleagues, the safety and efficacy of intraocular antibiotic injections are well established.[9–16] Several antibi-

Table 5-1. Recommended Dosages for Intravitreal Antibiotics

Antibiotic	Intravitreal Dose	Periocular Dose
Methicillin	2 mg	100 mg
Cefazolin	2.25 mg	100 mg
Gentamycin	200 (100–400) μg	20 mg
Tobramycin	450 μg	20 mg
Amphotericin B	5 μg	750 μg

otics and their recommended dosages are now well known (see Table 5-1), and each is usually diluted in 0.1 ml of normal saline. After obtaining vitreous aspirate, the syringe is disconnected from the intravitreal needle, and the solutions are then carefully injected into the mid vitreous cavity through the same needle. The intraocular pressure must be monitored as the injection of two or three agents each in 0.1 ml of fluid can raise the pressure considerably. The technique of vitreous aspiration and intraocular antibiotic injection can be repeated for diagnostic and therapeutic purposes 1 to 3 days later, though I have found this unnecessary in almost all the cases I have dealt with.

Vitrectomy

There is little doubt that vitrectomy plays a major role in the management of endophthalmitis, particularly when the infection is severe or advanced. Its role in clinically early or less virulent infection is somewhat less certain, and opinions vary depending on one's experience and training. Even in this group, however, the procedure is gaining in popularity as a safe, controlled method of obtaining a representative specimen for culture, introducing appropriate dosage of intraocular antibiotic, and dealing with some of the associated complications such as wound leak or disruption, pupillary membranes, and pupillary block. In fungal infections it is even more strongly indicated.

As a retinovitreal surgeon, my own bias is toward vitreous surgical intervention in most cases, but I recognize that many cases might have been adequately controlled without it. My bias is based on the experience that the surgery has low risk, and that apparently good results are achieved in most cases, but this is not an opinion based on controlled studies.

If a decision is made to do a vitrectomy, the surgery should be done immediately. My cases are usually in surgery within 1 to 2 hours after diagnosis if circumstances such as medical condition, location, and scheduling allow for it. Any longer delay should probably mandate that some form of antibiotic therapy be instituted in the interim. The pupil should be dilated before surgery if possible.

The surgery is often attended by much conjunctival and episcleral bleeding and edema because the tissues are congested. The eye is treated with extra caution due to the recent incision for surgery, and sclerotomy incisions are to be large enough to insert the instrument and fiberoptic system without undue pressure, which might disrupt the wound. Additional wound support with sutures may be necessary. I prefer to have traction sutures on lateral, medial, and superior rectus muscles to stabilize the eye and wound for insertion of instruments.

The infusion system is inserted early in the procedure, and usually balanced salt solution (B.S.S. Plus) is used, *without antibiotic*, at least until the specimen of material is obtained. Adrenalin (one part per million, diluted by adding 0.5 ml of 1:1000 in 500 cc B.S.S. Plus) may be added if pupillary dilation is a concern.

An anterior chamber aqueous specimen is aspirated with a fine cannula on a tuberculin syringe, either through the wound or through a separate paracentesis. At this time, if a pupillary membrane occludes the pupil or the view of the posterior segment, it can be removed from the lens implant with the cannula. I have occasionally injected viscoelastic material to help maintain the anterior chamber.

The vitrectomy instrument and fiberoptic probe are then inserted into the vitreous cavity and the vitrectomy begun, gently removing the central visible vitreous. Only that area able to be visualized can be cleared, and the procedure is often limited by poor visibility because of fibrin on the anterior or posterior lens implant surface. The lens is not manipulated or displaced. In most cases, by using the limited visibility and a degree of stereotactic technique, the central core of vitreous through the posterior hyaloid is removed. The inferior vitreous often contains more purulent material and is easier to visualize and remove.

One should never bring the instruments close to

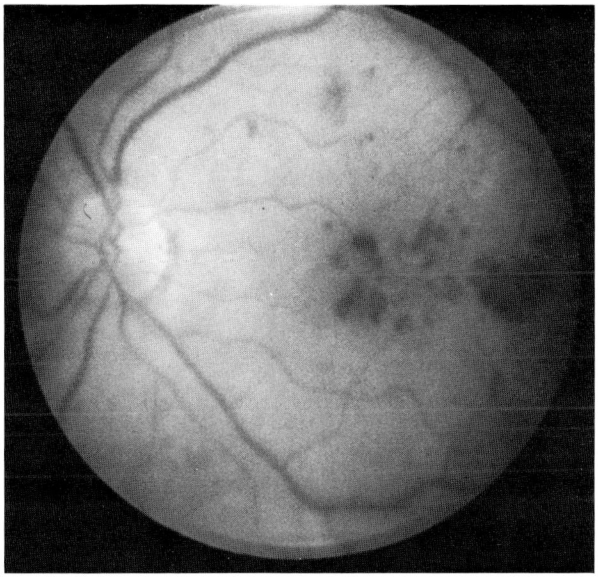

Fig. 5-10. Retinal hemorrhages still present in posterior pole in post vitrectomy eye, operated on for fulminating staphylococcal infection.

the retina or the vitreous base, as they are friable and congested and bleed profusely if traumatized.

Often the retina, when visible, shows hemorrhages (Figs. 5-10, 5-11) and a profuse white exu-

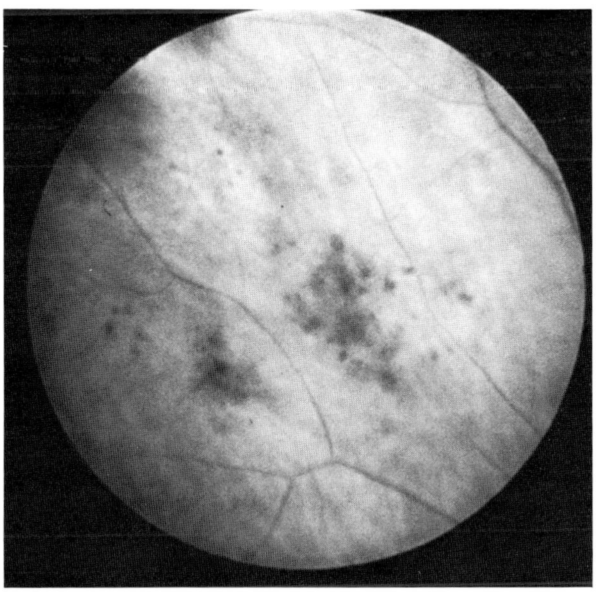

Fig. 5-11. Mid peripheral hemorrhages in same eye as Fig. 5-10.

date. No attempt should be made to "vacuum" the exudate as this, too, will traumatize the retina.

Once the material has been removed I allow the eye to soften a little to allow space for the upcoming preprepared antibiotic injections. The vitreous aspirate and aqueous specimen are carried to the laboratory for urgent Gram stain, culture, and sensitivity testing.

The sclerotomy incisions are closed, and the antibiotics injected carefully into the cavity through the incision with fine cannula or needle. The solution must not be injected in a strong jet stream as it may traumatize the retina.

GENERAL CONSIDERATIONS

The usual combination of antibiotics includes either methicillin or cefazolin for gram-positive organisms and Garamycin or tobramycin for gram-negative possibilities. The pharmacy preprepares the solutions so that desired dosage is contained each in 0.1 ml of normal saline. The pharmacist and microbiologists should be in-serviced as to your special needs and methods of dealing with the specimens.

Periocular antibiotics are usually injected using the same combination as used for intraocular injection, in the appropriate dosages.

Steroids

Opinions vary as to when to institute steroid therapy. The steroids are necessary to counteract the severe inflammatory reaction, and the toxicity of the infection on the retina.

Many begin steroids on the first day after institution of antibiotic therapy, but my own philosophy is that the steroids are so critical that I inject them intraocularly and subconjunctivally at the onset of treatment (Dexamethazone 400 mcg intravitreally, any depo steroid subconjunctivally). If the antibiotic spectrum is broad enough to cover the organism, the steroids will not negatively influence their action, whereas delay might result in con-

Table 5-2. Recommended Dosages for Systemic Antibiotics

Antibiotic	Spectrum	Dose for Average Build
Methicillin/Oxacillin	Gram positive Penicillin resistant	1 g IVI q4h
Cefazolin	Broader spectrum, mostly gram positive, penicillin resistant	1 g IVI q6h
Penicillin, soluble	*Streptococcus*	1 MU IVI q4h
Garamycin	Gram negative, broad spectrum	80 mg IVI q8h
Tobramycin	Gram negative, broad spectrum	80 mg IVI q8h

trolled infection but loss of function. Steroids are not used if fungus is suspected.

Systemic Therapy

The same combination of systemic antibiotics are used by intravenous route (Table 5-2). Full dosage is necessary in order to get adequate dosage into the eye. Gentamicin and other similar potentially toxic drugs are monitored for correct dosage in the standard protocols.

Antibiotic therapy is tailored according to Gram stain, culture, and sensitivity results. If gram-positive organisms are confirmed, the drugs for the gram-negative group can be discontinued, and vice-versa. If no organisms are seen, or if the results are uncertain, both drugs should be continued on the basis that the results may be false-negative. Change of antibiotics may be necessary if laboratory results and clinical progress so dictate.

Steroids are generally given by mouth if inflammatory reaction justifies it, initial dosage being Prednisone 60 mg daily.

Systemic therapy is continued for 7 to 10 days, depending on the organism (longer for gram-negative infections) and clinical course.

If the clinical course is unfavorable, it may occasionally be necessary to repeat the intraocular injections, and at that time a repeat culture can be taken. The more virulent infections may recover quite slowly, and it is generally not necessary to change plans unless there is apparent deterioration.

Topical Therapy

Traditionally, frequent use of eyedrops, especially antibiotics, has been ordered. It is my firm impression that, with the aggressive approach described, such frequent usage is unnecessary, and exhausting for the patient.

A topical antibiotic/steroid combination, combined with mydriatics, used 2- to 4-hourly in waking hours, is probably more than adequate. Topical hypotensive agents are frequently required for raised intraocular pressure.

LONG-TERM COMPLICATIONS

Phthisis bulbi may occasionally result from unsuccessful or delayed treatment. The only case of phthisis in my series occurred after *Staphylococcus*

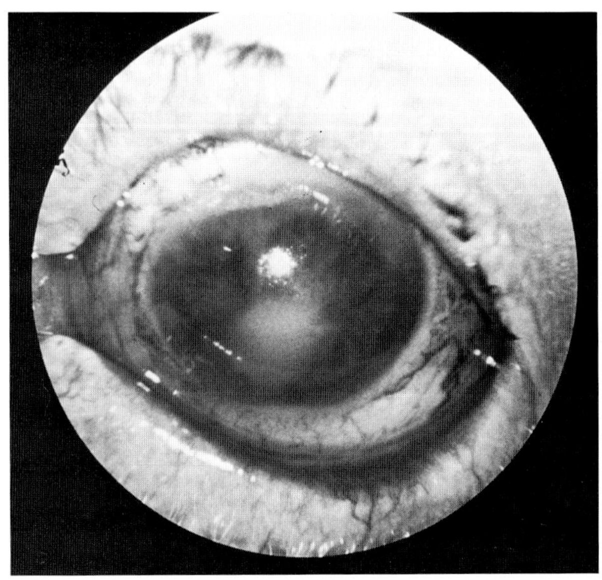

Fig. 5-12. Prephthisical eye 2 weeks after vitrectomy for neglected fulminating *Staphylococcus epidermidis* endophthalmitis. Note corneal edema and disorganized intraocular anatomy with fibrin in the anterior chamber.

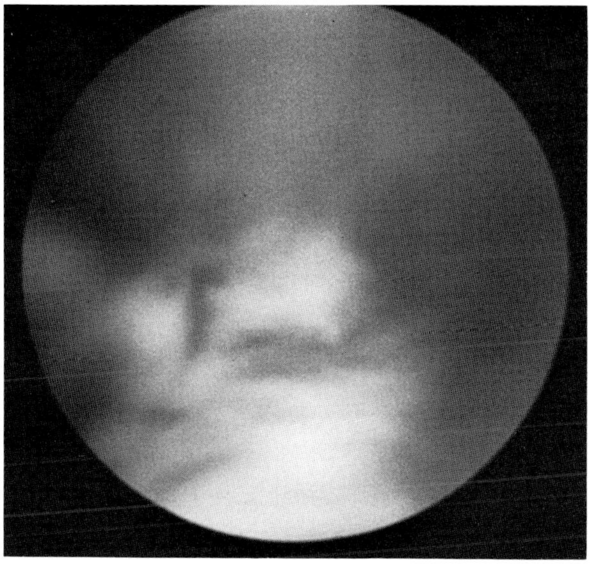

Fig. 5-13. Large dense mass of residual vitreous opacity inferiorly months following partial vitrectomy for exogenous staphylococcal endophthalmitis.

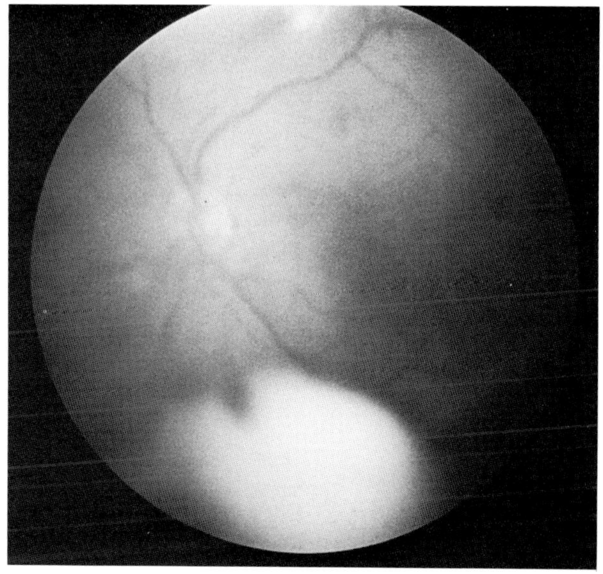

Fig. 5-15. Large vitreous aggregation of debris 4 weeks after limited vitrectomy for exogenous staphylococcal infection.

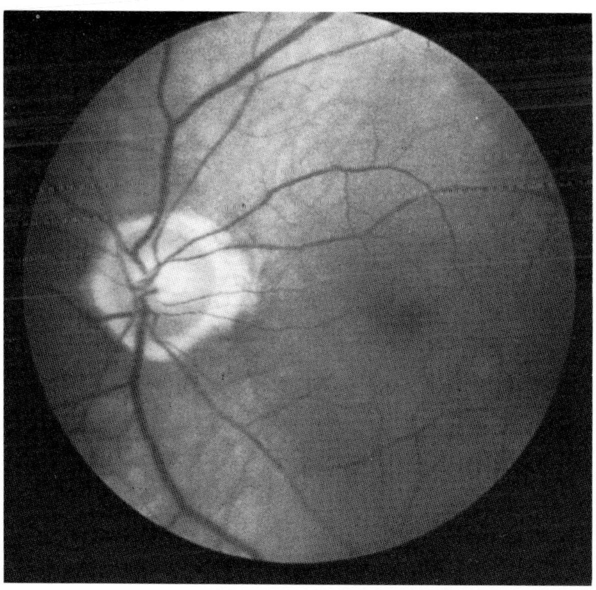

Fig. 5-14. Clear visual axis of same eye as in Fig. 5-13. Visual acuity is 20/20, but patient is disabled by large floater.

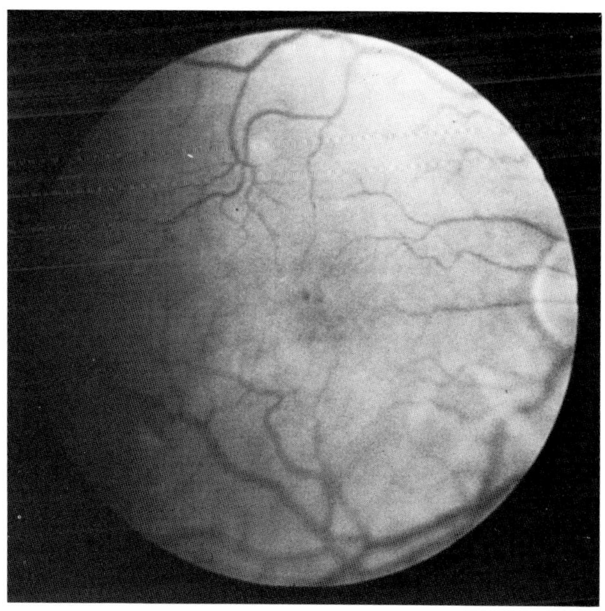

Fig. 5-16. Macular edema and hemorrhages 5 months after exogenous staphylococcal endophthalmitis. Visual acuity 20/100.

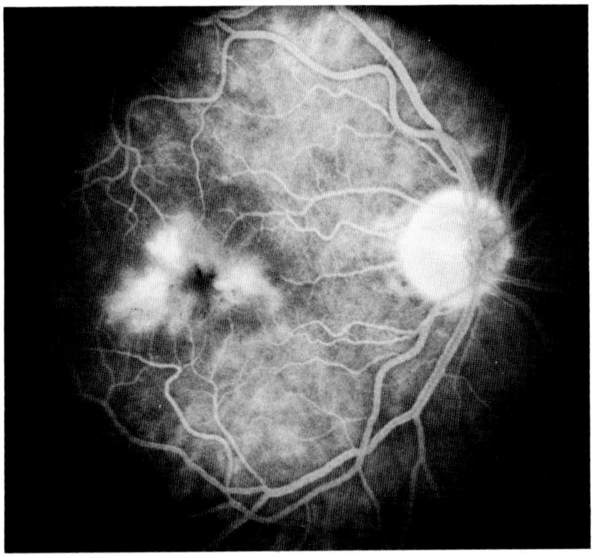

Fig. 5-17. Fluorescein angiogram of same eye as in Fig. 5-16. Macular edema is confirmed.

epidermidis infection and delayed treatment (Fig. 5-12).

Anterior segment complications such as corneal decompensation, pupil block, and pupillary membrane formation can be dealt with appropriately by surgical or laser techniques.

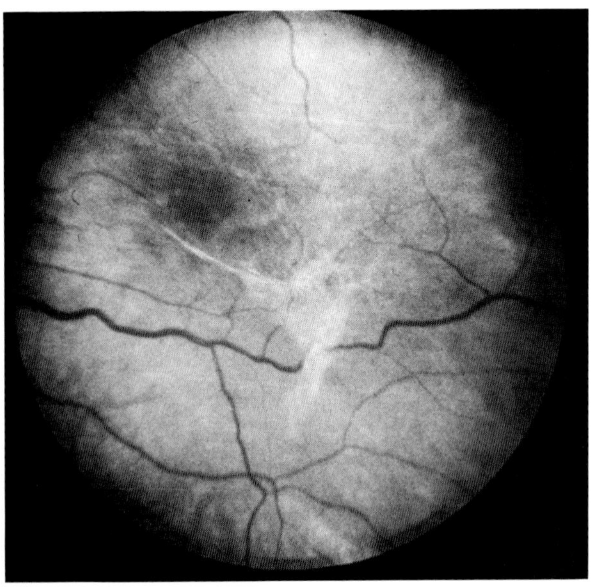

Fig. 5-18. Macular pucker 1 year after exogenous "bleb" endophthalmitis due to alpha hemolytic streptococcus. Visual acuity 20/200.

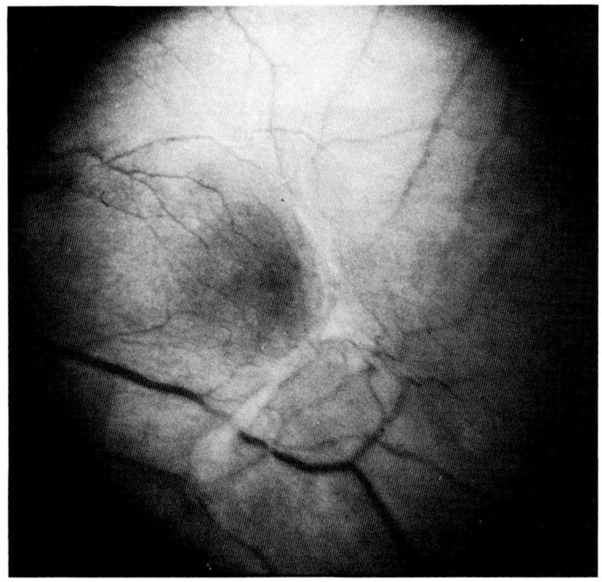

Fig. 5-19. Macular pucker 4 months after exogenous staphylococcal infection, treated by vitrectomy. Surgical removal of preretinal membrane improved acuity from 20/100 to 20/40.

Persistent vitreous opacity in cases where infection was cured may require an elective vitrectomy (Figs. 5-13–5-15).

Persistent maculr edema occurs not infrequently, with chronic decrease in visual acuity (Figs. 5-16, 5-17).

Macular pucker due to preretinal membrane formation is also not uncommon. Later elective surgery for the pucker may be done if indicated (Figs. 5-18, 5-19).

Retinal detachment is an occasional complication, usually quite late, and is dealt with on its merits.

RESULTS

Visual acuity may be as good as 20/20, but the eye also may not achieve normal vision and may even be blind. In general, infections are almost all cured, but occasionally the eye or vision completely lost. Some cases do as well as if there had never been any infective incident (Figs. 5-20–

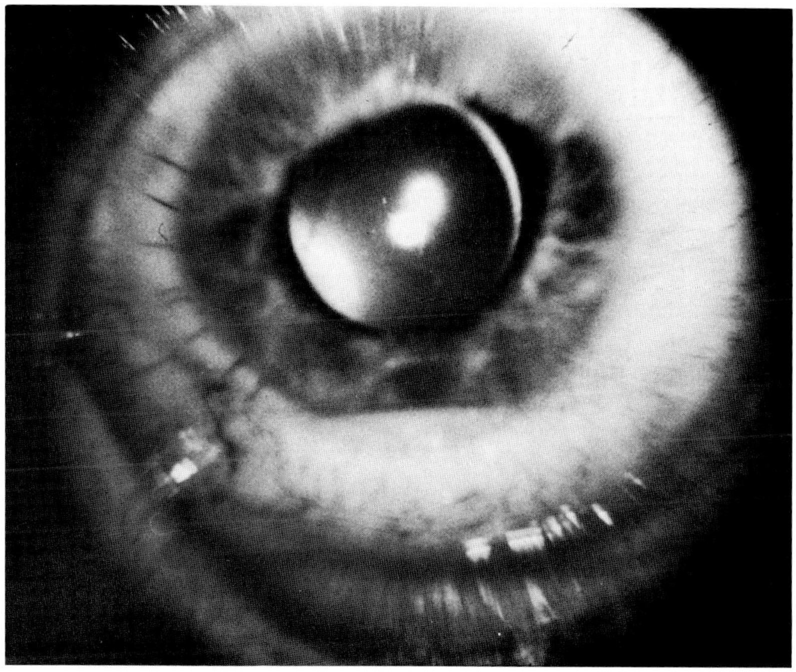

Fig. 5-20. Hypopyon due to staphylococcus epidermidis endophthalmitis following secondary implant through temporal incision. Treated by vitrectomy.

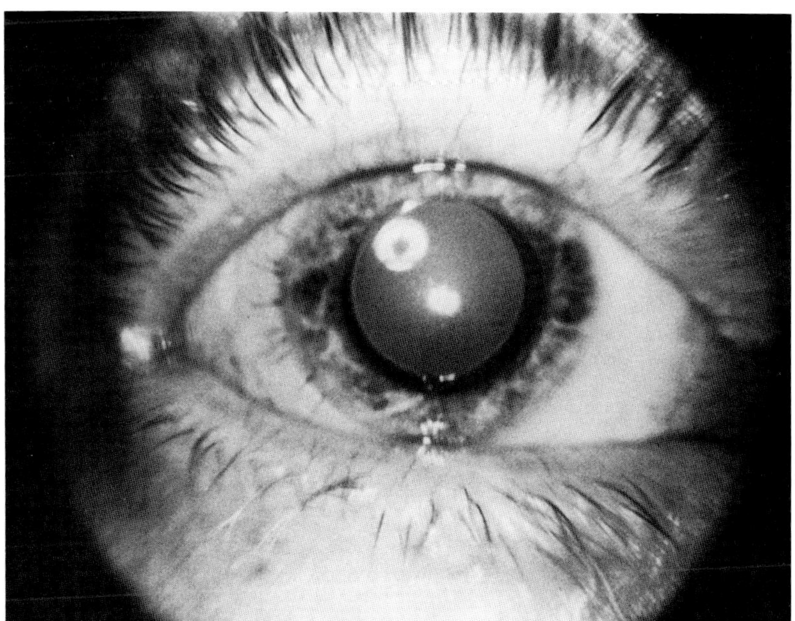

Fig. 5-21. Same eye as in Fig. 5-20 3 months later. Quiet eye with anterior chamber lens in good position.

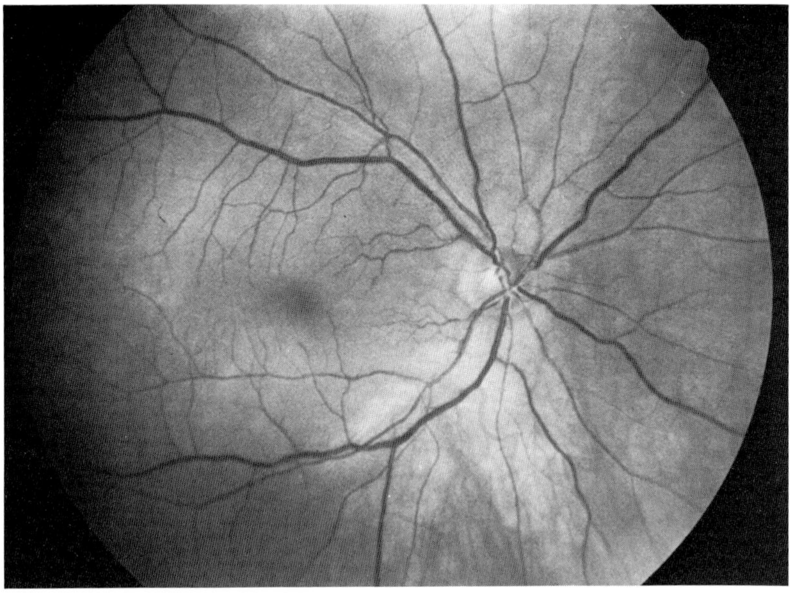

Fig. 5-22. Same eye as in Fig. 5-20. Wide-angle (60 degree) fundus photograph shows excellent clarity of media and normal retina. Visual acuity 20/16.

5-22). Much depends on the nature and virulence of the organism.

WHO SHOULD MANAGE THE CASE?

Anyone who is competent to do so should manage the case. In our local community the vast majority of infections are referred to the retinovitreal surgeons. For the usual range of organisms the drug therapy is relatively straightforward, but for unusual organisms requiring unfamiliar antibiotic therapy, we routinely request additional consultation from the infectious disease specialists.

The occurrence of endophthalmitis often adds a sour note to the relationship between patient and surgeon. In my experience, quick reaction and concern by the primary surgeon has generally helped to avoid the fracture of the relationship and many of the associated problems.

ENDOGENOUS ENDOPHTHALMITIS

There are significant differences in management when the origin of the infections is endogenous. The organism is often identified by blood cultures, and the infection not necessarily fulminating in the eye, or the patient may be so ill that it is difficult to give the eye priority.

These factors may lead to a more "conservative" approach, and management without invasive procedures on the eye. If there is any doubt, or if the infection is fulminating in the eye, the management is very similar to that described for exogenous cases.

PHAKIC ENDOPHTHALMITIS

For phakic patients who develop endophthalmitis through a bleb or following trauma, or in endogenous infections, it may be necessary to remove the lens (by fragmentation through the pars plana) as part of the surgical management, which is otherwise not any different.

SUMMARY OF MANAGEMENT OF ENDOPHTHALMITIS

1. High index of suspicion.
2. Hospital admission.
3. Vitreous biopsy or vitrectomy.
4. Intraocular antibiotics.
5. Periocular antibiotics.
6. Systemic antibiotics.
7. Steroids: intraocular, periocular, systemic.
8. Management of long-term complications.

REFERENCES

1. Leopold H: Management of intraocular infection. Trans Ophthalmol Soc UK 91:575, 1971
2. Maylath FR, Leopold IH: Study of experimental intraocular infection. I. The recoverability of organisms inoculated into ocular tissues and fluids. II. The influence of antibiotics and cortisone, alone and combined, on intraocular growth of these organisms. Am J Ophthalmol 40:86, 1955
3. Allansmith MR, Skaggs C, Kimmura SJ. The diagnostic value of anterior chamber paracentesis in 14 cases of postoperative endophthalmitis. Trans Am Ophthalmol Soc 68:335, 1970
4. Rowsey JJ, Newsom DL, Sexton DJ, Harms WK: Endophthalmitis: Current approaches. Ophthalmology 89:1055, 1982
5. Von Sallman L, Meyer K, DeGrandi JL: Experimental study on penicillin treatment of exogenous infections of vitreous. Arch Ophthalmol 32:179, 1944
6. Von Sallman L: Penicillin therapy of infections of the vitreous. Arch Ophthalmol 33:455, 1945
7. Von Sallman L: Penetration of penicillin into the eye: further studies. Arch Ophthalmol 34:195, 1945
8. Leopold IH: Intravitreal penetration of penicillin and penicillin therapy of infections of the vitreous. Arch Ophthalmol 33:211, 1945
9. Graham RO, Peyman GA, Fishman G: Intravitreal injection of cephaloridine in treatment of endophthalmitis. Arch Ophthalmol 93:56, 1975
10. Kasbeer RT, Peyman GA: Intravitreal oxacillin in experimental staphylococcal endophthalmitis. Albrecth Von Graefes Arch Klin Exp Ophthalmol 9:316, 1974
11. Koziol J, Peyman GA: Intraocular chloramphenicol and bacterial endophthalmitis. Can J Ophthalmol 9:316, 1974
12. May DR, Ericson ES, Peyman GA, et al: Intraocular injection of gentamicin: Single injection therapy of experimental bacterial endophthalmitis. Arch Ophthalmol 91:487, 1974
13. Paque JT, Peyman GA: Intravitreal clindamycin phosphate in the treatment of vitreous infection. Ophthalmic Surg 5:34, 1974
14. Peyman GA, May DR, Ericson ES, et al: Intraocular injection of gentamicin: Toxic effects and clearance. Arch Ophthalmol 92:42, 1974
15. Peyman GA, May DR, Homer PI, et al: Penetration of gentamicin into the aphakic eye. Ann Ophthalmol 9:871, 1977
16. Peyman GA, Nelson P, Bennett TO: Intravitreal injection of kanamycin in experimentally induced endophthalmitis. Can J Ophthalmol 9:322, 1974
17. Cottingham AJ, Forster RK: Vitrectomy in endophthalmitis: Results of a study using vitrectomy, intraocular antibiotics, or a combination of both. Arch Ophthalmol 94:2078, 1976
18. Ossoinig KC: Clinical echo-ophthalmology. p. 101. In Blodi FC (ed): Current Concepts in Ophthalmology. Vol. 3. CV Mosby, St. Louis, 1972
19. Diamond JG, Kefring SL, Ossoinig KC: Echography and vitrectomy. p. 971. In White D, Brown RE (eds): Ultrasound in Medicine. Vol. A. Plenum, New York, 1977

Medical-Legal Considerations

6

Philip A. Shelton

Most ophthalmologists are increasingly and uncomfortably aware of the impact of federal and state law on their medical practices. The law, in its broad generic sense, has always been present as the set of rules that groups of people live by. As our society has become more complex and more rights and responsibilities have been added, these rules or laws have become more numerous and intrusive due to the increasing diversity of interests between people.

While some honest attempts have been made to simplify paperwork requirements, codify laws using plain language, reduce court backlogs, and find alternate means of resolving disputes such as arbitration and mediation panels, little headway has been made against the tidal forces of increasing civil litigation and governmental regulation.

This chapter attempts to give the ophthalmologist some understanding of the current "hot spots" in the law along with a broad overview of the major areas of interface between the law and our medical practices.

The area of malpractice litigation is probably of most interest to individual ophthalmologists, although the broader questions of governmental and administrative regulation are of more long-term importance to the profession in general. This chapter considers only the issues of medical malpractice. Most of the cases cited are ophthalmic, but significant noneye cases are used for illustration of trends.

MALPRACTICE LITIGATION

The ultimate dispute mechanism in our civilized society is the adversary proceedings or court trial. Historically, its roots may be in the selection of individual or tribal champions who fought in mortal combat for the idea, land, and principle in contention. It has since become highly stylized and more complex but still consists of a referee (judge), two or more adversaries (parties), their champions (attorneys), and a jury or finder of facts. The rationale for this system is the conviction that it is the best way to discover the truth.

Unfortunately, the abrasive aspects of the adversary system often evoke angry, confused, and indignant responses from the physician who is not trained in its rules or familiar with its mechanisms. These responses are uniformly counterproductive. Our medical training will support us well if we remember to maintain a posture of equanimity when confronted by the unexpected or unfamiliar.

In order for a plaintiff to prevail in a malpractice suit, each of the four elements must be proved: (1) the physician had a duty to the patient, (2) the physician breached the applicable standard of care (negligence), (3) the negligent act of omission was the cause of damage, and (4) there was, in fact, damage. Failure to prove each of these elements should result in a nonsuit or verdict for the physician.

Duty to the Patient

This is usually not a problem area once the doctor–patient relationship has been established. The questions that sometimes arise have to do with the degree of contact necessary to establish or dissolve the relationship. This duty arises from the acceptance by physicians or their office staff of an appointment to see a patient with a specific medical problem. If after accepting such an appointment the physician decides not to see the patient, he or she should timely notify the patient in writing (registered, return receipt requested) to seek other medical aid and offer valid suggestions on where such aid can be found. In *Maltempo v. Cuthbert,*[1] the most recent extension of the physician's duty occurred when a physician covering for Mr. Maltempo's family doctor was called by the patient's wife. Dr. Cuthbert was told that Mr. Maltempo, a diabetic, was very ill and in jail, and the family was concerned that he was not getting proper care from the medical personnel in prison. Dr. Cuthbert assured the family that he would check the situation and call them if any problems arose. He called the jail and was told that Mr. Maltempo was being treated by the jail physician, Dr. Freeman. Dr. Cuthbert never called Dr. Freeman, never visited the jail and never called the Maltempo family again. Mr. Maltempo died by aspiration of vomitus shortly thereafter, and Dr. Cuthbert was found liable for breach of his duty to communicate with the Maltempo *family*—since he undertook a duty to a person not even his own patient.

The Virginia case of *Lyons v. Graether* (1977)[2] seems to outline the barest minimum contact necessary to establish the duty or doctor–patient relationship. A new patient made an appointment to see the doctor with a specific complaint (vaginal infection). When the patient arrived at the physician's office, he refused to see her because she was accompanied by her seeing-eye dog. He made no effort to recommend another physician for her. She delayed finding another gynecologist and suffered harm thereby. The court stated that the physician, by his employee, had accepted an appointment at a specific time for a specific problem and that at the least he was duty bound to refer her elsewhere for care that he had not provided. Thus, your staff can make you liable without your ever having seen or even spoken to the patient.

In those cases in which a physician speaks directly to a patient or even to another physician about the patient (e.g., emergency department physician) and either makes a diagnosis, suggests therapy, or makes a follow-up appointment, the duty to the patient is even more evident.

In a recent case[3] of cataract extraction with subsequent complications, an attempt was made by the patient to suppress the opinion of the second treating ophthalmologist, who failed to find that the defendant ophthalmologist's actions were the cause of the plaintiff's loss of vision. The patient claimed that since the second doctor had treated the patient, admission of his statement would breach the physician–patient privilege. The appeals court found the trial court's disallowance of this testimony to be in error, reversed the finding for the plaintiff, and remanded for a new trial on the grounds that (1) there was no longer an ongoing doctor–patient relationship, and (2) courts normally find a waiver of physician–patient privilege on health and medical history, which the patient–plaintiff has put into issue.

Breach of the Standard of Care

Establishment of the Standard of Care

The standard typically quoted is: That degree of skill and learning ordinarily used under the same or similar circumstances by members of the profession. For ophthalmology all jurisdictions use at least a statewide, and most now use a national, standard. In *McCormack v. Linberg*[4] and *Logan v. Greenwich Hospital Association,*[5] the court specifically held that the standard of care for a specialist is national, not local, and a specialist must be held to the same standard of care as other specialists in the field. It generally requires expert testimony to establish a breach of this standard, as such matters are beyond the competence of the lay jury. The major exception is called *res ipsa loquitor,* or "the thing speaks for itself". This doctrine, if applicable, will allow the case to go to the jury without expert medical testimony to support it. The general rule is that the circumstances must be of such a character whereby a layman is able to say, as a matter of common knowledge and observation, that the consequences of professional treatment were not such as ordinarily would have followed had due care been exercised. Thus the res ipsa doctrine generally applies to sponges left in operative sites. Res ipsa has specifically been ruled inapplicable in ophthalmology cases where a viral corneal infection occurred post-thyroidectomy *(Merritt v. Deaconess Hospital et al.),*[6] where endophthalmitis occurred following cataract surgery *(Adams v. EENT Hospital et al.),*[7] and *(Schofield v. Idaho Falls Latter Day Saints Hospital),*[8] and where a retinal detachment followed a cataract extraction with vitreous loss *(Stundon v. Stadnick).*[9]

In *Miller v. Scholl,*[10] the court ruled that failure to use phacoemulsification as an alternate procedure in 1973 did not constitute negligence:

> Mere evidence that the conduct of the surgeon did not measure up to the standards of a single member of the profession as opposed to the standards of the profession *as a whole* [italics added] does not support a submission of negligence in a malpractice action, for the basic and fundamental reason that standards of a single member of the profession may be higher or lower than the standards of the profession as a whole.

In the matter of timely referral to subspecialists, the Supreme Court of Wyoming in the 1981 case of *Siebert v. Fowler*[11] found for the defendant ophthalmologist in the absence of specific expert testimony that one with the requisite skill, diligence, and knowledge would have referred the diabetic patient to a retinal specialist for laser treatment at an earlier time.

In a most interesting 1983 case *(Sikorski v. Bell),*[12] the Court of Appeals of Georgia stated that unnecessary surgery may not be malpractice if a patient is fully informed and the surgery is adequately performed. In this case of a patient with advanced glaucoma, a surgical procedure was done with resultant suprachoroidal hemorrhage and a total loss of vision. The plaintiff's expert suggested that alternate nonsurgical procedures could have been used, but he did not adequately contradict the defendant ophthalmologist's proof as to his compliance with the applicable standard of care.

By far the most significant change in the standard of care is represented in the trilogy of Washington State cases: *Helling v. Carey* (1974),[13] *Gates v. Jensen* (1979),[14] and *Harris v. Groth* (1983).[15]

The Helling court concluded that failure to test for glaucoma in patients under age 40 was negligent in spite of uncontradicted expert testimony that this was not the standard of care. The court invoked a judicially determined standard of care based on the 1932 decision of *The T.J. Hooper*[16] (a tugboat that damaged its barges in tow in stormy seas because of failure to have a radio receiver that would have given an updated weather report). Tugs did not usually carry radio receivers, but Judge Learned Hand said in the opinion: "Courts must in the end say what is required; there are precautions so imperative that even their universal disregard will not excuse their omission."

Following the Helling case, the Washington State legislature redefined the standard of care to the exercising of that degree of skill, care, and learning *possessed* (emphasis ours) by other persons in the same profession. The court in *Gates* v. *Jensen*[14] held that this is a much broader standard than exercising the degree of skilled care and learning *practiced* (emphasis ours) by other persons in the same profession. This reasonable prudence test may therefore require a standard of practice that is higher than that exercised by the medical profession. Thus, the court found for the plaintiff where the defendant ophthalmologist failed to do visual fields and a dilated fundus examination in a patient whose tension was in the glaucoma suspect range and who subsequently suffered damage to her optic nerves.

The most recent case in this trilogy *(Harris v. Groth,*[15] 1983) was won by the ophthalmologist because the jury instruction requested by the plaintiff was overly broad and did not correctly state the law. It is questionable at best whether the angle-closure glaucoma in this case could have been detected by an intraocular pressure test. However, the court reiterated its view that a "reasonable prudence" standard is applicable in Washington State rather than an "average practitioner" standard.

In summary, there seems to be a tendency to extend the required standard of care beyond that ordinarily used by members of the profession locally to that level of skill, care, and learning possessed by other professionals often on a national level. In making this decision, the court will balance ability, impact and cost. This tends to accelerate the speed with which the standard of care approaches the state of the art.[17]

Informed Consent

In early malpractice cases, the touching of someone's body without their consent was a "battery." The modern view is that the standard of care requires the physician to inform the patient of the nature of the proposed treatment, alternate therapies including none, and the risks and reasonably expected benefits of each one and only then secure their consent. A growing minority of states has ruled that the disclosure should be such that a reasonable patient could make an intelligent choice on the basis of its contents. This standard does *not* require expert witness testimony as to the usual actions of the physicians in the specialty.

In most states, however, the standard of disclosure required is "measured by those communications a reasonable medical practitioner in the same branch of medicine would make under the same or similar circumstances."[18] In addition, these states require expert medical evidence to establish this standard.

The recent case of *Welch v. Whitaker*[19] concurred in the directed verdict in favor of the ophthalmologist who allegedly failed to warn the patient of the possibility of corneal scarring subsequent to the removal of a corneal foreign body and rust ring. No expert medical evidence was presented by the patient–plaintiff on the issues of the standard of disclosure, the standard of care of removal of the foreign body and the proximate cause of the corneal scarring.

In the vast majority of states, the patient–plaintiff must then prove that a reasonable patient as well as the individual plaintiff would not have given consent had he or she been informed of the risk or outcome that actually transpired.

There are exceptions to the informed consent doctrine that relieve the physician from the duty to fully disclose. Medical emergencies and patient incompetency (which may require guardian consent) are clear examples. Voluntary waiver, wherein a patient knowingly and intelligently declines to be informed in order to reduce anxiety upon disclosure is a rarely used but available exception. The most controversial is the therapeutic exception, where it is clearly poor medical practice and potentially harmful to the patient's health to fully disclose the risks. The problem with the therapeutic exception is to balance the individual patient's right to make informed decisions against society's policy encouraging procedures needed to maintain a health populace.

On a trial court level, the Massachusetts Superior court in *Precourt v. Frederick*[20] allowed a jury verdict to stand against the defendant ophthalmologist who was found negligent by failing to inform his patient with recurrent uveitis, that use of systemic steroids might cause aseptic necrosis of bones and joints. There was no expert evidence that this was usual practice, but Massachusetts joins a growing number of states following the reasonable patient standard of required disclosure. This case was reversed on appeal. The majority of the court held that the risk of aseptic necrosis was "so remote as to be negligible," and therefore Dr. Frederick did not have a duty to disclose this risk. The dissenting judge concurred in the result but only on the grounds that since the critical dose and time relationship for the causation of aseptic necrosis by systemic steroids is unknown, the plaintiff's statement of his potential unwillingness to proceed with only the second of two courses of prednisone had the risk of aseptic necrosis been disclosed was insufficient evidence on causation to allow submission to the jury.[20]

Contrasting the Precourt case is the 1979 North Dakota case of *Winkjer v. Herr.*[21] Here the defendant ophthalmologist did not notify the patient that the use of phospholine iodide could cause cataracts. The court found for the defendant and stated that "information does not indicate at what levels and over what length of time the drug has been shown to possibly cause cataracts. There can be no liability for a physician to disclose a risk that was unknown in the manner in which a particular drug or treatment was prescribed."

An interesting case of apparent invalidation of a signed consent form was found in New Mexico case of *Toppino v. Herhohn.*[22] In this case, involving plastic reconstruction of a woman's breast, the surgeon's statements that "we'll get this right" and "this will be right" were held to be an express warranty of results in spite of a signed consent form that said "though good result are expected they cannot be and are not guaranteed. . . ."

The court held that since the defendant did not raise the defense based on the alleged conclusiveness of the signed surgical consent at trial, he could not raise it on appeal.

In the North Carolina case of *Estrada* v. *Jaques*[23] the appeals court reversed the summary judgment of the lower court in favor of the defendant, based on the presumed validity of a signed consent form. The appeals court held that a signed consent form is not given conclusive weight. Rather it is only *some evidence* of valid consent and is not sufficient to grant automatic summary judgment under a North Carolina statute governing signed consent forms. Knowledge of procedures is not a broad enough disclosure. The patient must be informed of their usual and most frequent risks and hazards. Since the procedure in question was experimental (embolization technique), the patient must be in addition be told of the experimental nature of the procedure, any uncertainty regarding risks of the procedure and the known or projected most likely risks.

Another very important informed consent decision, although not an ophthalmological case, was *Logan* v. *Greenwich Hospital Association.*[5] In 1983, the Supreme Court of Connecticut held in Logan that *all* alternative modes of treatment, including those that might be more hazardous, had to be disclosed to the patient. In addition, the court stated that medical care in Connecticut was henceforth to be judged against a national standard rather than a local statewide standard.

Thus the trend seems to be toward the reasonable patient standard of disclosure with the physician having almost no relief from the requirement of an exhaustive recitation of all possible alternatives and complications, even those he may never have encountered. This pendulum has swung to the extreme; it is hoped that some counterforce is due and may be apparent in *Hook v. Rothstein,*[18] where the court pointed out that the physician should be concerned with the patient's best interests and not what a lay jury, untrained in medicine and employing perfect hindsight, might later conclude he or she should have disclosed [referral to dissent in *Scaria v. St. Paul Fire and Marine Insurance Company,* 227 NW2d 647,659 (1975)]. However, if a state-of-the-art alternative is safe, effective, and of reasonable cost and availability, it should be disclosed, even if not recommended.[17]

Causation

Once the plaintiff has demonstrated a breach (negligence) in the applicable standard of care, he or she must connect the negligent act or omission with the damage suffered.

The standard for proving causation is generally "reasonable medical probability," not simply possibility. In almost all cases, proof of causation requires expert testimony. In *Lazenby v. Beisel,*[24] the patient became blind following a retrobulbar hemorrhage. The defendant's expert suggested that failure to do a lateral canthotomy, to give intravenous acetazolamide (Diamox), or to give IV mannitol decreased the patient's chance to maintain his sight, which was lost due to increased intraocular pressure. The appeals court held that the trial court erred in instructing the jury that negligence is a legal cause of injury if it lessens a person's chance of complete recovery. No evidence was given that using a lateral canthotomy, IV Diamox, or IV mannitol would probably have salvaged the patient's vision.

In *Edwards* v. *United States,*[25] the plaintiff failed to prove that a flat anterior chamber following cataract extraction in his right eye, which spontaneously reformed within 5 days, was the cause of the patient's subsequent glaucoma, which was controlled on medication. The courts stated: "The decision to delay surgery was a judgment decision and the evidence is not persuasive that the judgment exercised was in error." Also, "since plaintiff's left eye has greater pressure than his right, it is illogical to ascribe the pressure in the right eye to the cataract surgery or treatment of the right eye. . . ."

There are some cases, chiefly those involving wrongful death, in which the standard of causation is altered to "if there was any substantial possibility of survival and defendant has destroyed it, he is answerable" (*Hicks v. United States*).[26] There does not seem to be a tendency for the courts to apply this doctrine of "best last chance" to eye cases, but the possibility always exists that in a truly desperate situation it may be invoked.

Damages

These are usually clearly evident and measurable by loss of visual acuity or field, diplopia, cosmetic defects, lost wages, and other factors. Pain and suffering, although subjective, can be objectively valued by the jury upon persuasive evidence.

An interesting eye case held that a patient does *not* have a duty to submit to cataract surgery in order to reduce the damages caused by malpractice. In a 1979 case (*Frisnegger v. Gibson*),[27] the patient sustained a cataract subsequent to the perforation of his eye by a defendant ophthalmologist who was injecting the eyelid preparatory to chalazion removal. The patient suffered severe depression and refused to have the cataract removed that had incapacitated him. This trial court properly approved a reasonable person test for the jury to determine whether damages should be reduced rather than the mandatory test requested by the defendant.

SUMMARY

It is often a traumatic and frightening experience for an ophthalmologist to be involved as a defendant in a medical malpractice suit. The initial shock should not precipitate irrational or angry behavior, which is counterproductive to the physician's interests. Cooperation with one's attorney is essential to secure the best possible defense. While even a careful ophthalmologist may be sued for nonmeritorious claims, avoidance of malpractice litigation is enhanced by following a few simple rules:

1. *Be kind to your patients.* Nothing breeds litigation like hostility.
2. *Keep good records.* They are essential to your defense and unparalleled as the best available evidence.
3. *Inform your patients of all the possibilities.* Only the physician can ask: "Do you understand what you have been told or read? If not, what are your questions?"
4. *Don't be afraid of second opinions.* They increase your stature in the patient's view.[28]
5. *Write lots of letters.* Document your records with return-receipt-requested letters discharging patients, following up on significant no-shows and explaining complex points to patients.
6. *Be careful what you say about others.* Careless words may entrap another physician in a needless malpractice suit. If your remark was malicious (e.g., that "butcher," "quack"), you may be sued for slander. Be wary of violating patient privacy and confidentiality by remarks over the phone while within another person's range of hearing.
7. *Train and control your employees.* They are your agents when acting within the scope of their employment. Document job descriptions and the protocols they must follow for all phases of their work. From telephone manners and questions to the technical aspects of fundus photography or other procedures, your staff's negligence will usually be viewed as your negligence.[29]

REFERENCES

1. *Maltempo v. Cuthbert*, US Court of Appeals 5th Cir, Nov. 21, 1974
2. *Lyons v. Graether*, 239 SE2d 103, Va, 1977

3. *Trujillo v. Puro,* 683 P2d 1963, 101 NM 408, 1984
4. *McCormack v. Linberg,* 352 NW2d 30, Minn App, 1984
5. *Logan v. Greenwich Hospital Association,* 465 A2d 294, Conn, 1983
6. *Merritt v. Deaconess Hospital et al:* 357 NE2d 65, Oh, 1975.
7. *Adams v. EENT Hospital et al,* La App, 346 So2d 327, La, 1977
8. *Schofield v. Idaho Falls Latter Day Saints Hospital,* 409 P2d 107, Idaho, 1965
9. *Studon v. Stadnick,* 469 P2d 16, Wyo, 1970
10. *Miller v. Scholl,* 594 SW2d 324, Mo, 1980
11. *Siebert v. Fowler,* 637 P2d 255, Wyo, 1981
12. *Sikorski v. Bell,* 307 SE2d 701, Ga, App, 1983
13. *Helling v. Carey,* 519 P2d 981, Wash, 1974
14. *Gates v. Jensen,* 595 P2d 919, Wash, 1979
15. *Harris v. Groth,* 663 P2d 113, Wash, 1983
16. *The T.J. Hooper,* 60 F2d 737, 2nd Cir., 1932
17. Shelton PA: State of the art v. the standard of care. Int J Cataract Surg. 1:7, 1984
18. *Hook v. Rothstein,* 16 SE2d 690, SC App 1984
19. *Welch v. Whitaker,* 317 SE2d 758, SC App 1984
20. *Precourt v. Fredericks,* SJC Mass S-3457 8/19/85; Dockett #41128 Oct, 1983
21. *Winkjer v. Herr,* 277 NW2d 579, ND, 1979
22. *Toppino v. Herhohn,* 673 P2d 1318, 1983
23. *Estrada v. Jaques,* 321 SE2d 240, NC App, 1984
24. *Lazenby v. Beisel,* 425 So2d 84, Fla, 1983
25. *Edwards v. United States,* 497 F Supp 379, Ala, 1980
26. *Hicks v. United States,* 368 F2d 626, 4th Cir, 1966
27. *Frisnegger v. Gibson,* 598 P2d 574, Mont, 1979.
28. Shelton PA: Second opinions—A guide for the perplexed. Int J Cataract Surg 2:3, 1985
29. Shelton PA: Vicarious liability and the employer/employee relationship. Int J of Cataract Surgery. 1:2, 1984

Section II

CATARACT

Richard H. Keates

Section Editor

Introduction to Cataract Surgery 7

Richard H. Keates

The skill, effort, and technology in perfecting a "modern" cataract extraction technique is truly staggering. The technology and information explosion has led to a quantum leap in techniques of cataract extraction and intraocular lens implantation.

One has only to look at the day's office mail to see the dramatic increase in journals devoted to one area of interest in ophthalmology. Beyond this there are services that provide audio and video tape cassettes devoted entirely to ophthalmology, not to mention satellite television programs sponsored by the American Academy of Ophthalmology. The message is clear: the field is undergoing rapid change that appears to speed up as one watches. Certainly, the practicing ophthalmologist is at risk of becoming seriously outdated regarding just cataract surgery in a matter of a few years. How did this come to pass?

The reader is certainly familiar with the evolution of the current intraocular lens, yet attention should rightfully be directed again toward the history of these devices. Dr. Harold Ridley deserves to stand with the other giants of ophthalmology for his ceaseless efforts to perfect a workable intraocular lens. The current generation of intraocular lenses is a reflection of the inspiration provided by Dr. Ridley. The list of those who followed reads like a page from *Who's Who in Ophthalmology:* Baron, Strampelli, Dannheim, Choyce, Barraquer, Epstein, Binkhorst, Copeland, Worst, and others. Yet this was not enough. Kelman was the first to introduce phacoemulsification in 1967; the surgical microscope came into common use shortly thereafter. Vitreous suction cutter devices were developed about the same time, while hyaluronic acid for eye surgery was finally used in anterior eye segment surgery in 1977. It was about that time that Daniele Aron-Rosa and Frans Fankhauser developed the Nd:YAG laser so that ocular tissues could be safely cut. Other more subtle advances in surgical instrumentation, techniques, and research were developed, but space precludes listing all these advances.

This awesome glut of information and hardware did not happen overnight, although it appears so. Today's triumph rests on the agonizingly slow and tedious work of many that was performed over decades. That is what the following chapters are based on. It is not just one surgeon's technique or solution to a problem that is presented here, but the expression of clinical experience that has been modified and improved upon since modern cataract surgery became a possibility.

In summary, the reader is urged to take the following techniques and to improve on them as experience dictates, for this is the true value of these chapters.

Ambulatory Cataract Surgery

8

Joseph L. Dowling, Jr.

Ambulatory surgery, also known as outpatient surgery, "in-and-out" surgery, and day care surgery, as the term is used in this chapter, is surgery performed in a free-standing facility or in a hospital setting without an overnight stay. The primary goals of ambulatory cataract surgery are to decrease the patient's anxiety to the lowest possible level and to disrupt his normal routine as little as possible. Secondary goals are enhanced patient satisfaction, increased efficiency, and lower cost. Ambulatory cataract surgery can be performed in various settings: a general hospital operating room, a separate hospital facility designed for ambulatory patient surgery, a free-standing ambulatory surgical clinic designed for various types of ambulatory surgery, a free-standing ophthalmic surgical clinic used by a number of ophthalmologists, or a private office operating suite.

This chapter is concerned primarily with cataract and intraocular lens implant surgery. However, most ophthalmic surgical procedures can be performed on an ambulatory basis. We have encountered no medical complications or problems in more than 10 years' experience with ambulatory strabismus surgery under general anesthesia. Essentially all anterior segment operations, including glaucoma procedures, corneal transplantation, and plastic procedures, are suitable for ambulatory surgery. A 1981 poll of the membership of the Outpatient Ophthalmic Surgical Society (OOSS) concluded that all ophthalmic procedures can be safely and effectively performed on an ambulatory basis except for three: exenteration of the orbit; repair of retinal detachment with air or gas tamponade, and transcranial orbitotomy.

In the past decade, free-standing general surgicenters have established an enviable record in regard to cost, quality, and physician and patient satisfaction.[1] Although ambulatory general surgery was reported as early as 1909, the first contemporary Surgicenter was founded in Providence, Rhode Island, in 1968. Despite vigorous support by many physicians, it encountered extraordinary opposition from Blue Cross and was finally forced to close after a long struggle. The concept succeeded, however, and there are now approximately 150 free-standing surgical centers across the country. They have achieved a remarkable safety record. The Surgicenter in Phoenix, Arizona, founded in 1970, is the oldest surviving free-standing operating facility. During its first 10 years in operation, 70,000 surgical procedures were performed, mostly under general anesthesia, without one single death or hospital transfer.[1] The Salt Lake City Surgical Center in its first $5\frac{1}{2}$ years of operation, cared for 26,000 patients ranging in age from 10 days to 91 years with no major surgical or postoperative complications.[2] In 1980, the Society for the Advancement of Freestanding Ambulatory Surgical Care reported on 369,528 surgical procedures with but one death.[3] This mortality rate of less than one death in a third of a million patients is remarkable. "One could conclude syllogistically that it is 400 times healthier to be a patient in such a facility than to be a young American adult" whose death rate is 443 deaths for a third of a million.[4] It is estimated that 40 percent of all operations traditionally performed on an inpatient basis could be performed in an ambulatory facility and the percentage is climbing.[5] The concept of ambulatory surgery has been considered and endorsed by various medical groups, including the American College of Surgeons and the American Medical Association (AMA). In 1971, the AMA House of Delegates passed a resolution stating that "The American Medical Association endorses the concept of outpatient surgery for selected procedures and selected patients as good medical practice."[6] The American Academy of Ophthalmology (AAO) has taken no official stand but has maintained a continuing interest in ambulatory eye surgery. Courses, papers, and symposia have been featured at its annual meetings. Through the Committee on Health Plans, the needs of the patient in safe and effective ambulatory surgery have been assessed, reimbursement procedures recommended, and a comprehensive set of recommendations for ambulatory surgery is currently being prepared.

As recently as 1948, the standard postcataract routine involved double eyepatches and shields in a darkened room. The unfortunate patient was kept flat in bed for 48 hours until the first dressing was applied. The eye was subsequently examined every other day; if all went well, the patient was permitted out of bed for half-hour periods twice daily with a gradual increase to the tenth day, when discharge was considered.[7] As recently as 1961, a poll of ophthalmologists in various parts of the country reported an average hospital stay following cataract surgery of 8.2 days; even into the 1980s, a 2- or 3-day or even longer hospital stay after cataract surgery was not unusual.[8]

The past 20 or more years have seen a marked change in the postoperative management of cataract patients. Ophthalmologists have gradually shortened the hospital stay and lessened the various physical restrictions imposed on their patients, a trend that has culminated in the development of ambulatory eye surgery. These changes have resulted from a variety of factors, including improvement in wound closure techniques, technologic advances in needles and suture material, escalating hospital charges, frequent hospital bed shortages, and recognition of the debilitating physical and psychological effects of hospitalization and inactivity, particularly on elderly patients. Perhaps the single occurrence that most focused the attention of ophthalmologists on hospital stay was Kelman's introduction of phacoemulsification in 1967.[9] This procedure, introduced with a wave of publicity previously unknown in ophthalmology, touted the advantages of a small incision and early ambulation (e.g., tennis the day after cataract surgery). Ophthalmologists performing standard intracapsular extraction responded by shortening their hospital stays and minimizing their postoperative restrictions, and they were delighted to find no adverse effect on the final outcome of surgery.

The evolution of cataract surgery to an ambulatory setting, often in a free-standing facility, and the elimination of virtually all postoperative restrictions are procedures still resisted by many ophthalmologists accustomed to time-honored conservatism in the care of their patients. Ironically, cataract surgery, which is one of the oldest operations known to humankind, was performed on an ambulatory basis without restriction in activity for several thousand years until "medical advances" mandated hospitalization with a prolonged and restricted convalescence.

There has been growing interest in ambulatory surgery for several years. Ophthalmology journals are replete with articles and notices of courses and meetings on ambulatory surgery. A recent poll of 33 prominent cataract surgeons in various parts of the country revealed that slightly more than one half of all their operations are performed on an ambulatory basis.[10]

To determine the prevalence of ambulatory surgery in the United States, a survey of 674 ophthalmologists selected at random from the membership list of the AAO was conducted in early 1984. Questionnaires were mailed to each participant in this sample, and a researcher phoned to record the responses. A second round of questionnaires was sent to those who did not respond to the initial request. The results were coded for computerization, checked for errors, and analyzed using frequency distributions and cross-tabulations. Of the 674 questionnaires mailed, 230 were addressed to ophthalmologists retired or deceased or others such as retina specialists who do not perform cataract surgery. Of the revised total, responses were received from 340, yielding an overall response rate of 79 percent. The results regarding ambulatory surgery are tabulated in Table 8-1.

Statistically, this survey accurately portrayed cataract surgery as practiced in the United States in 1984. There were several significant observations. First, 60.8 percent of ophthalmic surgeons in the United States performed at least some ambulatory surgery, but only 12.8 percent of cataract surgeons did ambulatory surgery routinely (90 percent or more). Second, of those surgeons who did not perform ambulatory cataract surgery, 62.1 percent believed that ambulatory surgery was safe and successful, and 82.3 percent of surgeons not performing ambulatory surgery expected to undertake ambulatory surgery in the future.

However, unbeknown to most ophthalmologists, the option of ambulatory surgery had become academic by the passage of the Tax Equity and Fiscal Responsibility Act of 1982 (TEFRA), which included the Peer Review Improvement Act of 1982. This act authorized the establishment of Peer Review Organizations (PROs) in each state and required them to determine which "services could, consistent with appropriate medical care, be provided more economically on an outpatient basis." Cataract surgery was determined to be such a procedure and the contracts negotiated by HCFA with each of the states have now made ambulatory cataract surgery mandatory on all Medicare patients except in certain specific instances such as when the nonoperative eye is legally blind, or when specific authorization is obtained in advance from the PRO. The guidelines for these exceptions vary from state to state.

Table 8-1. National Ambulatory Surgery Survey—1984

Surgeon Group	%
Cataract surgeons	
Perform ambulatory surgery	60.8
Do not perform ambulatory surgery	39.2
Frequency of ambulatory surgery by those surgeons who perform it	
Under one half	52.9
More than one half	25.2
90% or more	21.8
Nonambulatory surgeons	
Believe procedure is less safe	52.6
Believe procedure is safe	47.4
Nonambulatory surgeons	
May switch in future	77.3
Will not switch in future	22.7

But not everyone has accepted the concept of ambulatory surgery. Some conservative and conscientious ophthalmic surgeons still believe in hospitalization for their postoperative patients. The comments of surgeons responding to the survey who are opposed to ambulatory surgery expressed their concerns:

Many patients are older and need aftercare, which is often times not available at home.

There is adverse exposure to malpractice

There is a risk of endophthalmitis, postoperative glaucoma

Ambulatory cataract surgery is too dangerous to the patient; tissue does not heal in 24 hours

The special problems of the geriatric population make the hospital stay a necessity

Anesthetic risk requires local anesthesia.

It weakens the financial base of hospitals by screening off the easy cream of cases and leaves only the hard, expensive, unwanted cases.

Prefers to watch the patient more carefully after surgery

Passing ECCE and IOL off as a minor procedure is not acceptable.

The patient's welfare is at stake, and this is best served in the hospital.

Some resent that ambulatory surgery is being pushed on ophthalmology primarily as a cost-saving procedure.

Increased malpractice liability for the ambulatory cataract surgeon who experiences an unfavorable result is another concern. Fortunately, to date there have been no malpractice cases brought in which the performance of cataract surgery on an ambulatory basis was charged as negligence, and it appears unlikely that outpatient surgery increases a surgeon's malpractice liability.[11] To establish surgeon liability, plaintiffs must prove that their physician did not render competent care in a manner comparable to that rendered by ophthalmologists in general. The standards of care are constantly being redefined and "as long as there is room for an honest difference of opinion among competent physicians, a physician who uses his own best judgement cannot be convicted of negligence" *(Cebula v. Benoit)*.[11] Surgeons must be prepared, however, to defend the procedures that their best judgment has dictated.

In addition to the usual requirement for competent medical care, the ophthalmic surgeon who owns his or her own surgical facility has the added liability of responsibility for the facility and its employees. Hospitals have traditionally established the standards of care for surgical facilities; therefore, free-standing surgical enterprises must establish and maintain facilities and procedures at least equal to those of hospital standards. A free-standing surgical facility must have its own malpractice and liability insurance separate from that of the ophthalmologists using the facility.

The reality of ambulatory cataract surgery makes it encumbent upon every ophthalmologist to study and evaluate carefully the various aspects of ambulatory cataract surgery, with particular attention to its effect on recovery of the eye and the occurrence of postoperative complications, its medical and psychological benefits, the acceptance of the procedure by patients, the advantages to the ophthalmologist, and the cost.

AMBULATORY CATARACT SURGERY, WOUND HEALING, AND COMPLICATIONS

The concept of early ambulation after cataract surgery is not new. Sporadic reports describing the good results and lack of complications of early ambulation after cataract surgery have appeared for almost 100 years,[12] but they have been largely ignored. Moreover, there is very little, if any, documentation in the medical literature supporting the justification for the various restrictions traditionally imposed on cataract patients. The medical literature appears to contain no reports demonstrating adverse effects from early ambulation and outpatient cataract surgery. It has generally been assumed that the relaxation of postcataract restrictions has occurred as the result of corneoscleral suturing and meticulous wound closure. It is interesting to note, however, that reports of early ambulation following cataract surgery in the pre-corneoscleral suture days also showed no increased complications or any poorer visual results than those obtained with the standard methods and restrictions. Retrospective studies of thousands of patients undergoing ambulatory cataract surgery have shown no differences in postoperative complications and visual results from similar series of hospitalized cataract patients.[13,14]

Two excellent prospective studies on the safety of ambulatory cataract surgery have been published. In 1960, Norval Christy, operating at his mission hospital in Taxila, Pakistan, kept 1,000 consecutive cataract patients in bed for 8 days, 1,000 consecutive cataract patients in bed for 1 day, and 1,000 consecutive patients walked from the operating table with no subsequent restriction on their activities.[15] All these operations were performed by Dr. Christy himself, using essentially the same technique. No corneoscleral sutures were used. Apposition of the wound margins was maintained only by a bridge of conjunctiva and patching. Analysis of the complications and visual results in these 3,000 patients showed no significant differences among the three groups. Therefore, since 1960, all cataract patients at Christy's hospital have walked from the operating table and their activities have not been restricted. In 1975, Miles Galin and associates reported a well-designed, double-masked, randomized study.[16] A series of cataract patients, all operated on by the same surgeon using the same technique, were assigned to random postoperative convalescence groups that were not made known until the conclusion of surgery. One group was hospitalized for 3 days postoperatively, a second group was hospitalized for 1 day, and the patients in the third group were discharged immediately following surgery. The patients were followed postoperatively by ophthalmologists who were not involved in the surgery and who were not aware of the patient's treatment group. In this study, also, careful evaluation of the results in the three groups showed no differences in postoperative complications or final visual results.

The reintroduction of intraocular implants during the 1970s increased the need for accurate and secure wound closure. A shallow or flat anterior chamber occurring with an iris-supported lens was a potential disaster and a surgical emergency. The early years of implant surgery were associated with rapidly evolving surgical techniques and frequently increased surgical trauma, factors tending to encourage postoperative hospitalization, and more frequent observation of patients. Fortunately, modern wound-closure techniques adequately withstood the implant challenge; with time and advancing technology, ophthalmic surgeons have become as confident of their implant techniques as of their standard cataract procedures. Williamson[17] reported a retrospective series of 2200 outpatient intraocular implants using the intracapsular technique with iris-supported and anterior chamber lenses. Pierce and Sinskey[18] reported their technique in performing 500 extracapsular extractions with posterior chamber lenses performed in their office operating facility, of which about 20 percent were done under general anesthesia. Their complications were not analyzed, but their results were very satisfactory; nevertheless, three patients required transfer to a hospital, and they recommend that emergency transportation be readily available. Given the documented safety and the Medicare restraints on hospitalizations for cataract surgery, it seems unlikely that any further groups of patients will be subjected to prospective studies. In order to demonstrate the safety of ambulatory surgery, I have recently reviewed 500 consecutive cataract operations that I performed during 1985 and 1986 (Table 8-2).

Table 8-2. 500 Consecutive Ambulatory Cataract Operations Performed in 1985, 1986

Procedure	No. of Patients
ECCE with PC IOL	483
Secondary IOL	10
ECCE with AC IOL	4
ECCE with PC IOL & trabeculectomy	2
ICCE	1
	500

Table 8-3 lists all the complications observed during the period from surgery to the fifth postoperative day — an interval exceeding a maximum in-hospital stay. There were no cases of endophthalmitis, iris prolapse, or shallow or flat anterior chamber. Healon was used in every case and, although it was routinely removed following implant insertion, may account for the substantial incidence of postoperative elevated intraocular pressure. All patients with elevated intraocular pressure were treated with timolol (Timoptic) and acetazolamide (Diamox) and pressures returned to preoperative levels in all cases within 1 to 3 days. The hyphemas were small to moderate and all cleared within a few days without problems. The patient with acute iridocyclitis responded to local and systemic steroids and cycloplegics. The choroidal hemorrhage occurred at the time of nucleus removal. The eye was successfully closed and several weeks later the cortex removed, a posterior chamber lens inserted, and good visual result obtained. One patient developed acute pulmonary edema on the basis of a myocardial infarction in the middle of surgery. The eye was closed with difficulty and the patient admitted to intensive care — the only unplanned admission from the operating room in this series. One patient, a physician, developed severe pain during the night following surgery, was found to have an intraocular pressure rise to 58 mm Hg and was hospitalized, the only patient in the series admitted following discharge. During this same time period, 1985 and 1986, eight patients were hospitalized for elective cataract surgery, three because of blindness in the fellow eye, four because of severe medical problems, ischemic heart disease, kidney failure, and advanced diabetes, and one severely crippled from rheumatoid arthritis. The final visual results in this series of patients and the incidence of late complications

Table 8-3. Operative and Postoperative Complications to Fifth Postoperative Day

Complication	
Acute iridocyclitis	1
Choroidal hemorrhage	1
Acute pulmonary edema	1
Hyphema	16
IOP > 29	61
IOP > 40	20

were also not adversely affected in any way by outpatient surgery and early return to normal activities.

There are very few circumstances in which hospitalization is preferable to ambulatory cataract surgery. Some surgeons prefer to hospitalize patients undergoing surgery on an only eye. Most one-eyed patients, however, particularly those who are older and who have attentive relatives, are better managed at home. These patients have been accustomed to very limited vision, and they become less confused in a familiar environment. Concerned relatives, properly indoctrinated and devoted to only one person, will give better care than any hospital or private nurse can provide. Eye shields can be applied without an underlying patch and patients can use glasses as soon as lid movement returns.

Many surgeons consider cataract surgery under general anesthesia to be a reason for hospitalization. Although most general ambulatory surgical procedures and many outpatient cataract operations are performed under general anesthesia, there is justification for admitting at least some of these patients. General anesthesia has profound systemic effects, the very predicament that ambulatory surgery seeks to avoid. Hospitalization may be necessary for those with bilateral amputations, crippling arthritis, or morbid obesity who cannot easily come to the office for follow-up, and for some patients with mental illness who are unable to cooperate at home.

For several years we gave patients the option of either outpatient or inpatient surgery. Initially, about one-half of the patients chose hospital admission. As it became clear to us that most ambulatory patients tolerated the overall experience more easily, we investigated to determine why so many patients chose to be hospitalized. This revealed that most patients who chose inpatient surgery did so not of their own preference but because their families were insecure about being responsible from immediate postoperative care. Therefore, we expanded our preoperative counseling to include the patient's family and to emphasize to them the concepts of ambulatory surgery. The result was that essentially all patients then chose ambulatory surgery, and we have continued to find this counseling most helpful in the present era of compulsory outpatient surgery.

One of the principal points advanced by proponents of hospitalization for cataract patients is that a hospital and its facilities favor the early recognition and prompt treatment of endophthalmitis, a condition that is eye threatening and that can evolve rapidly.[19] It is essential for ophthalmologists performing ambulatory surgery to emphasize to the patients and their relatives that any moderate to severe ocular pain should be reported at once and to emphasize and reemphasize their availability. One direct call to the surgeon should insure an earlier diagnosis and more immediate treatment than the hospital procedure of the patient telling the nurse and waiting for the nurse to contact the surgeon. Moreover, without exposure to the risks of infection inherent in the hospital environment, the actual incidence of endophthalmitis may be less in patients who are not hospitalized.

GENERAL MEDICAL AND PSYCHOLOGICAL BENEFITS OF AMBULATORY CATARACT SURGERY

A basic precept of ambulatory cataract surgery is to disrupt the patient's normal physical and psychological routine as little as possible. Most cataract patients have elected surgery so they can continue functioning normally and improve the quality of their lives. They are frequently elderly and are frequently only marginally compensated in terms of physical and psychological adjustments. Their familiar environments and routines are important to their well being.

Elderly patients do not react well to change. They can often manage the ordinary stresses of life, but they are unable to manage additional pressure. Hospitalization and change in routine induce stress, alter metabolism, reduce muscle tone, interfere with circulation, and upset the gastrointestinal (GI) system. Patients with compensated medical problems such as hypertension, diabetes, and cardiovascular disease are particularly vulnerable to disruptions in normal routines. Familiar surroundings, customary food, and one's own friends and relatives are important in maintaining vitality. Our experience has shown that the more aged and more infirm the patient, the better ambulatory cataract surgery is tolerated and the more it is indicated. Only younger and stronger and healthier patients are able to withstand easily the various stresses induced by hospitalization.

Postoperative care has advanced considerably since the days of complete immobilization and sensory deprivation with double eye shields and the resultant "black mask psychosis." Nevertheless, the emotional and psychiatric effects of cataract surgery and hospitalization are rarely evaluated and infrequently understood. The incidence of overt psychiatric reactions associated with cataract surgery is generally reported to be between three and four percent.[20,21] Linn and associates[22] conducted an intensive, psychiatric study of hospitalized cataract patients. They specifically sought disturbances that would be missed by casual observation. Many disturbances occurred only at night or for transitory periods and would easily be overlooked by surgeons and nurses on morning rounds. Subtle alterations in mood and unexpressed delusions and hallucinations were frequently elicited by careful questioning. Ninety-five percent of patients in this series were found to display some form of abnormal behavior during hospitalization, and in 62 percent of cases the abnormal behavior was fairly evident. The patients studied in this report lived in a home for the aged and therefore may not be entirely representative of the cataract population. There is evidence, however, that many patients in the general cataract population have a high incidence of organic brain disease and a vulnerability to postoperative psychosis.[22] Moreover, patients with organic brain disease are known to react abnormally and unpredictably to sedatives. Studies have shown that the incidence of psychiatric reactions following cataract surgery are increased by general anesthesia, advancing age, and the degree of limited vision in the fellow eye.[21]

The cataract operation should be considered simply as one activity or event in an otherwise normal day. The surgery should not disrupt the normal routine much more than a shopping trip or an appointment with the dentist. On the day of surgery, the patient wakes in his or her own bed, takes his usual medications at the usual time (only anticoagulants and aspirin may be reduced), and has a breakfast of at least liquids. Diabetics take normal or slightly reduced medication, including insulin. At the hospital, the patient walks to the preparation room. In most instances, premedication is not required. After the drops are instilled, the patient receives a single injection of local anesthetic, and with the Super-Pinkie or other ocular decompressor in place, is free to sit up, walk around, and socialize with relatives or other patients. The patient can walk to the operating room. Following surgery he or she can walk back to the preparation room, get dressed, and almost immediately return to the normal environment and activities.

The hospitalized patient has spent the night in a strange bed in a strange room, separated from familiar sounds and people. The patient has probably required (or been given) a sleeping medication the night before and is probably kept quiet in bed in a dimly lit room until being transported to the surgical suite. The patient is aware of other patients, many of whom may actually be sick. There may be an incompatible roommate. This environment is clearly depressing for many and will undoubtedly heighten tension and anxiety for all, requiring substantial premedication that often produces unpredictable and undesirable effects. A similar level of tension and apprehension occurs on return to the hospital room from surgery. Hospitalized patients complain of more pain and require more pain medication than do ambulatory patients. They are more confined to bed; this inactivity with enforced bed rest tends to induce a variety of complications, such as phlebitis, pulmonary embolism, and acute urinary retention. There may be transient disorientation progressing to delerium. Side rails are sometimes required, frequently provoking a claustrophobic reaction. Many postoperative patients have tried, with some success, to climb over the side rails and have ended up on the floor.

Hospitalization has other dangers as well. A recent Centers for Disease Control (CDC) study reports that 5 percent of all patients admitted to hospitals acquire infections during their stay. Each year more than 2 million hospitalized patients in the United States acquire infections, and some 550 deaths result. In addition to the increasingly complex problems of nosocomial infections, there is a significant incidence of falls and other injuries occurring among hospitalized patients as well as possible medication errors, which can never be completely eliminated in a busy hospital. Clearly ambulatory cataract surgery affords patients physical and emotional benefits they would not attain on an inpatient basis.

PATIENT ACCEPTANCE OF AMBULATORY CATARACT SURGERY

Patients today are also health care consumers; they are, by and large, intelligent and selective in their choice of medical procedures. They insist on more information, more convenience, and more dignity and personal attention in their medical care. Hospitals are frequently perceived as alien and dehumanizing institutions. By contrast, a well-organized ambulatory surgery facility provides convenient access and parking, pleasant surroundings, and simplified preadmission procedures. Ideally, office personnel who are known to the patients are in attendance. All personnel are trained to allay anxiety and make the surgical experience as pleasant as possible for the patient. Patients are not repeatedly asked their names, medications, allergies, and which eye is to be operated on. The privacy of the patients is respected—only clothing tops are removed; dentures and hearing aids are not disturbed. Patients are not inappropriately called by their first names. Numerous surveys have shown that patients appreciate and search for such treatment. In one recent survey, 98 percent of respondents found outpatient cataract surgery to be a positive experience, 97 percent would prefer outpatient surgery for another operation, and 98 percent would recommend it to their families and friends.[23]

A new and more competitive medical care environment is emerging in which the successful ophthalmic surgeons will be those who are responsive to the preferences and choices of their patients. Surgeons performing ambulatory surgery in their own office operating facilities report significant and sustained increases in their surgical volume as word of mouth spreads from satisfied patients. It seems highly likely that for those ophthalmologists who do not perform ambulatory surgery in an appropriate facility, many of their patients will transfer to ophthalmologists who do.

BENEFITS OF AMBULATORY SURGERY FOR THE OPHTHALMOLOGIST

Ambulatory surgery is more efficient and convenient for the ophthalmologist. There are two basic models of ambulatory surgery, one hospital-controlled and one physician-controlled. Each model has its subvariations, and each has unique and distinct advantages and disadvantages.

The hospital-controlled ambulatory surgery subvariations are (1) a hospital-integrated facility (2) a hospital-adjacent facility, and (3) a hospital satellite facility. The hospital-integrated facility has the advantage of using existing facilities and personnel with relatively little additional investment or expense. The facility can be established quickly; it has great flexibility if the outpatient capability is not fully used. Transfer to more sophisticated surgical or recovery room facilities can be accomplished conveniently. But the disadvantages of this setting are considerable. The hospital is organized for inpatient care, and it is difficult to accomplish proper ambulatory care within the hospital bureaucracy. Ambulatory patients may be regarded as second-class citizens by hospital personnel, they may be bumped by emergency cases, and individual needs may be disregarded. The reception, preparation, and recovery rooms are often shared with inpatients, a situation not desirable for ambulatory surgery.

A hospital-adjacent facility eliminates many of the disadvantages of the hospital-integrated facility. An area specially designed for ambulatory surgery is provided. Personnel can be properly trained within the concept of ambulatory surgery. This area may be shared by a number of different specialties. Even with these advantages, however, the rigidity of hospital tradition and regulations remains difficult to overcome. Personnel inadequately trained in ophthalmologic techniques may be assigned. The hospital anesthesia department may not be knowledgeable of, or sympathetic to, ambulatory surgery.

The hospital-controlled satellite has essentially the same advantages and disadvantages as the hospital-adjacent facility. There are nevertheless, numerous advantages to hospital-controlled ambulatory surgery over inpatient surgery. Scheduling is convenient, there are no pre- and postoperative rounds, and record keeping is simplified. The first postoperative examination occurs in the office in which adequate and familiar equipment is available. The office counseling staff is available to explain and demonstrate postoperative procedures to patients and their families. Transfer to an inhospital status is easily accomplished, and all levels of medical backup are readily available. The hospital-controlled satellite has the advantages of no capital outlay, no increased expenses for supplies and personnel, and no increase in administrative responsibilities. In the final analysis, however, all three hospital models allow surgeons use of the hospital's facilities, but they are subject to the rules, regulations, inconveniences, and frustrations of dealing with a large institution.

The physician-controlled ambulatory surgery models offer the ultimate advantages to the ophthalmologist and the ultimate care for the patient. Subvarieties are (1) an office operating room, (2) an ambulatory ophthalmic surgical facility that may be individually or group sponsored, and (3) a free-standing Surgicenter. In the first two varieties, the ophthalmologist has control of the environment, of scheduling, of personnel, and of equipment. Approximately twice as many cases can be safely and conveniently done within the same time period in a private operating facility as in the usual hospital operating room.[24] The facility is designed for the comfort and convenience of both the patient and the ophthalmologist. Cases are scheduled at the convenience of the surgeon. No longer is there competition for hospital beds and operating room time. There are no last-minute cancellations or delays by preceding cases, emergencies, or a lunchtime shortage of operating room personnel. Surgeons have the loyalty and dedication of a skilled team that they have selected and trained themselves. The staff has incentive to be efficient. They know they will not be assigned to some other department or be given additional cases if they finish early. Surgeons select and get the equipment and supplies they want, when they want them. Requests for new equipment do not have to go on next year's capital equipment budget list to be considered many months hence. Conversely, there are serious disadvantages to the physician-controlled facility. A large initial capital investment must be made, followed by substantially increased operating costs for personnel, supplies, insurance, and so forth. Licensure and reimbursement may require a massive entanglement in federal, state, and local bureaucracy. Ophthalmologists must have a significant entrepreneurial spirit and a willingness to assume extensive administrative responsibilities, and they must have an exceptional surgical practice. The free-standing surgicenter is physician owned but usually not by the ophthalmologist and, being used by a variety of surgeons, has essentially the same advantages and disadvantages as the hospital-adjacent facility.

Ambulatory surgery, either in an established hospital setting or a free-standing general surgicenter, is within the reach of almost every ophthalmologist. Each must weigh the advantages and disadvantages of the various settings in light of his own personal needs and resources. Establishing an office operating facility or a free-standing ophthalmologic surgical facility is a major undertaking. Once the facility is completed, the ophthalmologist has a new business enterprise to manage and support. Only a small percentage of ophthalmologists are in a position to undertake such a risky and time-consuming project.

For those who are still uncertain about ambulatory cataract surgery, a certain basic fact needs to be recognized and appreciated. Outpatient ophthalmic surgery has ended the dependence of both the surgeon and the patient on the hospital. For the first time, patient and doctor are independent of hospitals and are therefore in a bargaining position because they have an alternative. Ophthalmologists must recognize that their patients will choose the medical facility they judge most appropriate for them; they must have a facility that is at least as desirable. To remain competitive in the rapidly evolving area of ophthalmic care delivery, a new partnership must be established between the ophthalmologist and the hospital. The goals and the problems of ophthalmologists and hospitals must be articulated and reconciled in a collaborative partnership that can benefit both. The hospitals are qualified by experience and law to provide and support medical facilities. They can easily offer proper facilities and equipment for ambulatory eye surgery; they do not want to lose the large segment of patients who can be managed on an ambulatory basis. Ophthalmologists, on the other hand, have the skill and knowledge to implement ambulatory surgery. They have the responsibility of attracting and satisfying their patients. To function effectively in a hospital setting, they must have control or an important voice in policies, procedures, personnel, and purchasing and the freedom to use their own personnel in the ambulatory center when desirable. If the hospital administrators and governing boards cannot be convinced of the necessity and advantages of this new relationship, the only reasonable alternative is for ophthalmologists or groups of ophthalmologists to consider their own free-standing operating facilities.

AMBULATORY CATARACT SURGERY AND MEDICAL COSTS

The medical profession generally does not like to consider cost as the primary reason for undertaking any particular medical practices or procedures. It is fortunate that ambulatory surgery, which has so many advantages to recommend it, produces substantial financial savings as well. As might be expected, third-party payers and government agencies have been slow to recognize and encourage ambulatory surgery and, often at the instigation of hospitals, have actively opposed it. Many insurance policies have required hospital admission to qualify for any reimbursement. The reasons for this opposition are not entirely clear. For those hospitals that are not fully occupied, ambulatory surgery would not generate any new dollars but would represent only a reallocation of existing revenues. For hospitals utilized to full capacity, cataract patients have probably been used to subsidize the costs of those with more complex and expensive illnesses. Third-party providers in locations with high hospital bed utilization consider ambulatory surgery an additional expense rather than a significant saving because the hospital beds not used by cataract patients are filled immediately with other sicker and more costly patients. From a community's point of view, there is also the possibility of duplicating resources when new ambulatory surgical facilities are built.

Nevertheless, many health care economists believe that ambulatory surgery offers the best opportunity for significant health dollar savings in the next decade. The OOSS has estimated that if all ophthalmic surgery that could be done on an ambulatory basis were done so, the annual savings would approach $1 billion—not an inconsiderable sum even in today's inflated economy. The insurance industry and the federal government have recognized these potential savings, and it seems likely that in the future ambulatory surgery will be compulsory for many procedures. The attitude of the government is evident from the fact that in 1980 Congress authorized 100 percent reimbursement of the usual and customary fee for Medicare procedures performed on an ambulatory basis to surgeons who accept assignment, rather than the 80 percent reimbursement rate allowed for inpatient surgery.

A brief 1984 survey of some 30 facilities demonstrates a wide range of charges for cataract and intraocular implant surgery depending on the type of facility (Table 8-4).

Some physicians who operate their own unlicensed private operating facility make no facility charge; others add $200 or $300 to the surgical fee, and some bill a modest fee of $125 to $250. Essentially, much of the cost of this type of facility is borne by the ophthalmologist as a tradeoff for increased efficiency, patient volume, control, and convenience. There is some possibility that reimbursement will be authorized for these facilities in the future. The licensed and certified ophthalmic surgical facilities receive Medicare reimbursements of $500 to $600 that must be accepted as full payment. Payments may vary slightly for other insurance plans. Ambulatory surgery charges by a general hospital are about one half that of inpatient

Table 8-4. Surgical Facility Charges—Cataract and Intraocular Implant Surgery

	Range ($)
Physician office operating suite not licensed	0–250
Ophthalmic surgical facility licensed, Medicare certified	500–600
Hospital outpatient	790–2,201
Hospital inpatient	1,325–2,878

charges and about twice those of free-standing facilities. Analysis of these charges — which include operating room, recovery room, equipment, supplies, medications, basic laboratory tests, and nursing services — indicate essentially identical charges for both inpatients and outpatients, with the major difference being the inpatient hospital room charge. There is a definite pattern of using less medication, fewer supplies, and less extensive preadmission testing by those ophthalmologists who are personally responsible or whose patients are personally responsible for payment of those items. Ophthalmologists who control the facility may be tempted to cut costs, to the detriment of the patient, whereas hospitals need to review periodically their procedures and regulations to be certain they are truly necessary and justified.

REIMBURSEMENT, FACILITY CONSTRUCTION, AND LICENSURE

The transition to ambulatory surgery from inpatient surgery is most easily made in the familiar hospital environment. Ideally, forward-thinking hospital administrators will grasp the underlying philosophy of ambulatory surgery, appreciate its benefits, and cooperate with the ophthalmologist in developing suitable procedures and facilities. If such cooperation is not forthcoming, the physician must consider the enormous task of developing a free-standing facility. The ophthalmologist who responds to this challenge must have a good deal of cash or credit, perseverance, resilience, and managerial ability.

Reimbursement of private operating facility expenses has been difficult to achieve. Although some private insurance carriers recognized the advantages of ambulatory cataract surgery early on, the major third-party payers were slow to support this concept, probably because of opposition by hospitals that feared loss of revenue. The major breakthrough in the recognition and reimbursement of ambulatory surgery in free-standing units was the passage by Congress of the Omnibus Reconciliation Act (P.L. 96-499, Section 34) on December 5, 1980. This act authorized payment of facility fees under Part B of Medicare (P.L. 89-97, Section 100, 111, 1965) in ambulatory surgical centers and in physicians' offices. The surgeon, assistant surgeon, and anesthesiologist are reimbursed in the usual fashion, since surgical fees are reimbursable regardless of where the surgery is performed. The passage of this act provided the stimulus for other providers such as Blue Cross and Medicaid to negotiate outpatient facility rates. After passage, the law came under the jurisdiction of the Health Care Financing Agency (HCFA) of the Department of Health and Human Services (DHHS) for establishment of regulations and implementation. It was not until August 1982 that these regulations were published. They provide for facility reimbursement for 12 specific procedures performed in ambulatory surgical centers. These regulations provide for a fixed facility fee to be accepted in full payment for use of the operating and recovery rooms, anesthetic supplies, nursing services, medication, and any laboratory tests done at the facility on the day of surgery. No mention or provision was made for the part of the act authorizing payment for procedures performed in physicians' offices. The procedures and payments currently authorized are listed in Table 8-5.

Comparable surgical procedures such as trabeculectomies and corneal transplants are not listed and are therefore not currently reimbursable. Both

Table 8-5. Authorized Procedures for Medicare Facility Reimbursements and Reimbursement Amount[a]

Group I: $231.00
Chalazion
Discission, lens
Foreign-body removal
Lacrimal duct probe/reconstruction
Group II: $275.00
Canthoplasty
Tarsorrhaphy
Group III: $296.00
Ectropion
Entropion
Group IV: $336.00
Cataract extraction
Enucleation
Iridectomy
Eye muscle surgery
Group V: $504.00
Cataract with IOL (multiple procedure)

[a] Will vary slightly according to geographic reimbursement factor.

the AAO and OOSS have submitted greatly expanded lists of ambulatory surgical procedures to HCFA. On April 6, 1984 HCFA published a tentative list of additional procedures for public comment but as of early 1987 no change in the original list or reimbursement schedule had been approved, nor had there been any update of the facility fees established in 1982, and based on 1979 and 1980 data. The "Omnibus Budget Reconciliation Act of 1986" (OBRA) mandates change in ASC reimbursement procedures. This legislation requires HCFA to review and update ASC facility rates yearly, with the first update no later than July 1, 1987, and to review and update the list of covered ASC procedures, with the first update no later than April 21, 1987, with subsequent updates required at least every 2 years. A further objective of this legislation is to equalize payments between ASCs and hospital outpatient departments (OPDs). OPDs have previously been reimbursed on the basis of reasonable cost, but for 2 years there will be a blend of hospital cost and ASC rate. Beginning on or before October 1, 1987, payments to OPDs will be 75 percent hospital cost and 25 percent ASC rate and during the second and subsequent years, the blend will be 50 percent hospital cost and 50 percent ASC rate. In the interim, the Secretary of Health and Human Services is to develop a prospective payment system for hospital outpatient ambulatory surgery that is to include facility, medical, and all other health costs except for physician services. The Secretary must submit a final report on this system to Congress by April 1, 1989. Other provisions of OBRA relating to ambulatory surgery change the facility reimbursement from 100 percent to 80 percent with the patient or supplemental insurance responsible for the other 20 percent and require Peer Review Organization (PROs) to conduct 100 percent preoperative review of certain ambulatory surgical procedures, of which cataract surgery is expected to be one. The details of how this review will be implemented have not been determed as of early 1987. OBRA does not change the ophthalmologist's surgical fee of 100 percent reimbursement for procedures performed in an approved ASC.

Two options are available for the ophthalmologist who contemplates developing a private surgical facility. The first is an unlicensed office operating room, and the other is a fully licensed ambulatory surgical center.

The physician's office operating suite is substantially less expensive and easier to develop than a fully licensed facility. The major drawback is that operating and capitalization costs are not reimbursed by most third-party payers. The first office operating rooms were built for the convenience of the surgeon with little concern for facility reimbursement. They were basically an extension of the minor surgical capability available in many ophthalmologists' offices. The additional costs were borne by the surgeon from revenues generated by increased efficiency, increased surgical volume, and perhaps a modest increase in the surgical fee. Salaries of operating room personnel, surgical supplies, and new equipment have increased tremendously in recent years, making the costs incurred by a nonreimbursed facility increasingly difficult to absorb. The Omnibus Reconciliation Act did authorize reimbursement for private office facilities, but HCFA has not and probably will not establish the enabling regulations in the foreseeable future.

The OOSS is attempting to develop a deemed in compliance status for office facilities when accredited by a national accrediting body without requiring full state licensure. It is not clear how these facilities presently or in the future will relate to federal, state, or local regulations. Typical state laws requiring licensure of free-standing ambulatory surgical centers define such facilities as establishments exclusively for ambulatory patients for the purpose of performing surgical procedures. Obviously, this definition could easily be construed to cover any office performing any surgery, even a chalazion excision. State health department officials frankly admit that they do not know where to draw the line in regard to private offices. If office facility reimbursement is finally authorized, it is likely that increased regulation will also be forthcoming. Space requirements for a one operating room private office suite vary from as few as 800 to as much as 1,500 sq ft. Construction costs utilizing existing space currently average about $60 per square foot, whereas new construction costs approximately $100 per square foot. Surgical equipment for a surgical suite with one operating room costs an additional $150,000, bringing the total investment for this type of facility into the $250,000 range.

The first question the ophthalmologist must consider is whether the undertaking is affordable. The financial feasibility of a private operating facility can be calculated from the following formula:

$$\frac{C + D + E + F}{A} + B = \text{cost per case},$$

where A is the number of cases per year, B is supply cost per case, C is staff cost, D is equipment cost, E is building cost, and F represents operating expenses. Since Medicare facility reimbursement is a fixed amount that is not likely to rise commensurate with future cost increases, and commercial carriers generally allow only 5 percent profit after taxes, a private surgical facility itself is not and will not be a money-making business. This formula, however, does not consider marketing implications and the considerable promotional leverage that can significantly increase market share. It is estimated that an office operating facility can be justified with as few as four to five surgical cases per week. The decision to proceed should be made in consultation with architects, lawyers, accountants, medical management consultants, and other advisors.

The alternative approach is a fully licensed, Medicare-approved ambulatory surgical center conforming to federal regulations. This approach involves considerably more red tape, expense, and uncertainty. Procedures vary widely in different states. Twenty-two states have laws pertaining to ambulatory surgical facilities that require them to be licensed. The first requirement is usually a certificate of need (or a declaratory ruling that one is not needed) which must be obtained from the local Health Services Administration or Health Planning Council and then from the State Health Facilities Commission.

The certificate of need is granted upon the recommendation of these advisory committees, which presumably represent the best interests of the community and the consumer in objectively determining the need for additional health facilities. In actuality, they are often dominated by hospital officials, executives of health insurance organizations, and others with a personal stake in the medical care delivery and facilities of their state. It is quite possible that, after expenditure of a great deal of time, effort, and money, the certificate of need will be denied and the project terminated. If a certificate of need is obtained, the next step is state licensure, which is granted by the State Department of Health after all provisions of state law and regulation are met and the facility has been inspected. Before construction, the local zoning and parking regulations should be investigated. The building plans must carefully observe the various federal, state, and local fire and building codes and the American national standard specifications for the physically handicapped. If a new ambulatory surgical facility has 6-foot-wide corridors, for example, it would be most unfortunate and expensive to discover at the time of state inspection that an 8-foot-wide emergency corridor was required through the length of the building. State licensure essentially requires construction, organization, and facilities identical to the requirements of hospitals.

A facility must have a legally constituted governing body, a written transfer agreement with a local hospital, written standards of administration, quality assurance, records that must be similar in content and form to hospital records, provision for drugs and radiographs, provision for periodic review of emergency training for personnel, and a detailed operating room manual. The OOSS has a prototype operating room manual available to its members. After a certificate of need and state licensure are obtained, an application must be made to Medicare. The cost of a certified ophthalmic surgery center with two operating rooms is about $1 million. Therefore, the surgical volume required to justify this type of facility is considerably greater than that for an office operating suite.

State licensed ambulatory surgical facilities must meet rigid and specific requirements and undergo periodic inspection for licensure. Office-based surgical facilities and ambulatory surgical facilities in states not requiring licensure are in need of an accreditation procedure to ensure the attainment and performance of the highest standards and to demonstrate the achievement of these standards to the public. The important development of ambulatory surgery could be seriously impaired if less than optimum surgical standards were maintained, if unnecessary and excessive surgery were done, or if increased malpractice suits resulted. Accreditation may be voluntarily sought from the Accreditation Association for Ambulatory Health Care (AAAHC), which is directed by representatives from a number of ambulatory health care organizations including OOSS, or the Accreditation Program for Ambulatory Health Care, a subunit of the Joint Commission on Accreditation of Hospitals (JCAH). The AAAHC views its role as that of consultant rather than inspector. The process involves peer review by trained surveyers who are practicing physicians and administrators. The team includes at least one ophthalmologist who is personally experienced in office-based surgery when an ophthalmology facility is being inspected. The Accreditation Handbook for Ambulatory Health Care describes the 15 survey standards and the survey process in detail. The accreditation process is designed to be ongoing, with continued improvement in the quality of the facility. The AAAHC is a nonprofit corporation, and fees are based on projected operating costs but nevertheless range between $1,000 amd $5,000 per survey. AAAHC accreditation has been recognized and accepted by various third-party payers and has helped reduce malpractice risks and the cost of liability insurance and has improved public image. For state-licensed ambulatory surgical facilities that undergo state inspection annually, this voluntary accreditation, although desirable, may represent an additional expenditure of time and money that may not be necessary.

THE AMBULATORY CATARACT SURGERY PROCEDURE

Ambulatory cataract surgery is not inpatient surgery that simply discharges the patient soon after the surgery. Whereas inpatient surgery is based on the science of medicine, outpatient surgery combines the science of medicine with the art of medicine.

Because of the lack of understanding and resistance to the principle of ambulatory surgery by hospital personnel, particularly nurse administrators and anesthesiologists, the caliber of outpatient surgery in a hospital setting is rarely equal to that achieved in free-standing operating facilities. A combination of training, teaching, and communication as well as administrative reorganization for ophthalmic facilities is absolutely necessary to overcome the standard hospital resistance to change. The important principles of ambulatory surgery are pre-operative counseling, implementation of the team concept, minimal interference with usual routine, and prompt return to normal environment and activities.

This section describes details of ambulatory surgery as carried out in my personal practice. The first step in the transition to ambulatory surgery is the opportunity and necessity to rethink and reevaluate all aspects of the cataract procedure. Different surgeons will prefer different but equally effective methods. All procedures must constantly undergo evaluation and change.

Presurgical Management

The key to successful ambulatory surgery is preoperative counseling, which minimizes or eliminates patient anxiety. The relaxed patient does not require sedatives, tranquilizers, and pain medications, all of which have undesirable systemic side effects and interfere with the patient's normal routine.

Preoperative counseling begins when the decision to schedule surgery is made. The counselor describes the entire procedure in detail, emphasizing the fact that this is major surgery for the eye, requiring advanced technology and considerable surgical skill, but minor surgery for the patient as a whole. Patients are encouraged to view video tapes describing cataracts, cataract surgery, and intraocular implants. The patient is provided with as much information as desired but not more. Some patients are interested in the fine details of the surgical procedure, whereas others have little interest in technicalities but are concerned primarily with what they will feel and experience. The purpose and necessity of informed consent is described and the patient is given a large-print copy of the informed consent form to review at home. The financial arrangements are reviewed in detail. A support network of patients who have undergone the procedure is available to talk to new patients. Postoperative patients who happen to be in the office at the same time can be particularly effective in counseling and in relieving anxiety.

Evaluation of the patient's general medical status is an important aspect of presurgical management. A general physical examination is strongly recommended at the time of counselling and reconfirmed in writing. The patient's primary care physician is given a form detailing the proposed procedure, the date, the type of anesthesia, and the location of the surgery. The physician is asked to evaluate the patient thoroughly and to record principle findings and suggestions or recommendations, including any preadmission tests to be obtained within the week before surgery. If the patient does not wish to have a general medical evaluation—and patients do have that right—that fact is recorded in the medical record, and a brief history and physical examination is performed by the ophthalmologist at the time of the preoperative visit and appropriate laboratory tests are obtained at that time.

Preadmission or admission laboratory tests and procedures are a standard hospital routine. Most textbooks of general surgery and ophthalmology recommend, and most hospital policies require, certain standard tests, which usually include a hemogram, urinalysis, chest radiography, ECG, and blood chemistries (serum electrolytes, blood glucose, and blood urea nitrogen). Despite the frequent repetition of these recommendations and requirements, no factual data are cited to justify or substantiate them. Since these tests can be expensive and unpleasant for patients, the tests used in free-standing facilities should be carefully chosen; unjustified, merely routine hospital tests should be eliminated. Robbins and Mushlin[25] have designed a set of criteria to be applied in recommending or requiring a particular test:

1. The condition tested for must be asymptomatic and not obvious on routine history and physical examination.
2. The condition must significantly affect the morbidity or mortality of surgery, or must represent significant risk to those associated with the patient's care.
3. Preoperative diagnosis must be more beneficial to management than a diagnosis established during the perioperative or postoperative period.
4. Tests must be of sufficient specificity and sensitivity to allow for detection of the condition.
5. Prevalence of the condition must be high enough so that efficient detection of an asymptomatic patient with the condition is possible.

The first three criteria require that recognition of the conditions being sought would affect the morbidity or mortality of the procedure. Sensitivity and specificity require that the test identify a high percentage of patients who have the disease without too high a percentage of false-positive results. The final requirement is that the test produce enough positive results to justify patient inconvenience and cost. The purpose of preadmission testing is to detect any disease that, left undetected, might affect the outcome of the surgical procedure and not to serve as a routine screening test. The most important preoperative medical evaluation is a thorough history and physical examination with appropriate laboratory data required only as indicated by that examination.

Using the Robbins–Mushlin criteria and applying known scientific data, the only reasonable routine preadmission test indicated for otherwise asymptomatic patients is the hematocrit. Anemia may be a contraindication to surgery, the patient is asymptomatic, the test is inexpensive, and the predictive value of the test is 100 percent.

Routine chest radiographs are usually included in the preoperative evaluation of cataract patients. But chest radiographs should be obtained on patients only when indicated from the history and physical findings. Various surveys and studies have demonstrated that routine chest radiographs in a healthy population are essentially useless and have an extremely high cost/benefit ratio. The cost of finding one asymptomatic patient with unsuspected interstitial lung disease by routine chest radiography is $500,000 per patient.[26] The Royal College of Radiologists, in a study of more than 10,000 patients undergoing nonacute elective surgery, found that preoperative radiographs ordered for no apparent indication did not alter the choice of anesthesia or the decision to operate and were of little value as a baseline study.[27]

An ECG is frequently ordered as a routine preoperative procedure. Electrocardiograms also should be performed only when indicated by the history and physical examination. When no particular indication is present, the information to be obtained from a routine ECG should be questioned. The data usually sought are the recognition of ischemic heart disease, the detection of conduction defects, and the existence of a silent myocardial infarction; they are intended to serve as a baseline study if any cardiac problem develops during the postoperative period. In fact, ECGs are poor indicators of ischemic heart disease, conduction defects do not carry an increased risk for surgery, and physical examination will reveal significant cardiac arrhythmias. There is no evidence to support the contention that baseline ECG studies are of any value, and studies have shown such a baseline test to be of little value.[28,29]

A nonfasting blood glucose determination, preferably 2 hours postprandial, is desirable in those patients in whom a serum glucose has not been performed within 6 months of surgery, as cataracts are particularly prevalent in patients with diabetes mellitus. Detection of a mild blood glucose elevation, however, would not be reason enough to cancel cataract surgery. The principal information obtained from routine urinalysis and BUN and creatinine determinations is the capacity to detect impaired ability of the kidneys to excrete systemic medications. Since systemic medications are not generally required in ambulatory surgery, these tests are not indicated in otherwise asymptomatic patients. A study of two groups of patients, one undergoing routine biochemical profile screening and another not screened, found no difference in either quality of care or length of hospital stay.[30] The total cost of hospital care in the screened group was 5 percent higher because of follow-up tests and consultations.

Counseling is done by trained office personnel who establish an ongoing relationship with the patient. The counselor usually calls the patient a week or so before surgery to determine whether there are questions or concerns. All systemic medications are continued without interruption except for aspirin and anticoagulants, which may be reduced in dosage or eliminated for a period before surgery.

Preoperative counselling is reinforced by the ophthalmologist at the preoperative visit a few days before the scheduled surgery. There are four components to this visit:

1. The eye is reexamined with careful attention to vision, pinhole correction, facial and particularly brow configuration, slit-lamp examination of the cornea, depth of the anterior chamber, iris color, the reactivity of the pupil, and intraocular pressure. The pupil is not dilated at this time in order to ensure full dilation at the time of surgery. Once dilated, a pupil may not regain its full capacity to dilate again for as long as a week. A dilated examination with description of the cataract type and fundus examination was recorded at the time the surgery was scheduled. Occasionally the preoperative examination will uncover conjunctivitis, a hordeolum, or other cause for cancellation of surgery, and the operating time can be filled by scheduling another patient. This examination imprints the characteristics of this particular eye in the surgeon's mind and permits planning for such problems as an overriding brow, a prominent eye, a shallow anterior chamber, or borderline elevation of the intraocular pressure. These findings are noted as the examination proceeds, and they are incorporated in both the office and hospital records. If there are any factors that jeopardize a normal visual result, such as a mild endothelial dystrophy or questionable macula, this should be brought to the attention of the patient and relatives at this point. A poor visual result on the basis of corneal decompensation, macular degeneration, or other pathology will always be ascribed to the surgery unless the possibility was clearly described preoperatively. The previous operative reports of those patients undergoing second eye surgery are reviewed. Any difficulties encountered at the first operation, such as backache, posterior capsular plaques, or scleral collapse, will likely occur with the second procedure and may be prevented or more easily managed when anticipated.
2. The informed consent form is witnessed and signed. The orders written and the time of arrival at the hospital reconfirmed. No premedication is usually ordered, except for extremely

anxious patients. The health questionnaire is reviewed and the patient reassured that any drug allergy, idiosyncracy, or other health problem is known to the surgeon.

3. The details of each step from the time the patient arrives at the hospital until he or she is ready to leave are described and the approximate time in the hospital and the operating room estimated. The single local anesthetic injection is described, patients assured that they will feel nothing during the operation, and reminded that they will be unable to move the eye. They are assured that an anesthesiologist will be present to monitor them and that if they must cough or sneeze, no harm will occur. Immediate pre- and postoperative instructions are reviewed and a printed instruction sheet given to the patient (Fig. 8-1). The telephone availability of the surgeon is emphasized and the patient is encouraged to call at any time, particularly if eye discomfort develops.
4. Finally, the patient is encouraged to ask any questions and to express any residual anxieties.

INSTRUCTIONS FOR OUT-PATIENT CATARACT SURGERY

1. On the morning of surgery, you may drink clear liquids, including tea or caffeine-free coffee, before going to the hospital. If your operation is scheduled after 11:00 AM, you may also have a piece of toast or a roll.
2. Unless instructed otherwise, take all your regular medications as you normally do, both in the morning of surgery, and after you get home.
3. When you return from the hospital, you may wish to rest, but feel free to walk around, read, watch television and eat. You may find a glass of wine or a cocktail relaxing.
4. You may feel some mild discomfort in your operated eye. This should be easily controlled by 1-2 Tylenol tablets which may be taken as necessary every 3-4 hours. If you have any moderate-to-severe pain, please call the office immediately (421-2277).
5. On the morning after surgery, you may remove your eye shield and patch and wear your glasses or you may wait to have the shield and patch removed at the time of your office visit.
6. Please bring your eye kit with you for your office appointment. it will also be helpful if the person who is to instill your eye drops can be with you at the first postoperative visit.
7. The doctors are available to talk to you at any time. Just call the office number (421-2277) which is answered 24 hours a day. Do not hesitate to call if you have any questions or concerns.

Fig. 8-1. A preoperative instruction sheet is given to the patient as part of preoperative counseling a few days before surgery.

Implementation of the team concept requires an organized and continuous program, which is more easily planned and carried out in a private facility. The effort is of even greater importance when ambulatory surgery is performed in a hospital environment and should include admission clerks, receptionists, nurses, surgical technicians, anesthetists, and particularly administrators and anesthesiologists. Unless the personnel involved with ambulatory surgery are separate and distinct from those involved with inpatient surgery, the standard hospital biases will prevail and patients will not get the full benefit of ambulatory surgery. Frequent communication among all people involved is a basic component of ambulatory surgery.

Surgical Management

On the day of surgery, an attempt is made to disrupt the patient's normal routine as little as possible. There are no restrictions on fluids orally. The patients are encouraged to have juice and tea or decaffeinated coffee in the morning and, if their surgery is scheduled for late morning or afternoon, breakfast is permitted. Diabetic patients are usually scheduled late in the morning so they can have their regular insulin, their usual breakfast, and lunch as soon as the surgery is completed. Policies regarding oral intake before surgery vary widely. The second edition of the OOSS facilities booklet includes the oral intake policies of 28 facilities for morning surgery under local anesthesia (Table 8-6). Fewer than one half the surgeons follow the tradition of NPO from the previous midnight. A recent study compared gastric volumes of two groups of surgical patients.[31] One group had NPO overnight, and the other group had tea or coffee and toast for breakfast. During surgery under general anesthesia, their gastric volumes were aspirated, and no significant difference was found in the gastric fluid volumes of the two groups. Their conclusion was that a light breakfast probably decreases gastric acidity without increasing volume.

Table 8-6. Oral Intake Policies—Local Anesthesia, Morning Surgery—of 28 Free-Standing Facilities

Policy	*N*
Nothing by mouth	12
Light breakfast	8
Liquids only	4
No restrictions	4

Surgery is performed under local anesthesia almost without exception because it is well tolerated by cataract patients and is conducive to rapid ambulation; there is also evidence that local anesthesia is safer than general anesthesia. Gills[32] reported five deaths in 20,000 cataract operations performed under general anesthesia and none in 20,000 cataract operations performed under local anesthesia.

Standby anesthesia is usually employed. Most ophthalmologists are not comfortable managing the occasional cardiac, pulmonary, or neurologic emergency while performing surgery. Anesthesiologists check patients medically and monitor them at the time of the retrobulbar block and during the surgical procedure. The anesthesiologist or anesthetist maintains hand contact with the patient throughout most of the procedure.

The monitoring process for eye surgery under local anesthesia differs significantly from the monitoring process for general anesthesia. There are four elements to be monitored in eye surgery: the retrobulbar block, oculocardiac reflex, pulse and blood pressure, and respiration. The time of greatest vulnerability for the cataract patient is when the retrobulbar block is given. Possible complications are retrobulbar hemorrhage, perforation of the globe, oculocardiac reflex, intravascular injection with side effects from epinephrine (Adrenaline), toxic reaction resulting in grand mal seizure, and respiratory arrest from bupivicaine (Marcaine) probably due to optic sheath puncture. The patient should be closely monitored by the anesthesiologist and the ophthalmologist both during and immediately after the retrobulbar block. The length of the danger period following injection of the local anesthesia is not clear but should not exceed 15 to 30 minutes. When the block has taken effect, the danger of an oculocardiac reflex is eliminated.

Pulse, blood pressure, and respiration are the other three parameters monitored during surgery. Pulse and blood pressure usually remain steady and constant during ambulatory cataract surgery because the patients have little anxiety and have taken their usual cardiac and antihypertension medications according to their normal schedule. A major indication for monitoring patients during surgery has been inadequate breathing under the drapes caused by the depressant effect inherent in all preoperative sedatives. This hypoventilation frequently did not occur until the patient relaxed and drifted into sleep. Since no preoperative sedation is necessary with well-prepared ambulatory patients, and if care is taken to make certain there is no impediment to airflow under the surgical drapes, this hypoventilation does not occur. It is therefore usually safe and proper for the anesthesiologist to leave as the case is finishing to monitor the next patient while the patient is receiving a retrobulbar injection. There is ordinarily no reason to monitor the patients after surgery. In a hospital setting, anesthesiologists and recovery room personnel frequently do not understand that eye local patients need to be monitored before surgery and not after.

The dilating drops for extracapsular procedures, usually cyclopentolate 1 percent and phenylephrine (Neo-Synephrine) 2.5 percent, are started on arrival. An intravenous access is inserted, preferably using a heparin lock. The heparin lock affords rapid access to a vein and is less expensive and less cumbersome than the usual intravenous apparatus; it also gives the patient greater mobility during the preoperative waiting period. Fluid intake is more controlled, so the patient has less chance of needing to void during the operation or developing pulmonary edema. The assistant surgeon drops out of surgery when the implant is in position to give the local anesthesia for the next patient. This consists of a single injection of 5 ml of a combination of 2% lidocaine (Xylocaine) and 0.75 percent bupivicaine (Marcaine) with 1/200,000 of epinephrine and an ampule of alidase given outside the muscle cone. No additional seventh nerve, skin, or muscle injection is usually necessary.

The discomfort of the retrobulbar injection is generally mild and well tolerated. Some ophthalmologists choose to eliminate all discomfort and produce amnesia for the injections by the use of nitrous oxide[33] anesthesia, methohexital (Brevital), or a fentanyl-diazapem (Valium) combination. The Super Pinkie or other orbital and ocular decompressor is applied for a minimum of 30 minutes. During this time, the patient is free to sit up and walk around, is encouraged to visit the bathroom, and, if facilities permit, to socialize with other patients and relatives. The patient can walk to the operating room. Activity and ambulation are encouraged during this waiting period before surgery to minimize the time during which patients must lie quietly on their back. Prolonged periods of immobility in elderly patients cause restlessness, backache, muscle cramps, and other symptoms undesirable during the course of a cataract operation. During surgery, music provided through earphones is pleasant for the patient and muffles operating room sounds and talk. At the end of the procedure, a patch and shield are applied, patients return to the preparation room where they have a snack, redress, and are promptly discharged in the company of relatives to return home with essentially no limitation of activities. If glasses are required for the other eye, they may be worn instead of the shield. No pain medication stronger than acetaminophen (Tylenol) should be necessary for postoperative discomfort. The need for stronger medication is a warning sign indicating a call to the ophthalmologist. During 10 years of ambulatory cataract surgery, not even one call has been received for stronger pain medication. The ophthalmologist or counselor telephones the patient at the end of the day to inquire as to well-being. This call is very reassuring and is very much appreciated by both patient and family.

Postoperative Management

A postoperative visit is routine on the day following surgery. A brief overnight history is recorded. The vision is checked without correction and with pinhole. The vision should be at least 20/70 and, if not, the reason should be determined. The cornea and anterior chamber reaction are evaluated by slit-lamp examination and the appearance of the pupil and implant observed. The intraocular pressure is measured. The patient's counselor then goes over the postoperative instructions with the patient and relatives and provides a written instruction sheet. Older patients have no restrictions of their normal activities. Younger patients are given modest limitations on physical activity, particularly in regard to lifting and vigorous activity for a period of 2 to 3 weeks. No patch is worn, but glasses are recommended for 2 weeks to protect the eye from trauma. A plastic shield without a patch is recommended for protection while sleeping during this period. The patient is allowed to drive as soon as he feels confident, provided the other eye has good vision. The patient is examined again in 3 to 5 days and usually 3 weeks later. A new lens prescription is ordered at 8 weeks.

SUMMARY

Ambulatory surgery is an emerging trend in ophthalmology. The surgical results are at least equal to those resulting from inpatient cataract surgery, but the adverse systemic and psychological effects of hospitalization are eliminated. Patient preference and well-being, together with significantly lower cost, make the consideration of ambulatory cataract surgery imperative in this increasingly competitive surgical environment.

Free-standing, physician-controlled ambulatory facilities have many advantages, but the development of an ambulatory surgical facility is an enormous undertaking for most ophthalmologists. It is hoped that the emergence of ambulatory surgery will forge a new partnership between ophthalmologists and hospitals that will develop hospital-based ambulatory surgical facilities combining the advantages of free-standing and hospital-based facilities.

Ophthalmic surgery is undergoing profound change. Until recently, technologic developments and elimination of complications were of primary concern. Today there is growing emphasis on developing a surgical experience for the patient that is as pleasant and free of anxiety as possible.

REFERENCES

1. Moxley JH, Roeder PC: New opportunities for out-of-hospital health services. N Engl J Med 310:193, 1984
2. Wong HC: General anesthesia for ambulatory surgery. Int Anesthesiol Clin 20:37, 1982
3. Bruns K: A statistical analysis of free standing outpatient surgical care facilities for the year 1979. Soc Adv Freestanding Surg Care Rep 4:5, 1980
4. Bruns K: Postoperative care and review of complications. Int Anesthesiol Clin 20(1):3, 1982
5. Olson LL: Establishing Free Standing Ambulatory Surgery Centers. American Medical Association, Chicago, 1982
6. Reed WA: Freestanding surgical care facilities. Int Anesthesiol Clin 20:109, 1982
7. Spaeth EB: The Principles and Practice of Ophthalmic Surgery. 4th Ed. Lea & Febiger, Philadelphia, 1948
8. Collected Letters of the International Correspondence Society of Ophthalmologists 6:66, 1961
9. Kelman CD: Phaco-emulsification and aspiration. A new technique of cataract removal. A preliminary report. Am J Ophthalmol 64:23, 1967
10. Consultation section: Am Intraocular Implant Soc J 9:344, 1983
11. Shelton PA: Outpatient cataract surgery and the evolving standard of care. Cataract 1:13, 1984
12. Chisolm JJ: The rational method of treating cataract patients to the exclusion of compresses, bandages, and dark rooms. Am J Ophthalmol 3:135, 1886
13. Galin MA et al: Immediate ambulation and discharge after cataract extraction. Trans Am Acad Ophthalmol 78:43, 1974
14. Williamson DE: One thousand consecutive outpatient cataract extractions. Ear Nose Throat J 54:52, 1975
15. Christy NE: Effect of early ambulation. On the incidence of postoperative complications of cataract surgery. Am J Ophthalmol 49:293, 1960
16. Galin MA, et al: Out-patient cataract surgery. Trans Ophthalmol Soc UK 95:42, 1975
17. Williamson DE: Outpatient ophthalmic surgery. Course notes. American Academy of Ophthalmology, San Francisco, 1983
18. Pierce JC, Sinskey RM: Office implant surgery. Cataract 1:14, 1984
19. Simmons RJ, Chandler PA: Early discharge after cataract surgery. p. 118. In Brockhurst RJ et al (eds): Controversy in Ophthalmology. WB Saunders, Philadelphia, 1977
20. Linn L: Psychiatric reactions complicating cataract surgery. Int Ophthalmol Clin 5:143, 1965
21. Karhunen U, Orko R: Psychiatric reactions complicating cataract surgery: A prospective study. Ophthalmic Surg 13:1008, 1982
22. Linn L, et al: Patterns of behavior disturbance

following cataract extraction. Am J Psychiatry 110:281, 1953
23. McMahan LB: Ambulatory surgery survey: More acceptance, quicker recovery. IOL Ocul Surg News 2:22, 1984
24. Tennant JL: Outpatient cataract surgery. Audio-Dig Ophthalmol 21:14, 1983
25. Robbins JA, Mushlin AI: Preoperative evaluation of the healthy patient. Med Clin North Am 63:1145, 1979
26. Rucker L, et al: Usefulness of screening chest roentgenograms in preoperative patients. JAMA 250: 3209, 1983
27. Royal College of Radiologists: Preoperative chest radiology. Lancet 2:83, 1979
28. Carson JL, Eisenberg JM: The preoperative screening examination. p. 16. In Goldmann DR et al (eds): Medical Care of the Surgical Patient: A Problem-Oriented Approach to Management. JB Lippincott, Philadelphia, 1982
29. Rubenstein LZ, Greenfield S: The baseline ECG in the evaluation of acute cardiac complaints. JAMA 244:2536, 1980
30. Durbridge TC, Edwards F, Edwards RG, et al: An evaluation of multiphasic screening on admission to hospital. Precis of a report to the National Health and Medical Research Council. Med J Aust 1:703, 1976
31. Miller M, et al: Gastric contents at induction of anesthesia. Br J Anaesth 55:12, 1983
32. Gills J: Anesthesia in outpatient cataract surgery. IOL Ocul Surg News 2:6, 1984
33. McMahan LB: Nitrous oxide analgesia for cataract surgery. Ophthalm Surg 13:307, 1982

Manual Extracapsular Cataract Extraction

9

David J. McIntyre

The popularity of the extracapsular cataract procedure in the United States has been growing at an astonishing rate over the past several years. The pendulum is swinging from intracapsular to extra capsular, and there is a rapidly growing body of statistics showing decreased rates of cystoid macular edema and retinal detachment along with apparent superiority of the postpupillary styles of intraocular lens. Likewise, lens implantation has reached a level of popularity that makes it an inseparable part of any discussion of cataract treatment.

In this chapter, techniques of cataract surgery, specifically the manual technique of extracapsular extraction, are discussed. But why manual? Manual because it's popular, popular because it's a simple, direct unencumbered method. Such a method can be undertaken without a major investment of machinery, or of time devoted to the maintenance of that machinery. It's a popular method worldwide.

Before we begin the discussion of technique—of instrumentation and the development of surgical skills—patient preparation is discussed.

PATIENT PREPARATION

Clearly, ultimate refinements of surgical success and patient satisfaction are achieved through the reduction of anxiety. Patient education and counseling results in a tremendous reduction of anxiety. Thus, in our practice, a great deal of energy is devoted to helping the patient understand as much about the reality of his disease and its treatment as possible.

Patient education is enhanced at every step throughout the treatment process. Printed materials are given to the patient during the examining visit and for later review at home (these may be mailed to the patient in advance of his first examination). Video counseling is used to provide basic information as the patient relaxes in the waiting room and/or in the limousine when transportation is supplied. But the ultimate counseling is personal counseling. Every individual who has direct contact with the patient and his family is able to appropriately answer questions. Later, the patient and family have a combined counseling session with a patient educator who covers the material with the amount of detail appropriate for each patient.

Diet

While we attempt to educate and counsel as much as possible, we try to interfere with the patient's daily routine as little as possible. In most cases, this means following a normal diet both before and after surgery. For those patients with metabolic disorders, such as diabetes, it is particularly important for them to follow their normal routine of medications and diet, come to the operating room for the surgical procedure, and then return home to resume near normal activities.

PROPHYLACTIC ANTIBIOTICS

There is no existing objective proof that prophylactic antibiotics alter the results of cataract surgery, but they are used anyway. Our recent routine has been topical tobramycin three times a day for the 2 days before and the morning of surgery.

PREMEDICATIONS

With a comfortable, confident educated patient, little or no premedication is needed. Still, many seem to be reassured by "getting something." Consequently, we use a small amount of chloral hydrate, a long established "old fashioned" hypnotic of known safety. The usual dose is 500 mg about 1 hour prior to the procedure.

DILATION

For satisfactory surgery, wide pupillary dilation is a major aid. We dilate the pupil in routine cases with cyclopentalate 1 percent and phenylephrine 2.5 percent. Three drops of each are instilled over a period of 10 to 15 minutes about 45 minutes prior to surgery. Secondary lens implantation is frequently an entirely different matter. Where sufficient peripheral posterior capsule exists to allow postpupillary lens implantation, dilation may be carried out as in the primary cataract procedure. On the other hand, for secondary implants following earlier intracapsular extraction, the pupil is constricted preoperatively with pilocarpine.

OCULOPRESSION

I regard oculopression as one of the major advances in intraocular surgery in our generation and feel we owe a great debt to Daniel Vörösmarthy of Hungary for his very fine basic study (see also Chapter 11). We include 45 minutes of oculopression in the preparation of our patient. The mercury bag we use is a modification of that originally described by Norman Buys. It is conveniently held in position by a Velcro attachment to a simple headband and creates a pressure of 30 mmHg. The mercury bag is applied to the preoperative eye when the patient first comes into the operating area. It is removed briefly during the injection of the retrobulbar anesthetic and then reapplied and left in position until the patient is skin prepped for surgery. External pressure of 30 mmHg over a period of 45 minutes produces a significant decrease in vitreous volume and in orbital tissue fluid. This "moderate" softening of the globe is appropriate to the surgical procedure we are describing. It certainly is possible to obtain a softer eye with the additional combination of intravenous osmotic agents and general anesthesia. However, extreme softness can require other changes in the operative procedure, particularly those involved with nucleus removal. So, we use 30 mmHg of oculopression for 45 minutes.

ANESTHESIA

Although the basic concepts of local anesthesia for intraocular surgery were established some years ago, there has been a renewed examination of this entire subject recently. The concept of akinesia for surgical safety was clearly established by Atkinson and appears to have been a basic landmark in the development of ophthalmic surgical technique. Although regional block approaches to the facial nerve have been popular and extremely successful, the combination of longer acting motor blocking agents and greater available preoperative time has resulted in a reexploration of peripheral local akinesia of the orbicularis muscle. Several practices have reported successful use of a modified retrobulbar injection with peripheral diffusion into the orbicularis fibers. However, to date, we have stayed with separate regional block of the facial nerve at the stylomastoid foramen by Nadbath technique and a traditional retrobulbar injection.

Anesthetic Agents

In the past several years, two new agents for local anesthesia have become well established. Bupivacaine (Marcaine) and etidocaine (Duranest) both demonstrate significantly longer effects than the commonly used lidocaine. The etidocaine demonstrates the longest motor blocking effect and at the same time the least sensory blocking effect. Although bupivacaine has been in more popular use, a significant complication has been reported: several episodes of respiratory arrest. The presumed mechanism is subarachnoid seepage through the optic canal. However, we are not aware of similar reports with the use of etidocaine, though it does seem reasonable that this might also occur.

For the past year, we have done 800 to 1,000 cases with 1.5 percent etidocaine. The major inconvenience of this drug is a prolonged retrobulbar motor block that commonly leaves the patient with paralytic strabismus at the 24-hour dressing. Consequently, we are currently evaluating a mixture of etidocaine and lidocaine. It seems that everything has both advantages and disadvantages.

TECHNIQUE

Anesthesia

It has been our practice for several years to inject local anesthesia during a very brief, fixed general anesthetic obtained with intravenous methohexital (Brevital). The methohexital is given in a graduated dose ranging from 15 mg in the very slight and aged patient to 45 mg in the normal, healthy 70-year-old patient, and upward to 70 mg in the robust healthy adult. The injection is given as a single bolus, but over a period of some 10 seconds. With sufficient venous circulation time, the patient will begin a brief period of fixed general anesthesia. The 2- to 3-minute period of anesthesia provides adequate time for injection of the local agents.

Local injections are made about 20 minutes before beginning the operation about halfway through the period of oculopression. Our preference for a local injection is currently a mixture of 2 percent lidocaine with equal part of 1.5 percent etidocaine. We have found that this provides a very strong, prolonged motor blocking effect with adequate sensory anesthesia. Because of the great importance of akinesia, we have continued to inject both the facial nerve by Nadbath technique and the retrobulbar muscle cone per conjunctiva.

Position

The position of the patient relative to the surgeon is extremely important if maximum convenience and comfort are to be ensured. In order to approach an optimum position, we have modified both the operating table and the surgeon's chair. It is ideal for the surgeon to be able to sit upright with both feet on the floor with his back supported in a balanced position. The patient's head is then positioned in the surgeon's lap with the surgical field at the appropriate height for his hands; arms thus may swing directly from the shoulder. In this position, the only support required is a gentle touch of the fingertips to the patient's brow. The microscope may then be brought into position with the appropriate objective length, angulation, and ocular tube length, to couple the eye with the surgical field. These positioning factors will allow one to work with relative comfort through the extended hours of a surgical day.

For those patients of considerable body weight, we use a reverse Trendelenberg position. The head is extended slightly on the neck to bring the orbital rim to a horizontal plane. In this position the head is firmly fixated by a strap of adhesive tape running across the forehead and down to the headrest on each side.

We use the barrier technique of draping the lid margins from the operative field with the vinyl drape. This is held in position with a lightweight modified Barraquer wire eye speculum, and when necessary, a superior rectus bridle suture is inserted.

Filtration

We are acutely sensitive to the risk of contamination during surgery, particularly that which may be caused by particulate and biologic material carried in irrigating solutions. Thus, we endure the inconvenience of terminal filtration of the infusion fluid used during cataract surgery. The disposable infusion set we use includes an appropriate in-line filter. The inconvenience of its use is minimized by the proper set-up technique. The tubing pinch clamp is closed while the spike and drip chamber are inserted into the fluid reservoir. With release of the pinch clamp, the fluid is allowed to enter the tubing in a single column. The filter capsule is held vertically so that the air column being pushed out by the advancing fluid rises through the filter. After the fluid has wetted the entire lumen of the tubing system, it is allowed to run at full flow for several seconds. Then with the vibration of a sharp rap on the filter capsule (administered with a heavy scissors or hemostat), the flow through the filter increases remarkably. With this set-up technique, balanced salt solution (BSS) flows through the filtered tubing system at some 50 to 60 drops per minute under a pressure head of approximately 24 inches. This has proven entirely sufficient for our surgical technique.

Surgical Technique

The surgical technique begins with division of the conjunctiva at the surgical limbus. This is done with the blunt Wescott scissors and Colibri forceps. The scleral vessels are then cauterized with the bipolar cautery, which is sufficient to obtain adequate hemostasis.

Using a trifacet diamond scalpel, a limbal groove is made with a single pass of the diamond blade (Fig. 9-1). The eye is fixed with only the tip of a sponge spear, and with careful visual control, the groove is intended to one-half to three-quarters of the limbal thickness. In most cases of senile cata-

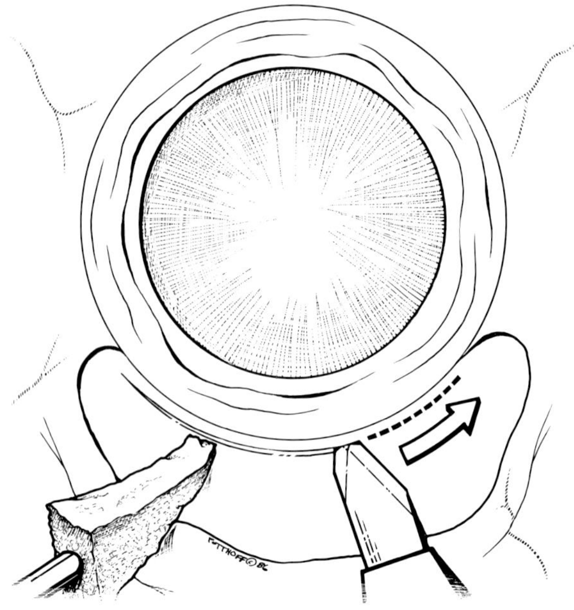

Fig. 9-1. Corneal scleral incision is begun with a groove made by the diamond scalpel.

ract, the final incision must be 9.5 mm or greater chord length. In a youthful patient with a very soft nucleus, the incision may be as little as 7.5 to 8 mm. On the other hand, with the senile brunescent cataract 10.5 mm is a more reliable dimension.

The depths of the groove at 12 o'clock are touched with the tip of the diamond blade to make a minimum puncture into the anterior chamber (Fig. 9-2). Through this puncture the anterior capsulectomy is done with a hooked cystotome (Fig. 9-3). Our preference has been to do the anterior capsulectomy under a large air bubble in order to hold the capsule surface against the lens material, minimize leakage of the anterior chamber volume, and enhance visualization of the capsule surface.

The cystotome is prepared as a disposable instrument for each surgical procedure. Using a $25 \times \frac{5}{8}$-inch needle, a very small hook is formed by simple pressure against a flat metallic surface. The hook is curved to approximately 90 degrees but needs only a length of one-third to one-half the size of the tubing diameter. A 45-degree bend is then made in the center of the needle length and the cystotome is mounted on a plastic handpiece. This is connected to an air-filled 5-ml syringe by a sterile extension set. During the procedure, the surgical assistant supplies air to fill the anterior chamber and replace any that may be lost.

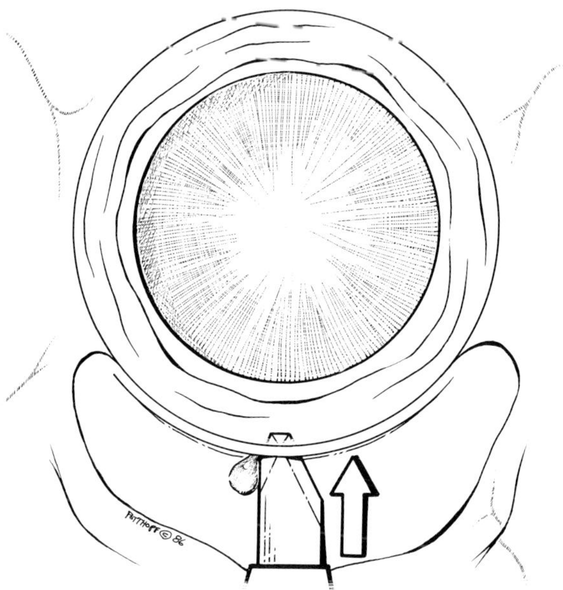

Fig. 9-2. A small puncture into the anterior chamber at 12 o'clock will allow entry of the cystotome.

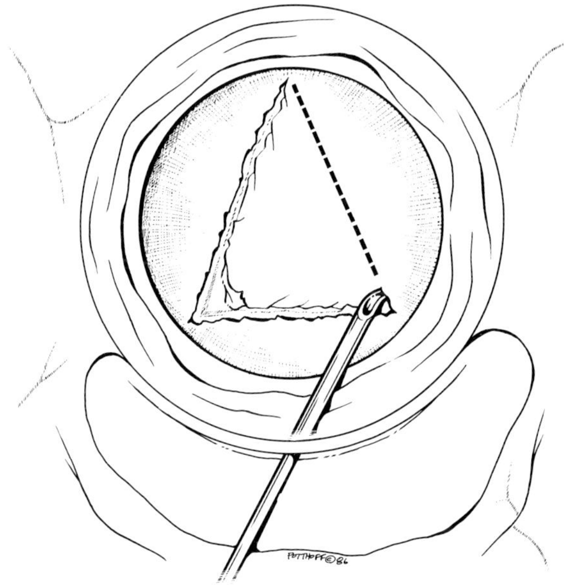

Fig. 9-3. Under a large air bubble the triangular anterior capsulectomy is made by multiple small punctures with the hooked cystotome.

The anterior capsulectomy is begun superiorly, making the horizontal upper base of a triangle. The capsulectomy incision is made by a series of very small punctures, each communicating with the previous. The triangular capsulectomy is a distinct aide in in-the-bag implantation of the intraocular lens (IOL). After completing the superior base, the nasal and temporal legs of the triangle are completed with their juncture at 6 o'clock. When the incision is completed the cystotome hook is used to ensure that the capsule fragment is free and to drag it toward the entry point as the instrument leaves the anterior chamber.

The incision is completed with the trifacet diamond blade (Fig. 9-4). A single pass in each direction is ordinarily sufficient. We do not attempt to create a multiplane incision. However, when making the entire incision with a super scalpel, such as the diamond, it is very important to lift the incision margin and inspect for any possible strands of intact Descemet's membrane. A small strand of Descemet's may be nearly invisible until expression of the nucleus is attempted; presence of vitreous then

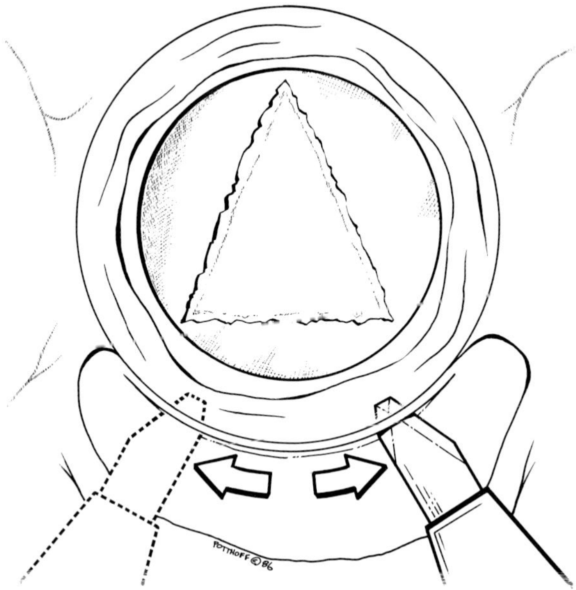

Fig. 9-4. Incision is completed to its full depth with the diamond scalpel.

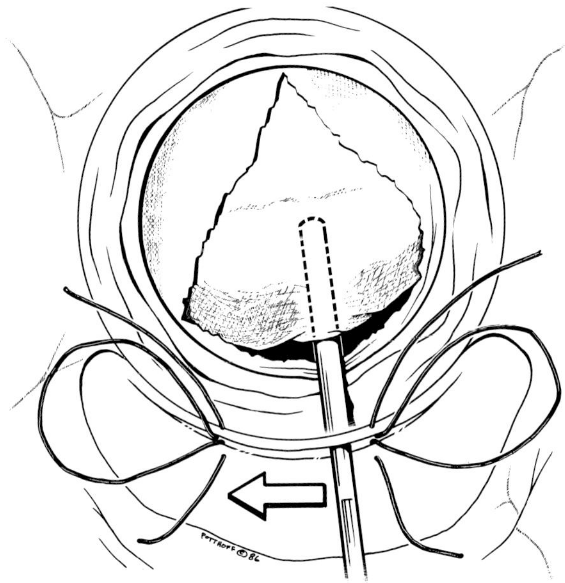

Fig. 9-5. Control suture loops are extracted from the anterior chamber and the superior equator of the nucleus is prolapsed with the tip of a 26-gauge anterior chamber cannula.

gives one startling notice of the condition of the incision.

Control sutures give me a great deal of peace of mind, and if they are to serve their purpose during a possible expulsive hemorrhage, they must be both strong and relatively large in diameter. We use 8-0 black silk to insert two control sutures dividing the incision into approximately equal thirds.

The loops of these control sutures are pulled from the wound and laid over the ends of the incision with the tip of a 26-gauge anterior chamber cannula. This cannula has a finely polished tip and is mounted on a BSS-filled tuberculin syringe. The same cannula is also used to prolapse the superior equator of the nucleus into the anterior chamber (Fig. 9-5). The tip of the cannula slides under the margin of the capsulectomy to my right hand side (by my own convention), and then with gentle simultaneous infusion of BSS, the tip of the cannula passes horizontally under the superior equator of the nucleus, lifting it forward in front of both the iris and superior anterior capsular leaflet.

The nucleus is expressed by a simple, gentle, and leisurely bimanual technique (Fig. 9-6). With toothed Colibri forceps in the left hand, the episclera is grasped just above the incision margin at 12 o'clock. With this forceps, a force is exerted superiorly, slightly tenting the incision open. Simultaneously, a force is directed to the center of the posterior segment, creating initial vitreous pressure that causes the nucleus to begin its extrusion movement.

With the right hand, the angle of the 26-gauge cannula is used to apply counterpressure through the peripheral clear cornea at 6 o'clock. I make a point to keep this instrument inside the scleral spur so that no sudden movement is likely to occur as the nucleus extrudes. With the two instruments, I prefer to alternate the force on the eye so that the nucleus is extruded in a slightly rocking movement, and my proprioception guides me in understanding which hand is supplying the most effective force. As the nucleus nearly completes one half of its slide out of the anterior chamber, the force is maintained with the cannula while the Colibri forceps lifts the nucleus out of the anterior chamber. With the 26-gauge cannula, the anterior chamber is then deepened while any iris prolapse that may have occurred is repositioned.

The control sutures are tied with a temporary knot consisting of a simple bow over a surgeon's loop. The residual cortex is then removed as com-

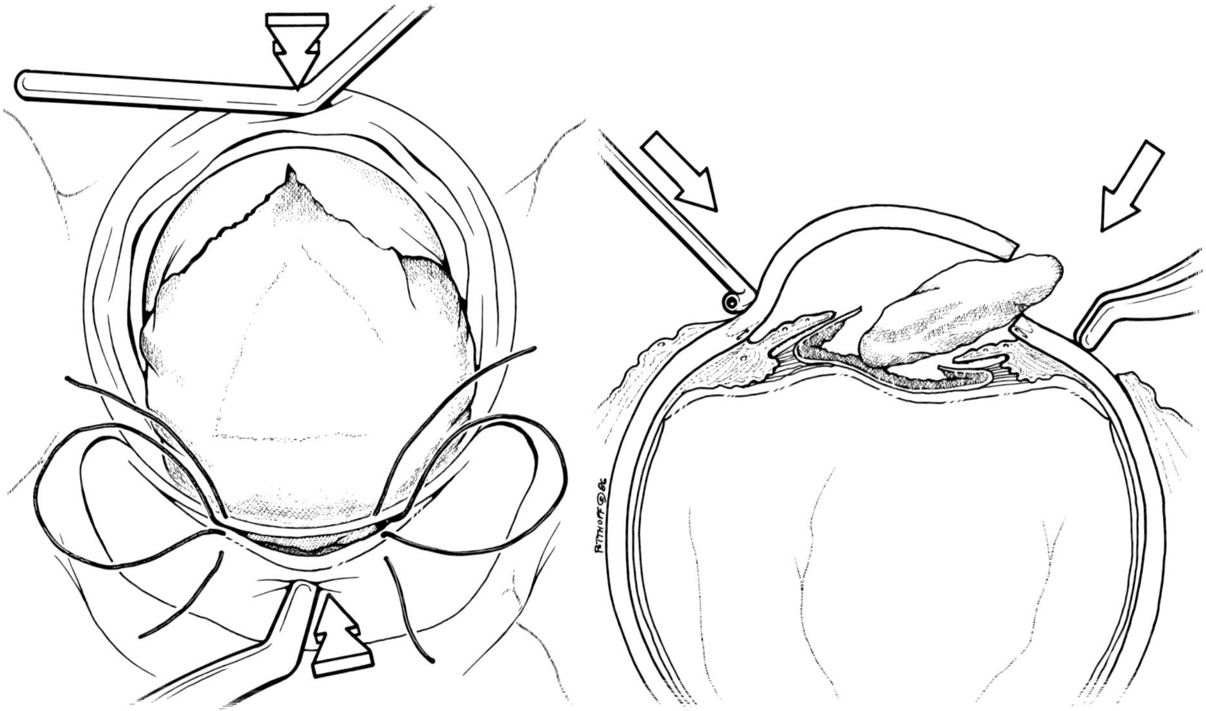

Fig. 9-6. Alternating forces with the Colibri forceps at 12 o'clock and the heel of the cannula at 6 o'clock cause a controlled expression of the nucleus.

pletely, gently, and safely as possible. I have used a manual system of cortex aspiration for the past 10 years and continue to feel that it gives maximum control and safety. The manual system is quick, easy, inexpensive, and reliable and allows a level of control of which machines are not ordinarily capable. However, there are a number of details in the technique of the procedure that are essential to its use.

Our coaxial cannula aspirating system is used with continuous gravity-fed infusion of filtered BSS. For most senile cataracts, the aspirating port of 0.2-mm diameter coupled with a 5-ml disposable syringe provides the most comfortable balance between force and vacuum pressure. On the face of it, 0.2 mm seems intuitively too small to many surgeons, but in point of fact, 0.3 mm is actually too large for optimum safety; this is where the details of technique are so important.

The mechanism of cortex removal is basically an occlusion of the aspirating port by a particle of cortex. This occlusion affords one a grip on that particle of cortex and allows it to be pulled or stripped from the peripheral capsular bag (Fig. 9-7). Aspiration is accomplished by an increased force on the syringe, which raises the aspirating pressure at the cannula port and causes an intrusion of the cortical material. When the particle of cortex has been completely aspirated, aqueous solution or BSS fol-

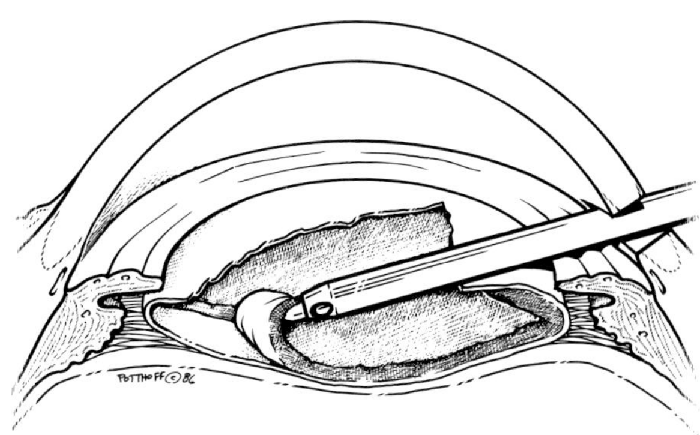

Fig. 9-7. Cortical fragments are gently stripped from the periphery of the capsular bag with the coaxial cannula.

lows it into the syringe. At this instant, the surgeon should stop aspirating and allow the anterior chamber to remain filled by the gravity-fed infusion fluid. However, with an aspirating port of more than 0.2 mm, there is very little restriction to the rate of aspiration of BSS and consequently, it is much more difficult for the surgeon to stop aspirating rapidly enough to avoid shallowing of the chamber.

The balance between force and pressure relies upon a nonelastic system and it is critically important to exclude air from the cannula and syringe. Thus, during the set-up procedure a small amount of BSS is placed in the syringe, allowed to wet the inside of the syringe barrel, and then used to expel any remaining air bubbles.

We begin aspiration of the residual cortex by removing those loose particles lying in the anterior chamber along with any small air bubbles that may remain from the anterior capsulectomy. Such air bubbles will disturb the pressure relationships within the syringe, so the instrument is removed from the anterior chamber and pointed directly upwards; then the syringe is tapped to coalesce and float any air bubbles to its tip where they will be expelled.

The peripheral residual cortex is then stripped and aspirated in the normal fashion. My convention is to begin at six o'clock, grasp a first particle of cortex within the capsular bag, strip it upwards into the pupillary space, and aspirate it when it is completely visible. All aspirating force ceases after that particle has been removed. I then return to an adjacent area in the peripheral capsular bag and grasp the next particle of cortex, strip, and aspirate.

Modern extracapsular cataract surgery is characterized by the most complete possible removal of lens material. This can be accomplished with a variety of instrument systems. However the mechanics of the procedure are very much the same regardless of the instrument used. My personal preference has been for the manual aspiration system, which gives me the greatest possible control over the procedure.

Cortex stripping and removal makes use of the anatomic structure of the lens. In most cases, there is a definite fibrillar structure to the most peripheral cortex in the immediate subcapsular area. Consequently, when this peripheral fibrillar cortex is grasped, it will strip from the periphery of the capsular bag all of the contained lens cortex. As particles of cortex are stripped from the periphery, they may be aspirated when visibly present within the pupillary aperture. In the manual aspiration system, it is my choice to have a cannula device directly attached to a syringe. Infusion fluid is continuously fed by gravity through the coaxial cannula system. Aspirating forces in the side-ported inner cannula are created by gentle fingertip forces on a simple disposable syringe. To have a full range of aspirating vacuum pressures available, I am most confortable combining a 5-ml syringe with a 0.2-mm aspirating port. Thus, a full continuum of pressures is available at the aspirating port, ranging from regurgitation to a nearly complete vacuum. The 0.2-mm aperture provides the full range of effects from occlusion, which grasps cortical material for stripping, to aspiration of all non-nuclear lens material. At the same time, the small diameter of the aspirating port significantly restricts the flow of aqueous solution or BSS, limiting the rate at which an anterior chamber collapse could occur. The final result makes available a full range of pressures to effect the stripping and aspiration of cortical particles; combined with restriction of aqueous flow, it allows normal human response time to minimize endothelial trauma.

We must emphasize and reemphasize that this system is functional only when the cannula and syringe are filled with fluid to the exclusion of all visible air bubbles. The elasticity introduced by vapor bubbles destroys the force-pressure relationship and will prevent proper function of the instrument system.

To prepare the coaxial cannula system for use, the infusion tubing is wet on the inside with BSS, its inline filter is stabilized by a flow of BSS and the vibration of several sharp raps with a heavy instrument, and the cannula and syringe are filled with a small amount of BSS to remove any air. With this instrument, I then directly enter the anterior chamber and aspirate any small air bubbles that may have remained following the capsulectomy, as well as any loose fragments of cortex present in the anterior chamber. After aspirating this material, the syringe and cannula are removed from the anterior chamber, held with the cannula point upwards and tapped several times with the fingertip. This will coalesce any air bubbles in the syringe, which then may be expelled forceably.

In the anterior chamber, the cannula tip is introduced into the peripheral capsular bag at six o'clock. With a very light aspirating force, fragments of peripheral cortex in this area are impacted. While they are obstructing the aspirating cannula port, sufficient grip can be established to allow the particles to be pulled or stripped from the periphery of the capsular bag into the pupillary space. When the particles are visible in the pupillary space, a greater force is applied to the syringe to cause their rapid aspiration. As they near complete aspiration into the cannula, the force on the syringe is completely stopped; this ensures that the anterior chamber depth is maintained by gravity infusion and that the surgeon's hands will be relaxed as he again introduces the cannula into the peripheral capsular bag. Beginning at six o'clock, I customarily work continuously around in each direction, aspirating each fragment of cortex in its turn.

When approaching the superior capsular bag, we have found it completely satisfactory to hold the instrument transversely, entering through the temporal or nasal third of the incision, reaching into the capsular bag at twelve o'clock, and impacting particles and stripping them downwards into the pupillary space. In most cases, the superior cortical fragments will be stripped and aspirated partly through the temporal and partly through the nasal portion of the incision. It has been a rare patient indeed in whom the bridge of the nose is a significant obstacle to this procedure.

During the stripping and aspirating of cortical particles, the inner cannula aspirating port is held anteriorly at all times. The aspirating forces are truly intermittent, while the gravity infusion is continuous with approximately 24 inches of pressure head.

Following complete removal of the cortical material, the coaxial cannula may be used as a polishing or vacuuming device for both the central posterior capsule and the inferior anterior capsular leaflets (Fig. 9-8). When small fragments of cortex are visibly clinging to the central posterior capsule, the aspirating port is turned posteriorly, and with exceedingly gentle aspiration the instrument is used as a small vacuum sweeper, simultaneously scraping and aspirating these particles. This procedure is so gentle that the "spider web" reflexes, which indicate impaction of the posterior capsule, are ordinarily not seen. If plaques of posterior capsular fibrosis are present, these may frequently be gently teased and stripped from the posterior capsule in the same fashion. Great care, of course, is required to avoid excessive forces that might tear the posterior capsule.

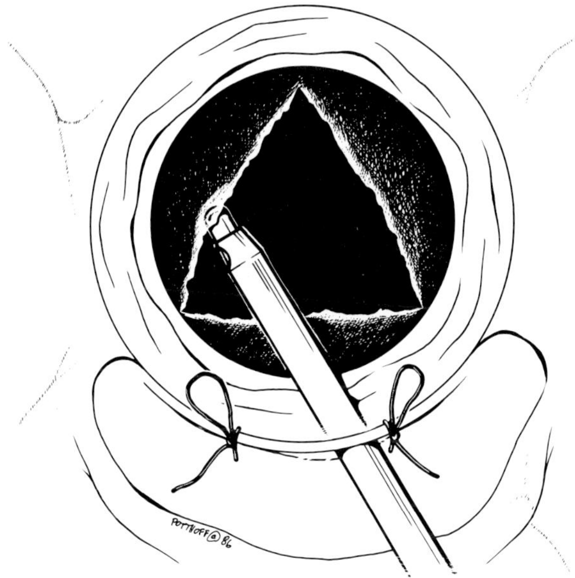

Fig. 9-8. The coaxial cannula is used to polish the central posterior capsule and remove epithelial cells from the anterior capsular leaflet.

The growth of secondary cortex and consequent clouding of the posterior capsule is one of the inherent inconveniences of extracapsular cataract surgery. It appears that the incidence of this problem may be reduced by physically removing the epithelial cell bodies from the inner surface of the inferior capsular flaps. Consequently, with the aspirating port anteriorward, the instrument is used to vacuum these cell bodies from the capsular surface. As this is done, an increased clarity is seen contrasting with the very slightly "ground glass" appearance normal in the anterior capsular leaflets.

INTRAOCULAR LENS

Intraocular lens implantation is now clearly established as the finest solution to the usually severe hyperopia of aphakia. Current data also strongly suggest that several varieties of posterior chamber implants placed within the capsule bag produce the least possible postoperative inflammation.

But which one? There are a great many styles of artificial lenses implanted behind the iris plane. It has been my view that essentially all of these are entirely satisfactory if they are comfortable for the surgeon to implant. Each of us has his own biases and habits, and each may find that a slightly different style of implant seems most comfortable in the context of his own surgical procedure and skill.

I began implantation of the Shearing-style lens in 1979. A specific technique of its use evolved and it has provided us with an extremely satisfactory optical result, minimum surgical complications, and a low incidence of requirement for postsurgical capsulotomy. Consequently, I have not found a reason for change.

The technique we have evolved includes

1. Implantation within the capsular bag.
2. The convex surface of the implant against the posterior capsule.
3. Ten- to 15-degree angulation of the fixation loops.
4. Final sizing of the tip-to-tip loop length at the time of insertion.

The basic technique is as described in the following paragraphs.

Inspection for apparent optical quality and cleanliness is done at the outset of the operation and the lens is soaked in BSS until insertion.

Alteration of loop length and angulation is made immediately prior to insertion. Lenses that have polypropelene haptic loops may be modified and expected to hold their configuration after insertion. Consequently, the lens is grasped at the center of the optic with a toothless Kelman-McPherson forceps. The haptic loops (at the point where they exit the optic) are gently bent forward with the plano surface of the lens upward. This forward bending is checked repeatedly until the resting position of the loop is in 10- to 15-degree anterior angulation. At the same time, the tip-to-tip loop length may be modified by bending at the point of exit from the optic. In the average patient with a lens power of 21 to 22 diopters, bending is continued until the tip-to-tip length is approximately 11.5 mm. However, in the high myope with a lens power of 8 to 12 diopters, the haptics are left full length. In these eyes with a larger capsular bag, stable positioning requires a larger tip-to-tip diameter.

The lens is then inserted directly into the capsular bag. This procedure may be facilitated by the use of sodium hyaluronate, or in a quiet eye with no evident vitreous pressure, by the use of a Sheet's glide and BSS. The lens is passed directly into the anterior chamber while held with the Kelman-McPherson forceps, so that the advancing inferior haptic loop passes directly under the inferior anterior capsular leaflet into the capsular bag at six o'clock. As the optic enters the anterior chamber, the tip of the superior haptic is grasped with a toothless Colibri forceps. The Colibri and Kelman-McPherson forceps then both proceed simulta-

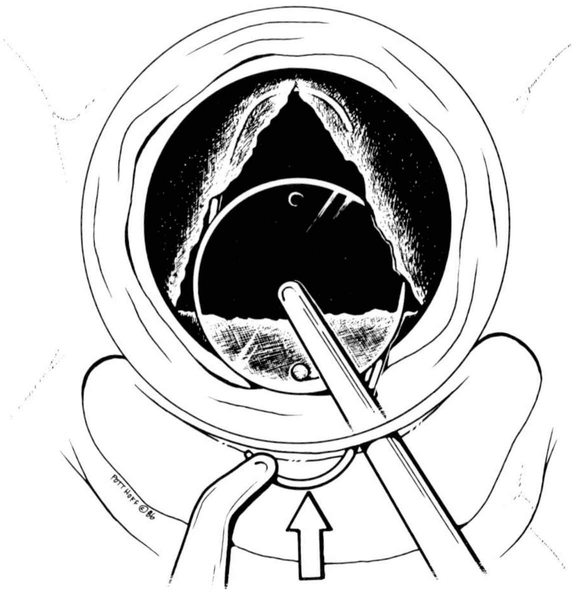

Fig. 9-9. The posterior chamber lens is implanted directly into the capsular bag.

neously into the anterior chamber where the Kelman-McPherson forceps release their grip and the lens position is maintained by the toothless Colibri (Fig. 9-9). If the Sheet's glide has been used, it is extracted from the anterior chamber with the Kelman-McPherson forceps, which are handed to the instrument nurse, and replaced with a prepared irrigating iris hook. This hook has BSS dripping under gravity flow at 24 inches pressure head. It is first used to dampen the surface of the cornea for clarity, then enters the anterior chamber posterior to the superior haptic, and grasps both the superior pupillary margin and the superior anterior capsular leaflet (Fig. 9-10). By lifting these structures, the upper haptic can be placed directly into the capsular bag. The irrigating hook may then be used to press the optic gently posteriorly against the central posterior capsule while the tip of the haptic is released by the toothless Colibri forceps. Finally, both instruments are removed from the anterior chamber. The anterior chamber is immediately deepened with BSS and the control is suture retied.

The position of the IOL within the capsular bag may be verified by the tip of the BSS cannula. When the chamber is fully reformed, pressure through the sclera over the tip of the haptic loop will cause direct immediate motion of the lens if the tip of the haptic is outside the capsular bag. A preliminary gentle movement of the pupillary margin will be seen if the haptic is properly positioned within the bag. If necessary, the lens can be rotated with a small hook or cannula tip to adjust its position within the capsule.

CLOSURE

After completing a very clean and complete extracapsular cataract extraction and in-the-bag insertion of a postpupillary IOL, the wound is closed in a manner that will produce the least possible postoperative astigmatism. We have confirmed the findings of others that the shortest, deepest corneoscleral sutures produce the least astigmatic effect, and thus use interrupted 10-0 nylon sutures placed with the Alcon CU-6 needle. These are ordinarily inserted in running fashion with the suture loops simultaneously divided and each separate bite tied as an interrupted suture (Fig. 9-11).

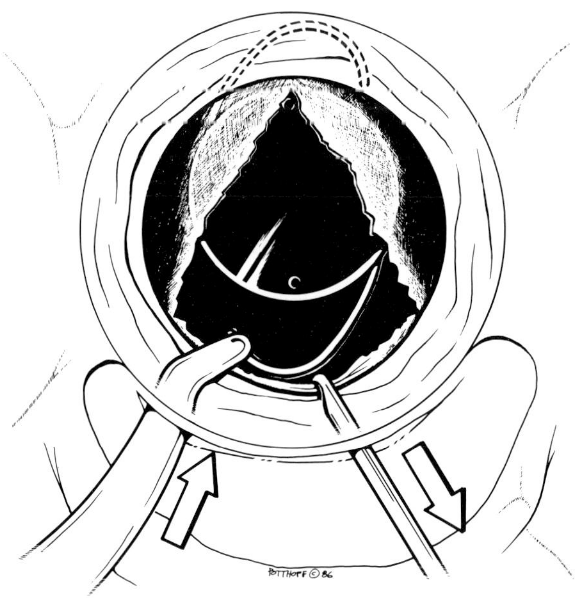

Fig. 9-10. Placement of the superior haptic is aided by the irrigating iris hook.

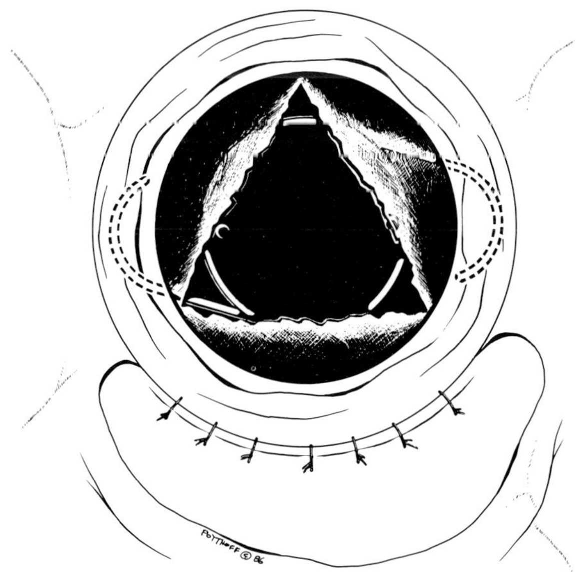

Fig. 9-11. Following permanent closure and prior to rotation of the sutures, the lens position is examined and rotated if necessary to ensure placement within the capsular bag.

Because it is difficult to rotate suture knots into the tissue in the short deep bite technique, we use the slip knot to minimize the bulk of the knots. The complete knot is a full square over a slip. This technique, while different from the usual surgeon's loop followed by square knot, is no more difficult and becomes automatic with a few cases' experience.

IRIDECTOMY

In our routine white patient with a negative history for intraocular inflammation or glaucoma, and where the surgical procedure has been entirely routine and uneventful, the case is terminated without iridectomy. However, there is no strong evidence at the present time to justify either routine iridectomy or its exclusion.

At the conclusion of the procedure, a final inspection is made to reconfirm the position of the IOL within the capsular bag and the absence of any residual cortex or significant blood within the anterior chamber. It has been our custom to inject subconjunctival soluble steroid and gentamycin and to instill a drop of combined corticosteroid and antibiotic. Once a protective dressing has been applied, the patient is discharged from the operating room.

POSTOPERATIVE CARE

Each patient is examined at 24 hours postsurgery. The dressing is removed and the patient allowed to resume essentially all normal activities, protected with glasses during the day, and the Fox shield while sleeping. At this 24-hour examination, antibiotic/steroid drops are instituted four times daily and normally continued for approximately 3 weeks.

The patient is examined again at 1 week, presuming that the course is normal. At that time, brief dilation is done for examination purposes. (In addition, the brief cycloplegia will help to reduce postoperative inflammation.) Most normal patients are then reexamined at approximately 3 months for prescription of final eyeglasses.

Phacoemulsification Associated with Intraocular Lenses

10

Richard P. Kratz
Paul F. Olson
Stephen H. Johnson
Michael K. Farley

Kelman[1] first reported the removal of the crystalline lens through a small incision in 1967. This was followed by case reports at the American Academy of Ophthalmology in 1969, and the first classes in phacoemulsification were taught in 1971. This new technique made a major impact on cataract surgery throughout the world. Intracapsular cases usually were hospitalized for 5 to 7 days in the United States and often for up to 21 days in Europe. This was followed by a very restricted physical activity for the next 2 months. The Kelman technique permitted outpatient cataract extraction with no physical restrictions. The rapid recovery allowed glasses or contact lenses to be fitted in just 3 weeks compared with the usual 9 weeks.

Other surgeons modified the original Kelman technique developing posterior chamber emulsification, the two-handed method, the scleral incision, and anterior capsulotomies designed to fit the individual intraocular lenses.[2-6] The equipment was also altered to include piezoelectric and autoclavible ultrasonic handpieces, some of which provided surgeon control over the ultrasound power and aspiration. The ultrasound tips included 15-, 30-, 45-, 60-degree round and oval as well as a dual tip (Fig. 10-1). The irrigation and aspiration added 0.2- and 0.3-mm port size tips to the 0.5- and 0.7-mm tips. Filters were added to the infusion tubing to prevent the introduction of particulate matter and bacteria into the anterior chamber.

ULTRASONIC EQUIPMENT

The ultrasonic handpiece consists of a hollow needle that is accelerated to 250,000 G to take advantage of the inertia of the nucleus. It has a stroke of 0.3+ mm and makes 27,000 to 40,000 strokes per second. The ultrasound is generated by magnetostrictive metal wafers or by a quartz crystal piezoelectric system. The original ultrasonic machine was made by Cavitron. Since then CooperVision-Cavitron, United Sonics, Fibrasonics, Surgical Design Systems, United Surgical Systems, Mid Labs, Phacosystems, Innovative Surgical Products, Site, and Staar have marketed phacoemulsification machines. The newer machines give the surgeon the option of controlling the cutting power and aspiration.

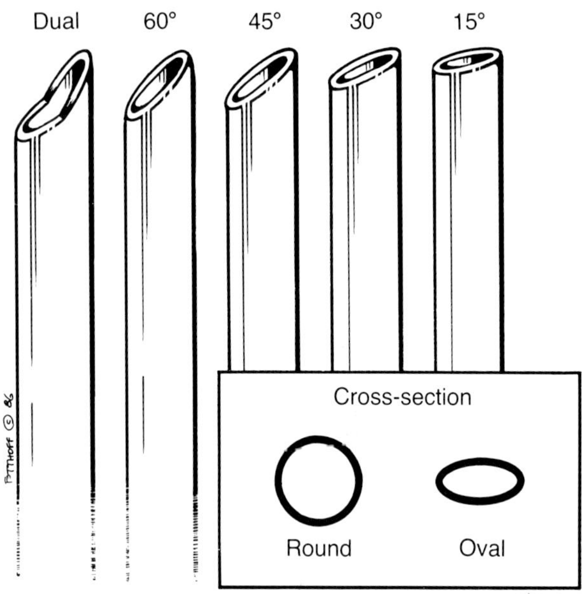

Fig. 10-1. Phacoemulsification tips are available from 15 to 60 degrees and can be either round or oval. The dual tip combines the cutting ability of the 60-degree tip with the aspiration ability of the 15-degree tip.

ADVANTAGES

Renewed interest in phacoemulsification has come with the introduction of foldable lenses that can be inserted through a 3-mm incision.[7] Most of the advantages of phacoemulsification are related to the small incision size. It allows the surgeon to be in control throughout all steps of the procedure. The small incision permits rapid healing with early return to full activity, including gainful employment, thus reducing the overall disability expense. The small incision resulted in less astigmatism and less chance of a wound leak and flat anterior chamber or peripheral anterior synechiae.

Other advantages of phacoemulsification lay in special cases in which it seems to offer advantages over intracapsular cataract extraction. These include one-eyed patients, especially those in whom the first eye was damaged after vitreous loss or retinal detachment. Phacoemulsification offers greater safety in patients with high myopia or retinal detachment or in those who might be at risk of vitreous loss, such as "bull-necked" persons. The small incision permits preservation of filtering blebs or combined trabeculectomy with cataract extraction. Patients with thin sclera are best treated with small-incision phacoemulsification.

DISADVANTAGES

Phacoemulsification requires special training and practice. A good intracapsular surgeon is not automatically a good phacoemulsifier. The technique requires meticulous attention to detail. For example, an incision that is 0.5 mm too long will cause loss of anterior chamber in phacoemulsification but will be unimportant in intracapsular cataract extraction. The expense of the required operating microscope, the ultrasonic machine, and the disposable pack limit its value in third-world situations. Machine failure may occur and the surgeon must be able to convert to a planned extracapsular cataract extraction if machine troubleshooting fails. The surgeon must have thorough knowledge of the machine.

Some cases are probably done as well or better by planned extracapsular cataract extraction. This would include extremely hard nuclei, subluxed nuclei, advanced corneal dystrophy, and very low endothelial cell counts, depending on the individual case and the experience of the phacoemulsification surgeon.

PREOPERATIVE PREPARATION

Preoperative pupil dilatation and medication are essentially the same as in planned extracapsular cataract extraction or intracapsular cataract extraction. Intraocular pressure reduction to about 15 mmHg is desirable, but very low pressure results in an excessively deep anterior chamber, making nucleus removal difficult. The reduction may be done by a Honan[8–10] or Varrosmarty balloon,[11] mercury bag, Super-Pinkie,[12] or digital compression.

ANESTHESIA

The procedure may be done under local, general, or combination anesthesia. The retrobulbar injection is painful, and it is helpful to have the anesthesiologist give a bolus of sodium pentathol through the in-place IV line just prior to the injection. The patient will be completely asleep for several minutes and have no memory of discomfort from the injection. It is helpful to have the anesthesiologist monitor the patient and give small increments of additional sedation if needed. Most cataract patients are elderly and have an increased risk of cardiac or pulmonary dysfunction. The presence of the anesthesiologist does much to avoid potential problems or correct them if they occur.

SURGEON POSITION

The surgeon is usually at the patient's head, and the section is made at the 12 o'clock position. Terry[13] recently challenged this by stating that corneal flattening always occurs in the healed state after cataract extraction. In order to minimize postoperative astigmatism, the incision would be at 12 o'clock when the plus axis is at 90 degrees, and the incision would be at 3 o'clock or 9 o'clock when the plus axis is at 180 degrees. Placing the microscope hand controls in a sterile glove across the patient's upper chest permits the surgeon, assistant surgeon, or nurse to change the focus zoom or x,y axis.

INCISION

Since 90 percent of cataract extractions also have an intraocular lens implanted at this same surgery, the incision size should be planned to match the optic size. Thus a 6-mm optic intraocular lens calls for a 6-mm conjunctival flap, usually fornix based unless it is to be combined with a trabeculectomy. The incision may be limbal in single, double, or triple planes. Some surgeons believe that a scleral pocket incision results in less astigmatism.[14,13] (Fig. 10-2). This incision calls for a one half scleral thickness cut 2 mm behind and parallel to the limbus, which is then dissected into clear cornea, terminating at the anterior edge of the limbal arcade. It is important to change the angle of dissection when the cornea is reached. This avoids the bleeding and iris prolapse that will occur if the incision is carried to the iris root. If carried to the anterior edge of the limbal arcade, it will form a good shelf for the support of an anterior chamber lens, should one be required. The initial entry into the anterior chamber is a 1.0-mm razor incision at 11 o'clock for the irrigating cystitome and a limbal puncture wound at 3 o'clock for the spatula when a two-handed technique is used (Fig. 10-3). The incision is enlarged to 3 mm to admit the ultrasonic tip and to allow irrigation and aspiration to be performed after completion of the phacoemulsification. When the nucleus and cortex are removed, Healon is usually injected into the anterior chamber and the section enlarged to the full optic size.

Surgeon interest in phacoemulsification has recently been stimulated by the introduction of fold-

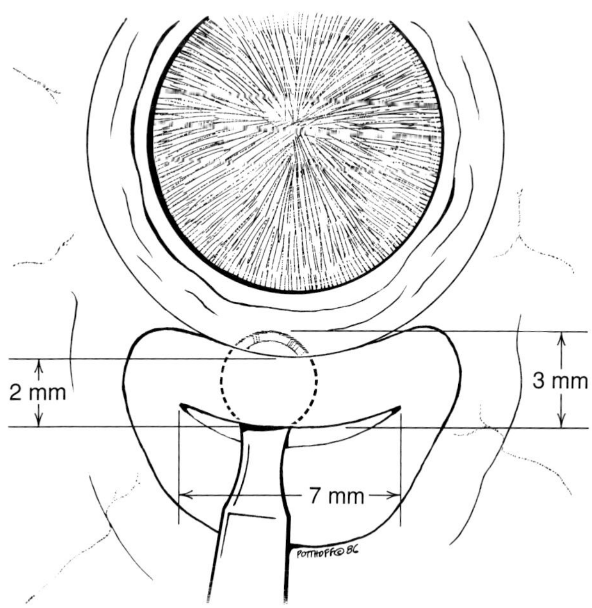

Fig. 10-2. The scleral pocket incision is made 3 mm behind the limbal arcade and 2 mm behind the limbus; it is 7 mm in length at one half scleral thickness.

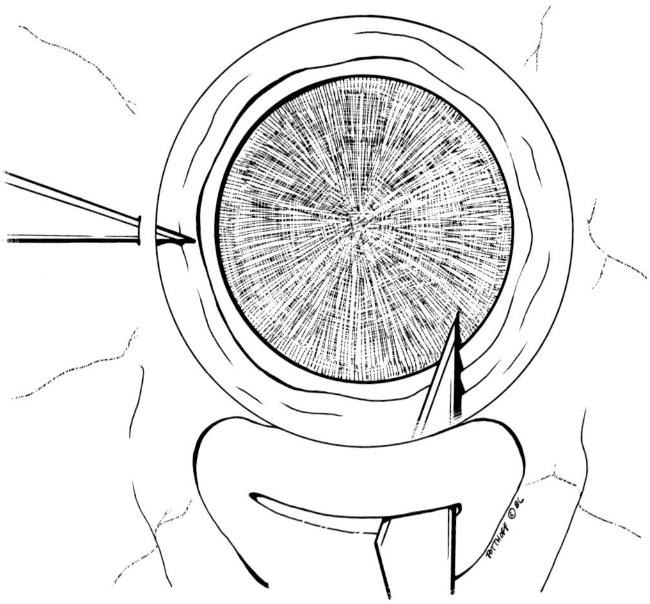

Fig. 10-3. A 0.5-mm puncture wound is made at the 3 o'clock position and a 2-mm puncture wound made at 11 o'clock.

able silicone intraocular lenses, which require only a 3-mm incision.[7] Studies are being done on a 1-mm incision to remove the cataract followed by injection of silicone into the capsular bag to produce an accommodating intraocular lens. Ophthalmic surgeons generally regard the incision size as a chord, whereas it is actually an arc. This means that intracapsular cataract extractions and extracapsular cataract extractions are large as compared with the phacoemulsification incision (Table 10-1).

ANTERIOR CAPSULOTOMY

The original "Christmas tree" capsulotomy would sometimes tear through the zonules and continue on to the posterior capsule. It has been chiefly replaced by the "can-opener" or D capsulotomy. Hara and Hara[15] recommended a superior linear capsulotomy and emulsification of the nucleus within the capsular bag.

The original irrigating cystitome was made from a 22-gauge needle and was difficult to use in a deep-set eye. This was modified to make the shape more like a cyclodialysis spatula. Some surgeons prefer to use a bent disposable needle that ensures a sharp point with each case. Dardenne et al.[3] use a Sato knife with no infusion into the anterior chamber. Clayman and Parel[16] developed a rotating cutter for the anterior capsulotomy, while Schlegel uses a mechanical needle that perforates the capsule. Mendez[17] developed an ultrasonic needle to do the capsulotomy and Kern[18] reported a cautery to incise the anterior capsule. Aron-Rosa and co-workers have done anterior capsulotomies with the Nd:YAG laser.[19,20] Actually, the entire anterior capsulotomy requires only about 30 seconds, and it is doubtful that the additional time required to set up more complex mechanical devices is fully justified.

Table 10-1. Comparison of Incision Sizes in Cataract Removal Procedures

Procedure	Chord (mm)	Arc (mm)
KPE	3.0	3.1
KPE/IOL	6.5	6.8
ECCE	10.0	13.0
ICCE	11.5	18.0

NUCLEUS REMOVAL

The original Kelman procedure called for anterior chamber nucleus emulsification preceded by nucleus subluxation. Subluxation is one of the hardest parts of the surgery for the beginning phacoemulsification surgeon. Often when repeated attempts fail, the iris is mildly traumatized and the pupil constricts making subluxation impossible. Properly performed, the technique calls for imbedding the cystitome into the nucleus; then, with a rocking motion, the nucleus is separated from the cortex. This may be done in a 6-12 or a 3-9 direction. After the loosening is accomplished, the equator of the nucleus is tilted in front of the iris so that anterior chamber emulsification may be performed. Sometimes an irrigating spatula is passed over the iris and under the nucleus like a "tire iron" to sublux the nucleus into the anterior chamber.

vitreous. This will require posterior vitrectomy and should be done before the eye becomes inflammed. If the surgeon is not comfortable with this procedure, the case should be referred to a vitreous surgeon before the media becomes cloudy, making visualization almost impossible. Postoperative increase in intraocular pressure, iritis, cystoid macular edema, and retinal detachment will be increased when vitreous loss has occurred. If the capsule is ruptured during the late stage of cortical aspiration, it is possible to instill Healon into the anterior chamber, preventing anterior chamber collapse and extension of the posterior capsular tear. Small amounts of cortex will easily be absorbed. If a posterior chamber intraocular lens is used, it should be placed in the ciliary sulcus and may be inserted over a Sheets glide to avoid herniation of vitreous into the anterior chamber. If vitreous fills the anterior chamber or is present at the incision, an anterior vitrectomy is indicated. This can be performed through the phacoemulsification incision. An intraocular lens is not contraindicated, but may have to be in the anterior chamber instead of in the posterior chamber.

POSTOPERATIVE COMPLICATIONS

Early postoperative complications such as wound leak or flat anterior chamber are rare. Microcystic edema or iritis may be present if the procedure has been difficult. The intraocular pressure may be elevated and is usually associated with incomplete removal of Healon. Postoperative use of a anhydrase inhibitor or a β-blocker may help. Hyphema is uncommon due to the small incision size. It clears promptly and as long as the posterior capsule is intact it will not get into the vitreous. Retained cortex is usually absorbed and only presents a problem if a large particle occludes the visual axis. If this occurs, it should be aspirated; otherwise a dense fibrotic membrane will develop in the visual axis. Retained nuclear chips or capsular scrolls in the anterior chamber should be removed if they contact the endothelium and begin to cause microcystic epithelial edema, otherwise the cornea may go on to complete decompensation.

The most common postoperative complication is clouding of the posterior capsule. This has been reported as occurring in as few as 6 percent and as many as 53 percent of cases followed up for 3 years. The posterior capsulotomy may be performed by a needle knife or a Nd:YAG laser.[23-25] The laser has the advantage of convenience and eliminates the possibility of endophthalmitis.

SPECIAL CASES

Marfan's syndrome usually presents a soft nucleus that may be removed with the irrigation-aspirating tip without ultrasound. If the edge of the capsule is in the visual axis, it may be necessary to remove the entire capsule as well. Hypermature lenses will release a milky fluid with the first capsular puncture, making further capsulotomy a blind procedure. It is better to aspirate the turbid anterior chamber and proceed with caution, as the anterior and posterior capsules may be in contact with each other. It is well to remember that the nucleus of a young person is very thin, and it is possible to tear both the anterior and posterior capsules with the cystitome. A small pupil and posterior synechiae with a shallow anterior chamber are common in long term narrow-angle glaucoma. Healon may be used to deepen the chamber and assist in freeing posterior synechiae. If the pupil is small, i.e., less than 3 mm, a peripheral iridectomy and an iridotomy may be used to give sufficient room for emulsification. The pupil may be reformed by prolene sutures. If a filtering bleb is present the incision may be placed to one side with preservation of bleb function. If this is impractical, the conjunctiva and Tenon's capsule may be incised posteriorly to the bleb and the entire unopened bleb dissected forward to the point it enters the sclera. The emulsification incision is placed 1 mm posterior to this and made one-half scleral thickness. It is tunnelled toward the limbus and into the bleb and anterior chamber at one-half scleral thickness. Phacoemulsification may be combined with trabeculectomy in poorly controlled glaucoma patients who have cataract.

REFERENCES

1. Kelman C: Phacoemulsification and aspiration. A new technique for cataract removal. A preliminary report. Am J Ophthalmol 64:23, 1967
2. Thrasher B, Keller D: Extracapsular cataract extraction, phacoemulsification and posterior chamber intraocular lens implantation. p. 255. In Cataract and Intraocular Lens Surgery. Aesculapius, Birmingham, AL, 1984
3. Ohrloff C, Dardenne K, Konen C, Sherif A: Erfahrungen mit den erstern 1.400 Hinterkammerlinsen-implantationen nach Phakoemulsifikation. Klin Mbl Augenheilkd 181:253, 1982
4. Davison JA: Modified J-loop intraocular lens insertion after posterior chamber iris-plane phacoemulsification: A safe, easy method. Am Intraocul Implant Soc J 7(4):368, 1981
5. Cozean CH Jr, Waltman SR: The effects of posterior chamber phacoemulsification and secondary Kelman anterior chamber lens implantation on the corneal endothelium. Am Intraocul Implant Soc J 7(3):237, 1981
6. Johnson SH: Emulsification of the nucleus: The Bimanual technique. p. 55. Cataract Surgery. McGraw-Hill, New York, 1986
7. Mazzocco T: Update: Silicone compressible intraocular lens. Presented at Contact Lens Association of Ophthalmology, January 1984
8. Honan PR: New safety valve for Honan balloon. Am Intraocular Implant Soc J 8(2):163, 1982
9. Davidson B, Kratz RP, Mazzocco TR, Maloney WF: An evaluation of the Honan intraocular pressure reducer. Am Intraocul Implant Soc J 5:237, 1979
10. Honan P: Preoperative reduction of intraocular pressure. p. 101. In Cataract and Intraocular Lens Surgery. Aesculapius, Birmingham, AL, 1984
11. Varosmarty D: Okulopressor, ein instrument zur erzeugung intraoculorer-hypotenie. Klin Monatsbl Augenheilkd 151:376, 1967
12. Gills JP: Constant mild compression of the eye to produce hypotension. Am Intraocul Implant Soc J 5:52, 1979
13. Terry CM: Incision and wound closure to reduce astigmatism. p. 134. In Cataract Surgery. McGraw-Hill, New York, 1986
14. Colvard DM, Kratz RP, Mazzocco TR, Davidson B: The Terry surgical keratometer: A 12 month follow-up report. Am Intraocul Implant Soc J 7:348, 1981
15. Hara T, Hara T: Subcapsular phacoemulsification and aspiration. Am Intraocul Implant Soc J 10(3):333, 1984
16. Clayman HM, Parel J: The capsule coupeur for automated anterior capsulectomy. Am Intraocul Implant Soc J 10(4):480, 1984
17. Mendez A: Anterior capsulotomy with ultrasound cystotome. Am Intraocul Implant Soc J 10:363, 1984
18. Kern R: Anterior capsulotomy by Diathermy. Presented at the Fourth Meeting of the European Intraocular Implantlens Council, Cannes, France, October 1985
19. Aron-Rosa D: Use of a pulsed neodymium-YAG laser for anterior capsulotomy. Am Intraocul Implant Soc J 7(4):332, 1981
20. Aron-Rosa D, Aron J, Cohn HC: Use of a pulsed picosecond Nd:YAG laser in 6,664 cases. Am Intraocul Implant Soc J 10(1):35, 1984
21. Johnson S, Kratz R: A simple device to augment irrigation and aspiration. AIOIS J 8:168, 1982
22. Terry CM: Introduction to a surgical keratometer. p. 27. In Emery JM, Jacobson AC (eds): Current Concepts in Cataract Surgery: Selected Proceedings of the Sixth Biennial Cataract Surgical Congress. CV Mosby, St. Louis, 1980
23. Lewicky A, et al: Six percent incidence of secondary posterior capsule opacification using the extracapsular technique in 100 intraocular lenses. p. 536. In Current Concepts in Cataract Surgery. CV Mosby, St. Louis, 1978
24. Knolle G Jr: Management of the posterior capsule. In Cataract and Intraocular Lens Surgery. Aesculapius, Birmingham, AL, 1984
25. Kratz, R: Clean posterior capsule. p. 118. In Current Concepts in Cataract Surgery. CV Mosby, St. Louis, 1978

Intracapsular Cataract Extraction with Intraocular Lenses

11

Jerald L. Tennant

PATIENT EDUCATION

Cataract surgery should begin with the education of the patient. Many of the problems encountered during and after surgery can be traced to patients' lack of understanding of what is expected of them. The education process begins when the patient first contacts your office. The telephone receptionist must respond to the patient with consideration and must accommodate the anxiety of the patient who is already worried that surgery must be performed.

Upon arrival to the office, a spirit of cooperation and trust must be initiated. An environment must be created in which the patient is made to feel important. Only after patients begin to feel comfortable about the physician and staff will they be able to concentrate on the cataract operation itself and the important role played by the patient in the overall success of the surgical event.

Next, one should consider the use of videotapes and written booklets to explain the nature of cataracts, when surgery should occur, what complications can occur, and what it will cost the patient in both money and effort. It is very important that the complications be discussed in lay terms. It is of little value to discuss the incidence of "expulsive hemorrhage." One must discuss the "loss of the eye due to uncontrollable bleeding" or similar terms that an elderly patient can comprehend.

There is currently consideration in Congress to make it a felony for a physician to involve a Medicare patient in any care or to order any treatment without first discussing the cost with the patient. There should be no need for such a law. Physicians should give their patients written estimates of the total and out-of-pocket costs. None of us likes to be committed to any expense without knowing if we can afford it, even if we need it.

PREPARATION IN SURGERY

The evaluation of macular function and of intraocular lens (IOL) calculation is beyond the scope of this chapter. After it is determined that surgery should be performed, a complete history and physical examination should be done. Special attention should be given to the control of hypertension and to any tendency toward bleeding. We have had more trouble with bleeding during the surgery than with systemic organ system dysfunction. Patients on anticoagulants, including aspirin or other antiprostaglandins, should be considered at additional risk for troublesome bleeding during surgery.

Since outpatient eye surgery has been found to be safe and 46 percent less expensive than inpatient surgery, most eye surgery in this country will soon be performed as outpatient surgery. This will encourage the use of local anesthesia.

LOCATION OF SURGERY

According to a study by the Department of Health and Human Services, the most common Medicare diagnosis in 1983 was cataract extraction. In each state surveyed, it accounted for about 15 percent of Medicare surgeries. The average hospital stay was about 3 days.

Another interesting event to occur, in 1984, was the refusal of Medicare to pay for cataract surgery performed in the hospital because it could have been performed in an outpatient setting. Clearly most cataract surgery in the future in the United States will be performed in an ambulatory surgery center. We have performed 99 percent of cataract surgery in an outpatient setting since 1976. Of 4,500 such patients, only five have required hospitalization:

1. Development of bigeminy; admitted for medical control
2. Development of bigeminy; admitted for medical control
3. Development of abdominal pain after surgery, admitted for evaluation; no abnormality identified
4. Expulsive hemorrhage in uniocular patient admitted for pain control and psychological support
5. Asthmatic attack precipitated by timolol

SEDATION OF THE PATIENT

We do not give the patient any sedation prior to arrival at the surgicenter. When outpatient surgery is to be performed, the patient should receive medication and undergo the recovery process beforehand. After recovering from the medications given, the patient is taken to surgery. In addition, it is important to use short-acting medications, which will be worn off before the patient is expected to go home.

We have used the narcotic fentanyl (Sublimaze) for outpatient cataract surgery. Although the half-life of Demerol is not the same as that of fentanyl, comparable active drug levels of fentanyl to meperidine can be determined (Table 11-1). With a half-life of 30 minutes, the patient goes home with an active drug level of fentanyl comparable to 2.5 mg meperidine, which will not adversely affect the thinking or mobility of most patients. Since fentanyl is given in a dosage that is unfamiliar to most surgeons, the equivalent dosage of meperidine (Demerol) has been used here for understanding. The surgeon should remember that 0.1 mg (2 cc) of fentanyl is equal to 75 mg of Demerol.

We have noted that an occasional patient will have muscular rigidity with fentanyl. Our anesthesiologist, Dr. Wayne Hellman, discovered that 1 mg of Valium given intravenously before admin-

Table 11-1. Comparison of Active Drug Levels (Fentanyl to Meperidine)

Injection Time (min)	Fentanyl/Meperidine Level (mg)	Stage of Surgery
	0.03/20.0	Injection prior to surgery
+30	0.015/10.0	Completion of orbital compression
+30	0.0075/5.0	Completion of surgery
+30	0.00375/2.5	Completion of postoperative care
		Observation and departure

istration of fentanyl prevents this troublesome side effect.

Complications of Sedation

The most frequent problem encountered is oversedation of the patient. It is important that patients not fall asleep during the surgery. If they do, they will often awaken with a start and try to get up. If they stay alert during the surgery, this never occurs. In addition, it is common for surgeons and anesthesiologists to overmedicate patients. The use of such drugs as barbiturates and long-acting tranquilizers will not wear off in time for the patient to safely go home.

The use of nitrous oxide was promoted for cataract surgery by Corboy[1] at the last Outpatient Ophthalmic Surgical Society meeting. We have found N_2O very useful in younger patients. However, older patients have a tendency to become confused and to develop abdominal distention with N_2O. We therefore prefer the Valium–fentanyl regimen in older patients and to reserve the N_2O for the patients under 50 years of age.

RETROBULBAR BLOCK

It is preferable to use a long-acting anesthetic for eye surgery. The principal ones available are bupivacaine (Marcaine) and etidocaine (Duranest). We have found Marcaine to give more predictable and profound blocks than Duranest. We therefore use Marcaine 0.5 percent for our blocks.

Since all the nerves desired to be blocked exit through the superior orbital fissure, we prefer to place a 25-gauge needle into the posterior orbit when injecting Marcaine. We try to avoid entering Tenon's capsule. Placement of about 3 ml Marcaine into the posterior orbit is followed by application of the Super-Pinkie. This causes the anesthetic to diffuse throughout the orbit, giving a profound and predictable block in most cases. Usually even the orbicularis oculi is blocked, eliminating the need for a lid block (Fig. 11-1).

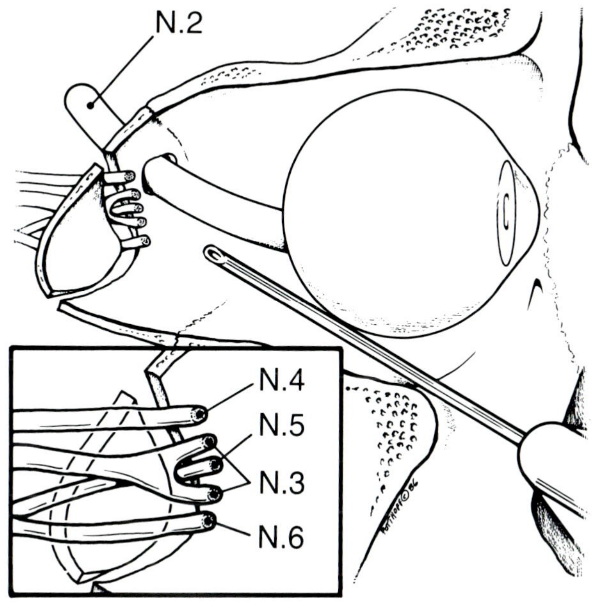

Fig. 11-1. The nerves that need to be blocked pass through the superior orbital fissure.

Complications of Retrobulbar Block

Gills and Loyd[2] recommended that the block be performed per conjunctiva rather than per cutaneous. It is true that it is easier to be sure that one is inside the cone with the per conjunctival approach, but we have had severe complications using this approach. Gills and Loyd recommend injecting 3 to 5 ml Marcaine into the cone, but have found a 10 percent incidence of respiratory arrest using this technique. The patients were artificially supported and their breathing returned in about 30 minutes. It was evident from the associated neurologic defects that accompanied the respiratory arrests that the Marcaine was intracranial.

From cadaver measurements, we determined that the average volume of the cone is 1.6 ml. Thus if one is injecting 3 to 5 ml into a 1.6-ml space, the anesthetic fluid must go someplace outside the cone.

Studies performed during the time it was popular to inject dye into the orbital veins to look for orbital tumors revealed that this dye would sometimes enter the subarachnoid space via the optic nerve sheath.[2] These studies confirmed the existence of a potential space around the optic nerve into the brain. We therefore postulate that injection of 3 to 5 ml Marcaine into the cone will force the material to enter the subarachnoid space when Tenon's capsule is strong and intact. We suspect that in the 90 percent of cases that do not go into respiratory arrest with this technique, the Tenon's capsule is weak and allows the anesthetic to leak into the orbit before the potential space into the subarachnoid space is blown open.

Lawton Smith[3] wrote of the problems with respiratory arrest with Marcaine, and the use of this material was restricted at Bascom Palmer because of respiratory arrests. However, we have not had a single respiratory arrest with Marcaine in more than 3,000 cases, except when using the intraconal injection recommended by Gills and Loyd. We therefore believe it is not the drug per se that is at fault but the method and volume of injection that is responsible for the respiratory arrests. If one insists on injecting into the cone, the volume injected should be restricted to 1.5 ml.

One of the complications that can occur with the injection of the retrobulbar block is to penetrate the eyeball with the needle. In the days where we were trying to place the injection into the cone, we penetrated two eyes with the needle. I was taught that injection of the anesthetic into the eye would be recognized when the cornea turned white during the injection and that the retina and endothelium would likely be destroyed by the injection. This did not happen in my cases. Instead, the accident was not identified until I began the surgery. The eyes were mushy soft with almost zero pressure. It was very difficult to make the groove for the incision, but the surgery went well otherwise. However, at the end of surgery, it was impossible to keep the eye at normal pressure. Injection of fluid into the anterior chamber simply caused the eye to inflate; then it would run out the scleral hole, leaving the eye soft again. Postoperatively, the eyes gradually became normotensive. One could see the site of scleral and retinal penetration. However, no therapy was needed. The holes pigmented themselves as if cryotherapy had been applied, and retinal detachment did not occur. In one case, penetration was just below the macula. The pigmentation was just below the macula and caused macular distortion with 20/200 vision. The other case was more peripheral and did not affect the acuity at all. Obviously, the recommended technique of trying to inject outside the cone eliminates this complication.

Since respiratory arrest and drug reactions can occur, it is important that the person giving the block be skilled at endotracheal intubation and have the necessary instrumentation available and in working order (have you checked the batteries in your intubation scope lately?)

Retrobulbar hemorrhage used to be a feared complication of retrobulbar injection. It does indeed occur. However, the Super-Pinkie has made this occurrence a very manageable problem. Quick application of the Super-Pinkie when a hemorrhage is recognized will stop the bleeding and proceed to decompress the orbit. We have not had to cancel a case for retrobulbar hemorrhage since we began using the Super-Pinkie.

ANTIBIOTICS

It is a curious thing that ophthalmologists tend to give their prophylactic antibiotics after surgery when it is well known that antibiotics need to be

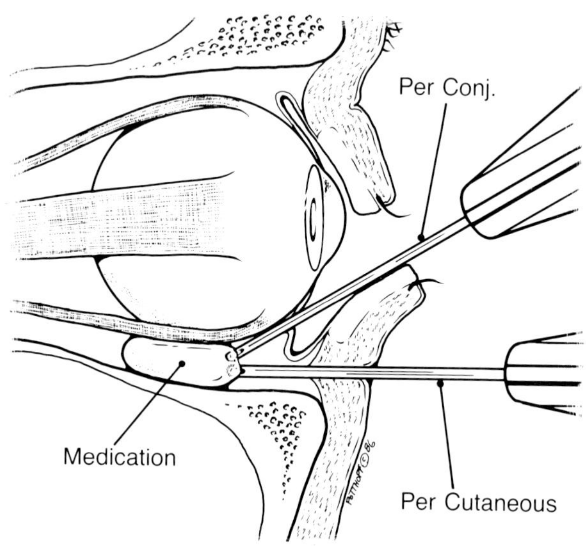

Fig. 11-2. The location of medication after per cutaneous injection and per conjunctival injection is the same.

present at the time bacteria are introduced if they are to be effective. In addition, it is the habit of most ophthalmologists to place the antibiotics and steroids under the conjunctiva by the per conjunctiva route. It should be recognized that placement by the per cutaneous route puts the medication at the same ultimate site without the irritation and scarring caused by placing the medication under the conjunctiva (Fig. 11-2).

It has been shown that 1 cc Garamycin given percutaneously gives cidal doses in the aqueous in 15 minutes.[4] We therefore inject this into the inferior orbit after the retrobulbar injection.

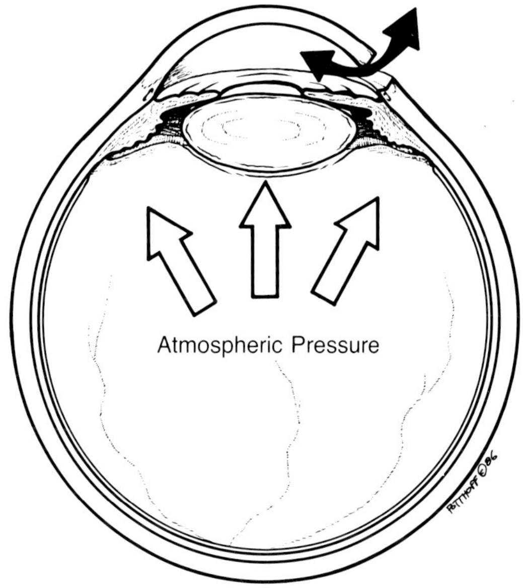

Fig. 11-3. When the eye is surgically opened, it assumes atmospheric pressure.

PREVENTION OF VITREOUS LOSS

The traditional teaching in ophthalmology has been to treat the symptom of a forward movement of the vitreous by using various chemicals to shrink the volume of the vitreous body. It should be realized, however, that there is no such thing as positive vitreous pressure—there is only positive pressure on the vitreous. When one approaches the subject in this manner, one begins to understand and better control the forward displacement of vitreous.

It is also important to realize that the eye goes to atmospheric pressure as soon as the eye is opened. Certainly such agents as Diamox, glycerin, mannitol, and urea, reduce the volume of the vitreous, but they cannot approach bringing the eye to atmospheric pressure without killing the patient. Thus their use only treats the symptom but not the cause of positive pressure on the vitreous (Fig. 11-3).

Extraocular and intraocular events can press on the vitreous. Extraocular causes include (1) pressure from lid speculum, (2) retrobulbar hemorrhage, (3) medications injected into the orbit, and (4) orbital fat and vascularity.

Note that the last three causes force the globe to be pressed forward. The insertions of Tenon's capsule through the muscle insertions into the sclera form a ring around the globe. In addition, the thinnest part of the sclera is beneath the muscles. Thus, anything that pushes the eye forward causes the muscles to become tight bands against the thin sclera. This presses in turn on the vitreous, tending to press the vitreous out of the eye. Decompressing the orbit to decrease orbital volume and retroplace the globe releaves this pressure of the muscle against the globe and reduces pressure on the vitreous (Fig. 11-4).

Vörösmarthy of Hungary[5] was the first to develop an orbital decompressor. However, his work went unnoticed in this country for years. The first to develop an orbital decompression unit in this country was the nurse who worked with Gills.[6] She suggested that a toy ball sold under the name Super-Pinkie be applied to the orbit to soften the eye. A rubber drain was passed through the center of the ball and clamped around the patient's head to create pressure on the orbit. Tennant[7] learned the technique from Gills and wrote the first paper on the subject. Honan[8] then developed an apparatus almost identical to that of Vörösmarthy, in which a balloon is applied to the eye by a rubber strap and inflated with a gauge similar to a symphgmomanometer.

The main concern all of us have had with these devices was the theoretical possibility of central artery or vein occlusion. However, these devices have now been used in hundreds of thousands of

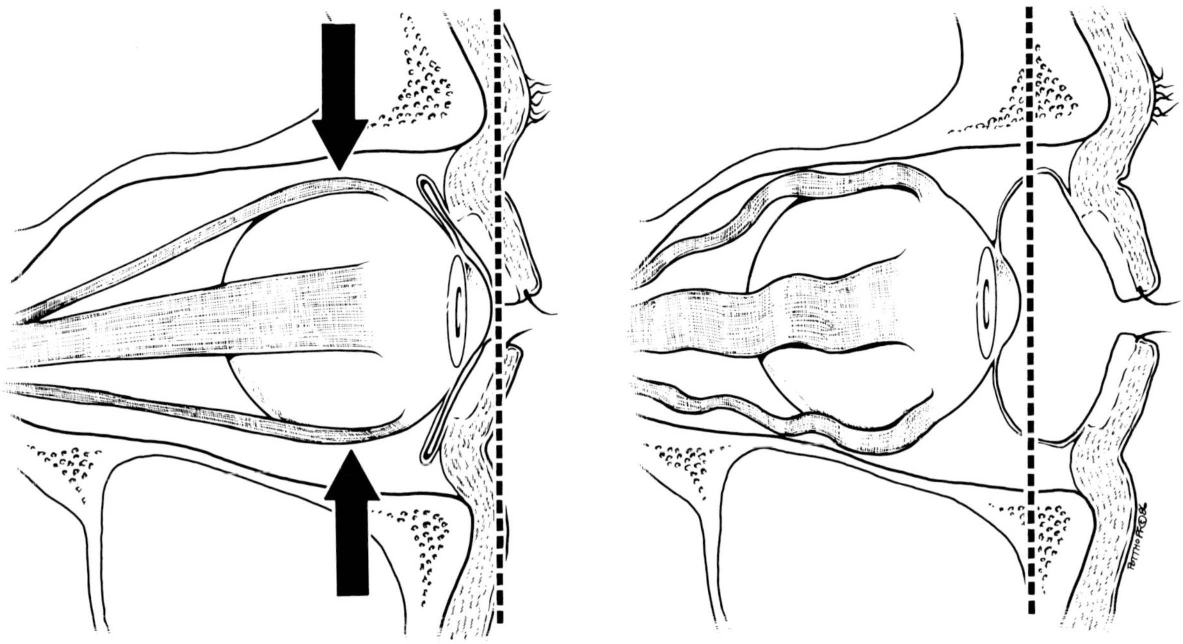

Fig. 11-4. Pressing on the orbit with a sphere decompresses it.

operations, and it is clear that the incidence of vascular occlusion is no greater than the reported incidence when the devices are not used.

Anecdotally, there have been reports of choroidal wipeout after the use of pressure devices; however, it is not known how high a pressure caused the problem (Figs. 11-5, 11-6).

We studied the vitreous loss when we used Diamox and glycerin and compared that with the vitreous loss when these drugs were abandoned and only the Super-Pinkie was used. We found that our incidence of vitreous loss was 14 in 200 (7 percent) when Diamox and glycerin was used and 18 of 716 (3 percent) when only the Super-Pinkie was used. The chi-square value of these numbers is 0.0028 showing that this was statistically very significant. Thus, treating the symptom of vitreous pressure with Diamox and so forth is much less effective than treating the cause of vitreous pressure with orbital decompression using the Super-Pinkie.

It is possible to have intraocular as well as extraocular causes of vitreous loss. The intraocular causes are bleeding and fluid blockage; the fluid blockage is either at the trabeculum, the pupil, or the ciliary processes. Intraocular pressure (IOP) should be measured immediately before surgery is

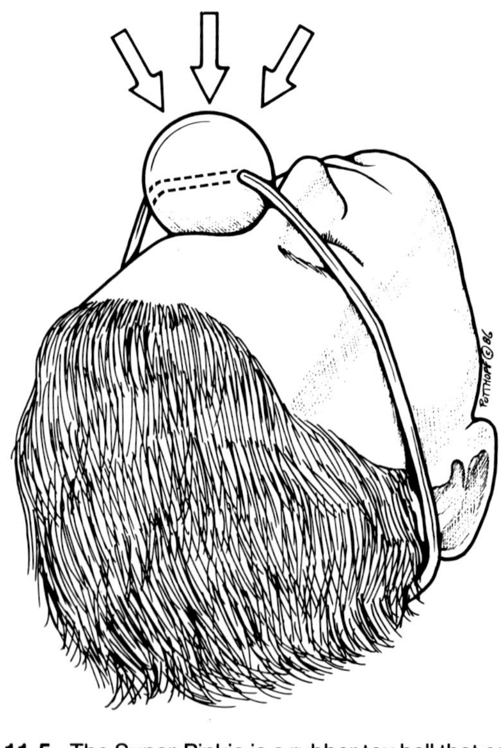

Fig. 11-5. The Super-Pinkie is a rubber toy ball that can be used to decompress the orbit.

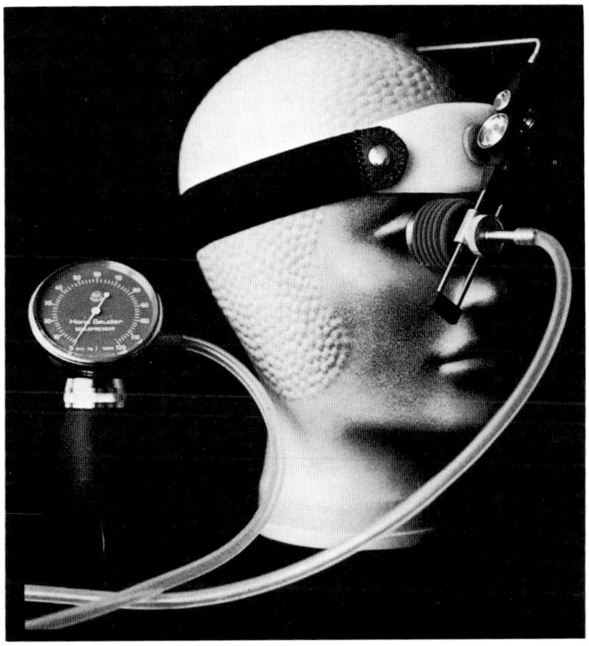

Fig. 11-6. The balloons designed by Vörösmarthy and Honan press on the eye after being inflated. (Photo printed with permission, International Ophthalmic Industries Corp.; Weston, MA; USA agent for Hans Geuder Instruments and Systems, West Germany.)

begun. If the eye is 5 Schiotz units or less, the eye is abnormally hard. Before the eye is opened, sclerotomies are made at the 10 and 2 o'clock positions, about 3 to 5 mm behind the limbus. If blood is present, the diagnosis is obvious. If no blood is present, the cause is fluid blockage or the bleeding is at the bottom of the eye, where it cannot exit these sclerotomies. To differentiate between these two, 0.1 ml liquid vitreous is aspirated with a 30-gauge needle through one of these sclerotomies. This volume will cause the eye to become very soft. After waiting about 60 seconds, if bleeding is present, the eye will be observed to have become very hard again. Two more sclerotomies must then be made at the 5 and 7 o'clock positions to provide exit ports for the blood. The sclerotomy sites should be cauterized to shrink the lips of the incisions so that they will stay open to allow the blood easy egress. If the eye does not become hard, it means that a fluid blockage was present and corrected by the fluid aspiration.

Complications from the Prevention of Vitreous Loss

When I was a resident, I saw a patient regurgitate glycerin, aspirate it, and develop severe pneumonia. In addition, I saw a patient develop a cerebrovascular accident after repeated administration of glycerin. I have also seen many patients develop renal stones and lassitude from Diamox as well as rashes and nausea from single dosage. It is therefore pleasing to realize that these drugs are no longer necessary or desirable with orbital decompression.

The only complication we saw from the Super-Pinkie occurred when we failed to understand its true function and were trying to soften the globe with it instead of using it to achieve orbital decompression. In a few cases, we placed folded gauze beneath the ball to place more pressure on the globe, with undesirable results. First, necrosis of the skin of the upper lid occurred with severe lid edema and sloughing of the skin, about the size of a dime. In addition, most of these patients had suprachoroidal bleeding requiring sclerotomies during surgery. It is important to remember that the Super-Pinkie is only intended to give orbital decompression and that the ball should rest on the orbital rim as the globe is retroplaced. Continuous pressure on the globe is undesirable.

The disadvantage of the Honan (Vörösmarthy) balloon is that it is designed to enter the orbit and place continuous pressure on the globe. If a pressure level above the recommended 30 mmHg is used, choroidal wipeout is possible. We have modified the balloon so that it is the same diameter as the Super-Pinkie. This prevents the undesirable complication of continuous high pressure on the globe.

POSITIONING THE PATIENT FOR SURGERY

It has been traditionally taught that the patient's head should be higher than the heart to prevent an increase in venous pressure, causing vascular en-

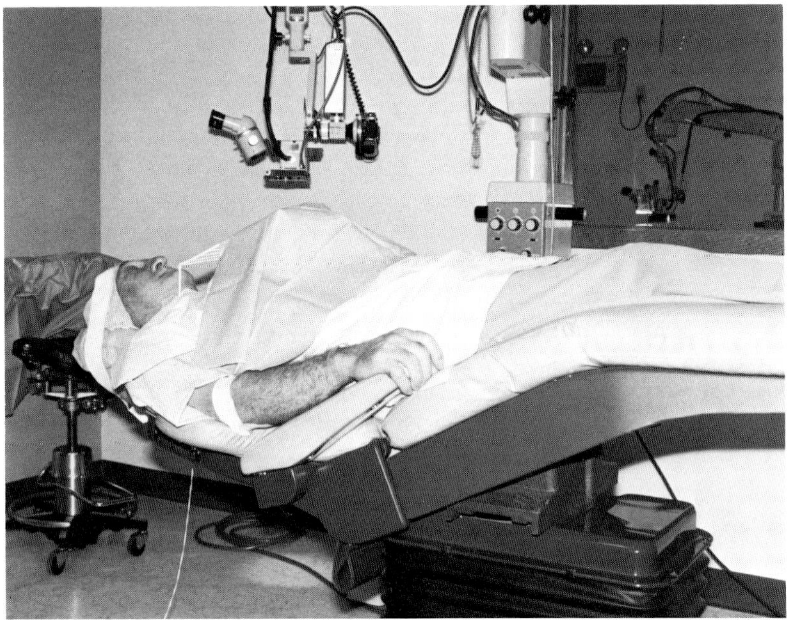

Fig. 11-7. The patient should be positioned so that both the legs and the head are higher than the heart.

gorgement in the choroid. Since we used a flat table, this meant that the patient's feet were lower than the heart, causing the patient to be restless due to stasis in the legs. The decrease in blood return to the heart can be significant. Thus, the proper position for patients undergoing eye surgery is with the head and the feet higher than the heart. This prevents the undesired effects in the eye and promotes adequate circulation. The heart and the lungs are the pressure-control mechanisms that prevent elevation of the legs from affecting eye pressure. This position can easily be accomplished with a dental chair. It can also be accomplished on a flat table by placing several pillows under the patient's legs.

It is desirable for the orbit to be parallel with the floor. Patients have a tendency for the chin to be lower than the forehead. This position makes the surgeon constantly work over the elevation of the superior orbital rim. This makes the entire operation more difficult and reduces the red reflex. Thus, one should place the orbital rims parallel with the floor and use 2-inch tape to secure the patient's head in this position.

It has also been traditional in ophthalmology to pipe oxygen under the drapes during local anesthesia. However, the oxygen has exploded as the cautery is used, severely burning many patients. Room air is quite satisfactory when the patient has not been oversedated. A convenient method of elevating the drape to allow exchange of air is shown in Figure 11-7.

PREVENTION OF INFECTION

Because endophthalmitis is such a disaster (see Chapter 5), a lot of theoretically beneficial events traditionally take place to prevent infection. This is not in keeping with what is known about eye surgery, especially under third-world conditions. Thousands of cataracts have even been removed in open-air theaters with no appreciable infection. Almost none of the European ophthalmologists wear gloves during surgery. Most cases of endophthalmitis are caused by organisms carried by patients themselves, and it is almost impossible to cause intraocular infection after the first 24 hours, even with innoculation of virulent bacteria into the cul-de-sac. Nevertheless, many of us are forced by hospital and Medicare policy to continue the rituals that have been dictated because someone thought it was a good idea.

We have allowed patients to wear their street clothes for the past 3,000 surgeries. A disposable cap, gown, and shoe covers are used. Patients walk into surgery, sit on the operating table, have the surgery, walk to the lounge, have a sandwich, and walk to their cars. We have had one endophthalmitis in those 3,000 cases. In that case, the organism was cultured from the patient's lids and nasopharynx. That particular organism was sensitive to the antibiotics we used; however, since they were not started until 24 hours postoperatively, the dosage was inadequate. We therefore begin the antibiotics immediately after surgery and give them hourly for the first day after surgery.

SELECTION OF AN EYELID SPECULUM

The use of the wire lid speculae, such as the Barraquer speculum, has become popular in the last few years because it permits placement of the needles of the phakoemulsifier or the other I and A instruments between the wires. However, this speculum does not work well with a globe that is markedly retroplaced from the Super Pinkie, as the lids are too relaxed to permit adequate tension to be placed on them by the wire speculum. We therefore prefer the Smirmaul lid speculum when the Super-Pinkie is used.

PLACEMENT OF THE BRIDLE SUTURE

It is important to have a good bridle suture, particularly if an IOL is to be used. The ability to position the eye properly during the insertion is dependent on a good bridle suture. If it will be difficult to rotate the eye easily, the suture should be replaced until it functions satisfactorily.

Complications Associated with the Bridle Suture

It is possible to place the needle through the sclera unless care is taken. Some believe that a round needle instead of a cutting needle helps prevent this complication. The Tennant Bridle Suture Forceps (Storz) helps in placement of the suture.

Occasionally, a hematoma will develop after placement of the suture. If this occurs, the conjunctiva should be quickly incised over the hematoma so the blood can exit. Otherwise, the blood will dissect to the limbus and interfere with visualization throughout surgery.

MAKING THE CONJUNCTIVAL FLAP

I prefer to make a fornix-based flap. The conjunctiva is grasped with the 0.3 Girard forceps at the 10 o'clock position. Blunt Wescott scissors are used to make a radial cut at this location. The scissors are placed under the conjunctiva for blunt dissection. The scissors are then pressed to the limbal attachment and used to cut the conjunctiva from its insertion. When the 2 o'clock area is reached, another radial cut is made to relax the conjunctiva and produce a flap that can be pulled over the incision at the end of the procedure (Fig. 11-8).

Complications of Making the Conjunctival Flap

If the scissors are not placed firmly at the insertion of the conjunctiva before the cut is made, the flap will be dog-eared. Should this occur, a rounded knife blade, such as Beaver #64, can be used to remove the "dog ears" from the limbus.

Some surgeons prefer to use a knife blade to make the conjunctival flap. However, I have seen novice surgeons penetrate the globe with this maneuver. Care is indicated if one elects to make the flap with a sharp knife.

Buttonholing the flap is a common complication when the conjunctiva is pulled with forceps while

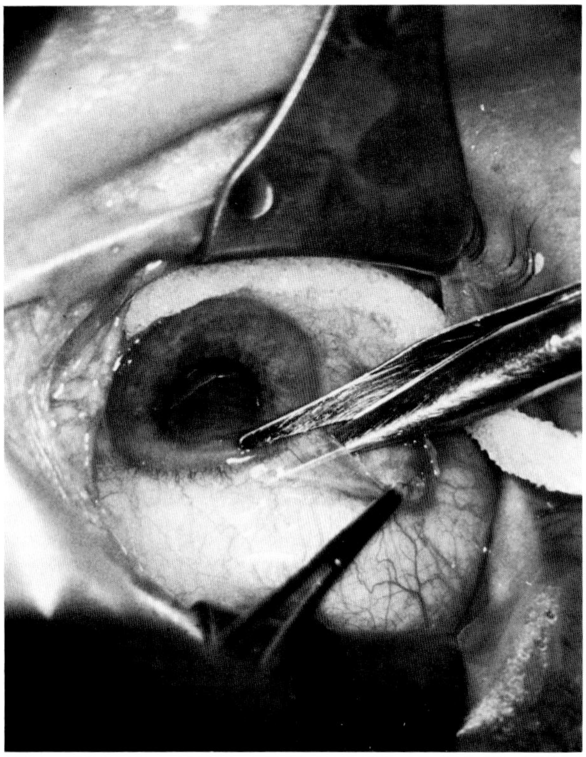

Fig. 11-8. The conjunctival flap is made at the limbus.

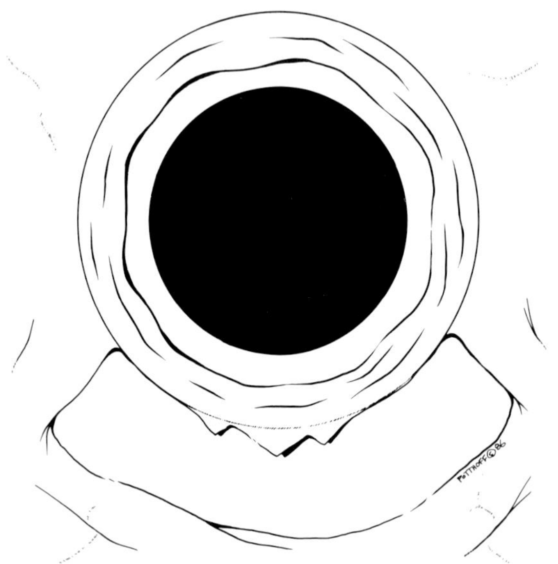

Fig. 11-9. The conjunctival flap becomes dog-eared if the scissors are not pressed tightly into the crotch of the last incision.

dissecting with a knife. It is more common with a limbus-based flap than with a fornix-based flap. It is a rare occurrence when the flap is developed as described above. Some buttonholes can simply be ignored; very large ones require suturing (Fig. 11-9).

MAKING THE INCISION

There are two very good reasons one should make a three-plane incision. First, this self-sealing incision makes control of the operation much easier, since any increase in IOP tends to cause the incision to close and seal. In addition, such an incision allows the tissue to slide, so that adjustment of the astigmatism is possible.

We prefer to make the groove with the guarded Neumann radial keratotomy diamond knife set at

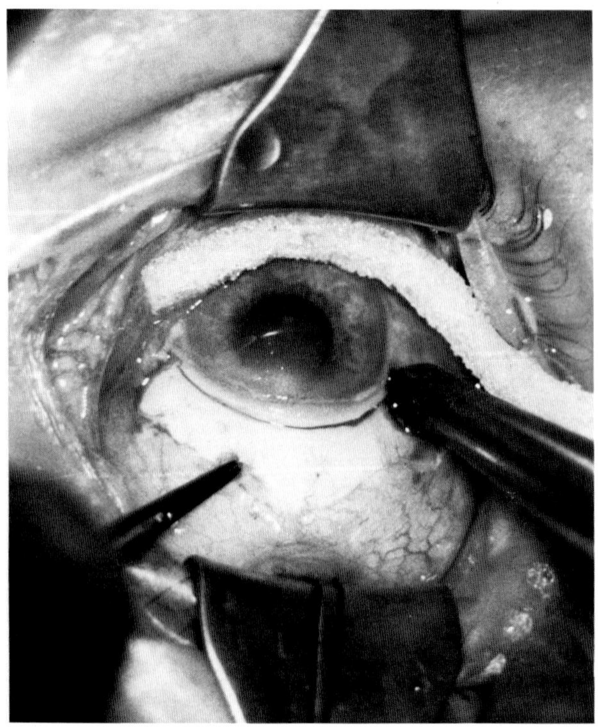

Fig. 11-10. The groove is made behind the limbus with the radial keratotomy knife set at 400 μm.

400 μm. The bevel is then formed with the round Greishaber blade. The cornea is lifted slightly with the Tennant Corneoscleral Forceps (Storz). A white band can be visualized. The rounded blade is placed just under the band about 1 cm from the right end of the incision. The blade is pushed away from the operator to the end of the incision. Now the blade is pulled toward the operator, who begins to make the bevel for the rest of the incision, moving toward the left. As this maneuver is carried out, the knife is lifted slightly toward the ceiling to hug the bottom of the white band, in order to stay within this space and not penetrate deeper into the globe. When the left end of the incision is reached, there will be a smooth bevel, about 2 to 3 mm in width. If it is not this wide, the rounded blade should be used to dissect until this wide bevel is achieved.

Safety sutures of 7-0 black silk are placed at the 2, 12, and 10 o'clock positions. These sutures should be radial, as they will position the wound for final closure and will dictate whether rotational and oblique astigmatism occurs.

The anterior chamber is entered using a razor-blade to enter at the central portion of the bevel. The scissors are then used to complete the section. The scissors are positioned to create a bevel 2 to 3 mm in width (Figs. 11-10, 11-11, 11-12, and 11-13).

Complications of Making the Incision

It is generally assumed that the sclera is about 1 mm thick at the limbus. However, if the R-K knife is set at 500 μm, penetration will occur in most

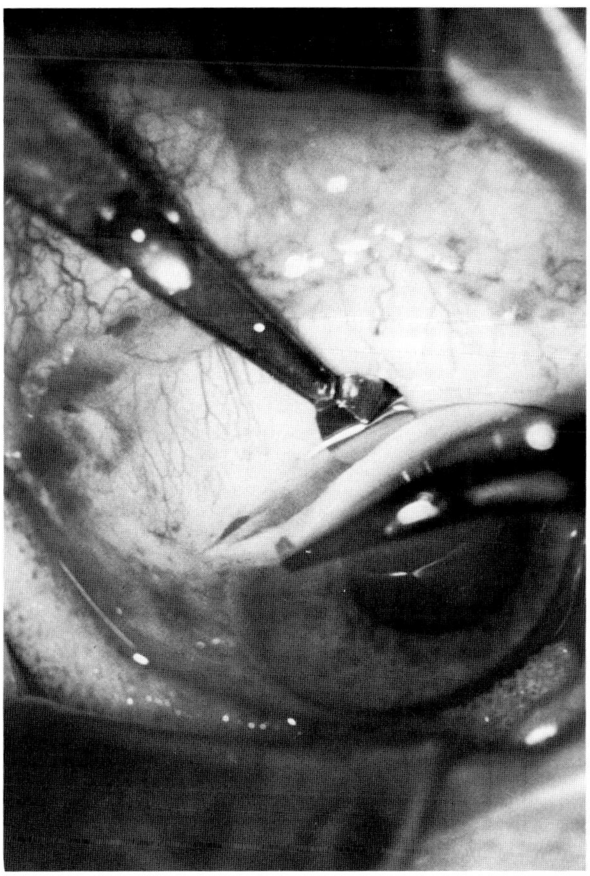

Fig. 11-11. The bevel is made about 2 mm into the cornea with the Grieshaber blade.

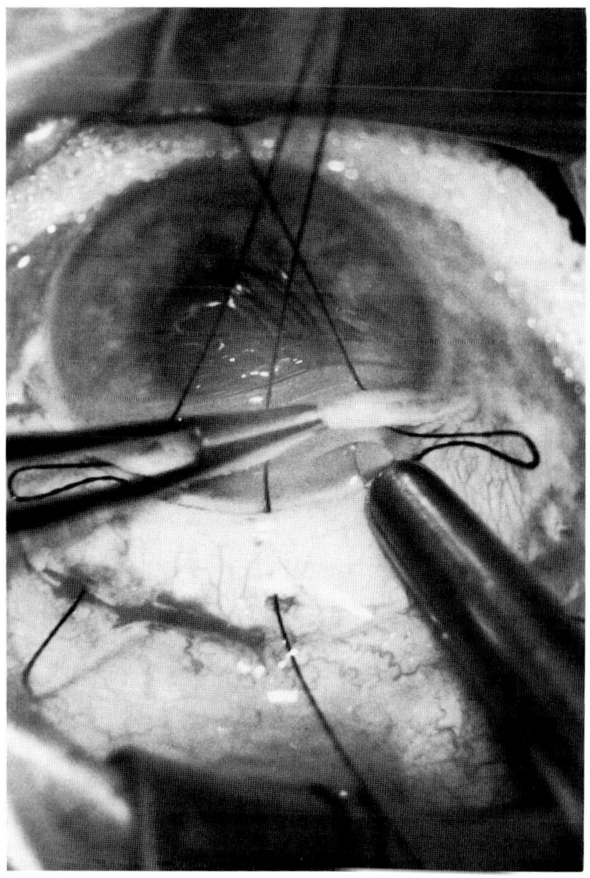

Fig. 11-12. The anterior chamber is entered with a 30 to 45 degree blade.

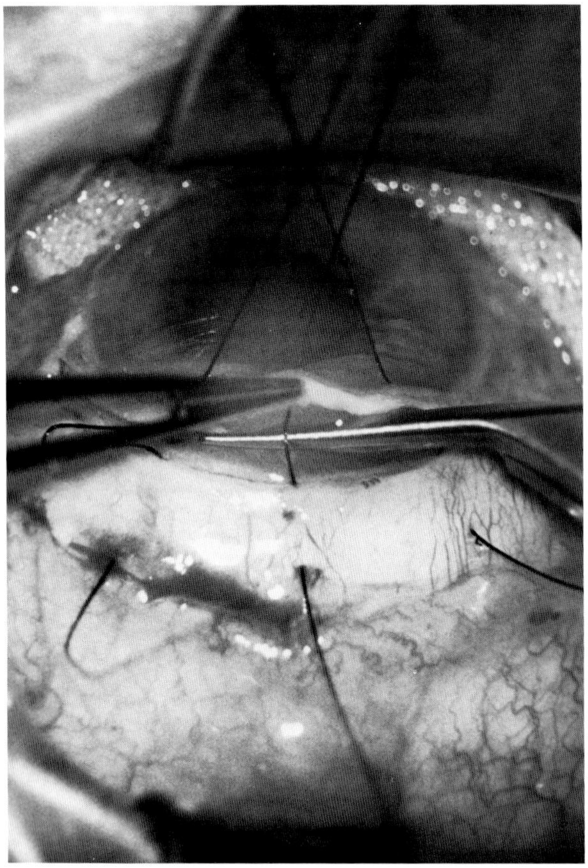

Fig. 11-13. The incision is opened with corneoscleral scissors.

cases. It was found by trial and error that 400 μm is a level that will not cause penetrations. Apparently the sclera is thinner at the limbus in cataract patients than in younger patients.

I have attempted to use diamond and ruby knives to make the bevel. However, these knives are too sharp for this job and tend to pass out of the dissection plane. Inadvertent penetrations are common. We have therefore returned to the Grieshaber blade for this purpose. We prefer the Grieshaber blade over other models because its fiber handle allows the use of acetone sterilization, whereas plastic-handled blades do not. The diamond knife and the Grieshaber blade are sterilized in acetone awaiting use in the next case.

Inadvertant penetration often causes localized bleeding and loss of the self-sealing aspect of the wound. Obvious points of bleeding must be cauterized. It is often necessary to place an additional 7-0 silk suture at the site of the penetration to ensure hemostasis and stop wound leakage (Fig. 11-14).

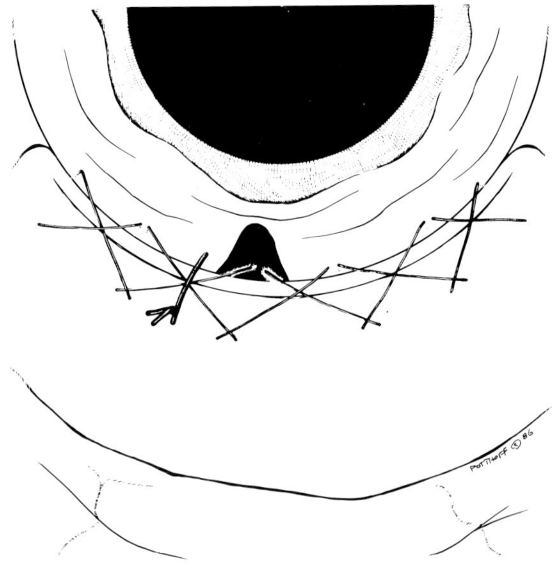

Fig. 11-14. An inadvertent penetration causing leaking of the wound can be closed with 7-0 silk.

PLACEMENT OF α-CHYMOTRYPSIN

We use α-chymotrypsin in all intracapsular cases. We tried previously to identify an age above which it was not necessary but found that some patients in their 80s still had very strong zonules. We therefore believe it is best to use α-chymotrypsin in all cases. The medication should be injected under the iris, using a blunt 30-gauge air cannula. This can be accomplished with the wound closed. This technique prevents damage to the endothelium (Fig. 11-15).

Complications with α-Chymotrypsin

Many surgeons were taught to use an olive-tipped needle to place the α-chymotrypsin under the iris. This was appropriate before microscopes

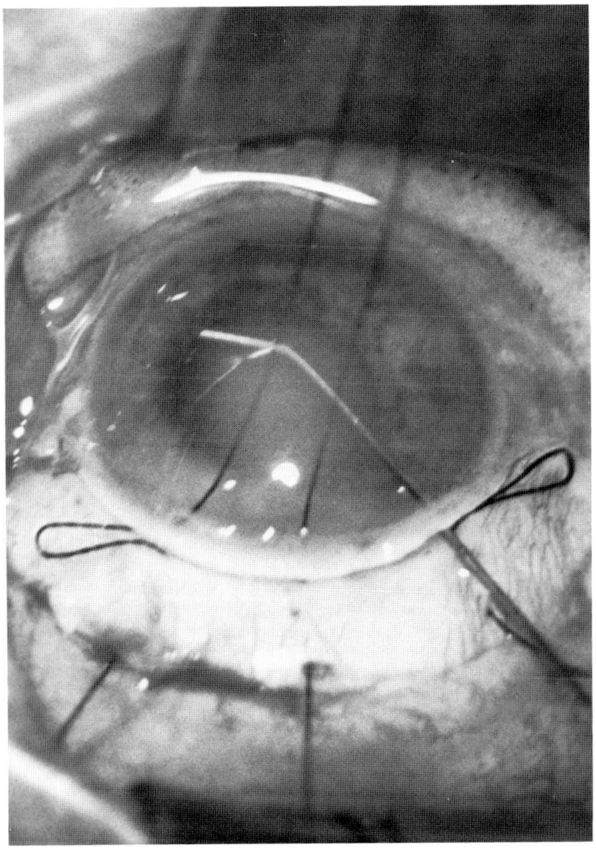

Fig. 11-15. α-Chymotrypsin is instilled under the iris with a 30-gauge air cannula.

were used. However, the olive tip is too thick and usually hits the endothelium. In addition, when the tip is passed through the incision, its thickness allows the chamber to leak and become flat. The 30-gauge air cannula is a much better choice with microsurgery. It is important to use a Micropore filter with α-chymotrypsin. This drug contains many impurities that will be injected into the eye unless it is filtered.

α-Chymotrypsin causes glaucoma because the zonules become small spherical fragments that float into the anterior chamber and clog the trabeculum. The glaucoma can be prevented if the chamber is irrigated around an air bubble as described below several times during the procedure.

MAKING THE IRIDOTOMY

Before the widespread use of implants and the availability of the laser to make iridotomies, many surgeons believed that iridectomies had to be basal and the larger the better. Some still hold to these old dictums. However, the laser has shown us that small nonbasal iridotomies work as well as or better than the traditional basal iridotomies. If a basal iridectomy is made, both anterior and posterior chamber lenses have a nasty habit of dislocating through them. In addition, lenses have taught us that just because an iridectomy looks wide open does not mean that any aqueous is flowing through it. It seems that the larger the iridectomy, the more likely the vitreous will try to pass through it and thus occlude it from the passage of aqueous. Thus, the purposeful creation of a very small, nonbasal iridotomy is desirable.

The iridotomy is made by lifting the iris away from the lens with the Tennant Corneoscleral Forceps (Storz) and making the incision with the sharp scissors (Vannas or Tennant–Weck) (Fig. 11-16A,B).

Complications of Making the Iridotomy

Making the iridotomy too large or too basal has been discussed. In addition, if the iridotomy is too large and too close to the implant, the lens will cause the lips of the iridotomy to roll open. Vitreous very often presents through the iridotomy under this condition, requiring that a vitrector be placed through the iridotomy and a vitrectomy performed (Fig. 11-17). Thus one must be sure to place the iridotomy at least 1 clock-hour or more away from the planned location of the edge of the implant.

If the iridotomy is inadvertently made too large, it can be sutured closed with 10-0 polypropylene. If that seems not to be required, one may be able to overcome the problem by covering the iridotomy with a bolus of Amvisc or Healon.

Occasionally, iridotomies will bleed when they

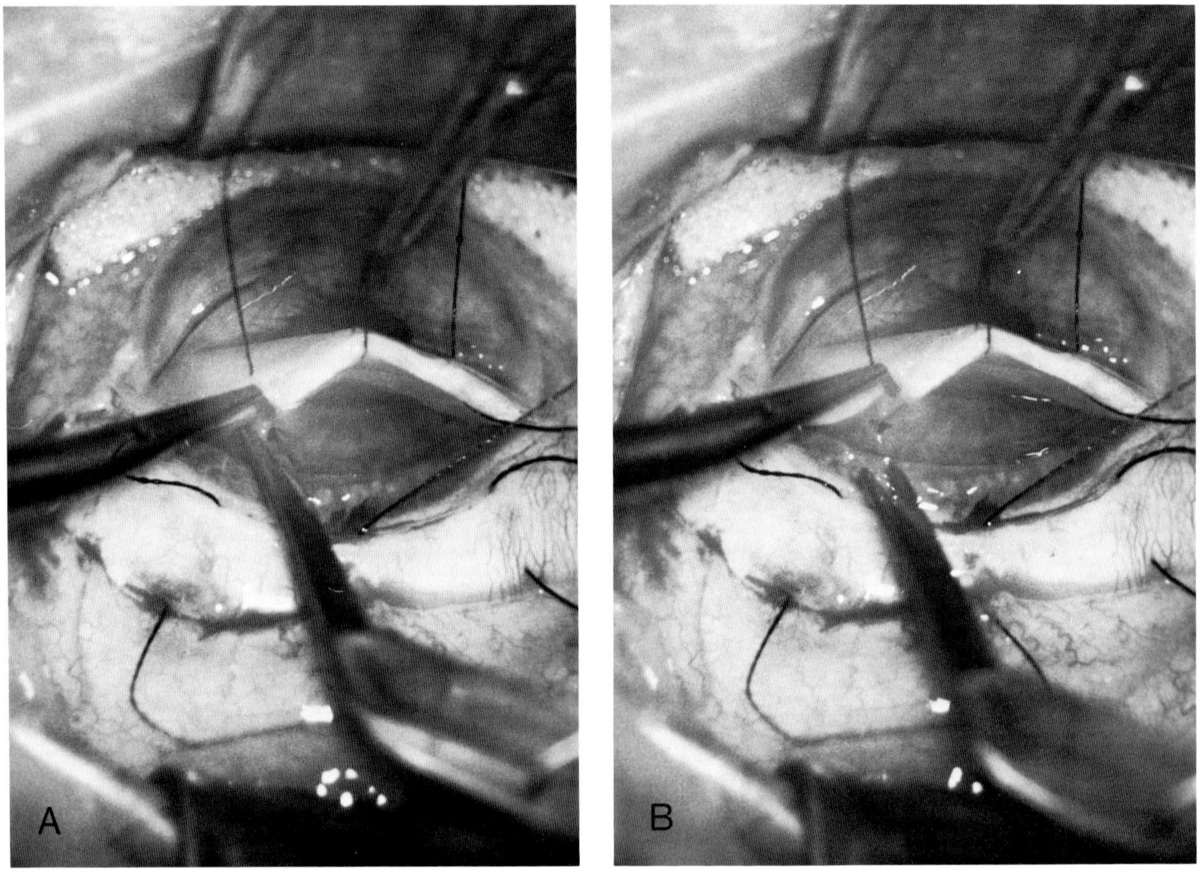

Fig. 11-16. (A,B) The iridotomy should be made as small as possible and near the base without being truly basal to avoid the implant entering the iridotomy.

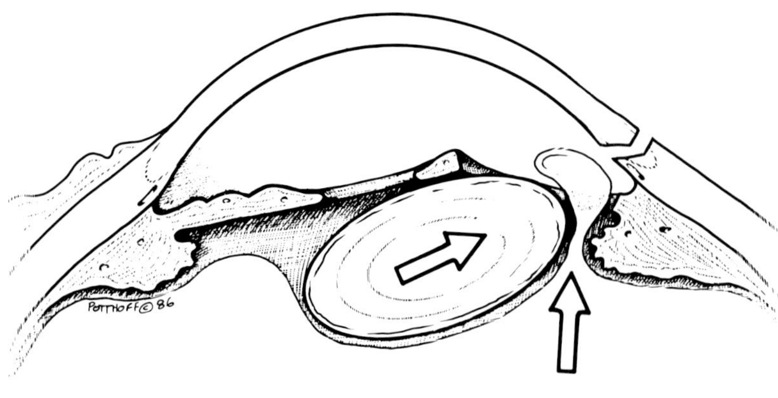

Fig. 11-17. If the iridotomy is either too large, too basal, or both, the implant can dislocate through it or vitreous can present through it.

are made. In an attempt to stop the bleeding with the cautery, one must be sure that it is turned down to zero and carefully raised in power. If the iris is cauterized with the cautery much above the minimal level, more bleeding occurs from the cautery instead of less. It is often desirable to use air tamponade to stop the bleeding.

INTRACAPSULAR EXTRACTION OF THE LENS

Before beginning the extraction of the lens, one must first check to see that nothing is pressing on the globe. The bridal suture is checked to see that it is free. The speculum should not be pressing on the eye. The patient should be awake and be told not to move for a few seconds. Only then can the extraction begin.

The assistant lifts the cornea enough to gain exposure but not so high that tension is placed on the globe. With a cellulose sponge in the right hand, the pupil is engaged. The sponge is pulled toward the incision and pressed gently toward the floor. This expresses aqueous from the posterior chamber so that a large ice ball will not form. The Rosenbaum-Drews iris retractor is now placed into position. Next, the warm cryoprobe is placed onto the surface of the lens and activated. The probe is held in this position for a few seconds until the ice ball has had time to extend into the cortex. It is then slowly lifted with the cryoextractor until the 12 o'clock pole of the lens is delivered. One should stop and look to determine whether there are stress lines around the upper pole of the lens. If they are present, the probe should be thawed and replaced, since zonules are frozen into the ice ball. If they are not present, the lens will deliver easily in most cases. The lens is moved gently from right to left to break the rest of the zonules and the lens is gently slid out of the eye.

If stress lines are present around the upper pole of the lens, zonules are frozen into the ice ball. One should therefore use the cartwheel maneuver to deliver the lens to prevent capsular rupture. It is important to remember that zonules tend to be tough and strong when pulled end-on but are rather easily broken when torqued with a sheering action. The cartwheel maneuver consists of reapplication of the probe at the 2 o'clock position with rotation of the lens about its axis. This causes the zonules to sheer off the lens. The cataract is then gently pulled from the eye. When the ice ball is defrosted, the zonules are on stretch and the lens will spring back into the posterior chamber unless it is supported from below. This is accomplished by placing the iris retractor on the six o'clock cornea to support the lens. Since the 12 o'clock zonules are ruptured, one must not presss hard enough to cause vitreous pressure, or vitreous will be lost. (Fig. 11-18).

Complications of Lens Extraction

If the pupil is not pulled toward the incision with the sponge as described, the endothelium will be damaged by the insertion of the iris retractor. If the aqueous is not absorbed by the sponge as described, it will come forward when the cryoprobe is placed on the lens. This will create a large ice ball, which will engage either the iris or the cornea, or both.

It is common for the novice to stab at the lens with the cryoprobe and quickly pull it from the eye in fear that the iceball will engage the iris. The capsule is not strong enough to permit cryoextraction unless the cortex is also frozen into the iceball. If only the capsule is engaged, it will tear, leaving the cortex and nucleus in the eye.

If the capsule tears with the nucleus still in the eye, one should not attempt to remove it by expression as one would do with planned extracapsular extraction, since the zonules are likely broken at the 12 o'clock position. Instead, two small spatulas or two 25-gauge needles should be used (Fig. 11-19). These are passed into each side of the nucleus so that it is grasped as if by a pair of tongs. The nucleus can then be pulled from the eye.

If vitreous presents and there is a considerable cortex, one should proceed directly to the use of a vitrector to clean up the mess. However, if the vitreous face has not been broken, a vitrector or an I and A unit should be avoided. Their infusion system will usually break the vitreous face, since many

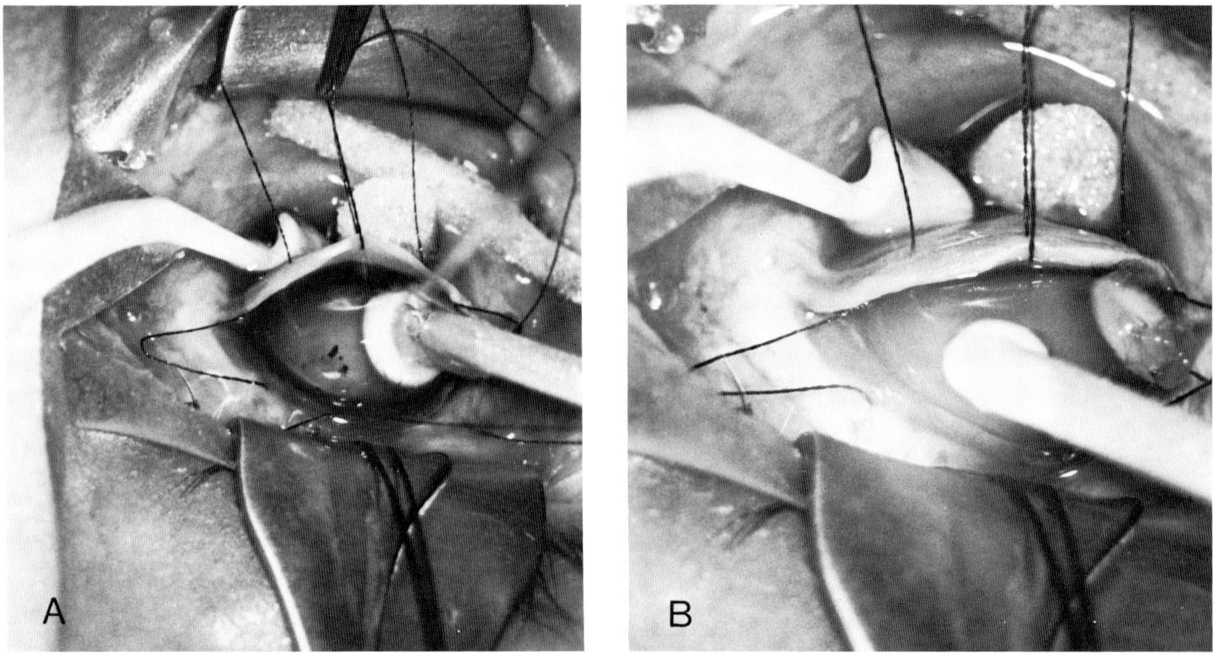

Fig. 11-18. (A,B) Stress lines near the ice ball indicate that anterior zonules have been frozen into the ice, and the probe must be thawed and replaced. When stress lines form or when the zonules seem tough, the probe is replaced and the lens is rolled from the eye to break the zonules with an oblique rather than a straight pulling motion.

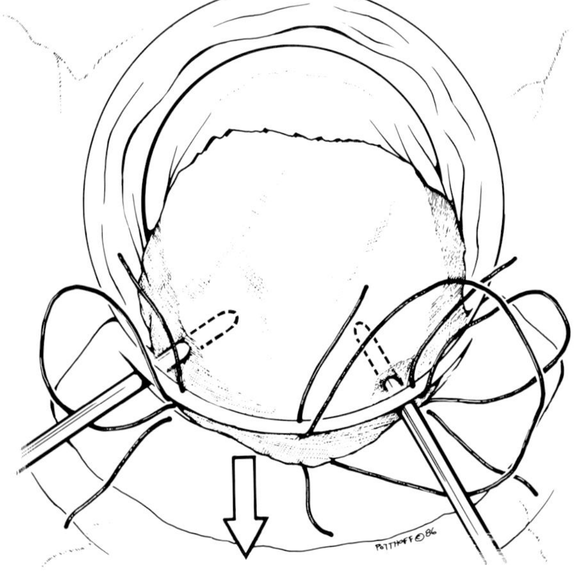

Fig. 11-19. The nucleus may be removed with a spatula.

zonules are already broken. One should instead use the Gills system,[6] since there is no infusion except as needed by the surgeon to maintain space. The Gills needle looks like a 30-gauge air canula except the bent end is about 8 to 9 mm long and the bore is 23 to 25 gauge. The length permits the needle to reach the inferior portion of the capsular bag, and the bore is large enough to engage cortex. The concept is to engage the cortex in the capsular fornix and then strip it from the eye. It is not intended that the cortex be aspirated into the 6-ml syringe attached to the needle. With diligence and patience, it is often possible to convert an unplanned extracapsular extraction into an eye that looks like a planned extracapsular extraction. However, the zonules are often broken at the 12 o'clock position, and any thought of a posterior chamber lens should be abandoned for a diaphragm anterior chamber lens (Fig. 11-20).

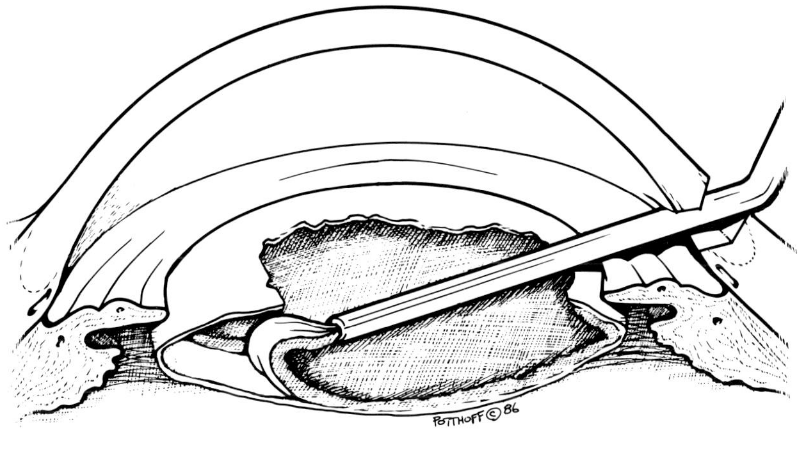

Fig. 11-20. The cortex may be removed with a Gills needle without breaking the vitreous face.

REPOSITIONING OF THE IRIS

Often the iris will be left in the wound at the conclusion of the lens-extraction maneuver. The novice will be tempted to lift the cornea and brush the iris back inside the eye. This is acceptable if the eye is very soft; however, if the vitreous is attempting to exit the eye, such a maneuver will certainly cause vitreous loss. The recommended procedure is to use a syringe with acetylcholine (Miochol) or carbachol (Miostat) solution coupled to a 30-gauge air cannula (Fig. 11-21). One begins a gentle stream of solution exiting from the needle. The flow of fluid is started before the wound is approached, to avoid a sudden surge of fluid with the needle in the eye. The solution is aimed parallel to the incision instead of toward the pupil to avoid filling the chamber until the iris is back inside the eye. The iris is brushed back inside the eye with the side of the needle. Once the incision has been brushed, the pupil becomes round; this is the signal that the iris has been properly repositioned into the eye. Gentle irrigation of miotic is continued until the pupil has achieved maximum constriction.

Complications of Iris Repositioning

The greatest risk associated with repositioning of the iris is vitreous loss. If one places either balanced salt solution (BSS) or air into the chamber with the iris out of the wound, vitreous will likely be forced from the eye. Since syringes have a tendency to be sticky and move quickly when the plunger does begin to move, it is important to begin plunger movement before the needle approaches the eye. In addition, it is important that the fluid not be injected toward the vitreous face, or the pressure of the injection can rupture the face. If vitreous is lost during this maneuver, it is essential that a generous anterior vitrectomy be performed.

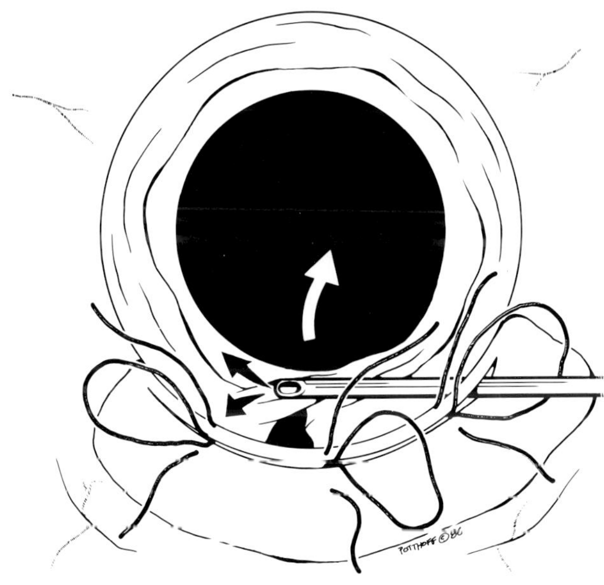

Fig. 11-21. Reposition of the iris is best done with the 30-gauge air cannula on a syringe.

It is important to realize that a small pupil is important for the insertion of an anterior chamber lens. Rupture of the vitreous face and tucking of the iris is likely if the pupil is large during placement of the anterior chamber lens.

ESTABLISHING THE CHAMBER

It is important to establish the chamber and to be sure that the pupil is centered at this point. The chamber is established by tying up the silk sutures at the 10 and 2 o'clock positions. The chamber is then deepened with sodium hyaluronate. This puts the surgeon in control of the eye and prepares it for insertion of the lens. It also brings the eye back to normal pressure. This approach reduces the tendency for choroidal effusion or hemorrhage. Noting that the pupil is central also informs the surgeon that the iris has not been left in the wound (Fig. 11-22).

TIGHTENING THE BRIDLE SUTURE

Pulling the bridle suture will now roll the eye downward, facilitating insertion of the IOL. Without this maneuver, it is often a struggle to begin insertion of the lens because of the incision being near or under the upper lid speculum. This is particularly true if the eye has been severely retroplaced by the Super-Pinkie and/or the chin is downward so the surgeon is working downward over the brow (Fig. 11-23).

SELECTION OF LENS IMPLANT

With intracapsular surgery, most agree that iris-supported lenses are less desirable than anterior chamber lenses. Anterior chamber lenses may conveniently be divided into three groups:

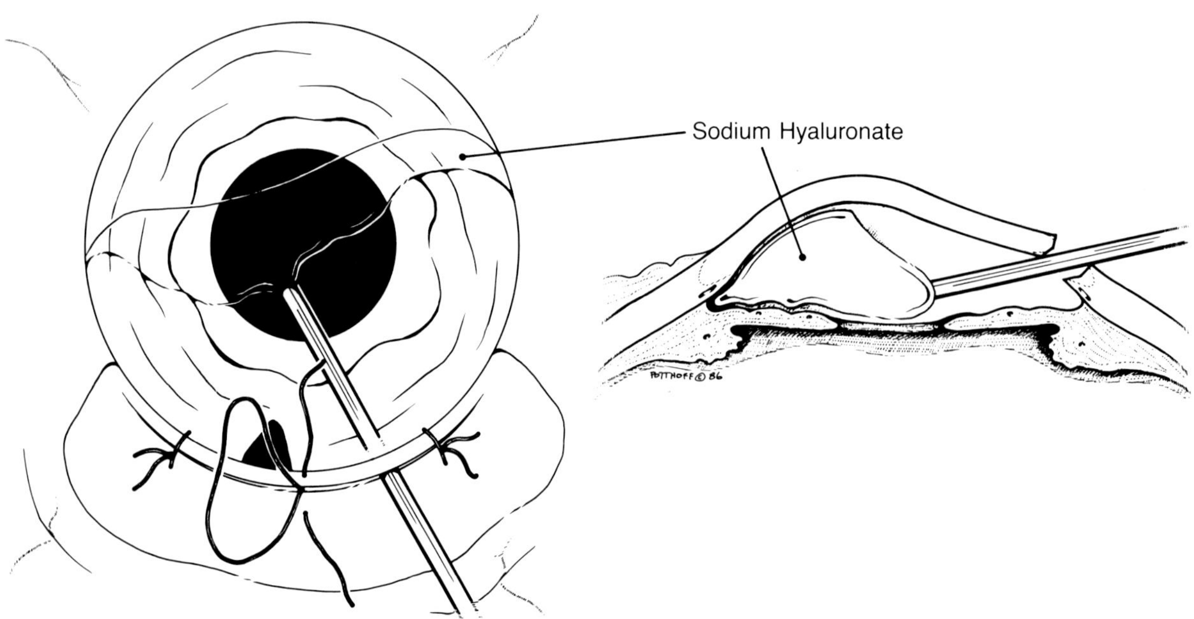

Fig. 11-22. The chamber is established by inflating it with balanced salt solution (BSS) or sodium hyaluronate.

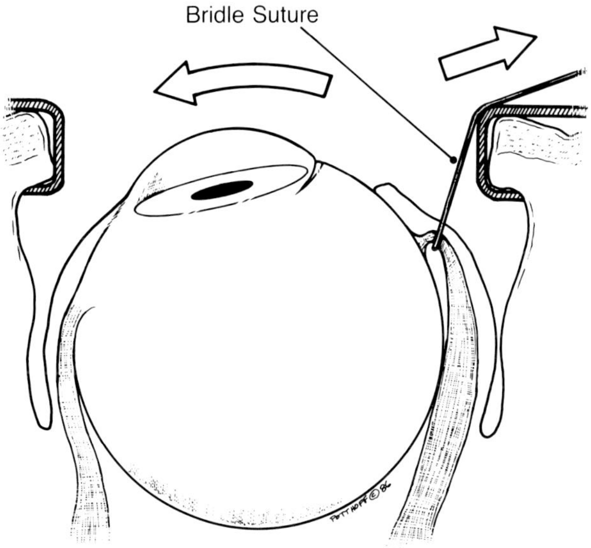

Fig. 11-23. The bridal suture should be tightened to rotate the eye downward.

Rigid (diaphragm) lenses: These lenses not only focus the eye but provide mechanical (diaphragm) support to the eye. This is very beneficial in some cases. Examples are Standard Tennant, Choyce Mark VIII, and Choyce Mark IX.

Semi-flexible lenses: These lenses were part of the evolution of anterior chamber lenses. Since they do not provide mechanical support and are not sizable, they should be abandoned. They were an important contribution to the advancement of lens design. Examples are Tennant Anchor, Kelman II, Hessburg, and Leiske.

Flexible lenses: This is really not the best terminology to lead one to the correct lens design. What happens with a truly flexible lens is that the lens moves in the eye. Any lens that moves in the eye eventually will destroy the eye. Thus, what we really desire is a sizable lens, which adjusts itself to the size of the chamber without losing stability. Examples of flexible lenses are Shepard Universal, Simcoe, Stableflex, Tennant Anchorflex, and Kelman Omnifit. It is my personal belief that no lens offers the stability while retaining the sizability offered by the Anchorflex.

If the eye has any of the following conditions, the flexible lenses should be avoided and the diaphragm lens selected:

1. Vitreous loss
2. Large iris coloboma
3. Positive vitreous pressure (insistance on putting in a flexible lens with the use of sodium hyaluronate will invite vitreous loss when the sodium hyaluronate is removed)
4. Marked guttata, when the likelihood of a future corneal transplant is evident
5. Younger patients when it is unreasonable to put in a flexible lens that has not withstood the test of time (as the rigid lenses have)

I prefer the Standard Tennant or the Choyce Mark VIII because the narrower optic of the Mark IX does not provide as much diaphragm support.

INSERTION OF THE LENS IMPLANT

The lens is grasped with the lens insertion forceps. The lens should be inspected for defects. Particularly important with anterior chamber lenses is to look for roughness of the posterior surface of the lens (this is the main cause of uveitis-glaucoma-hyphema (UGH) syndromes). The lens should be neutralized with a piezoelectric crystal gun.

Once the chamber is filled with sodium hyaluronate, the lens is placed into the chamber. The distal footplates are put into the distal angle. Gentle pressure is placed on the lens toward the distal angle while observing the pupil. If iris is tucked under the distal angle, the pupil will distort. If the iris is not tucked, the pupil will remain round and central (Fig. 11-24).

Complications of Lens Insertion

The smooth surface of the implant will not detach Descemet's membrane. However, the tips of the toes or the exposed edge of the optic in flexible lenses can detach Descemet's. Therefore, the lead-

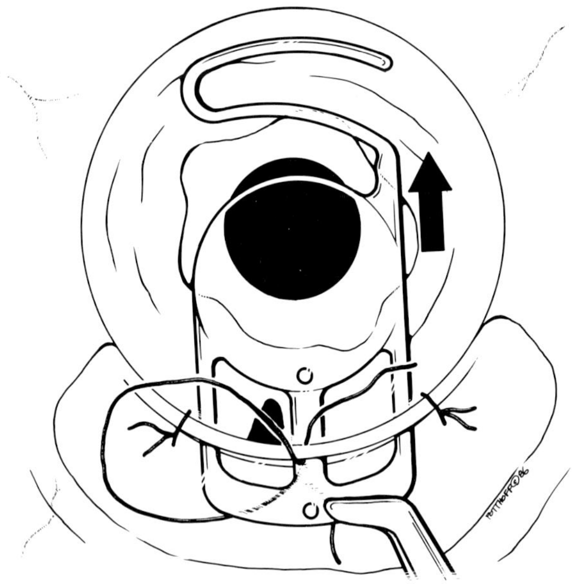

Fig. 11-24. The distal footplate of the lens is placed in the distal angle.

ing end of the implant must be dipped until it is past the cut edge of Descemet's. This is particularly important in the very elderly. It is fairly common for Descemet's to detach in patients over age 90; special attention to this problem should be given in these patients. If Descemet's does detach, it is repaired as follows: First, the chamber is deepened with air to press Descemet's into position. Next, a 10-0 polypropylene suture is used. The needle is passed through the cornea, through the area of detached Descemet's, and back through the entire cornea. This places a stitch to hold the detached Descemet's to the stroma. The knot is then tied and cut, and finally the knot is rotated into the stroma.

The iris is tucked with insertion of the lens as noted earlier. It is important with all lenses to correct the tucking of the distal feet before insertion of the proximal feet. It is much more difficult to correct the problem after the lens has been totally inserted. If the pupil indicates a tuck, the lens is pulled gently back from the distal angle and is moved side to side; the pupil is then observed. As the lens is moved gently from side to side, the tuck will unfold and the pupil will indicate that by becoming round. The feet are then gently placed back into the angle.

Insertion of the Proximal Foot

The sclera is pulled toward the surgeon at the center of the footplate about to be inserted. This is best done by turning an angled forceps upside down so that the angle of the jaw can pass under the plastic foot to grasp the scleral edge. Once the sclera is pulled back to make room for the footplate, an insertion instrument is placed to press the footplate into the chamber. With the Standard Tennant lens, the insertion forceps works well for this job. With the Anchorflex lens, the Sinskey hook is preferable (Fig. 11-25).

Complications of Insertion of the Proximal Foot

If the Standard lens is pushed toward the distal angle to insert the footplates, the angle will be torn and bleeding will occur. With flexible lenses, some pressure toward the distal angle is necessary and desirable. Bleeding almost always occurs when a torquing action is employed. Generally, one can press a couple of millimeters without tearing if the lens is simply pressed straight into the angle. However, if the lens is twisting while pressed into the

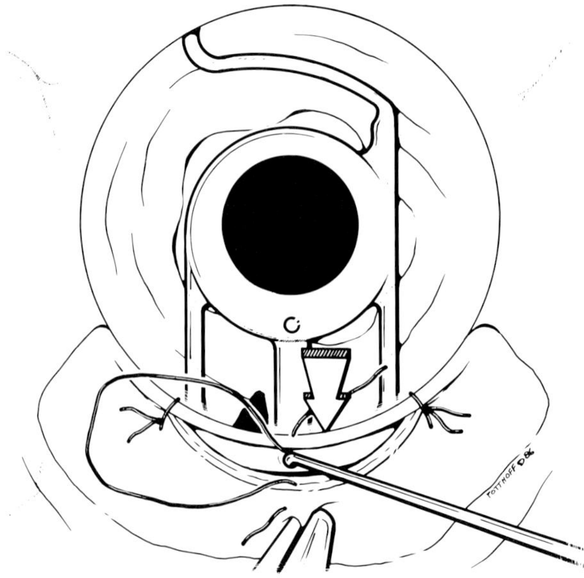

Fig. 11-25. The proximal footplate is placed into the angle.

angle, bleeding is likely. If bleeding begins, the eye should be closed and gentle irrigation begun with the 30-gauge needle and BSS. If the tear is small, this prevents clotting in the chamber and the bleeding stops. If the tear is larger and bleeding more pronounced, the lens is left in place and the IOP elevated until bleeding stops. An effort is then made to remove the excess clot so that the eye does not have to reabsorb it postoperatively. In some cases, this causes rebleeding, and the clot must be left in the eye. However, if some of the clot can be removed, the postoperative course will be better. Leaving the lens in the eye does not seem to interfere with resolution of the bleeding.

Tucking of the Standard lens at the 12 o'clock position generally occurs when the lens is pressed too far into the eye. As the footplates snap up into position, tucking occurs. This is noted by a pointing of the pupil. If the iris is simply stretched because the lens is slightly too long, a general ovalling of the pupil toward the 6 and 12 o'clock positions will occur, whereas tucking results in pointing toward the tuck.

Tucking of the Anchorflex is much more common. It should be ignored until the central suture is tied and the chamber is deepened. With the chamber deep, the Sinskey hook is place in the hole at the 12 o'clock position of the optic (or a Graether hook is placed in the angle where the haptic attaches to the optic). Gentle movement toward the 6 o'clock position followed by a right and left movement of the lens will release the tuck. This is noted by rounding and centration of the pupil. This maneuver is easiest to perform with the chamber filled with BSS. It is sometimes more difficult for the iris to unfold with the chamber filled with air or sodium hyaluronate.

With lenses that have an exposed optic, pupillary capture sometimes occurs at the time of insertion of the proximal feet or while the sutures are being placed. This should be ignored until the wound can be secured if the chamber is filled only with BSS. After the wound is closed, air is used to force the iris back into position. Alternatively, sodium hyaluronate can be used to reposition the iris. However, pupillary capture sometimes occurs when the sodium hyaluronate is removed. If that occurs, the wound should be closed and the eye then filled with air.

SUTURING THE WOUND

If the operating keratometer is used, I prefer to use 9-0 nylon and a shoelace suture. The 9-0 tends to stay where it is left, as there is less elasticity. If the keratometer is not used, I prefer 10-0 nylon interrupted sutures. The 10-0 suture has more elasticity which allows a greater margin of error in tying, and the interrupted technique allows one to cut the sutures earlier if astigmatism is excessive. Control of astigmatism is beyond the scope of this chapter.

REMOVAL OF THE SODIUM HYALURONATE

Most of the sodium hyaluronate must be removed to prevent the rise in postoperative pressure that will occur if it is left in the eye. The easiest way to remove it safely is with an I and A tip. However, this is usually not assembled during intracapsular surgery. One may force the sodium hyaluronate from the eye with either air or BSS. If air is selected, the tip of the 30-gauge needle is placed at the 6 o'clock position. The wound is held open as air is instilled. The air pushes the material from the eye. If BSS is used, one may use a technique similar to the use of air. However, I find it easier to place a cyclodialysis needle on the BSS bottle. This larger needle mechanically holds the wound open as an exit port while irrigation procedes to irrigate the material from the eye. The needle should not be placed across the chamber but simply placed just into the eye.

Complications of Removal of Sodium Hyaluronate

The principal problem during the removal of the sodium hyaluronate is vitreous loss. If the chamber suddenly shallows, the pupil will stretch around the edge of the optic and the vitreous face will rupture. One should therefore always watch the pupil. If the pupillary margin approaches the edge of the lens, one must reestablish the wound and use fluid or air to reposition the iris.

POSTOPERATIVE CARE

Antibiotic drops are given q3h for 1 week. Steroid drops are given as dictated by slit-lamp examination. Cycloplegic drops are not given. The pupil is bounced at the office visits with 2.5 percent Neo-Synephrine. If the pupil is dilated regularly with cycloplegics, rupture of the vitreous face with herniation into the anterior chamber is a frequent nuisance. Although I find ophthalmologists hesitant to stray from the traditional training that patients be given cycloplegics postoperatively, experience with 3,000 patients has shown us that this is unnecessary. (A possible exception to this rule is the use of the Mark VIII lens, where there is minimal clearance between the iris and the lens.)

COMMENTS ON SELECTION OF LENS TYPE

The following conditions must be present for an IOL to last over a period of years:

1. *The lens must not move within the eye:* Even microscopic movements cause damage. The lens acts like a piston in a hydraulic system. Movements of the lens with eye movements transmit push–pull forces to the endothelium, causing corneal dystrophy, and to the macular, causing macular edema.
2. *The lens surface must be smooth:* This is particularly true in areas in which the iris or ciliary body rubs over the lens. Otherwise the tissue is gradually abraded and a partial or total UGH syndrome results.
3. *The lens materials must last the life of the patient:* Many materials have been used that work well for a few years and then biodegrade. During biodegradation, the surface of the material is rough and UGH syndromes, partial or total, are common. Examples are nylon and polypropylene.
4. *The lens materials and the sterilization technique must be nontoxic:* Early lenses damaged many eyes because of the detergent Cetrimide, used to sterilize the lenses and monomer from poorly cured acrylic. There have been periodic questions about N_2O sterilization, injection-molding plastic, and additives for ultraviolet filtration. Some of these questions linger in the industry. Only the original Perspex remains unchallenged year after year as a suitable nontoxic material.
5. *Execution of the surgery must be excellent:* It is well known that a good surgeon with a bad lens will obtain a bad result; a bad surgeon with a good lens will obtain a bad result, and a good surgeon with a good lens will obtain a good result. The problem is that most bad surgeons and other surgeons who see their patients blame the bad results on the lens rather than on the surgeon. In addition, surgeons tend to pick lenses that are easy to use, not necessarily lenses that have been designed with the best features in mind. The problem is complicated by the fact that almost any lens manufactured today will look good for at least a year. Thus, a large number of poorly designed lenses may be inserted before it is recognized that the design or its materials are faulty. An example is the episode of the Azar 91Z.

Most lenses have specific features and peculiarities. If these are known, the system works well. If they are ignored, the system fails. An example is the Tennant Anchor lens, which worked very well as long as nonbasal iridotomies were made. However, with large basal iridectomies, the lens could be manipulated and dislocated by rubbing the eye. The lens developed a bad reputation simply because surgeons ignored the recommended technique of using the lens. Another example is the Kelman series of lenses. Placement of the distal footplates is not automatic but a learned skill. Kelman has made a great effort to teach how to place the footplates of his lenses, but few take the time to learn or heed his warnings.

The following features should be evaluated before selecting any lens:

- Lenses with very thin haptics become scarred into the angle.
- Lenses with closed loops vault toward the cornea when the eye is rubbed.
- Lenses with polypropylene loops will biodegrade. They are difficult to remove because they are generally scarred into the angle.
- Lenses with C-shaped or circular-shaped flexible contact points slide across the tissue in the angle when the eye is rubbed. One must have a double folded loop or S shape so that the compression energy is absorbed by the loop without transmitting the energy to the tissue.
- If both loops of the lens are flexible, there is a tendency for the lens to move in the eye. We want a lens that is self-sizing but stable in the eye. Thus one of the haptic members must be of sufficient strength to prevent motion.
- If a lens that is very flexible is present during a pupillary block, the optic will be pushed against the cornea. The ideal lens will have a member strong enough to prevent this disaster.

To my knowledge, the Tennant Anchorflex (T) is the only flexible lens that clearly fills these criteria. The Kelman Omnifit, the Kelman Multiflex, and the Feaster lens have copied the S-shaped haptic originally found only on the Anchorflex. It is questionable whether the opposite end of the lens is strong enough to prevent micromovements of the lens. I have seen photos of these lenses with pupillary block and the optic against the cornea. However, if the strength of the haptics of these lenses is adequate, they will indeed function as good lenses as well.

Some surgeons have questioned whether it is better for the haptic to engage the tissue in a few spots (with footplates the size of the original Choyce lens) or with a large arc of contact, as is present on the Tennant Anchorflex and the Feaster lens. The theory behind the wider arc is that tissue is less damaged when the mg/mm is reduced by spreading the force over a larger area. The criticism is that the footplates damage the angle and may damage the trabeculum. In reality, the footplate rests behind the trabeculum and should not involve the filtration mechanism. We looked at Anchorflex lenses present in the eye for 1 year and used posterior chamber lenses as a control. The incidence of eyes requiring antihypertensive medication was not statistically different in the two groups. Thus, the theory seems to be correct at 1 year.

It should be remembered that all anterior chamber lenses cause ovalling of the pupil. This has not caused glaucoma and is principally a cosmetic defect. A few, however, have photophobia. Also, most anterior chamber lenses have some tenderness to touch. These problems have stimulated many to use posterior chamber lenses. Posterior chamber lenses work vey well but also have hazy capsules, produce decreased vision in bright light due to dazzle on the capsule, and have a tendency for the optic to decenter. There is no perfect system.

Many surgeons now use anterior chamber lenses only as a backup lens to insert when the case goes poorly, in the face of ruptured capsule, vitreous loss, or bleeding with poor visibility. Thus the results with anterior chamber lenses look generally bad. In addition, many surgeons select flexible lenses for these complicated cases. Vitreous bands easily find spaces on flexible lenses to which they can attach. In addition, the vitreous is strong enough to move the flexible lenses. Therefore, I recommend that the diaphragm lenses be used instead of flexible lenses in these cases.

Finally, those of us who are relatively new in the design and use of anterior chamber lenses owe gratitude to Dr. Ridley, Dr. Strampelli, and particularly Dr. Peter Choyce for their pioneering work. Only those who try something new can know the cost of being first.

REFERENCES

1. Corboy J: Nitrous oxide analgesia for outpatient surgery. J Am Intraocul Implant Soc 10:1232, 1984
2. Gills JP, Loyd TL: A technique of retrobulbar block

with paralysis of orbicularis oculi. J Am Intraocul Implant Soc 9: 1983
3. Smith J: Retrobulbar bupivacaine can cause respiratory arrest. Ann Ophthalmol 14:1005, 1982
4. Golden B, Coppel S: Intraocular penetration of gentimycin. Arch Ophthalmol 84:792, 1970
5. Vörösmarthy D: Oculopression. Adv Ophthalmol 17:42, 1966
6. Gills JP: Techniques of controlling intraocular pressure and reducing vitreous loss. p. 260. In Emery J, Jacobson A (eds): Current Concepts in Cataract Surgery. CV Mosby, St. Louis, 1980
7. Tennant JL: Super-Pinkie for super soft eyes. p. 316. In Emery J (ed): Current Concepts in Cataract Surgery. CV Mosby, St. Louis, 1978
8. Honan P: Honan balloon. J Am Intraocul Implant Soc 9:342, 1983

Lensectomy and Vitrectomy for Infantile Cataracts

12

Creig S. Hoyt

CLINICAL PICTURE

For the removal of all lens opacities in children under the age of 18 months, I currently use the lensectomy–vitrectomy approach. I also use this technique in special circumstances, such as removal of dislocated or partially dislocated lenses and removal of persistent hyperplastic primary vitreous (PHPV) lens opacities at any age.

Until recently, most investigators had considered the monocular cataract a nearly hopeless clinical problem, in which successful visual rehabilitation is virtually unknown. Failure to obtain good visual acuity in these eyes has been attributed to the high incidence of associated ocular anomalies, including microphthalmus, nystagmus, foveal dysplasia, and strabismus. Surgical technique, timing, and complications have also been considered significant factors in determining the final visual outcome.

Recently several investigators have suggested that surgery performed during the neonatal period followed by immediate optical correction and amblyopia therapy may result in favorable visual outcome in these patients.[1–4] This work correlates well with experiments in the animal models disclosing that unilateral eyelid closure causes irreversible neural changes in several visual centers after only several weeks of visual deprivation.[5] The precise duration of this critical period for initiation of therapy in children has yet to be defined, but it seems unlikely that good visual results would be obtained in infants treated after 6 months of age,[6] although this view has been challenged by BenEzra and Paez.[7]

Although visual acuity results in the treatment of binocular congenital cataracts have always been better than those in the treatment of monocular congenital cataracts, improvement in this area has also been dramatic. There is a general consensus that maintenance of a good clear visual axis during the early months of life is essential in the rehabilitation of both monocular and binocular congenital cataracts. Moreover, the rapid change in aphakic refractive error during the first year of life[8,9] necessitates frequent, careful retinoscopy, preferably in the awake, alert child. Lensectomy vitrectomy produces a clear pupillary aperture that does not become opacified and permits an accurate refraction in the critical first months of life, during which the deleterious effects of a defocused image on the developing visual system are maximal.[10]

One of the persistent problems that confounds the ophthalmologist evaluating infantile cataracts is the lack of objective criteria in deciding which lens opacities require surgery. Many lens opacities are incomplete, leaving large areas of the lens either clear or only partially involved. Although general rules are cited as to those types of lens opacities that will invariably result in visual deprivation, an objective criterion for the evaluation of infantile lens opacities and their effect on developing visual systems remains an unfulfilled need. Parks[4] offered the guideline that all lens opacities that interfere with more than 3 mm of the retinoscopic reflex should be surgically removed in order to prevent severe visual deprivation.

SURGICAL ANATOMY

Infant eyes with developmental cataracts are frequently smaller than normal, both in corneal diameter and in axial length. Furthermore, clear definition of the corneal scleral junction is not always possible. Careful attention must be paid to the anatomy of the corneal scleral junction in all such cases. Moreover, it should be recalled that the infant cornea lacks the tensile strength of the adult cornea. It is easily torn if an instrument too large is inserted into a tight wound. Moreover, an induced corneal distortion can be produced by a single suture pulled too tightly at the close of surgery and can produce a significant astigmatic error that may preclude successful contact lens fitting.

Anomalies of the iris and the dilator muscle are commonly associated with congenital cataracts. All too frequently, it is difficult to dilate completely the pupil of a patient with an infantile cataract. This has been attributed to the histologic and pharmacologic immaturity of the dilator muscle in these patients.[11] Cycloplegic agents are frequently more effective in producing pupillary dilatation than are sympathomimetic agents in this situation.

The size and the shape of the lens in infantile cataracts is commonly abnormal. It may be hypoplastic in its anterior to posterior dimension, or it may be frankly microspherophakic. Clear attention must be paid to the size and shape of the lens to avoid inadvertent penetration of the posterior capsule early in the cataract procedure. Some forms of infantile cataracts exhibit either calcification of the lens or involvement with nonregressed blood vessels, or both. These lenses require special techniques in order to avoid problems with lens removal.

If a lensectomy–vitrectomy approach is to be performed through the so-called pars plicata, it should be recalled that a well-defined demarcation of the pars plana and pars plicata does not occur until at least 6 weeks of age.

INDICATIONS AND CONTRAINDICATIONS

No consensus has been reached concerning the indications for lensectomy–vitrectomy versus lens aspiration in the treatment of congenital cataracts. Authorities advocating the lensectomy–vitrectomy approach cite two major advantages for this technique. First, a single surgical procedure suffices in the vast majority of patients greatly reducing, if not eliminating, the need for secondary procedures.[10,12] Second, the large opening in the visual axis created by this operation without any potential for secondary opacity formation on the posterior capsule allows for frequent retinoscopic examinations during the first year of life, when rapid changes in the refractive error take place. These examinations can be performed in the awake, alert, uncooperative child in a clinic or private office.

Opponents of the routine use of this procedure suggest that the long-term complications of routinely violating the vitreous cavity in a young eye have not been adequately documented. Moreover, the frequent adherence of small strands of vitreous to the corneal–scleral wound seen in a limbal approach with the anterior vitrectomy technique may predispose to the development of macular edema or late retinal detachment.[10] I use the lensectomy–vitrectomy approach in all infants under 18 months of age in whom a cataract removal is to be performed. It is during this first year and a half of life that visual form deprivation may so quickly become irreversible. It is also during this period that the refractive error of the growing infant eye changes rapidly, and the aphakic correction must be accordingly adjusted. The advantages of the lensectomy–vitrectomy approach in this setting seem to me to be warranted despite the fact that the long-term risks of this procedure have yet to be defined.

In older children, I still prefer to use a standard lens aspiration approach with posterior capsulotomy. In these patients the need for a completely clear visual axis in order to prevent form-deprivation amblyopia and to allow for frequent retinoscopy is not nearly so compelling.

ALTERNATIVE PROCEDURES

Alternative procedures for the lensectomy–vitrectomy technique in the management of infantile cataracts include the many variations on standard lens aspiration with or without a posterior capsulotomy. Although some authorities have advocated the use of phacoemulsification in the treatment of infantile cataracts, this procedure does not seem to be indicated, since most of these lenses are soft and easily aspirated. In those lenses that are more difficult to aspirate, the potential for inadvertent damage to the posterior capsule with violation of the vitreous cavity early in the procedure makes use of a vitrectomy instrument preferable to phacoemulsification.

RECOMMENDED TECHNIQUE

I use a limbal approach with a Peyman vitrector when I believe that lensectomy–vitrectomy is indicated. This surgical technique entails using an operating microscope. The eye is immobilized by a single 4-0 silk suture passed beneath the superior rectus muscle, which is then secured to the drapes with a curved hemostat. The anterior chamber is then penetrated with a 25-gauge butterfly needle

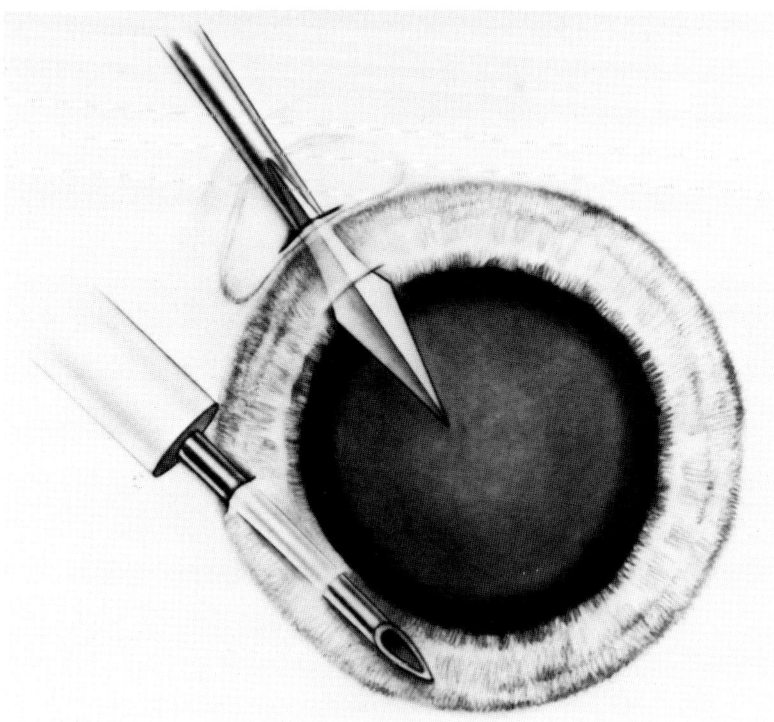

Fig. 12-1. A 26-gauge needle is used as a separate infusion line to maintain the anterior chamber. A limbal incision is made with a MVR blade.

that serves as the infusion line to maintain the anterior chamber during surgery. A long intracorneal course for this 25-gauge needle with completed penetration into the anterior chamber only by the very tip of the needle ensures stability for this infusion line and prevents inadvertent damage to the iris, lens, or vitreous from the needle (Fig. 12-1). An infusion solution of normal saline is used without supplemental epinephrine. The infusion line is not opened until the eye is penetrated by the MVR blade.

A corneal–scleral wound is made after a small conjunctival flap has been created in the superior temporal quadrant of the eye. I prefer to use an MVR blade for this incision (Fig. 12-1). After the infusion line has been opened and the height of the infusion bottle adjusted so as to maintain an adequate anterior chamber, a bent 23-gauge needle on a 2-ml syringe is used to perform an anterior capsulotomy. A can-opener technique is preferred over the Christmas treelike opening created by a single slash of the needle (Fig. 12-2). Following the creation of the anterior capsulotomy, the MVR blade is reintroduced into the anterior chamber and is used to break up the lens cortex mechanically. Following this procedure, the vitrector is introduced into the anterior chamber of the eye. Suction is produced by a hand-held syringe operated by the assistant. Using the cutting mode of the vitrector instrument, the anterior capsule is sharply cut away and aspirated (Fig. 12-3). The hydrated lens material can now be aspirated through the vitrector with little difficulty. When residual lens capsule or large lens fragments occlude the aspiration port of the vitrectomy instrument, a low cutting speed is used to remove these obstacles. A complete lens aspiration is obtained with the posterior capsule intact (Fig. 12-4). Any remaining fragments of the anterior capsule visible through the dilated pupil are now cut away. The vitrectomy instrument is now used to create a hole in the posterior capsule and the cutting speed is increased to a vitrectomy cutting speed of approximately 150 cuts per minute and a moderate anterior vitrectomy completed (Fig. 12-5).

Filtered air is now introduced through the infusion line, filling the anterior chamber. Withdrawal of the vitrectomy instrument through the filtered air can now be accomplished without dragging strands of the vitreous to the corneal–scleral wound. A single 10-0 nylon suture is used to close the corneal–scleral wound, paying particular at-

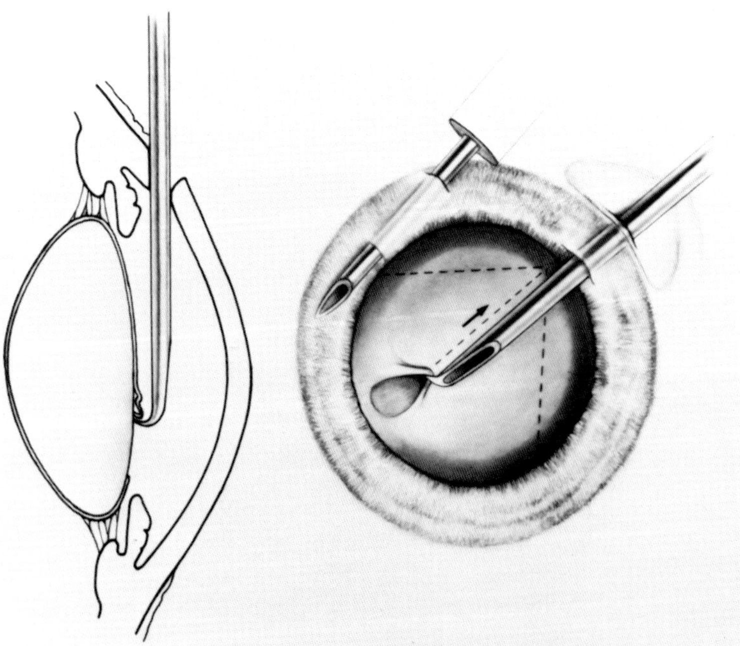

Fig. 12-2. An anterior capsulotomy is performed using a 23-gauge needle that has been bent to produce a sharp hook at its end.

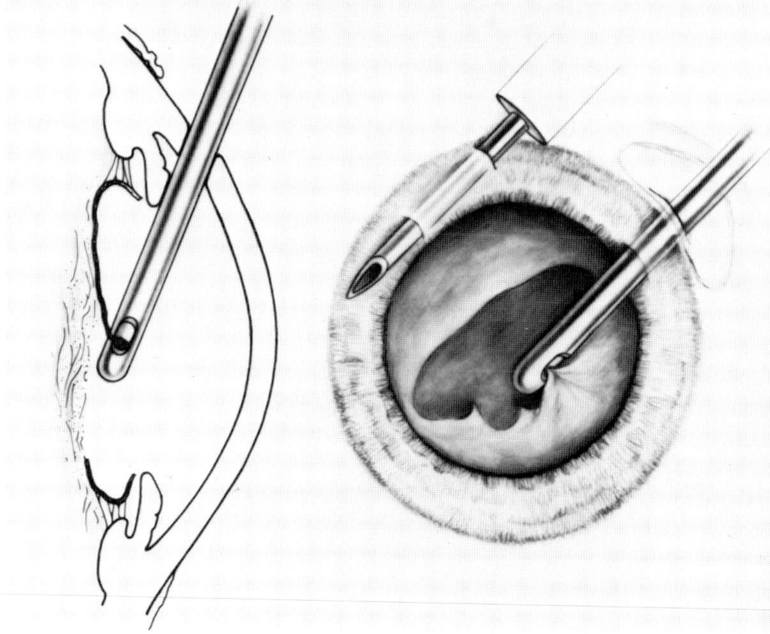

Fig. 12-3. The vitrectomy instrument is used to remove the anterior capsule.

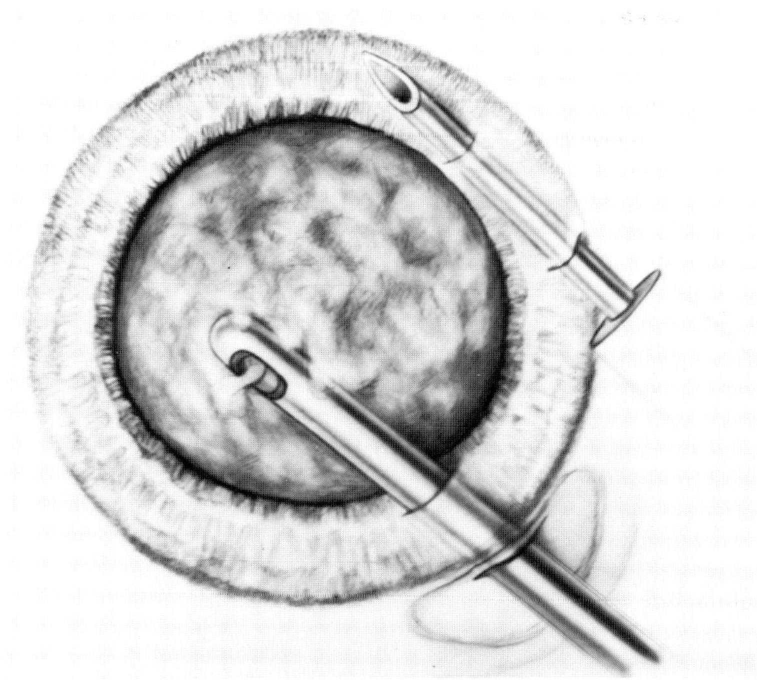

Fig. 12-4. Lens aspiration is performed using the vitrectomy instrument.

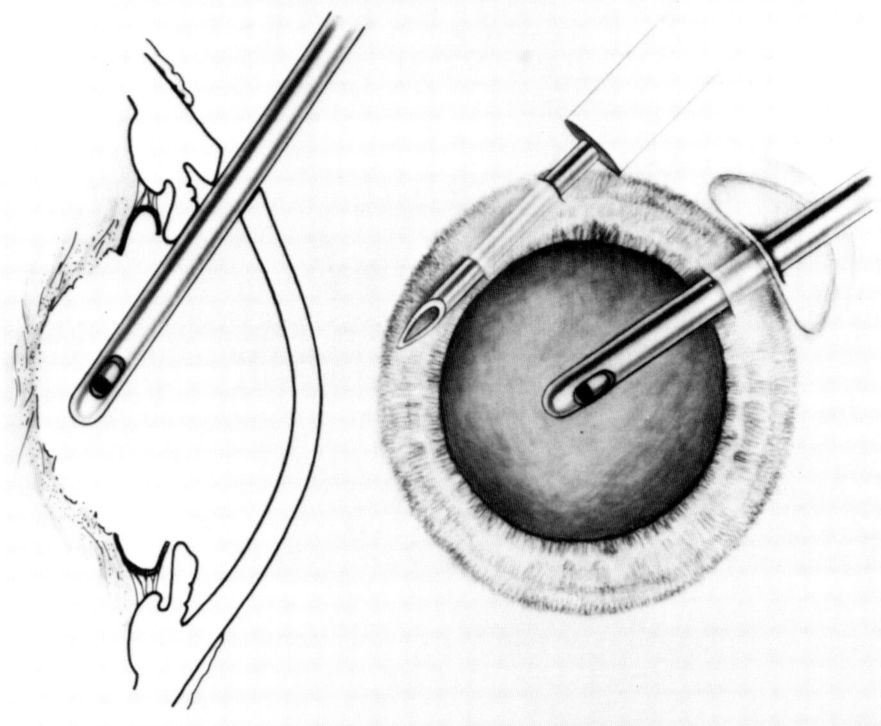

Fig. 12-5. A shallow anterior vitrectomy is performed and care is taken to be sure no vitreous strands extend across the iris to corneal wound.

tention to avoid pulling this wound too tightly closed, as severe errors of astigmatism may be caused in the infant eye. The infusion line is withdrawn from the eye and the corneal–scleral puncture site occluded with a Wec-cell sponge until corneal stromal swelling occurs and no further leakage from the wound is noted. No suture is used to close this site in most circumstances. A sub-Tenon's injection of gentamycin and Celestone is then completed. Atropine ointment is applied to the eye and a patch and shield taped in place.

PROGNOSIS AND COMPLICATIONS

No long-term prospective study has yet evaluated the lensectomy–vitrectomy approach and contrasted it to currently used lens aspiration procedures. Several studies, however, have already documented that the incidence of secondary procedures using the lensectomy–vitrectomy approach is greatly reduced in comparison with the standard lens aspiration procedures.[10,12]

A recent study presented by Parks and colleagues[12] at the American Academy of Ophthalmology in 1983 suggests that the incidence of aphakic glaucoma is no greater using the lensectomy–vitrectomy approach than in patients treated with lens aspiration. The follow-up period for this study was relatively short, however, and the incidence of glaucoma may increase with the passage of time. It is important to recall that the general incidence of glaucoma in aphakic children has dramatically decreased with the lowered incidence of rubella embryopathy.[12]

No information is yet available concerning the long-term risk of retinal detachment following lensectomy–vitrectomy in the treatment of congenital cataracts. Poyofuku and co-workers[13] have emphasized, however, that retinal detachment may occur in aphakic children more than a decade after the initial surgery. It will therefore be some time before we have a true estimate of the risk for retinal detachment following lensectomy–vitrectomy.

Whether macular edema is a significant complication of congenital cataract surgery remains controversial.[14–16] Nevertheless, it is clear that macular edema does occur in some circumstances. It would seem prudent to make all attempts possible to reduce the incidence of vitreous strand adherence to the corneal scleral wound. In our hands, this complication has been greatly reduced by insisting that the vitreous instrument be withdrawn only after the anterior chamber has been filled with filtered air.

REFERENCES

1. Enoch JM, Rabinowicz IM: Early surgery and visual correction of an infant born with unilateral eye lens opacity. Doc Ophthalmol 41:371, 1976
2. Pratt-Johnson JA, Tillson G: Visual results after removal of congenital cataracts before the age of one year. Can J Ophthalmol 16:19021, 1981
3. Beller R, Hoyt CS, Marg E, Odom JV: Good visual function after neonatal surgery for congenital monocular cataracts. Am J Ophthalmol 93:559, 1981
4. Parks MM: Visual results in aphakic children. Am J Ophthalmol 94:441, 1982
5. Von Noorden GK, Dowling JE, Ferguson DC: Experimental amblyopia in monkeys. Arch Ophthalmol 84:206, 1970
6. Vaegan, Taylor D: Critical period for deprivation amblyopia in children. Trans Ophthalmol Soc UK 101:114, 1981
7. BenEzra D, Paez JH: Congenital cataracts and intraocular lenses. Am J Ophthalmol 96:311, 1983
8. Enoch JM: The fitting of hydrophilic soft contact lenses to infants and young children. 1. Mensuration Data on aphakic eyes of children born with congenital cataracts. Contact Lens Bull 5:3, 1972
9. Jacobson SC, Mohindra I, Held R: Development of visual acuity in infants with congenital cataracts. Br J Ophthalmol 65:777, 1981
10. Taylor DI: Choice of surgical technique in the management of congenital cataracts. Trans Ophthalmol Soc UK 101:114, 1981
11. Korczyn AD, Laor N, Nemet P: Autonomic pupillary activity in infants. Met Ophthalmol 2:391, 1978
12. Chrousos G, Parks MM, O'Neil JF: Incidence of chronic glaucoma, retinal detachment, and secondary membrane surgery in pediatric aphakic patients. Presented at the American Academy of Ohpthalmology, Chicago, Illinois, 1983
13. Poyofuku H, Hirose T, Schepens CL: Retinal detachment following congenital cataract surgery. Arch Ophthalmol 98:669, 1980
14. Chandler PA: Surgery of congenital cataracts. Am J Ophthalmol 65:663, 1968
15. Hoyt CS, Nickel B: Aphakic cystoid macular edema: Occurrence in infants and children after transpupillary lensectomy and anterior vitrectomy. Arch Ophthalmol 100:746, 1982
16. Gilbard SM, Peyman GA, Goldberg MF: Evaluation of cystoid macular edema after pars plicata lensectomy–vitrectomy for congenital cataracts. Ophthalmology 90:1201, 1983

13 Indications and Techniques for Removal of Intraocular Lenses

Richard H. Keates

The use of intraocular lenses has increased greatly over the past several years. Approximately 700 to 800 thousand cataract extractions are performed in the United States annually. The latest reports indicate that approximately 85 percent of these patients will receive an intraocular lens (IOL). The same statistics indicate that at least 95 percent of these patients will experience good vision with no evidence of intolerance to the intraocular lens. Unfortunately, there have been IOLs that were not well tolerated. A variety of reasons such as inflammatory reactions against the IOL material, edge manufacturing techniques, and polishing materials have led to their intolerance. Other problems associated with lens designs allow for inappropriate lens movement, causing injury and incarceration by the surrounding tissue.

This chapter discusses the indications and surgical techniques for removal of intraocular lenses in addition to the medical management.

INDICATIONS FOR REMOVAL OF AN INTRAOCULAR LENS

Absolute Indications

There are seven absolute indications for removal: extrusion; dislocation up against the cornea, through the iris or into the vitreous cavity; iritis uncontrolled by topical steroids; endophthalmitis; incorrectly sized IOL; corneal decompensation clearly related to lens movement; and dense pupillary membrane enveloping IOL.

Extrusion

An obvious cause of extrusion occurs with ocular trauma. In these cases, a portion of the lens usually presents through a rupture of the globe. This is

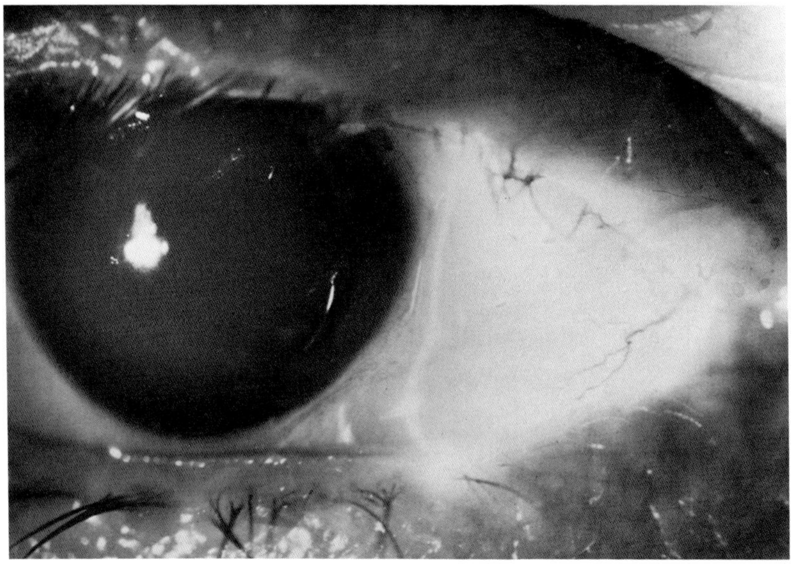

Fig. 13-1. Partially extruded intraocular lens.

most likely to occur in those patients who have a solid uniplanar lens that is in a vertical 12 to 6 o'clock position. This may also occur with flexible-looped lens with the same orientation. More frequently, IOL extrusion is seen following blunt trauma during the early postoperative period when the patient fails to wear a Fox shield or glasses to protect the eye. The immature surgical wound separates with partial prolapse of intraocular contents (Fig. 13-1).

With minimal extrusion, it may be possible to replace a loop or a partially prolapsed lens, along with iris tissue. With massive extrusion externalization of intraocular contents, this is not possible due to the extent of the trauma. The timing of replacement is important. Generally, if the iris does not appear necrotic or has been prolapsed for less than 12 hours, it need not be excised. All vitreous present in the wound must be excised with vitrectomy instruments. One must not forget about the

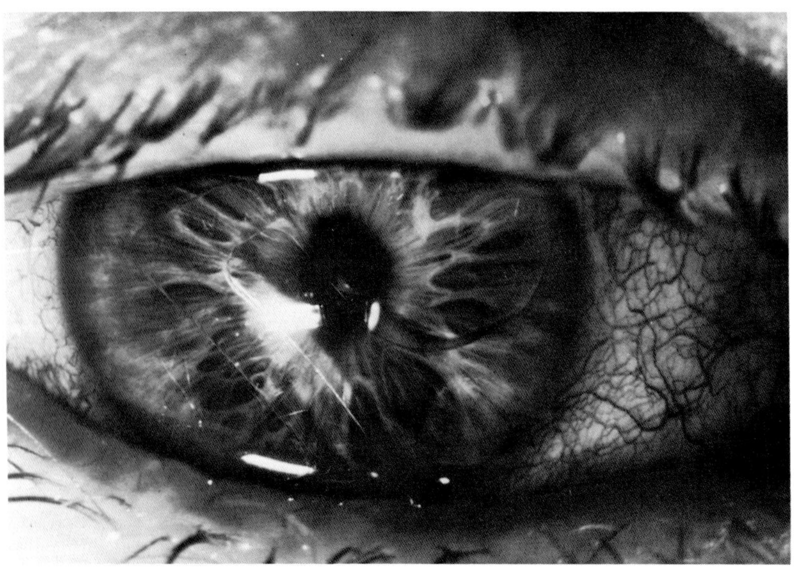

Fig. 13-2. Dislocated anterior chamber intraocular lens.

possibility of secondary intraocular infection or even sympathetic ophthalmia. Every effort to evaluate the full extent of the ocular injury must be made prior to surgery. In this manner the best possible surgical strategy may be formulated.

Dislocation

Most nontraumatic dislocations occur with incorrect sizing of the anterior chamber lens. Although the initial postoperative appearance is generally good, it soon becomes apparent that the lens is too small. The intraocular lens frequently demonstrates pseudophakodonesis. Movement of the lens may cause excessive currents in the aqueous humor, which contributes to the endothelial decompensation. Clinically, the spectrum of dislocation of an anterior chamber IOL ranges from minimal pseudophakodonesis to dislocation up against the cornea, through the iris or into the posterior chamber (Figs. 13-2 and 13-3). When minimal pseudophakodonesis with "propellering" occurs, the surgeon should observe the eye. If no gross movement occurs, surgical intervention is not required. When propellering occurs, the surgeon should observe the eye for a short period. During this time, the IOL may lodge in one position, since the anterior chamber is not perfectly round. If movement persists, the lens must be removed to prevent further damage. A small lens when propellering may come in contact with the cornea causing endothelial injury. A typical case presents with a lens that comes to rest with one haptic against the cornea, causing a focal area of corneal edema (Fig. 13-4). Under this circumstance, the lens must be removed. In those cases in which the IOL has come to rest with one haptic elevated, but without cor-

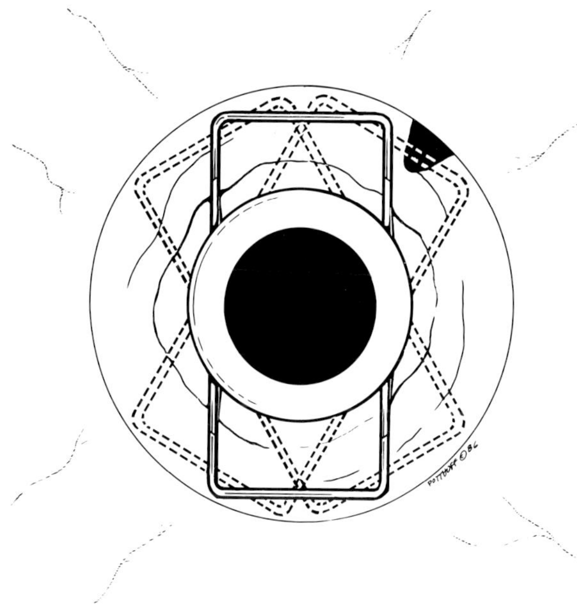

Fig. 13-3. Pseudophakodonesis resulting from a too small intraocular lens.

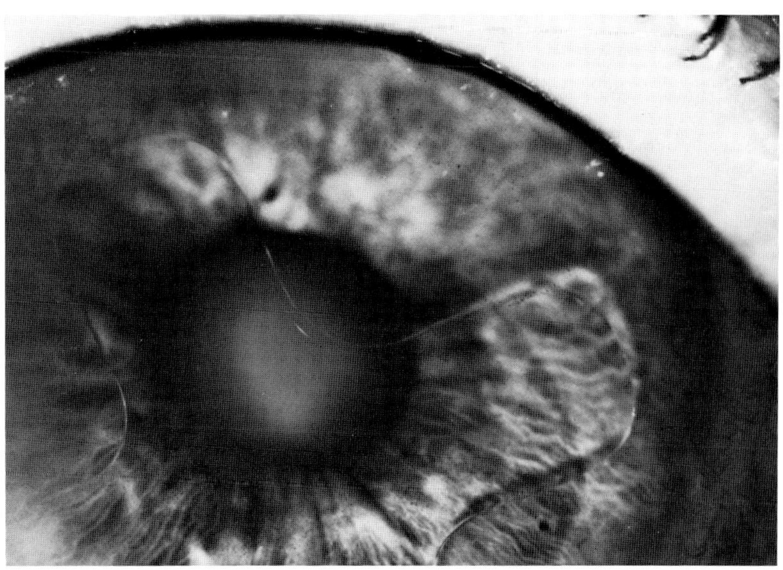

Fig. 13-4. Anterior chamber intraocular lens resting against the cornea.

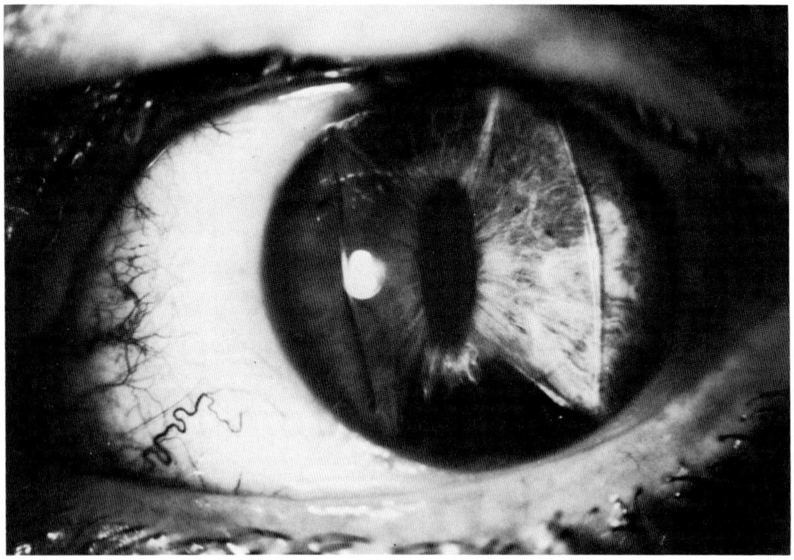

Fig. 13-5. Anterior chamber intraocular lens eroding into the iris.

neal touch, observation is advised to determine whether there is progression of endothelial decompensation.

Some rigid anterior chamber lenses have been observed to slowly erode through the iris, creating defects in the iris and ciliary body (Fig. 13-5). Also, the haptic of an anterior chamber lens may drop into an iridectomy causing erosion of the iris and ciliary body. This type of damage may result in chronic iritis, hyphema, and glaucoma, necessitating its removal. It is well known that the Azar 91 Z can cheesewire through the iris, causing recurrent iritis and secondary glaucoma (Fig. 13-6).[1,2]

Patients who have had herpes zoster with resultant iris atrophy may be unable to support an anterior chamber IOL. The author has observed several anterior chamber IOLs that eroded through ocular structures within days of an uncomplicated surgery.

Some posterior chamber lenses have been ob-

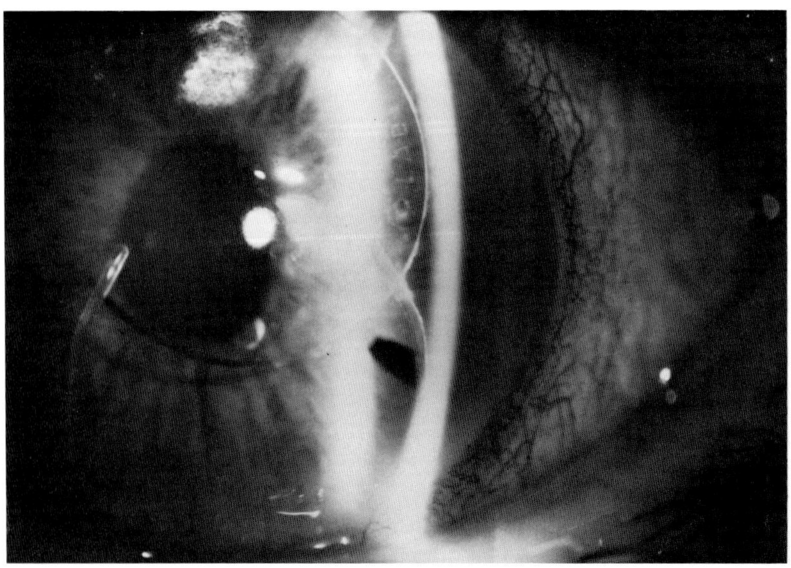

Fig. 13-6. Damage to iris resulting from the Azar 91Z.

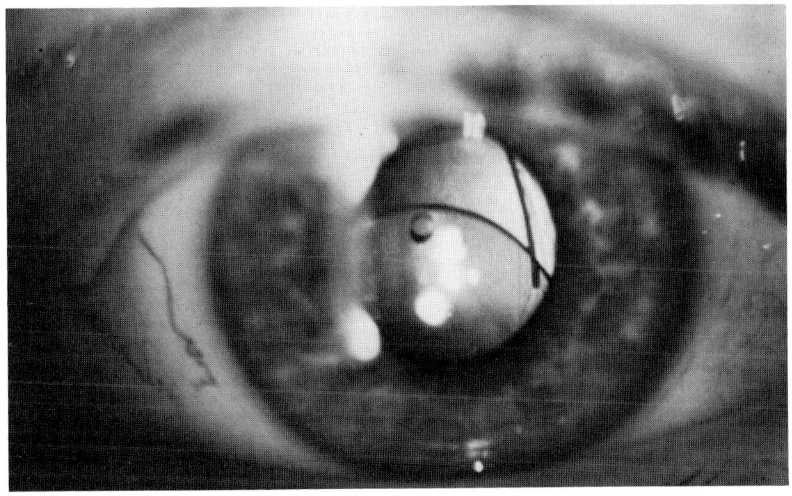

Fig. 13-7. Posterior chamber intraocular lens dislocated into the anterior chamber.

served to present a haptic through the iris into the anterior chamber. Varying degrees of dislocation can occur with and without progressive endothelial decompensation or iritis (Fig. 13-7). Similarly, if there is progressive damage, the lens must be removed.

Pupillary capture of a posterior chamber lens that is not vision threatening should not require surgical intervention. During the early postoperative period an attempt to alleviate the capture should be attempted. After widely dilating the pupil, scleral pressure applied over the point of contact by the haptics may shift the lens posteriorly. The pupil should be constricted if the maneuver is successful.

Iritis Uncontrolled by Topical Steroids

There is a group of patients who display a postoperative, recurrent iritis in excess of what would normally be expected.[3] The differential diagnosis includes a reaction to retained cortical materials, that is, phacoanaphylaxis, and infectious endophthalmitis. The reaction may also be directed against the polypropylene loops, to residual polishing compounds or even sterilizations techniques.[4,5] In the face of vision-threatening iritis, after an adequate trial of medical therapy, these lenses should be removed. At the time of removal, any remaining cortex should be removed along with appropriate samples for culture and sensitivity.

Endophthalmitis

Most causes of infectious endophthalmitis have been divided into an acute and late presentation. Most bacterial endophthalmitides will occur within 72 hours after surgery. The surgeon must be suspicious of any eye that presents after surgery with more than the expected reaction (Fig. 13-8). With the popularity of ambulatory surgery, the patient should be instructed to notify the surgeon immediately if increasing edema, redness, pain, or decreasing acuity develop.

Fungal endophthalmitis classically presents several weeks or even months after ocular surgery. The ocular inflammatory response typically is low grade, although some may present as a fulminant endophthalmitis. For the obvious case of endophthalmitis, whether bacterial or fungal, the surgeon is obligated to perform diagnostic tests, remove the IOL along with the abscess, and institute appropriate antibiotic therapy.

The surgeon must also be concerned with a small group of patients who present with a postoperative iritis requiring increasing amounts of steroids. These patients may actually have a smouldering endophthalmitis secondary to a less virulent organism. Again, in the differential diagnosis one must consider a reaction to the lens itself. Clinically, a fibrinous reaction may suggest the possibility of endophthalmitis. In this specific case, appropriate aqueous and vitreous taps should be performed. If organisms are recovered, the lens must be re-

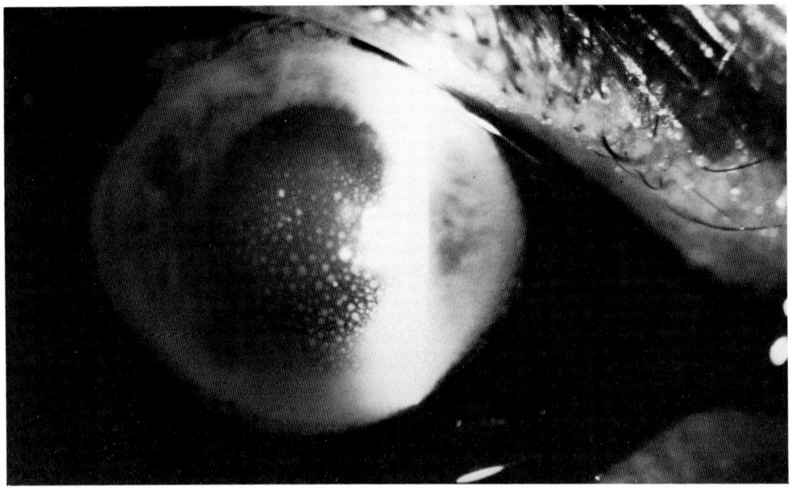

Fig. 13-8. Suspected endophthalmitis prior to tap.

moved. If no organisms are recovered, the problem becomes a clinical decision. The author recommends removing the lens and any remaining cortical material at that time. Since the possibility of endophthalmitis is still present, the patient should also be treated with appropriate measures.

Incorrectly Sized IOL with Pain

A small percentage of anterior chamber IOL patients show tenderness to touch, particularly over the upper lid. As long as the pain is well tolerated, the lens should not be removed. If the pain is not tolerated or persistent as a low discomfort, the lens must be removed.

Corneal Decompensation Clearly Related to Lens Movement

Endothelial touch may lead to focal decompensation. A mobile lens will cause increasing areas of endothelial decompensation. As soon one realizes that there is increasing decompensation, this is an absolute indication for removal of the offending IOL.

Dense Pupillary Membrane Enveloping IOL

In some patients one may observe an angle-closure chronic inflammation and a membrane slowly covering the IOL. Although the surgeon may be tempted to use a Nd:YAG laser to open some of these membranes, increasing vascularization and progressive encroachment by the membrane are sufficient cause for removal of the IOL (Fig. 13-9). At the time of lens removal, the membrane must be dissected from the lens to avoid iris or ciliary body damage during the course of extraction. Finally, the membrane can be cleared from the visual axis if necessary.

RELATIVE INDICATIONS FOR REMOVAL OF INTRAOCULAR LENSES

There are four relative indications for removing an intraocular lens. low-grade iritis controlled with topical steroids, recurrent hyphema, dislocation and repositioning, and removal of intraocular lenses during another procedure.

Low-Grade Iritis Controlled with Topical Steroids

Post-operatively, some patients may have a low-grade iritis that may be due to discontinuing the topical steroids too quickly. These patients usually respond very well to a few weeks of additional topical steroids. Rarely, other patients with iritis ultimately require topical steroids chronically once a day.

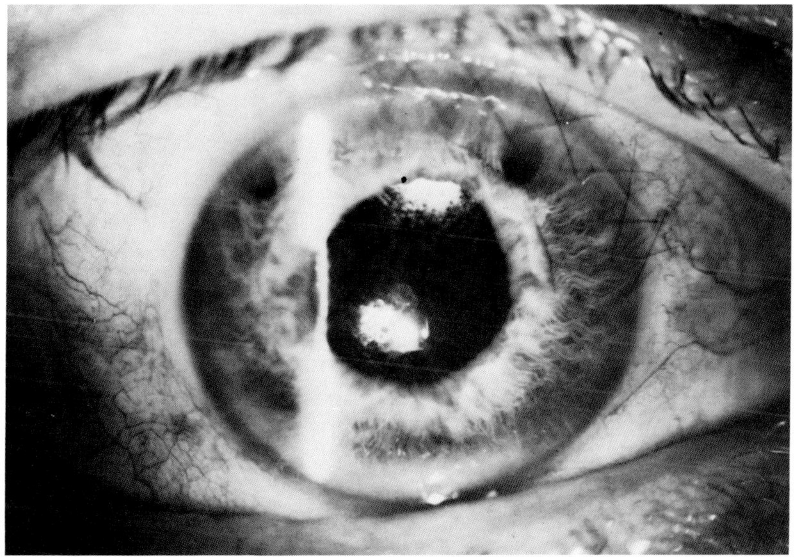

Fig. 13-9. Dense pupillary membrane enveloping the intraocular lens.

In the patient whose chronic iritis is well controlled with minimal topical steroid therapy there is no reason to remove an intraocular lens. However, if the patient requires increasing amounts of topical medications or develops a steroid induced glaucoma, removal of the offending intraocular lens should be considered. In the author's experience, the patients most likely to have chronic iritis are those with dermatosis such as acne rosacea.

Recurrent Hyphema

Recurrent hyphema syndrome may be seen with flexible-loop anterior chamber, iris fixed, and posterior chamber lenses. The flexible-loop anterior chamber lenses cheesewire into the iris, while the haptics of the posterior chamber lenses may erode into the iris or ciliary body. This erosion occasionally causes recurrent hyphemas. Similarly, the iris-fixed lens produces iris damage from continuous friction. Chronic friction eventually leads to vessel breakdown. With a history of red-outs or white-outs, in which the patients report hazy red or white vision, one should inquire about the use of anticoagulation or aspirin therapy. Minimal blood dyscrasia may tip the scale toward hyphema in a patient with lens-induced ocular damage.

Frequently, the dose of anticoagulation can be decreased, resulting in the resolution of the hyphema. The argon laser may also be used to coagulate the bleeding site or perform iridoplasty to prevent continual iris erosion. If after medical and/or laser therapy the hyphema persists, the surgeon must remove the lens.

Dislocation and Repositioning

In patients presenting with a dislocated posterior chamber lens, the surgical intent is to reposition and stabilize rather than remove the lens. After repositioning, the lens may be sutured into place. When the posterior capsule has been sufficiently disrupted to prevent adequate support for the posterior chamber lens, the lens may be removed and replaced with an anterior chamber IOL.

Total dislocation of the IOL into the vitreous is a rare occurrence. Although one may feel compelled to remove the lens, this is not a requirement as long as the lens is not causing more damage. There have been cases in which the IOL has been left in the vitreous. A contact lens or even a secondary IOL may be implanted. Often attempts to remove an otherwise well-tolerated IOL meet with disaster. Generally, these are not free-floating IOLs, but they are anchored in place by a vitreous strand.

Removal of Intraocular Lenses during Another Procedure: Penetrating Keratoplasty

In pseudophakic bullous keratopathy the question often arises as to whether the IOL should be removed. In the past, our philosophy was that if the lens left us alone we would leave it alone. We believed that the presence of the IOL may prevent the loss of vitreous or the need for a vitrectomy. We no longer feel this way. The deciding factor in this situation should be the stability of the IOL, the presence of progressive endothelial decompensation, chronic unexplained iritis, or massive vitreous investiture of the lens. In general, all iris-fixed lenses should be removed.

For these reasons, there is an increasing tendency to remove lenses such as the Copeland, Binkhorst 4-loop, and Azar 91 lens at the time of keratoplasty. If there is no endothelial decompensation however, directly attributable to the IOL, iritis, or vitreous investiture, there is no reason to remove the lens. In fact, the increasing tendency is to place a secondary intraocular lens at the time of keratoplasty in many patients who have aphakic bullous keratopathy.

TECHNIQUE FOR REMOVAL OF ANTERIOR CHAMBER INTRAOCULAR LENSES

A Preoperative Evaluation and Documentation

The surgeon must give the patient a realistic assessment of the quality of visual recovery. Often, the patient understands that the surgery is to relieve chronic discomfort, avert the possibility of infection, or maintain anatomic appearance. To predict visual recovery, a complete preoperative evaluation must be performed.

EVALUATION

Visual acuity should be documented by refraction. If not correctable to 20/20 or J1, a visual acuity by the potential acuity meter should be performed. A slit-lamp examination to record pathology should also be performed. Gonioscopy is extremely important to document the position of the haptics, vessels, angle structures, peripheral iridectomies, and vitreous adhesions. These details are most important in planning an approach to removing the lens. Fundus examination is important to document preoperative cystoid macular edema, retinal holes, and unsuspected retinal detachment. Fluoroscein angiography is a useful adjunctive study to look for cystoid macular edema. Specular microscopy is indicated to help determine the prognosis for corneal clarity following surgery.

SURGICAL TECHNIQUES FOR REMOVAL OF AN INTRAOCULAR LENS

The precise technique for removal of an IOL is dependent on its location. Specific techniques are discussed in this section. The following general comment should be considered for all lens types.

As with any other intraocular surgery, a soft eye and adequate anesthesia is required. The surgeon should have a viscoelastic material as well as heavy scissors with which to cut haptics and an automated vitrectomy device available.

Patients with traumatic wound dehiscense should be treated as any ruptured globe. General anesthesia should be administered to avoid the potential complications of retrobulbar hemorrhage. Care must be taken to avoid raising the intraocular pressure with the use of depolarizing muscle relaxants such as succinylcholine. Frequently a 360-degree peritomy is required to assess the extent of the surgery adequately. Total wound reconstruction is often required.

Once the decision to remove an IOL is made, the lens should be removed gently under the cover of a viscoelastic material. The viscoelastic material will protect the endothelium and help maintain the anterior chamber. This has greatly improved the success of lens removal and secondary implants.

Some IOLs are held in place with clips or sutures. One must remember to look for these attachments in order to prevent damage to ocular structures during lens removal.

Similarly, if one finds resistance to removal of the lens due to incarceration of the lens, further pressure should be avoided. Continued traction could result in iridodialysis and cyclodialysis or hyphema. It is safer to cut the optic from its haptic rather than cause ocular damage (Fig. 13-10). The removal of the cut haptic by gently twisting or backing it out of the tissue should be attempted (Fig. 13-11). It should be remembered that it is safer to leave a cut haptic than cause damage from aggressive attempts at removal.

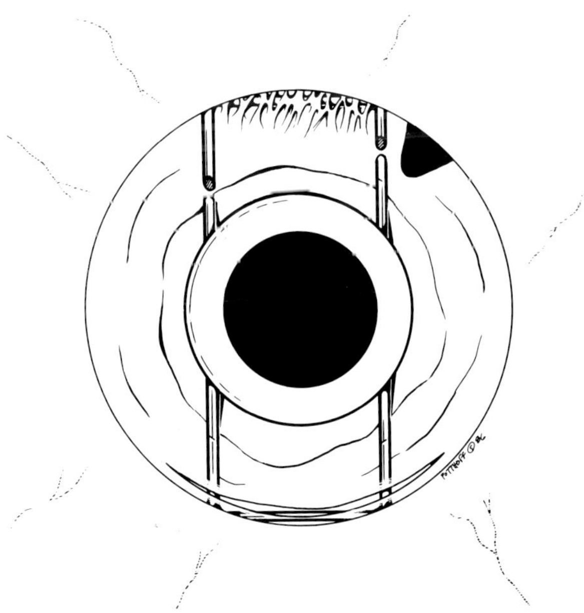

Fig. 13-10. Cutting the optic from the haptic during removal.

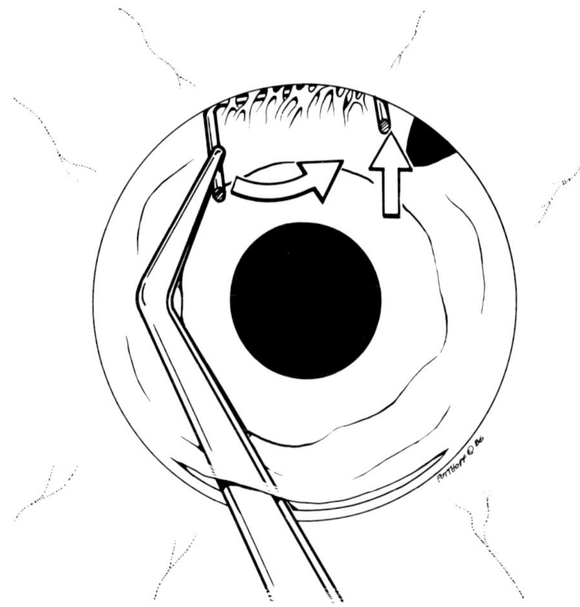

Fig. 13-11. Removal of cut haptic by twisting or backing out.

In nontraumatic cases, after thorough preoperative evaluation, a plan can be formulated as to what will be required to remove the lens. It must be decided whether the incision should be through the initial wound or through a separate site.

Finally, the surgeon must ensure that vitreous is not incarcerated in the wound. A vitrectomy should be performed when necessary to prevent a vitreous wick syndrome, chronic inflammation and possible endophthalmitis.

ANTERIOR CHAMBER INTRAOCULAR LENSES

Anterior chamber IOLs fall into two categories: rigid and flexible anterior chamber lenses. The technique for removal of both types is similar. It should be remembered that both rigid and flexible lenses may become incarcerated.

After thorough preoperative evaluation, the site

of incision can be decided. Factors to consider in making this decision include the position of the lens and the old incision site. Generally, the more posterior the incision, the easier it is to remove the lens. The trouble with a posterior incision is that one usually ends up in the old incision site, resulting in more bleeding than usual. Also, a secondary stab incision is required so that one can place a hook into the anterior chamber to manipulate the lens. The author recommends a more anterior incision of at least 7 mm in length. This will easily accommodate a 6-mm optic. A key to success is removing the lens without undue pressure.

Initially, a stab incision is made at 90 degrees away from the intended anterior incision site. Next the anterior incision should be made, but the incision should not be enlarged to 7 mm until a viscoelastic material has been injected into the anterior chamber. This will coat the front surface of the intraocular lens and will prevent collapse with contact between the IOL and the corneal endothelium. It is useful to place viscoelastic material over iridectomies and the pupil to prevent vitreous prolapse. The wound is then enlarged to 7 mm, and a lens hook is placed into the anterior chamber. If there are no adhesions, one edge of the lens is elevated and grasped with forceps, and more viscoelastic material is added at this time. Adhesions should be checked for by gently wiggling the lens. The spatula may be used to dissect weak adhesions bluntly from the lens (Fig. 13-12). The IOL is then slid out of the anterior chamber. A correctly sized anterior chamber lens may be inserted at this point through the same incision.

When adhesions are present, lens removal is more difficult. With Azar 91 anterior chamber lenses, the haptics cheesewire into the peripheral iris and become incarcerated. These lenses frequently have extensive adhesions along the superior and inferior haptics. Frequently, one can cut one side of the superior haptic near the optic and cut the other side of the superior haptic near the iris. The severed haptic now has one long end and one short end. This then permits the cut haptic to be dialed or backed out rather than direct traction applied, which could cause ocular damage (Fig. 13-11). The same procedure may be followed for the remaining haptic. If bleeding should occur during the procedure, it is best to try and increase the pressure in the eye temporarily by using viscoelastic material to tamponade it. The wound is then closed and subconjunctival steroids and antibiotics are administered. After closure of the wound, it is important to sweep the wound edge carefully through the peripheral stab incision to ensure there is no vitreous to the wound.

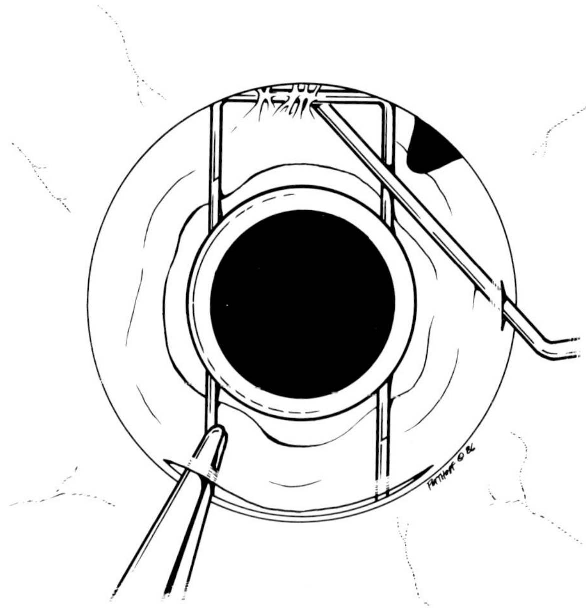

Fig. 13-12. Use of spatula to dissect weak adhesions bluntly from the intraocular lens.

REMOVAL OF IRIS-FIXED LENSES

For safety, some iris-fixed lenses had either metal clips or McCannel sutures to hold them in place. The surgeon must remember to look for these attachments prior to removal.

Deciding on the incision site for removal of an iris-fixed lens is similar to that on an anterior chamber lens. Again an anterior incision of a least 7 mm in length is suggested. Also the peripheral stab incision is very helpful for manipulation of an incarcerated haptic. Once the anterior chamber has been entered a viscoelastic material should be placed into the anterior chamber to coat the lens,

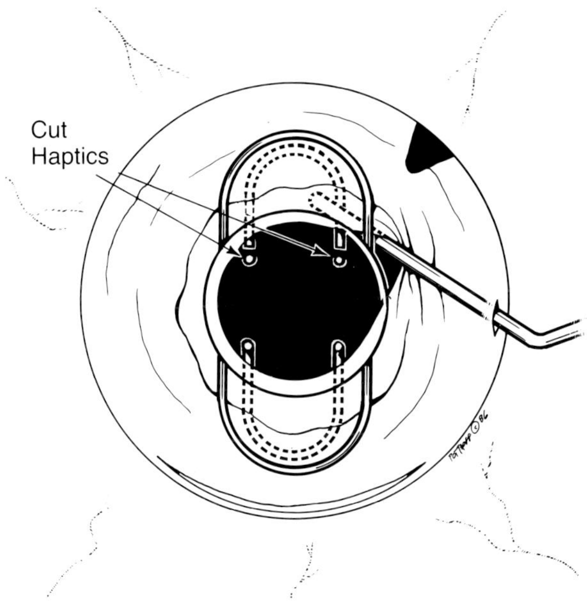

Fig. 13-13. Cutting of metal loop from the optic and breaking posterior adhesions with a spatula.

iridectomy site(s) and pupil. This will hold vitreous back and help protect the endothelium.

Once this is done, the wound is enlarged to 7 mm. The metal loop should be cut from the optic. There are usually adhesions to the loop that must be massaged free with a spatula loop once it has been cut from the optic (Fig. 13-13). A loose haptic may drift back into the vitreous. Each metal loop should be removed in this fashion. Next, the optic can be grasped and gently wiggled to be certain there are no adhesions. When it is freed of an adhesion it can be removed.

Two-looped Binkhorst lenses may require a slightly different approach, since the haptics may be incarcerated in the capsular bag. In these cases, it is important to divide the haptic and consider leaving them in place rather than tearing the capsule or iris.

Most four-looped lenses were placed following intracapsular surgery. The surgeon must be careful not to apply pressure on the lid speculum, which will force vitreous into the anterior chamber. After the lens has been removed and the wound partially sutured closed, air should be placed into the anterior chamber to demonstrate any vitreous adhesions. Vitreous adhesion should be cleaned up with an automated vitrector at this time.

REMOVAL OF POSTERIOR CHAMBER INTRAOCULAR LENS

If a lens has been placed in the sulcus and is mobile, it is relatively easy to fill the anterior chamber with viscoelastic material and dial the lens out of the posterior chamber. One should look for an adhesion along the haptic and be prepared to cut the haptic if necessary (Figs. 13-14 and 13-15). There is probably little danger in leaving haptics in the posterior chamber in these cases, unless it is the haptic material that is causing the inflammation. In that case it is imperative to remove the haptic.

It is very important to determine whether a vitreous strand is adherent to the IOL prior to removing it. If one were simply to pull on a lens with a vitreous strand attached to it, one could create a retinal tear. For this reason, if vitreous surrounds a lens, the surgeon must be prepared to clear it away with vitrectomy instruments.

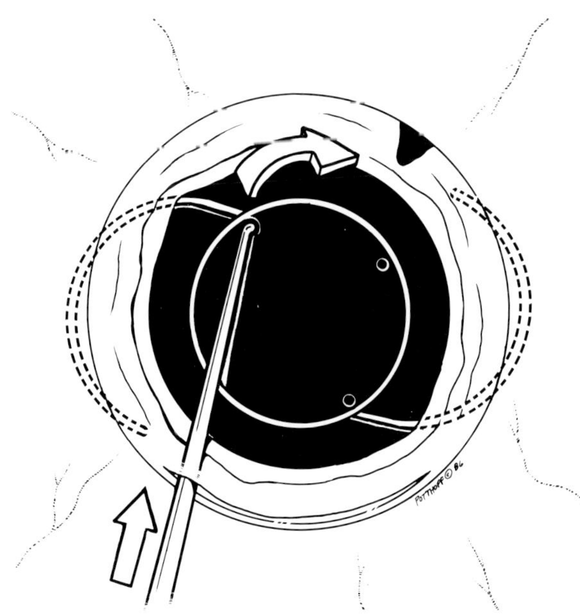

Fig. 13-14. Push-and-lift method of dialing an implant out of the sulcus.

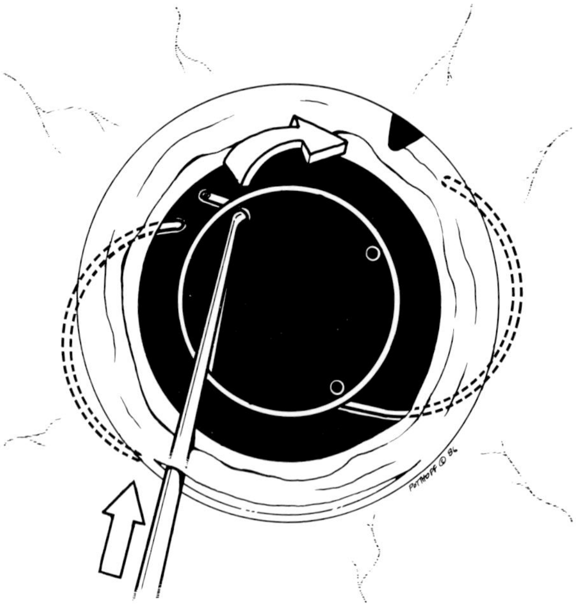

Fig. 13-15. Cutting of haptic adhesion prior to push and lift.

POSTOPERATIVE CARE

The medications generally include topical steroids and an antibiotic of choice four times a day plus scopolamine bid. Postoperative glaucoma usually responds rapidly to timolol and/or carbonic anhydrase inhibitors. Routine follow-up care is given in our office at 1 day, 1 week, and then 6 weeks later for final correction or a contact lens. Refractive procedures such as epikeratophakia have given good results for some of these patients. It is usually better to wait until the eye is quiet and one is sure that the inflammatory response has subsided before proceeding with an epikeratophakia.

REFERENCES

1. Azar RF: Complications of anterior chamber implants. Contact Intra-ocular Lens Med J 4:173, 1978
2. Hagan JC III: Complications while removing the IOLAB 91Z lens for the UGH–UGH+ syndromes. J Am Intraocul Implant Soc 10:209, 1984
3. Ellington FT: Complications with the Choyce Mark VIII and Mark IV anterior chamber implant (uveitis, glaucoma, hyphema). J Am Intraocul Implant Soc J 3:199, 1977
4. Drews R: Polypropylene in the human eye. Am Intraocul Implant Soc J 9:137, 1983
5. Maynor RC Jr: Five cases of severe anterior chamber lens implant complications. J Am Intraocul Implant Soc 10:223, 1984

Secondary Intraocular Lens Implantation and Intraocular Lens Exchange

14

Richard P. Kratz
Paul F. Olson
Stephen H. Johnson
Michael K. Farley

In 1985 1.1 million cataract extractions were performed in the United States, 90 percent of which had primary intraocular lens (IOL) implantation. In 1985 there were 120,000 secondary IOLs implanted in the United States; their numbers will rise over the next few years and will then fall to almost zero because primary implantation will reach nearly 100 percent.

INDICATIONS

The indications for secondary IOL implantation are failure to provide success with either aphakic glasses or contact lenses. The indications have become increasingly more liberal as technology has improved the quality of the lenses; it has also been recognized that the IOL must be well fixed in the eye. Improved surgical techniques, including vitrectomy and the use of sodium hyaluronate, have increased the success rate. However, in each individual case the risk–benefit ratio must be carefully evaluated in relationship to the life-style of the patient.

CONTACT LENSES

Subjective indications for secondary implantation include decrease comfort or contact lens intolerance, excessive loss or breakage, and trouble with contact lens manipulation. Objective symptoms include dry eyes, difficult-to-fit eyes, giant papillary conjunctivitis, corneal neovascularization, recurrent corneal erosion, and corneal ulceration.

SPECTACLES

Subjectively aphakic spectacles are thick in all but the high myopes, a few people tolerate the image magnification, jack-in-the-box phenomenon, barrel distortion, ring scotoma, or loss of peripheral vision without complaints. If the fellow eye still has useful phakic vision, both anisometropia and anisophoria reach unacceptable levels. These failures all become reasons to do secondary IOL implantation.

CONTRAINDICATIONS

There are probably no absolute contraindications. If the contact lenses or aphakic spectacles are well tolerated, there is little reason for secondary implantation. Caution should be exercised in patients with a low endothelial cell count or diabetes, in patients on anticoagulants, or in those with a history of retinal detachment. Special consideration has to be given to one-eyed patients and to young patients because they have a long life expectation. A shallow anterior chamber, peripheral anterior synechiae, angle neovascularity, controlled glaucoma, or filtering bleb may rule out an anterior chamber IOL, but not one in the posterior chamber. Posterior synechiae of the pupil and iris to the posterior capsule may preclude a posterior chamber lens implant but not one in the anterior chamber. Rubeosis, uncontrolled glaucoma, and recently active uveitis probably constitute the strongest contraindications.

INTRAOCULAR LENS EXCHANGE

Intraocular lens exchange is a special form of secondary IOL implantation when the first IOL has failed, but there are still valid reasons to use an IOL. One of the most common reasons is incorrect power. This is most apt to happen in the very long and very short eyes and to some degree cannot be avoided. As lens-power calculation formulas are improved, this error will become more rare.

SECONDARY POSTERIOR CHAMBER INTRAOCULAR LENSES

Posterior chamber IOLs have less chance of corneal trauma. The optical effects of glare, glitter, dazzle, loop, and edge exposure in the visual axis are minimized. The physiologic pupil response is maintained, and the image size is normalized. The posterior chamber lens may be used in the presence of a shallow chamber and filtering blebs. There is an absence of pseudophakodenesis. Posterior synechiae of the pupil margin and the iris to the posterior capsule are difficult to separate. In secondary posterior chamber IOLs, placement is in the ciliary sulcus rather than the capsular bag. The bag must be sufficiently present to support the IOL. The loop should be long enough to ensure fixation (about 14 mm) and should have a low compression force. If in doubt, a McCannel suture may be added. The compression force of the loop should be kept about 100 mg/mm with a rapid force decay. High compression forces erode into the uveal tissue, and excessively low forces, as found in some of the early silicone lenses, have been extruded from the capsular bag, resulting in a severe tilt of the optic. The optic should be large enough to cover the pupil in scotopic conditions without the presence of a posterior hole or laser spacer in the visual axis.

SECONDARY ANTERIOR CHAMBER INTRAOCULAR LENS

Anterior chamber lenses may be used in the presence or absence of the posterior capsule. Rigid anterior chamber lenses require a large inventory, as they have to be obtained in both power and length. Choyce[1] recommended "white to white plus 1 mm." Others have developed dipsticks in an attempt to be more accurate.[2–4] Lerman and Hockwin demonstrated a technique using a Schiemflug camera.[5] It has also been shown that the sulcus is often irregular and, while 3 feet of a tetrapod IOL may be at the scleral spur, the fourth foot may be traumatizing iris or passing through a basal iridectomy. It is best to put the iridectomies in midstroma to avoid this problem as well as pupil block. Rigid anterior chamber lenses may be too short, resulting in propellering and increased risk of corneal touch and decompensation. Excessively long rigid IOLs cause long-lasting tenderness with iris erosion, oval pupils, ectropion uveae, and iritis. A fracture of a Choyce-style footplate has been reported, and the authors have seen one case of fractured polymethyl methacrylate loops in both a flexible and a semiflexible IOL.[6] Prolene loops do not fracture but are believed to undergo ultraviolet degradation. Some of the thin-loop flexible-anterior chamber IOL have developed cocooning of the angle, making removal quite difficult.

The semiflexible and flexible anterior chamber lenses have minimized sizing problems as compared with the rigid lenses. However, a fair percentage develop peripheral anterior synechiae over the thin loops. This occludes some of the functioning angle and creates a potential removal problem of bleeding and iridodialysis. Unless the loops are cut short within the eye and then straightened out using two instruments within the eye before they are slid out of the cocoon, bleeding and iridodialysis may occur. This tendency to occlude the angle raises some questions about the use of anterior chamber lenses in an eye with a shallow anterior chamber or glaucoma.

IRIS-SUPPORTED INTRAOCULAR LENSES

Very few iris-supported secondary intraocular lenses have been used in the United States during the past 5 years. The iris supported lenses prior to that frequently subluxed unless sutured. Some sank into the vitreous, but more frequently they intermittently touched the cornea and caused progressive loss of endothelial cells and corneal decompensation. Some caused iris erosion; this was particularly common when metal loops were used.

PLANNING SECONDARY IMPLANTATION

If there is a 1-year time lapse between the cataract extraction and a secondary IOL implantation procedure, the incidence of cystoid macular edema appears to be less.[7] Hard contact lenses should be discontinued until stable keratometric readings are obtained.[8] The ultrasound tissue velocity should be 1,548 m/sec for phakic eyes and 1,532 m/sec for aphakic eyes. It is possible to calculate the required power from the refraction, but it may not be as accurate as the ultrasound A scan. Special formulas take into account extra-long and extra-short eyes. It is important to select a power that will match the fellow eye, if it has good vision. This will avoid anisometropia and anisophoria.

ANTERIOR CHAMBER EVALUATION

The cornea should be carefully inspected by slit lamp, and it is helpful to examine the endothelium or to obtain an endothelial cell count. If an anterior chamber lens is to be used, gonioscopy of the angle will reveal peripheral anterior synechiae or angled neovascularity that may be present. If a posterior chamber IOL is to be used, the pupil should be dilated so that posterior synechiae may be identified. If the posterior synechiae are extensive, it may be wise to use an anterior chamber lens instead. While the pupil is dilated, it is possible to evaluate the condition of the posterior capsule in relationship to the potential support of the posterior chamber IOL. If an iris coloboma is present, a plan should be developed either to avoid it or close it. Basal iridectomies should be identified as potential areas to avoid having the haptic enter the iridectomy and cause a decentration. Sometimes pupils are eccentric, and a plan should be developed to free synechiae or do some form of iris surgery to restore the pupil to a central position. A well-centered intraocular lens fails to give good vision if the pupil is at the margin of the lens. An extremely shallow anterior chamber will not offer sufficient room for an anterior chamber IOL; thus an alternative must be considered. Usually it is best to plan an anterior vitrectomy in the presence of vitreous herniation into the anterior chamber. This approach avoids vitreous to the wound with a resultant peaked pupil.

TECHNIQUE

A soft eye is very helpful, as is some preoperative pressure reduction such as a Honan balloon. Operating on the + axis gives the best results in minimizing astigmatism. A horizontal incision may be considered to avoid 12 o'clock peripheral anterior synechiae, the probable area of lowest endothelial cell count or the probable area of thinnest sclera resulting from the previous incision. A scleral pocket incision seems to minimize the astigmatism. If a rigid anterior chamber lens is to be used a dipstick or a white-to-white plus 1 mm is used to select the proper lens size. A semirigid lens may be less tender if white-to-white plus 0.75 mm with suturing of the haptic to the iris is done. Flexible anterior chamber intraocular lenses do not require such precise sizing.

Repair of an iris coloboma may be accomplished by passing a straight needle through the limbus, then through both halves of the iris, exiting at the opposite limbus. Both ends of the suture are retrieved from the anterior chamber by a Bonn hook and are then brought out through a 1-mm limbal incision located at the axis of the coloboma, where they are tied and cut. Sometimes two or three sutures are required to close a coloboma. If the coloboma is too large, closure may not be justified. If the pupil is eccentric, a plan should be followed to restore it to a near-central position. Sometimes cutting a vitreous strand preoperatively by a Nd : YAG laser or at the time of surgery will correct the pupil. Often this fails, as synechiae of the posterior iris to the vitreous face have developed or the iris has developed a segmental fibrosis that will not allow the pupil to regain its original position. In that case, the previously described suture technique will return the pupil to a more central position.

Vitreous herniation into the anterior chamber often may be reversed by air or sodium hyaluronate instilled into the anterior chamber. If this fails, an anterior vitrectomy by automated equipment should be considered. After the iris becomes scaphoid, a Bonn hook will identify and a Vannas scissors will cut any remaining vitreous strands that would otherwise result in a peaked pupil.

A Sheets glide with the end bent up slightly like a ski is passed to the opposite angle and light pressure put on the glide. If it causes pupil distortion, the iris has been tucked and needs repositioning. The anterior chamber lens will be guided into the correct position over the glide. A Sheets glide may also be used to insert a posterior chamber IOL, where the glide will hold back the vitreous and prevent the inferior loop from passing behind the posterior capsule. The glide is placed between the iris and the posterior capsule in this case. It is possible to suture the haptic of most anterior and posterior chamber lenses to the iris or even to the sclera, if indicated.

The use of a keratometer such as the Terry will help minimize the postoperative astigmatism.[9–11] It is important not to overinflate the anterior chamber, as an aqueous diversion may be created, causing the balanced salt solution to go posteriorly and the vitreous to move anteriorly, producing a severe shallowing of the anterior chamber.

RESULTS

The results of secondary IOL and IOL exchange have been generally encouraging. The visual acuity has been reported by Stark as 85 percent, giving 20/40 or better in 1983 and 91 percent, giving 20/40 or better if preexisting pathology was excluded. Kraff et al.[12] reported 87 percent within one line of preoperative vision. Mazzocco gave a similar report,[13] and Brown achieved 83 percent.[14] Lindstrom et al.[15] reported 94 percent at 20/40 or better in secondary implants or exchange. Shammas and Milkie[16–18] found 55 percent improved one line or more, while 42 percent were the same and only 3 percent decreased one line or more. Heslin reported 20/40 or better vision in 81 percent preoperatively and 91 percent postoperatively.[19] Patients with anterior vitrectomy had the same postoperative vision in 54 percent and improved vision in 41 percent.

The cornea decompensated in 2 of 23 cases in Brown's series. Johnson reported 2 of 75 eventually decompensated. This was not really a surprise, as the preoperative cell counts in the two patients were 673 and 1,009 respectively.

Iritis was less of a problem in secondary implants than in primary implants, presumably because of the smaller incision and less intraocular manipulation. Patients with glaucoma did not get worse according to Shammas and Milkie. In the series reported by Johnson, 10 patients of the 75 he studied had medically controlled glaucoma. None of these worsened after secondary IOL implantation.

Lindstrom and co-workers[15,20] recommended peripheral retinal examination with scleral depression and preoperative therapy, if indicated. Mazzocco reported that in his series of 40 patients, 1 had a late retinal detachment with counting fingers as the final visual result. Johnson reported no retinal detachment in 75 cases.

Shammas and Milkie[21] recommended preoperative intravenous fluorescein angiography to detect preexisting cystoid macular edema; they believed that the secondar IOL implantation might be made more severe from the second surgery. With a series of Choyce implants, these investigators listed 8 percent cystoid macular edema in primary cases, but 25 percent in secondary IOL implantation cases. Lindstrom et al.[15,20] reported 3 percent cystoid macular edema in their series of secondary IOLs and IOL exchanges. Johnson found 9 patients of 75 with preoperative cystoid macular edema, and 6 patients still had cystoid macular edema postoperatively.[19] Two new cases of cystoid macular edema developed but cleared within 8 weeks. None of these cases of cystoid macular edema showed a decrease of visual acuity from the preoperative level.

REFERENCES

1. Choyce DP: The Sixth Binkhorst Medical Lecture: Anterior chamber implants—past, present and future. Am Intraocul Implant Soc J 8:42, 1982
2. Johnson SH, Kratz RP: Improved technique for secondary anterior chamber lens insertion. Am Intra-Ocul Implant Soc J 8:267, 1982
3. Roberts JC: A method for anterior chamber lens size determination. Am Intraocul Implant Soc J 7:171, 1981
4. Choyce DP: Healon in anterior chamber lens implantation. Am Intraocul Implant Soc J 7:138, 1981
5. Hales RH: Dislocation of the Kelman II anterior chamber intraocular lens. Am Intraocul Implant Soc J 8:376, 1982
6. Shammas HJF, Milkie CF: Traumatic fracture of a Choyce-style anterior chamber lens. Am Intraocul Implant Soc J 7:46, 1981
7. Cobble CR: Traumatic expulsion of an intraocular lens. Am J Ophthalmol 94:263, 1982
8. Brown DC, Snead JW: Intraocular lens implant exchanges. Am Intraocul Implant Soc J 11:376, 1985
9. Terry CM: Incision and wound closure to reduce astigmatism. p. 134. In Cataract Surgery. McGraw-Hill, New York, 1986
10. Lindstrom RL, Destro MA: Effect of incision size and Terry keratometer usage on postoperative astigmatism. Am Intraocul Implant Soc J 11:469, 1985
11. Colvard DM, Kratz, RP, Mazzocco TR, Davidson B: The Terry surgical keratometer: A 12 month follow-up report. Am Intraocul Implant Soc J 7:348, 1981
12. Kraff MC, Sanders DR, Lieberman HL, Kraff J: Secondary intraocular lens implantation. Ophthalmology 90:324, 1983
13. Kratz RP, Davidson B, Colvard DM: Secondary posterior chamber intraocular lens implants. Am Intraocul Implant Soc J 7:342, 1981
14. Reidy JJ, Apple DJ, Googe JM, et al: An analysis of semiflexible, closed-loop anterior chamber intraocular lenses. Am Intraocul Implant Soc J 11:344, 1985
15. Lindstrom RL, Harris WS, Lyle WA: Secondary and exchange posterior chamber lens implantation. Am Intraocul Implant Soc J 8:353, 1982
16. Shammas HJF, Milkie CF: Secondary lens implantation in aphakia: Visual results and complications. Am Intraocul Implant Soc J 4:180, 1978
17. Shammas HJF, Milkie CF: Secondary implantation of anterior chamber lenses. Am Intraocul Implant Soc J 9:313, 1983
18. Shammas HJF, Milkie CF: Secondary lens implantation in aphakia: visual results and complications. Am Intraocul Implant Soc J 4:180, 1978
19. Heslin KB: Is "white-to-white" right? Am Intraocul Implant Soc J 5:50, 1979
20. Lindstrom RL, Nelson JD, Neist RL: Anterior chamber lens implantation. Am J Ophthalmol 95:55, 1983
21. Shammas HJF, Milkie CF: Cystoid macular edema following secondary lens implantation. Am Intraocul Implant Soc J 7:40, 1981

Section III

CORNEA

Stephen R. Waltman

Section Editor

Penetrating Keratoplasty

15

Stephen R. Waltman

Penetrating keratoplasty involves full-thickness replacement of the patient's diseased corneal tissue with suitable donor material. The procedure is performed primarily for optical reasons in an attempt to improve visual acuity. It may also be used therapeutically to restore an intact globe if corneal necrosis or melting results in impending or actual perforation. With improvements in medical therapy, the development of soft contact lenses and other adjuvants, and the utilization of conjunctival flaps, the vast majority of penetrating keratoplasties are now done for optical rather than therapeutic indications.

Seventy-five percent of the refractive power of the eye (45 of 60 diopters) is located at the air–corneal interface. This results from the small radius of curvature of the cornea and the marked difference in the indices of refraction between the cornea and air.[1] Therefore, any interference with regularity of the corneal surface may markedly denigrate the retinal image even with little stromal opacity. This is exemplified by early Fuchs' endothelial dystrophy when early morning corneal epithelial edema may significantly reduce visual acuity. Conversely, visual acuity may be quite good in patients with deep stromal opacities that do not completely occlude the visual axis if the anterior corneal surface is regular. Surgeons may overestimate the degree to which stromal opacification interferes with vision and underestimate the effect of epithelial edema or irregularity on vision. The refractive power of the cornea is slightly reduced at the posterior corneal surface. Because of the small difference between the indices of refraction of the cornea and the aqueous, however, this effect is less than 10 percent of the total refractive power of the cornea. Therefore, posterior surface irregularities, such as may occur with extensive guttata, may not seriously reduce the clarity of the retinal image.

CLINICAL PICTURE

The clinical picture usually encountered is that of corneal scarring or edema seriously reducing visual acuity and not responsive to topical medications or the use of soft contact lenses. These include cases of endothelial dysfunction, such as primary Fuchs' dystrophy, or aphakic or pseudophakic bullous keratopathy. Keratoconus or corneal scarring due to trauma or secondary to fungal, bacterial, or viral (usually herpetic) infections are also indications for keratoplasty. Patients with previous failed keratoplasties (regrafts) may also constitute a significant proportion of a corneal surgeon's referral practice.

CORNEAL ANATOMY

The cornea is composed of six separate layers[2] having a total central corneal thickness of approximately 0.52 mm. In the mid-periphery of the cornea, where most keratoplasty incisions are, the thickness approaches 0.70 mm. Maintenance of normal corneal thickness depends on the activity of the limiting cell layers; the epithelium and endothelium. Failure of either one of these cell layers results in increased thickness.

The epithelium consists of five to seven layers of nonkeratinized, nucleated cells that rest on the epithelial basement membrane. The surface squamous epithelial cells have surface projections called microvilli, which bond with the mucoid layer of the precorneal tear film to help retain it. These superficial cells exhibit rapid turnover. The middle layer is composed of wing cells, and a single basal layer is attached to the epithelial basement membrane by hemidesmosomes. Mitosis starts at the basal layer with cells continuously migrating forward until they are shed into the tear film on a daily basis.

The epithelial basement membrane is a product of the basal epithelial cells and interdigitates with Bowman's membrane. If it is destroyed by trauma, it can be regenerated in several weeks by the actively metabolizing basal epithelium. During these several weeks, and for some time thereafter, the epithelium is more loosely adherent to the basement membrane, and recurrent erosions may occur. Bowman's membrane represents a localized part of the anterior corneal stroma. It is composed of interdigitating collagen fibrils and is resistant to most trauma. If destroyed, it is replaced by less well-organized scar tissue.

The corneal stroma, which constitutes 90 percent of the normal corneal thickness, is made up of collagen fibrils of uniform thickness arranged in a highly organized, regular manner and suspended in mucopolysaccharide ground substance. There is more potential for separation between the individual lamellae posteriorly than in the anterior corneal layers. Because of the mucopolysaccharide ground substance, the stroma is hydrophilic and will swell when immersed in isotonic saline or serum. In vivo, this tendency to swell is reversed by the active metabolic pumping process present in the endothelium and epithelium. If the stroma is damaged by trauma or infection, it is replaced by collagen fibrils of varying diameters that are irregularly arranged. This leads to replacement of the normally transparent stroma with a scar of reduced transparency.

Applied against the posterior border of the stroma is Descemet's membrane. This highly elastic resilient layer is the basement membrane of the corneal endothelium. In infancy it is of uniform thickness, and this thickness increases with age. Also with aging or with trauma to the endothelium, Descemet's membrane may become irregularly thickened with the presence of visible corneal guttata centrally. These guttata are indicative of corneal endothelial dysfunction and repair and are present in a significant part of the population over the age of 40 years. The corneal endothelium is a single cell layer separating Descemet's membrane from the aqueous. The adjacent cells are held together by occluding zonules at their apices, which form tight junctions. In adults endothelial cell division probably does not occur. If endothelial cells are lost by aging or trauma, the adjacent cells much therefore enlarge to cover Descemet's membrane completely; otherwise, corneal edema results. The endothelial cell density may be approximated with a slit-lamp microscope or measured with a corneal specular photomicroscope. The average endothelial cell density in adults is approximately 2,000 to 2,500 cells/mm^2. Below a certain cell density, somewhere between 500 and 1,000 cells/mm^2, corneal edema occurs.

The endothelial and epithelial cell layers have an active metabolism. In humans cell mitosis and turnover occur in the epithelial layers but not in the endothelium.[1] Oxygen for the epithelium comes primarily from the tear film, and oxygen in the aqueous humor is used by the endothelium, which is the most active metabolic layer. Glucose and other nutrients for both cell layers come from the aqueous humor. The cornea is hydrophilic and will swell to approximately four times normal thickness if the metabolic activity of the epithelium and endothelium is prevented. Increases in corneal thickness are therefore most indicative of dysfunction of the limiting cell layers, primarily the endothelium, and may be the first clinical sign of endothelial dysfunction.

INDICATIONS

Penetrating keratoplasty involves replacement of full-thickness corneal tissue with adequate donor tissue. The diseased endothelium is replaced by donor endothelium, which probably remains in place for the duration of the clarity of the keratoplasty. A clear stroma without opacity is also provided, perhaps with some active, live fibroblasts. In penetrating keratoplasty, the epithelium may also be transplanted, but this is usually replaced with host epithelium over a given period of time. Penetrating keratoplasty is more than just a technical procedure; thus, the indications depend on patient factors but also to a considerable extent on the experience of the surgeon (Fig. 15-1).

Most corneal transplants are done for optical reasons, to improve visual acuity. The most common indication is corneal endothelial dysfunction. This is either in the form of primary Fuchs' dystrophy (Fig. 15-2) or for endothelial dysfunction after cataract surgery with or without an intraocular implant. Cataract surgery leads to a reduction in endothelial cell density, with the loss being determined by the complexity of the case and by the type of implant inserted.[3] Some patients with clinically normal-appearing corneas may have reduced endothelial cell density; these corneas may decompensate with apparently uncomplicated cataract surgery. Keratoconus is a prime indication for keratoplasty if the patient is unable to wear a contact lens and has an expanding cone with poor visual acuity. Corneal scarring due to trauma or microbial infections is an indication for keratoplasty. This is especially common with herpetic keratitis after the active viral disease has been controlled and visual acuity is reduced due to corneal scarring. Patients with certain of the corneal stromal dystrophies may require keratoplasty if vision is sufficiently reduced. This occurs early in life in the autosomal recessive condition, macular corneal dystrophy, and much later in life in the presence of lattice or granular dystrophy. Interstitial keratitis and trachoma are rare indications.

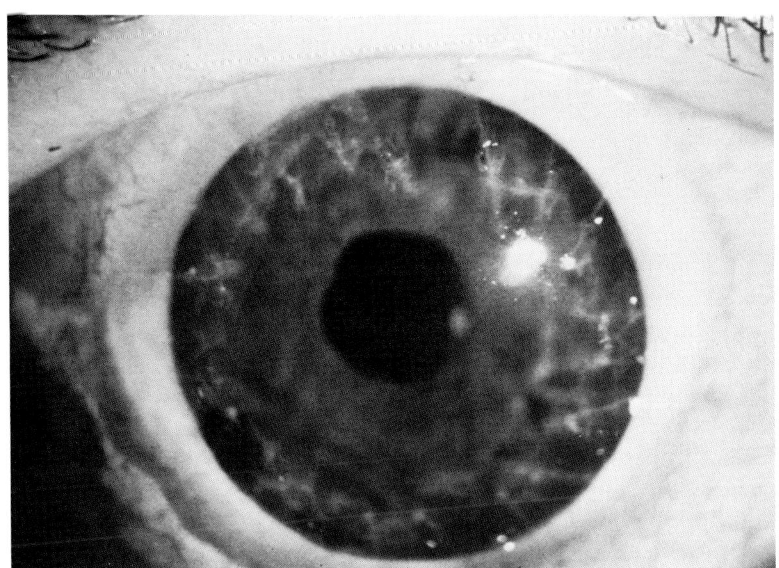

Fig. 15-1. Clear penetrating keratoplasty in a patient with extensive corneal scarring.

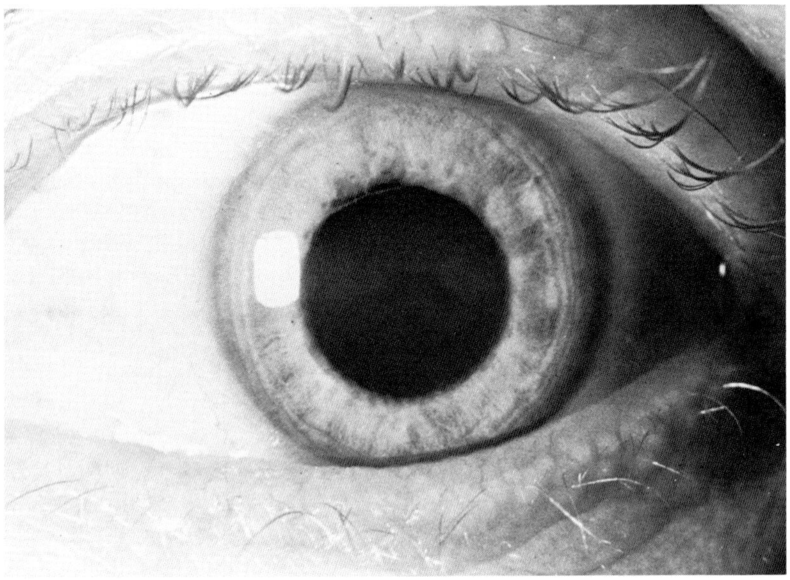

Fig. 15-2. Fuchs' corneal dystrophy with epithelial edema.

Therapeutic penetrating keratoplasty may be done for corneal necrosis or large central descemetoceles. These usually occur secondary to an infectious process, such as with bacterial, fungal, or herpes simplex or zoster infection. In general, it is best to try medical means or soft contact lenses, so that the eyes may be operated on when they are not actively inflamed. Sometimes, however, this is not possible due to the extensive damage to the central corneal stroma.

CONTRAINDICATIONS

Certain factors worsen the prognosis for successful keratoplasty, making them relative contraindications. It may be possible to treat these successfully prior to the keratoplasty and thus improve the prognosis for optical keratoplasty.[4,5] Corneal transplants fail due to epithelial or endothelial malfunction. Conditions that are detrimental to continued function of these cell layers must be corrected, if possible.

A normal tear film is crucial to epithelial healing and function. Therefore, all related components, such as continuity of the lids and conjunctiva and normal tear secretion, should be in the best possible condition. Patients with lid defects, which will result in postoperative exposure keratitis, should have these repaired, if at all possible. Marked conjunctival scarring with reduced tear function such as occurs in trauma, lye burns, ocular pemphigoid, or Stevens-Johnson syndrome is a relative contraindication. Reconstruction of the lids and cul-de-sacs with conjunctival grafting may permit keratoplasty to be undertaken. Otherwise, a keratoprosthesis, which may be placed through the lids, should be considered.

Uncontrolled glaucoma is a contraindication to penetrating keratoplasty, as the elevated intraocular pressure (IOP) will damage the donor corneal endothelium as well as the optic nerve. Furthermore, surgical therapy of the glaucoma, such as a filtering procedure or cyclocryotherapy, which may be required postoperatively after the keratoplasty, may damage the donor corneal endothelium.[6] Laser trabeculoplasty may become possible with a clear keratoplasty when it was not possible with a scarred cornea, but these cases are rare. Glaucoma should be controlled medically or surgically; if surgically controlled, a period of 3 to 4 months should elapse prior to attempting keratoplasty.

Patients with vascularized corneas may have a lessened prognosis for keratoplasty, but this is only a relative contraindication. Frequently, removing the diseased central cornea that has stimulated the vascularization will prevent further vascular ingrowth. In these patients, more topical, and occasionally systemic, corticosteroids may be used; sutures are removed relatively early, as these tissues heal quite rapidly.

Poor patient compliance can doom even the most technically successful keratoplasty. Patients who for various reasons will not use medications or who may continually traumatize their eyes are not good candidates for keratoplasty. Social factors must be taken into account so as not to deny good candidates visual rehabilitation, but also to prevent operating on those who are poor candidates.

EYE BANKS

The operation of penetrating keratoplasty is unique to ophthalmologists in that they depend on the availability of living donor material supplied by an eye bank. Although the surgeon may not be actively involved in managing or running the eye bank, the ophthalmic surgeon must be aware of the criteria used in donor selection and the applicability of such standards to donor materials. This is so, as the operating surgeon is ultimately responsible for determining the suitability of the donor tissue to be used. Many eye banks in the United States are members of the Eye Bank Association of America, which has set certain medical standards with regard to donor suitability, training of technical personnel, and the physical facilities involved in eye banking.[7] Some donor-suitability guidelines follow.

Age

Corneas from donors under the age of 2 years are thinner and may be more steeply curved and more floppy. They have an extremely high endothelial cell count and are suitable for keratoplasty under certain conditions. Some surgeons may find these corneas difficult to work with, and the corneal diameter may be smaller in these eyes. The upper acceptable age limit is somewhat variable, as numerous studies have shown that donor eyes from older patients may be extremely usable.[8] Since there seems to be some reduction in endothelial cell count with aging, many surgeons prefer not to use corneal tissue if the donor is over 65 years of age. The availability of specular microscopy of donor tissue may allow us to choose those eyes from older donors that are most suitable for keratoplasty.

Disease Exclusions

It is the purpose of keratoplasty to transplant viable corneal tissue from donor to recipient without the possibility of transmitting any disease process. There have been reports of the transmission of Creutzfeldt-Jakob disease,[9] rabies,[10] and possibly an intraocular infection.[11] The exclusion criteria are therefore designed to try to prevent the transmission of a disease of the donor to the recipient. Corneas from septic donors are not considered suitable for transplantation, whether the sepsis is bacterial, fungal, or viral. External ocular infections of the donor mean exclusion as well. Also excluded are those donors who die of unknown causes and those who die of slow neurologic disease of possible viral origin. Donors with blastform leukemia, and possibly chronic leukemia, are also excluded. Some eye banks and surgeons prefer not to use donor eyes from patients who died of other neurologic diseases, such as multiple sclerosis, for which a viral etiology has never been proved. Patients on long-term chronic immunosuppressive therapy who may have latent infections appear not to be suitable donors for elective keratoplasty. Some surgeons will not use corneas from patients dying of carcinoma or those with previous eye surgery or disease. These criteria are for elective surgical procedures, and the criteria for the use of donor material for emergency procedures may vary somewhat under certain conditions. In all cases, the surgeon must be aware of all pertinent factors, since he or she has the ultimate responsibility for determining the suitability of the tissue.

It is now mandatory that all corneal donors be screened for the presence of both antibodies to

HTLV III virus and Hepatitis B surface antigen. This will reduce the risk of transmitting acquired immune deficiency syndrome (AIDS) and hepatitis B.

Storage Conditions

The interval from death to enucleation to placement in storage conditions should be as short as possible. It is usually considered acceptable if the eyes are removed from the donor's body within 6 to 12 hours postmortem, depending on the ambient temperature during storage. If the donor remains at room temperature, retrieval of the tissue must be more rapid than if the remains are refrigerated at 4° to 8°C. After removal, donor tissue should be evaluated with a slit lamp, either as a whole globe or following placement into storage solutions. The person processing the tissue should evaluate the condition of the epithelium, stroma, and endothelium, listing the assessment of each tissue. Donor tissue for penetrating keratoplasty may be stored as whole globes, in short-term storage media, in organ culture or after cryopreservation. Corneas stored on a whole globe are refrigerated and should be used within 24 to 36 hours.[12]

Most donor material in the United States is placed in short-term storage medium. The most popular medium used is McCarey-Kaufman (MK) medium.[13,14] This is a combination of TC-199 medium high-molecular-weight dextran, a suitable buffer, and antibiotics. The cornea is removed from the donor tissue with an approximately 2-mm rim of sclera. The donor tissue is then placed in approximately 20 ml MK medium and stored at 4° to 6°C. Such donor material should be evaluated with a slit lamp, while it is in the storage container, by both the eye bank and the operating surgeon. Under these conditions, donor storage times may range from 2 to 5 days. Many ophthalmic surgeons believe that the donor tissue should be used within 3 to 4 days after preservation. Before working with such tissue, the surgeon should be sure that the medium in which the material has been stored is crystal clear and not turbid. Any turbidity is suspicious of bacterial infection, and the material should not be used. It is important at the time of surgery to culture either the storage solution or preferably a piece of the residual corneoscleral rim; thus, if an intraocular infection does become apparent some clue to its origin and nature may be obtained. It is possible that the addition of certain substances to the storage medium, such as chondroitin sulfate, may permit storage of the material for longer periods of time, yet still be suitable for keratoplasty. K-Sol storage media uses 2%-chondroitin sulfate and may extend the storage time beyond 1 week for certain corneas.

At certain centers, corneas are stored under organ culture conditions. This involves storage of the corneoscleral rim in suitable media at 37°C with frequent changes of media to supply nutrients.[15] When stored at 4°C in MK medium, metabolization is essentially suspended, and the medium does not need to be changed. At 37°C there is active metabolic activity, and nutrients and additional oxygen must be supplied to the donor tissue. Conditions for culture are rigorous because of the possibility of bacterial or fungal contamination and increased growth at 37°C compared with 4°C.

Cryopreservation

Donor corneal tissue may be cryopreserved[16]; following thawing of the cryopreserved material, the endothelial cells resume functioning. Capella and co-workers[16] originated and successfully used cryopreserved corneas. The donor corneoscleral rim is processed through a series of cryoprotective solutions composed of albumin, DMSO, and sucrose. It is then frozen at a controlled rate and, after complete freezing, stored in liquid nitrogen. Storage time in the liquid nitrogen may exceed many months. When ready to be used, the tissue is thawed at a controlled rate, and the DMSO and sucrose are washed out by placing the tissue in pure 25 percent human albumin. Excellent results have been reported with this technique with long-term preservation of the donor endothelium. However, the procedure requires an experienced technician, much more so than in preparing the corneoscleral rim, and requires several hours for processing. Therefore, it tends not to be used frequently. Nevertheless, it would appear to be an excellent method for preserving tissue on a longer-term basis and perhaps for preserving tissue-typed corneas for use in the appropriate recipient.

RECOMMENDED TECHNIQUE

Preoperatively the patient may be given a hyperosmotic agent such as glycerin. Topical pilocarpine is instilled in phakic patients. This is followed by 5 to 15 minutes or oscular massage using digital pressure or a super pinky after the local anesthetic. I perform this technique in most cases under local anesthesia with an anesthetist in attendance. The retrobulbar injection of 0.75 percent bupivacaine (Marcaine) is given while the patient is breathing an analgesic nitrous oxide–oxygen mixture. This markedly reduces the pain of the injection as well as the memory of it. Marcaine has a long duration of action; akinesia, anesthesia, and sometimes optic nerve depression may occur for as long as 24 hours. General anesthesia is used for children or for uncooperative or highly nervous adults and for patients with perforated eyes. If the eye is perforated, specialized anesthetic techniques must be used with appropriate muscle relaxants to prevent cocontraction of the rectus muscles and expulsion of the intraocular contents.

Fixation

In phakic patients, 4-0 silk superior and inferior rectus bridle sutures are used following placement of a lid speculum. This is done under direct visualization using a tapered rather than a cutting or reverse-cutting needle. Fixation is especially important for trephining. In aphakic patients, in pseudophakic patients and those having combined keratoplasty and cataract extraction, as well as in certain children and young patients with keratoconus, a Flierenga ring is sutured to the eye (Fig. 15-3). The ring is usually 15 or 16 mm in diameter and is sutured to the episcleral tissue at 4-point fixation using Dacron sutures on a half-curved scleral spatula needle. The type of sutures is not of critical importance, since they will be removed after the keratoplasty, but the type of needle is important so as to get episcleral bites without cutting into the eye or pulling through the episcleral tissue. A suture is then looped beneath the 6 and 12 o'clock positions of the ring and clamped to the drapes. I sometimes use a double Flierenga–LaGrange ring, in which the sutures may be left

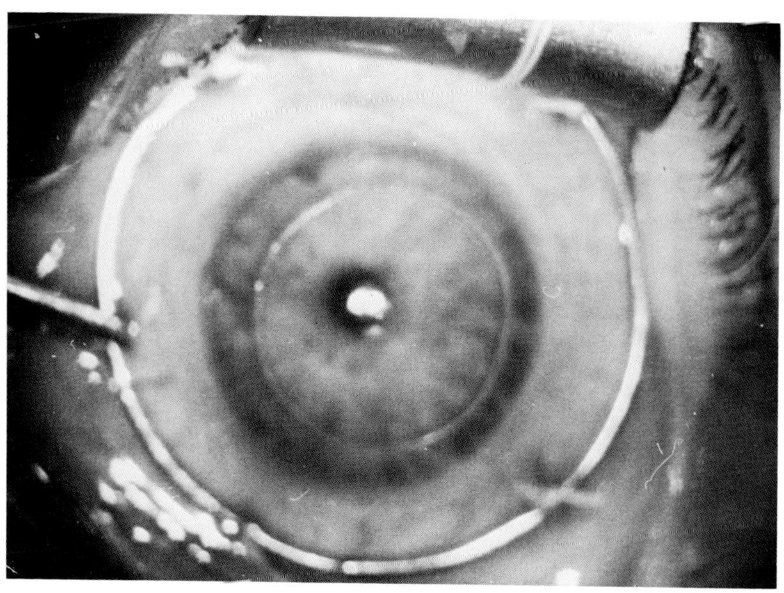

Fig. 15-3. A single ring is secured to the episcleral tissue with Dacron sutures.

long and pulled inferiorly and superiorly against the struts connecting the two rings. Combined rings and blepharostats are available.

Donor Preparation

Following the retrobulbar anesthetic, prepping and draping, and insertion of the lid speculum and fixation device, the patient's eye is covered to protect it from light exposure and drying as the donor tissue is prepared. The donor tissue, usually in MK medium, is removed from the medium and placed endothelial side up on a Teflon block (Fig. 15-4). Using a permanent trephine handle with a disposable trephine blade, the plunger is retracted, leaving sufficient clearance. The donor trephine size must be decided on, either after gently marking the host tissue or depending on the surgeon's preference for graft size. The Teflon block is held in the left hand beneath the microscope at low magnification; holding the trephine in the right hand, the trephine blade is gently applied 360 degrees to the donor tissue. A sharp downward movement then cuts through the donor tissue (Fig. 15-5). The trephine cannot be twisted or rotated, as the donor tissue is not fixated except by pressure between the trephine and the Teflon block. It is crucial to have an exceptionally sharp trephine for this part of the procedure. If the trephine is not sharp, damage to the endothelium may occur. If done correctly, the donor tissue is usually left on the Teflon block after the trephine blade and handle are removed from the field. Using a Paton spatula, the donor tissue is then handled from the epithelial surface, great care being taken to avoid the endothelial surface (Fig. 15-6). The donor tissue is inspected to ensure that the cut is perpendicular and centered, as well as for any other defects. It is then placed endothelial side up into a Petri dish; MK medium is used to cover the endothelium to prevent drying during the preparation of the host tissue. The Petri dish is then covered. The corneoscleral rim is inspected and a portion of it sent to the microbiology laboratory for culture. If the button remains in the trephine, the plunger may be carefully advanced, and the air between them compressed and the donor button elevated, which is then grasped with a forceps from the epithelial surface. On occasion, when a whole eye is the available donor tissue, it is preferable to remove the anterior segment as one would in preparing a corneoscleral rim and still do the trephining from the posterior corneal surface. Some surgeons prefer an anterior approach, especially in whole eyes. The use of an anterior approach frequently necessitates use of scissors, however, which may damage the peripheral endothelium. After successful completion of the trephi-

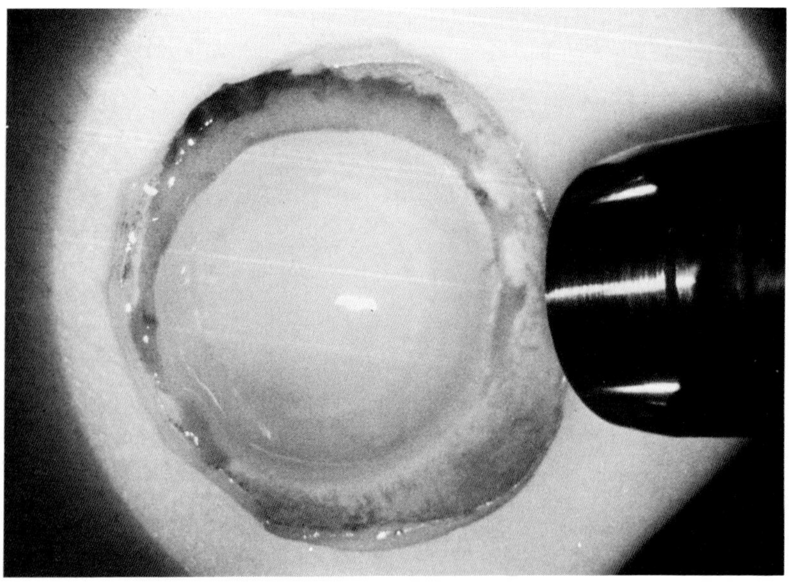

Fig. 15-4. Donor corneoscleral rim positioned on a Teflon cutting block. The trephine has the plunger retracted.

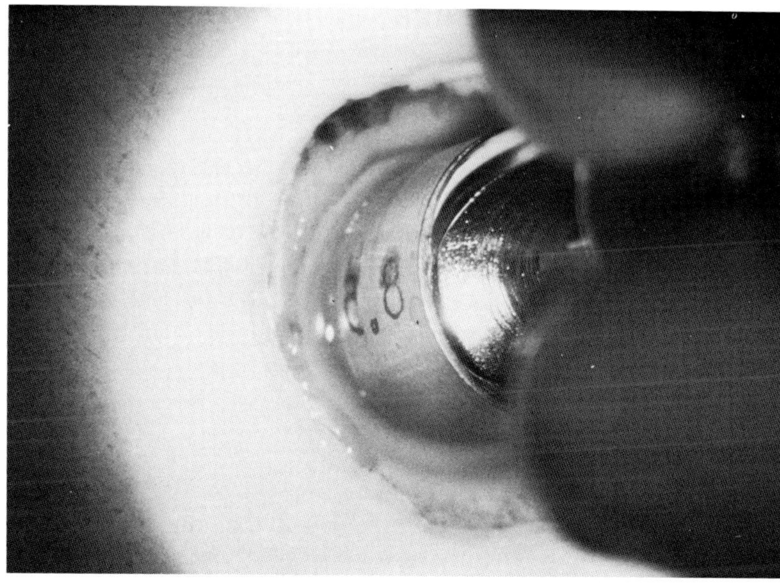

Fig. 15-5. The donor tissue is trephined from the posterior corneal surface.

nation and preparation of the donor material, attention can be directed to the host. In this way, if there is irreversible damage to the donor tissue, the host has received the retrobulbar injection only and avoided having the eye entered.

Trephining

The phakic eye is fixated with the two rectus bridle sutures and a Lester forceps, which grasps the insertion of the appropriate horizontal rectus muscle. The trephine is set at a depth of 0.2 mm and is used to make a scratch mark on the epithelium for centration. Centration is usually done by looking at the pupil or by measuring the distance between the edge of the trephine and the limbus in the four quadrants. The trephine is then set at 0.5 to 0.7 mm, depending on the condition being treated. After being sure the trephine is in contact 360 degrees, it is rotated back and forth, 90 degrees, in a cutting motion. A dull trephine will cause slippage with multiple shallow, irregular cuts. In this case, the trephine penetrates the host tissue by a cutting rotational movement rather than by the pressure used in the preparation of the donor material. Some surgeons prefer continuous clockwise or counterclockwise movement. In patients who have protuberant corneas, such as keratoconus, it may be necessary to retract the plunger gently to a much greater depth in order to engage the trephine 360

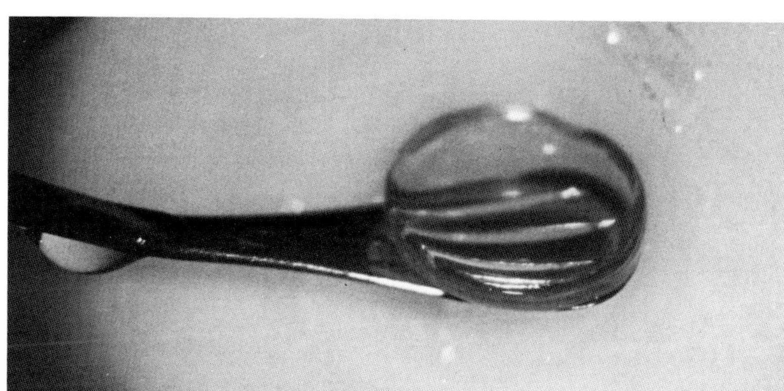

Fig. 15-6. A Paton spatula manipulates the donor corneal button from the epithelial surface.

degrees. In these cases, it may be possible to heat the tip of the cone gently and shrink it to enable the trephine to come into more even contact with the base of the cone and normal corneal tissue. If a patient is aphakic and a ring has been attached to the eye,[17] the ring is usually grasped firmly at one of the suture points and is used for fixation while doing the trephination (Fig. 15-7).

Using a razorblade knife, the patient's anterior chamber is then entered between the 8 and 10 o'clock positions after making sure there is a good, deep cut with the trephine. If the trephine cut is shallow along one area, it may be deepened with a razorblade knife so that the amount of tissue that has to be cut with scissors is kept to a minimum. After entering the chamber and being sure the incision is large enough to introduce scissors, the right Katzen corneal scissors is inserted into the anterior chamber (Fig. 15-8). Great care must be taken to avoid damage to the underlying iris and lens. The blade of the scissors is kept perpendicular, which to most surgeons feels as if the hand position for holding the scissors is greatly exaggerated. The incision is extended between 180 and 230 degrees with a right-cutting scissors. The left-cutting scissors is then used to complete removal of the diseased host tissue. If the cut is not relatively perpendicular, the deeper edges may be trimmed using a 0.12-mm Bonn forceps and either of the corneal scissors. This may be more difficult and treacherous if there is considerable bulge of the lens–iris diaphragm. Since scissors are crushing instruments, it is ideal to keep the amount of manipulation with the scissors to a minimum; this means deepening the original cut with the trephine or redeepening it with the appropriate blade prior to entering the anterior chamber. In the presence of a perforated cornea, the trephine is used only to outline the recipient opening, which is deepened with a razorblade and then completed with scissors.

Iris Surgery

Iridotomies are done in some phakic patients, specifically those who have lens changes, those with shallow anterior chambers, and those who have had previous inflammatory disease with or without the appearance of posterior synechiae. Some surgeons advocate iris surgery or iridotomies for all patients; one must balance the benefits to be gained in preventing pupillary block against the risks. These include damage to the lens and possible iris bleeding, at the point of iridotomy, or from the angle due to tension on the iris. It is advisable to try to keep the iridotomies out of proximity to the incision, which means making them beneath the shelf of the host corneal tissue. This is best done

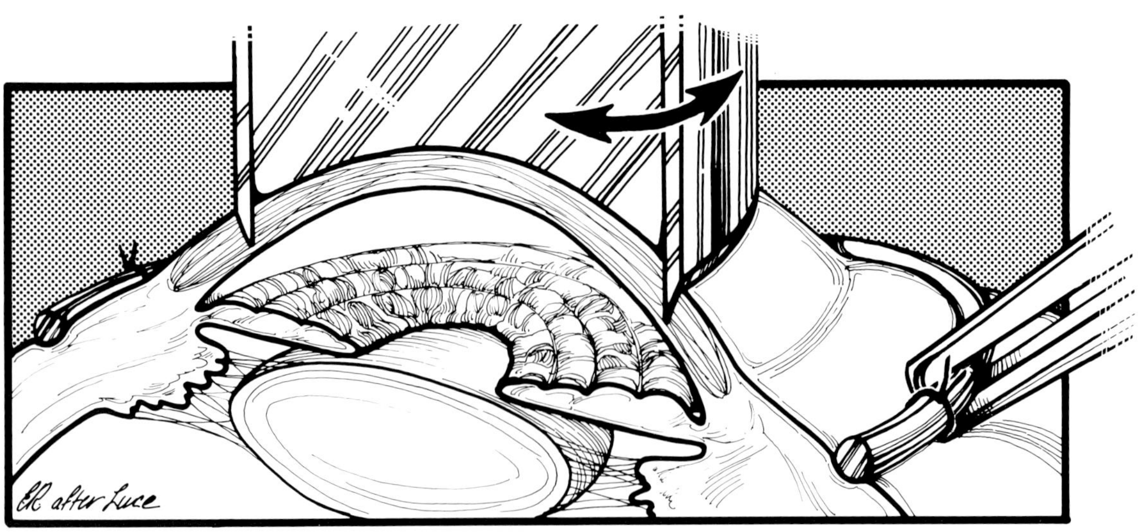

Fig. 15-7. The trephine is used to make an incision to approximately 80 percent depth.

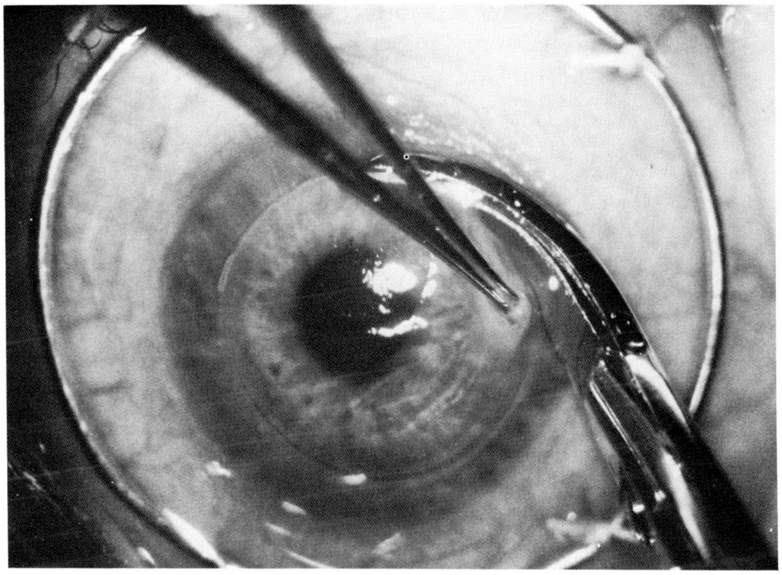

Fig. 15-8. A Katzen scissors is used to divide the deeper corneal lamellae.

using a nontoothed forceps to tent-up the iris gently, cutting along the tented-up edge beneath the residual host corneal tissue. One or two iridotomies may be done, and, if the patient is aphakic or pseudophakic, it is ideal to place at least one small iridotomy in the interior half of the eye. This will prevent pupillary block should air find its way behind the iris. In the phakic patient, the mid-peripheral iris may be coated with a viscoelastic material[18,19] to prevent contact between the iris and the donor endothelium. The donor button is handled from the epithelial surface, with a Paton spatula in the right hand (Fig. 15-9). The donor tissue is then placed endothelial side down into the recipient opening and grasped with a 0.12-mm Bonn forceps held in the left hand. During this procedure, an attempt is made to match up the individual aspects of the donor material with the host to try to get as

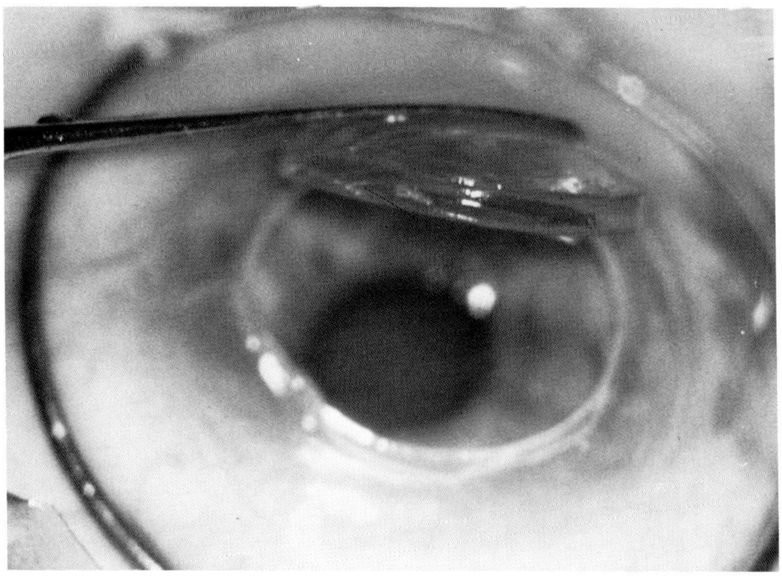

Fig. 15-9. Using the Paton spatula, the donor tissue is placed into the recipient opening.

good a fit and as circular an incision as possible. Endothelial trauma is to be avoided.

Suturing Technique

Placing the first suture at the 12 o'clock position is usually the most difficult. It involves grasping two thirds to three quarters of the thickness of the anterior corneal stroma, and without rubbing the endothelium on the iris or surrounding tissue, placing a 10-0 nylon suture directly adjacent to the forceps at three-quarters depth (Fig. 15-10). The forceps is then used to grasp the host tissue as the suture is passed through it. The suture is tied tightly with four individual knots. Since these sutures will eventually be removed before completion of the case, the precise depth of placement is not critical. The 6 o'clock position is then sutured with a backhand technique, and once again a forceps with a tying platform and a needle holder are used for suturing and tying. The 3 o'clock meridian is then sutured with an interrupted 10-0 nylon suture. The 9 o'clock suture may be placed either backhand or forehand, depending on the surgeon's individual preference, or may be placed using the needle holder in the opposite hand. The suture is tied. The sutures are cut relatively short with scissors. Air or saline is used to reform the chamber further and to assess the match between donor and recipient and the appropriate placement of the interrupted sutures. With the four cardinal sutures in place, a diamond-shaped figure results from the tension lines. For most patients, double continuous sutures are then used. The first suture is always of 10-0 nylon on a half-curved needle. The initial suture placement is in the inferior one half of the eye, facilitating postoperative removal of the knot. Between six and eight suture passes are placed in each quadrant in a clockwise rotation, each as deep as possible, usually three quarters or more depth. I do not like to use through-and-through sutures. The sutures are approximately 1 mm in the host and donor tissue. Approximately 24 to 32 suture passes are then placed around the circumference of the eye. Forehand suture passes are made from the 8 to 2 o'clock position and backhand passes from 2 to 8 o'clock. Slack is removed from the running suture using two McPherson forceps (Fig. 15-11). Care must be exercised not to squeeze or twist the nylon and to pull the suture parallel to the forceps. A triple throw is placed and the chamber deepened with liquid. Additional slack is taken out (avoid

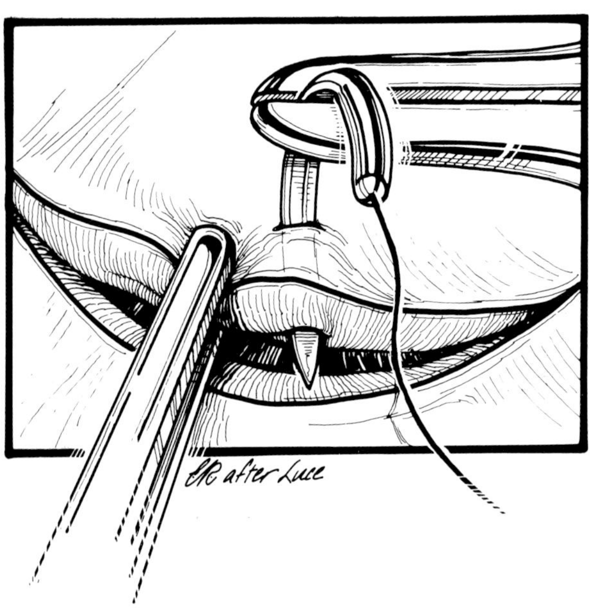

Fig. 15-10. The initial 10-0 nylon suture is placed adjacent to the Bonn forceps in the donor tissue.

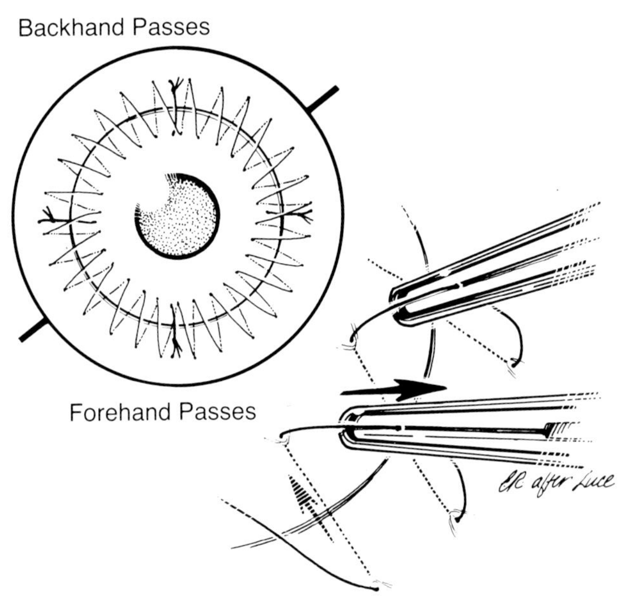

Fig. 15-11. The 10-0 nylon suture is tightened with smooth tying forceps.

excessive tightening), and two additional single throws complete the knot. The suture ends are removed with a razorblade knife, and the knot is buried. The interrupted sutures are removed, and the running suture may be adjusted. It is crucial to avoid endothelial trauma during suture placement, which may occur by dragging the endothelium in contact with the iris. This is facilitated by firmly grasping the donor tissue prior to placing the needle through it. Additional interrupted sutures may be placed if there is some area that is not as secure or if there is some leak along the suture track or along the wound. A second running suture of 11-0 nylon[20,21] with four to six suture passes in each quadrant is put in place. This is a more superficial suture, and it is not possible to place it to the depth of the original suture, as the wound remains approximated. The slack is taken out and the knot is cut short and buried. Great care must be taken to avoid cutting the original running suture with the very sharp needle of the 11-0 nylon. Furthermore, an effort should be made to space the 11-0 adequately with respect to the 10-0, so that when the 10-0 nylon suture is removed at 3 to 4 months postoperatively, there is minimal chance of dividing the 11-0 suture. I always prefer to suture using a single-arm suture in a clockwise fashion and, if the needle becomes dull or the suture breaks, to splice in another piece of suture and leave two knots in the running suture. Tightening is done in both directions away from the repair knot to allow both knots to be buried. If the suture does break during tightening of the 10-0 nylon suture, occasionally one loop may be left out or an additional piece of suture spliced in. The knot should always be buried on the host side, so that when attempting to remove the knot, trauma will not cause excessive wound separation. In certain instances, 12 to 16 interrupted 10-0 nylon sutures may be used with or without a running 11-0 suture. This is done in vascularized corneas, in corneas of unequal thickness, and perhaps for selective astigmatic control. It is also done when the keratoplasty has to be decentered somewhat. Because suture bites near the limbus may include conjunctiva or fascia, and because the part of the incision closest to the limbus may heal rapidly, these sutures may loosen and have to be removed. After the final suturing, the fixation sutures are removed, the sclera and muscles are inspected, and the patient receives a subconjunctival injection of short-acting steroids and an antibiotic, usually gentamicin.

Aphakic Eyes

Aphakic eyes require scleral support during the procedure, and the anterior segment should be cleared of formed vitreous. Vitreous in the incision will prevent adequate apposition of the posterior corneal surface, may lead to epithelial downgrowth or fibrous outgrowth, and may result in cystoid macular edema. After the ring is placed and the anterior chamber entered, formed vitreous presents in more than 90 percent of aphakic eyes. Occasionally, this can be prevented if the vitreous face is intact and back. Preoperatively topical pilocarpine is instilled and hyperosmotic agents are given. The anterior chamber is slowly entered and filled with air. After the diseased corneal tissue is removed, an iridotomy is done in the inferior one half the eye. If necessary, the anterior segment is then cleared of formed vitreous,[22] generally using a mechanical vitrector or cellulose sponges (Fig. 15-12). Every attempt should be made to ensure that the vitreous is behind the iris diaphragm and will not come into contact with the incision. If the iris diaphragm has been damaged, an attempt may be made to reconstruct it with sutures. Viscoelastic materials are not needed during aphakic keratoplasty, as air is kept in the chamber, and the same suturing technique is used as for phakic eyes. In some aphakic patients, especially those who have been intolerant to wearing a contact lens, it may be preferable to place a secondary intraocular implant. This may be placed in the anterior or posterior chamber, depending on the status of the posterior capsule. Most are placed in the anterior chamber; I prefer a single-piece, all-polymethylmethacrylate, uniplanar lens (Fig. 15-13). This keeps the iris diaphragm back and usually does not come into contact with the donor endothelium. The intraocular implant is coated with Healon to prevent contact between the endothelium and the implant during surgery (Fig. 15-14). If there has been loss of part of the iris structure but the angle appears capable of supporting an implant, occasionally one leg of the implant may be sutured to

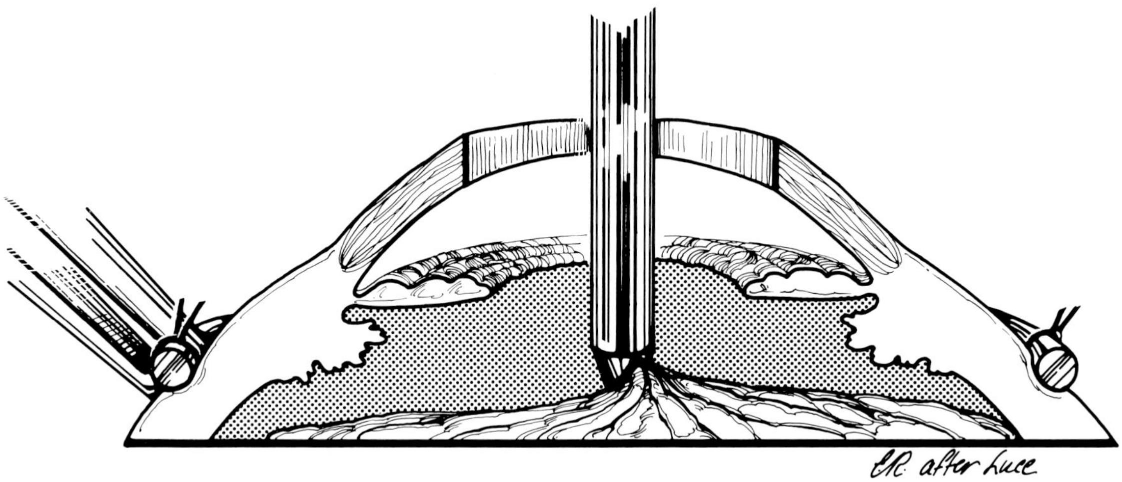

Fig. 15-12. An anterior vitrectomy may be performed with a mechanical vitrector.

the iris using 10-0 prolene to prevent its torsion and disappearance into the vitreous.

It may be necessary to remove an intraocular implant as part of the keratoplasty, whether or not it is replaced.[23,24] We have found this most useful in eyes that have iris-plane or medallion-type lenses and in those with certain of the more flexible, forward-vaulting anterior chamber lenses. When possible, iris synechiae should be freed from the intraocular implant. The medallion lens is relatively easy to remove by taking out the suture holding it in place and then sliding it from behind the iris. If it is encapsulated in a partially intact posterior capsule and lens remnants, the posterior loop should be divided and gently slid out through the tunnels present within this material. Every attempt should be made not to pull vigorously on any lens remnants or posterior capsule that may connect with the ciliary body.

For the most part, posterior chamber lenses do not need to be removed unless they have caused a significant amount of disruption of the anterior

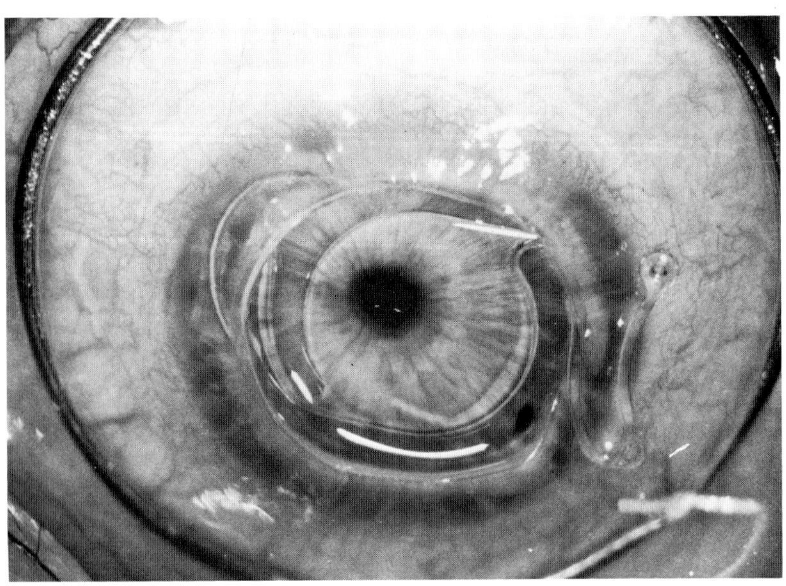

Fig. 15-13. Insertion of a flexible anterior chamber lens.

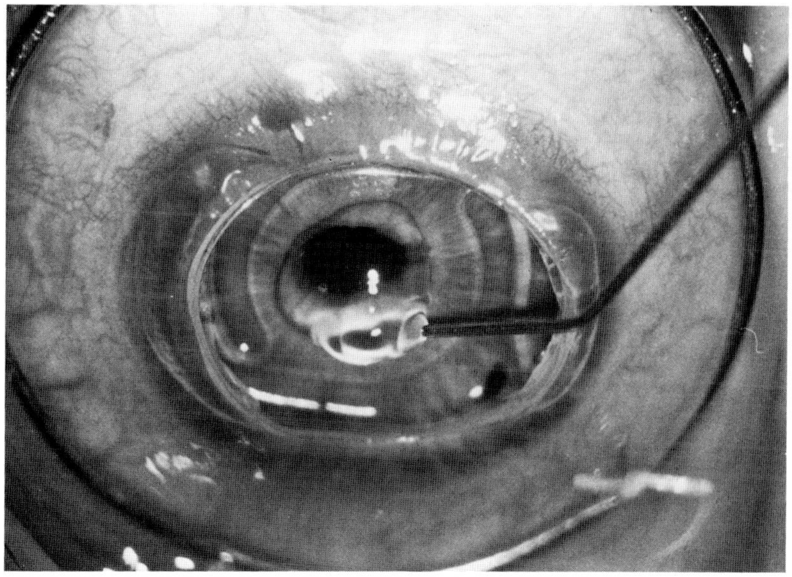

Fig. 15-14. The anterior chamber lens is coated with Healon to protect the donor endothelium.

segment. They are usually well back behind the iris, and coating the central part of the implant with Healon will prevent its contact with the donor endothelium during the procedure. Occasionally posterior synechiae between the posterior iris and the posterior capsule may distort the pupil. If the lens is relatively well centered with a good optical portion, this is probably left as is. If not, the iris may be freed gently from the posterior capsule and used to re-form a more normal pupil. However, there is great chance of disturbing the vitreous with this procedure. If vitreous comes up and around the posterior chamber lens, but the lens appears to be well centered and fixated, a vitrectomy may be done through the pupil and the iris diaphragm reconstituted.

Flexible anterior chamber lenses, especially those with prolene loops and those thought to have caused endothelial decompensation, should be removed. In these it is important to divide the supporting loops and gently slide them out of their fibrous encapsulated tunnels rather than pull them from the angle. Many of these lenses have irises that have wrapped around and fibrosed the intraocular implant in position. In some cases, it may be necessary to leave part of the loop within the angle rather than risk iridodialysis and anterior chamber bleeding. Choyce anterior chamber lenses are usually left in place unless there is some evidence that continued contact between the implant and the patient's endothelium was responsible for endothelial decompensation. If a Choyce solid anterior chamber lens has to be removed through the keratoplasty incision, one leg of it has to be pushed into the vitreous prior to its removal. Alternatively, a separate limbal incision is made and the lens slid out.

It is our conviction, from studies showing accelerated endothelial cell loss in the presence of an iris-plane lens,[25] that all metal-loop and probably most other iris-plane lenses should be removed at the time of keratoplasty. Vitrectomy is usually necessary at that point, followed by some decision as to whether a flexible anterior chamber lens made entirely of polymethylmethacrylate should be placed. Healon is used to coat the anterior surface of the flexible anterior chamber lens prior to the suturing technique.

Combined Keratoplasty and Cataract Extraction with or without Intraocular Lens Implantation

Patients who have simultaneous corneal disease and cataracts should have both entities dealt with at the same time. Sometimes the status of the cataract behind the cloudy cornea is difficult to assess preoperatively, but it may be even more difficult during the intraoperative phase. If the patient is elderly and if there are lens changes in the other eye and suspicion of lens changes in the operative eye from previous examinations, cataract extraction is frequently indicated.[26,27] If the lens is quite clear in the other eye, the lens should be left if preoperatively it appears to be relatively clear. We would like to perform only the appropriate surgery but not have to subject the patient to another procedure very soon. In most cases, an extracapsular cataract extraction is combined with keratoplasty. After placing the fixation ring and doing the corneal trephination, the anterior lens capsule is removed by making multiple cuts with a knife. This is done after preoperative pupillary dilatation. Cryo may be applied to the lens nucleus, which is then gently dislocated from the peripheral cortex. I personally prefer to grasp the lens nucleus with a widely open fine-tooth forceps and gently rock it out of its attachment to the peripheral cortex. Irrigation is then used to loosen the peripheral cortex. An automated irrigation-aspiration device is then used to remove the residual cortical material. This is best done by gently holding up the anterior lens capsule and removing all the cortical material from the fornices. It is easier to control the lens capsule and iris during keratoplasty, but visualization may be difficult due to the changing curvature of the anterior surface as more or less fluid builds up in the anterior segment. Care should be taken to avoid damaging the posterior capsule, and the posterior capsule should be polished with an appropriate instrument at the end of the procedure. For highly myopic patients and patients who are aphakic in the other eye, the donor tissue is then sutured in place, frequently not necessitating the use of Healon. Once the cataract has been removed from the eye, the iris diaphragm frequently falls back. After performing an iridotomy, the suturing technique is as before. If there is some bulge of the posterior capsule and iris diaphragm, Healon may be used to coat the mid-peripheral iris and central posterior capsule, followed by suturing.

If an intraocular implant is placed, the soft J-loop type lens is preferred. This may be placed in the capsular bag or in the anterior ciliary sulcus. The angle of placement of a posterior chamber lens is quite different than following cataract extraction, and care must be exercised as regards tension on the zonules (Fig. 15-15). Miochol is put in place to constrict the pupil, the iridotomy is done, Healon is used to coat the intraocular implant, and the suturing technique is as before. If the posterior capsule is not intact or vitreous presents, a one-piece, all-polymethylmethacrylate anterior chamber lens may be used after constricting the pupil. The placing of a multiflex lens is somewhat more difficult than following a standard cataract extraction, as the lens has to be lowered into the eye parallel to the iris diaphragm and then positioned. Visualization into the angle is frequently difficult during this procedure; one gets a clue as to the position of the implant by gently moving the feet of the intraocular implant until there is no pupillary peeking. The intraocular implant is then coated extensively with Healon or other viscoelastic material and the suturing technique performed. Once a watertight

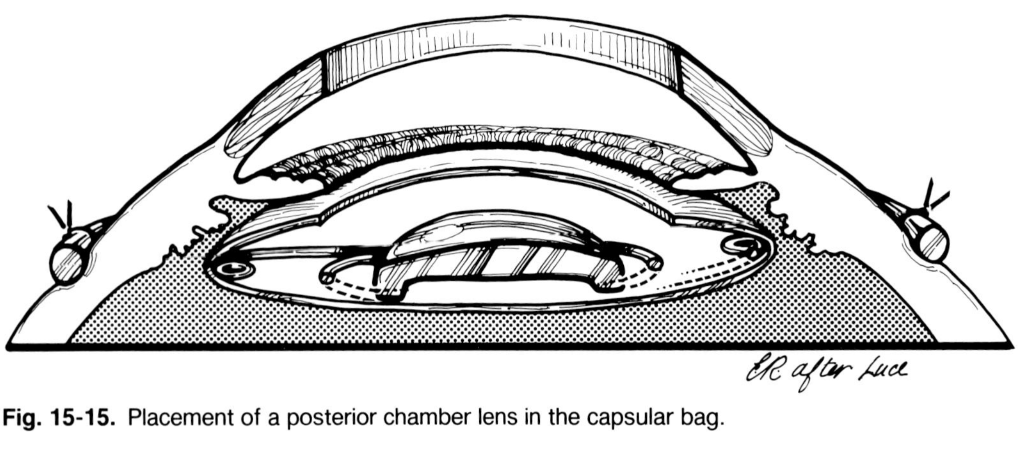

Fig. 15-15. Placement of a posterior chamber lens in the capsular bag.

double-running suture has been established, the ring is removed and the sclera inspected to make sure there is no uveal prolapse. The patient is then given subconjunctival antibiotics and corticosteroids.

Postoperative Care and Suture Removal

Patients are treated with topical corticosteroids. Topical antibiotics are used until the epithelium is completely healed and inflammation reduced. Careful monitoring of IOP is important. Postoperative care is critical to the success of the procedure, and experience is important. Small changes in the postoperative course may indicate possible future difficulties that may be avoided. Suture removal is dictated by clinical appearance and the suturing technique. If a single-running 10-0 nylon suture is used, it should be left in place for at least 6, and preferably 12, months. If two running sutures are used, the first one is removed after 3 to 4 months. Alternate loops are divided with a sharp razorblade fragment, and the uncut loops are lifted up with the dull back edge of the blade and removed with forceps. The epithelium should be disturbed as little as possible.

COMPLICATIONS

Certain unexpected events and difficulties may occur during the operative or postoperative period that, if handled correctly, may still allow good visual results. The surgeon must therefore be aware of the possible complications that occur intraoperatively and postoperatively to be prepared to make adjustments in the technique to compensate. Also, since donor tissue is transplanted, the surgeon must carefully assess the donor tissue before entering the operating room and then after its preparation but prior to the operative procedure on the recipient eye. If some irreversible fault occurs in the preparation of the donor tissue, or the donor tissue for some reason does not appear to be satisfactory at the time, the operative procedure can be halted before any incisions are made into the recipient cornea.

Intraoperative Complications

Donor Tissue

Most donor tissue for penetrating keratoplasty is preserved in MK media. The tissue arrives as a corneoscleral button consisting of the cornea and 2 to 3 mm of sclera immersed in tissue culture medium, usually kept at 4°C. Before entering the operating room, and once again in the operating room, the surgeon must assess the clarity of the medium in which the donor tissue is stored. If it is turbid or the pH value has changed, it is indicative of possible bacterial infection, and the tissue should not be used. If the medium is clear, the tissue is removed from its container and trephined. If the plunger of the trephine has not been retracted, the donor endothelium will be seriously damaged and in most cases the tissue should not be used. Similarly, if the trephine is dull, there may be compression of the peripheral endothelium and Descemet's membrane prior to penetration. The degree of damage must be assessed but in most cases will not prevent continuation of the procedure. Since the peripheral endothelium comprises much of the endothelium transplanted, however, this factor must be taken into account. Every effort should be made to prevent drying of the donor endothelium. This involves placing the donor tissue in a moist chamber and covering the endothelium with MK medium.

If the cut is irregular and slanted, it may be possible to trim the tissue to give a more perpendicular edge. If the cut is only slightly irregular, it may be possible to compensate by altering the cut in the host tissue to match it. An excess of Descemet's in the host tissue will thus correspond to an area of relative deficiency of Descemet's in the donor. Once the donor tissue has been prepared, attention is then paid to the host.

Retrobulbar Hemorrhage

A recognized retrobulbar hemorrhage should lead to cessation of the case prior to entering the eye. Even though this means occasionally sacrificing excellent donor material, if the retrobulbar hemorrhage is of any magnitude and is definitive, it is best to cancel the case. Extension of the retrobulbar hemorrhage after opening the eye makes the procedure extremely difficult and complicated.

Scleral Perforation

The globe is fixed with superior and inferior rectus bridle sutures for phakic patients or with a scleral ring for aphakic patients. The sclera may be penetrated with the needle, especially if a cutting needle is used beneath the rectus muscles. If this is the case, the eye becomes markedly soft, and it is necessary to remove the rectus muscles, suture the area of perforation, and apply cryotherapy to the retina while visualizing the retina, if possible, with an indirect ophthalmoscope. Occasionally when placing a scleral support ring, the globe may be penetrated. Since this is within 4 or 5 mm of the limbus, it enters through the pars plana. If there is uveal prolapse, the sclera should be sutured and cryotherapy may be applied.

Trephining and Cutting the Host Cornea

With adequate fixation, the host tissue is usually trephined to a depth of 0.5 or 0.6 mm. Since this occurs in the mid-periphery where the tissue is 0.7 mm, the anterior chamber is usually not entered with the trephine. Attempts should be made to keep the trephine perpendicular and achieve as uniform a cut as possible. Occasionally the cut may be angled. If the dissection is still superficial, the trephine may be reapplied, neglecting the previous superficial incision, and a full-depth, perpendicular incision made. If the dissection is deep and additional donor material is available, it may be necessary to enlarge the recipient opening slightly to achieve a perpendicular incision. Occasionally, because of unequal pressure, the trephine will enter the anterior chamber in one area before cutting to any depth in the other areas. If this occurs and the trephine mark is visible, a sharp razorblade knife may be used to deepen the incision mark and then scissors used to complete the excision of the host tissue. Scissors are crushing instruments rather than cutting instruments, and it is best to make the initial cut with a trephine or a razorblade knife as deep as possible and down to Descemet's membrane. It is also best to avoid entering the eye with the trephine, as damage to the iris or lens may occur if this is not recognized. Damage to the lens may be minimized by using miotics in phakic patients; thus, if any injury does occur, it is to superficial iris rather than to the lens capsule. Some authorities have advocated deepening the anterior chamber with air or viscoelastic material prior to trephination in an effort to prevent damage to the underlying structures. This is not usually necessary, however.

When trephining the host, especially with a very edematous cornea, it is possible to separate the edematous stroma from underlying Descemet's membrane without recognizing this problem. The scissors may slip in very easily beneath the edematous stroma and separate it from Descemet's membrane. The presence of a glassy membrane on the iris surface should alert the surgeon to this possible complication. Failure to recognize this and to excise Descemet's membrane and the damaged endothelium will result in keratoplasty failure. If there is any doubt as to the presence of Descemet's membrane, a fine, nontoothed forceps may be used to pick up the iris gently. This will not cause any damage to the iris tissue or underlying lens but will alert the surgeon to the presence of Descemet's membrane.

After removal of the diseased host tissue, attention is paid to any additional intraocular procedures that may be necessary. Hemorrhage does not generally occur in the anterior chamber unless the iris is manipulated or an attempt is made to remove an intraocular implant. Any bleeding from the iris will frequently stop with irrigation. Similarly, any bleeding from the angle caused by tugging on the iris also stops with time and irrigation. After the bleeding has ceased, it is best to remove as much of the clot as possible, leaving a small clot, if present, on the iris or angle so as not to disturb the underlying vessels. If an anterior chamber lens is to be removed, the struts holding it in place should be divided, and it should be slid out of the fibrotic tunnel, which usually holds it in place. Attempts to remove the implant by pulling will result in iridodialysis, cyclodialysis, and extensive anterior chamber hemorrhage, which may be extremely difficult to stop. Occasionally, if an iris is markedly vascularized and bleeds persistently, wet-field cautery may be done. All bleeding should stop prior to the use of viscoelastic materials, such as Healon, as the blood may otherwise mix with the Healon and take an excessive period of time to absorb.

Handling of the Vitreous

All vitreous must be cleared from the anterior segment so it does not become incarcerated in the wound and disrupt wound healing. This may be done with mechanical or automated vitrectors.[22] If, during the process of cataract extraction, the posterior capsule is opened to any extent and vitreous presents, a vitrectomy should be performed and as much of the residual capsule and cortical material removed as possible. If the opening in the posterior capsule is small, frequently a posterior chamber implant may be placed and then miosis achieved to prevent migration of vitreous into the anterior segment. Also during keratoplasty, attempts should be made to reconstruct the anterior segment as much as possible by freeing as much of the iris synechiae as may be present from previous operative procedures. Great care must be taken to avoid bleeding. Since corneal graft rejection may occur where the iris is in contact with the peripheral host tissue, however, it is best to free this, if possible. Healon may be used locally to keep the iris back from the corneal tissue during the immediate postoperative period. Excessive Healon may cause a drastic rise in IOP, and its judicious use is advised. Viscoat may be less likely to cause a rise in IOP.

Expulsive Hemorrhage

Expulsive choroidal hemorrhage at any stage during any intraocular procedure represents a therapeutic challenge. During penetrating keratoplasty, expulsive hemorrhage usually results in a disastrous complication.[28] Attempts should be made to do a sclerostomy and drain as much of the blood as possible; great skill and speed are required in suturing in a donor button. When this does occur in the middle of an operative procedure, the eye is usually lost, as it is impossible to close the eye quickly enough to prevent complete extrusion of the retina and intraocular contents. Once the intraocular contents have been extruded above the surface of the corneal opening, the blood may be drained intraocularly and the button secured in place to permit appropriate procedures, such as enucleation, at a later date.

Suturing

Suturing techniques may consist of interrupted or continuous sutures of silk, nylon, or other synthetic material. It is imperative that at the end of the operative procedure the wound be watertight and not merely airtight. An airtight wound may leak aqueous once the air has been absorbed from the anterior chamber. If the leak was not repaired intraoperatively, it may have to be fixed the following day. If an interrupted suture is loose and is not doing the appropriate job, it should be removed and replaced. When a running suture is tightened to take up slack and secure the wound closure, every effort should be made not to break it. This is best done using smooth tying forceps and pulling the forceps parallel to the wound so that if there are any burrs or irregular edges on the forceps, they never meet the suture at right angles. If a running suture is found to be loose after it has been tied, it may be divided, retightened, and tied again. If this is not feasible, an additional piece of suture may be spliced in and tightened and both knots buried. If there is leakage along the incision, additional interrupted sutures may be placed across the area. If there is leakage along a suture track, this usually results from deep suture placement or gaping of the posterior aspects of the incision. Occasionally, these leaks seal themselves during the immediate postoperative period, but it is preferable to correct any detectable leaks during the operation. This may be done using an interrupted suture to compress the corneal stroma around the suture track. This approach prevents leakage along the track and permits Descemet's membrane to heal over the posterior aspect of the incision.

Immediate Postoperative Complications

Wound and Suture Problems

A running suture that breaks during the immediate postoperative period necessitates repair. Depending on the extent of unraveling of the suture and the patient's cooperation, this may be done with topical or general anesthesia. Retrobulbar anesthesia is contraindicated, as the eye is potentially open and a retrobulbar hemorrhage may be disastrous. If the patient is not suitable for general anesthesia, quadrant blocks and topical anesthetic may be used. It usually will not be possible to retie the original running suture to itself, as this will leave a gap of two or three suture passes and frequently will lead to wound separation. An additional piece of suture is spliced in, the iris is reposited if necessary, and both knots are tied and buried. If there is a leak along the suture track rather than along the wound, sometimes placing a soft contact lens or a pressure patch may allow this to heal. If it does not heal within 24 to 48 hours, the same technique as used intraoperatively to compress the stromal tissue around the suture tract may be useful. This can frequently be done with topical anesthesia, great care being taken not to divide the running suture with the sharp side-cutting needle when placing the interrupted.

Anterior wound separations without detectable leaks may be left as is, although sometimes high astigmatic errors may occur. A soft contact lens may facilitate wound healing and permit the epithelium to fill in the very anterior area of wound separation.

Iris Complication

If the iris becomes incarcerated in the wound during the immediate postoperative period, this should be carefully evaluated. Incarceration prevents complete healing of the posterior surface, may lead to edema, and may be the area of graft rejection due to vascular ingrowth from the iris. The risks of reoperation must be assessed. Frequently in the immediate postoperative period it is possible to sweep this area and, by placing a viscoelastic material such as Healon, prevent its recurrence. If the area is small, however, and the iris is atrophic and tenuous, this is probably best left without further intervention. Should the iris incarcerate through the entire thickness of the wound or through the deeper two thirds to three quarters, surgical intervention is indicated.

A syndrome of a fixed, dilated pupil with a shallow chamber may occur after keratoplasty for keratoconus. The cause is unknown and has prompted some surgeons to use only short-acting mydriatics.[29]

Flat Anterior Chambers

Flat anterior chambers occur because of wound leak, pupillary block, or a very adherent iris that comes into contact with the peripheral host cornea. A wound leak may be diagnosed by a very low IOP and a positive Seidel test and a typical clinical appearance. Pupillary block may be diagnosed by a higher than normal IOP and bowing forward of the iris diaphragm. Pupillary block may be reversed by moving the pupil, usually by dilation. If air is the cause of the block, it will sometimes resorb. This may be prevented in most aphakic patients by placing an iridotomy in the inferior half of the eye. Thus glaucoma is prevented even if the pupil and the previous superior iris openings are occluded by the air bubble. Laser or surgical iridotomy may be required.

In some cases, if inflamed eyes are operated on, such as following a perforation or a recent bout of intraocular inflammation, the chamber may become flat as the iris becomes quite sticky and adheres to the peripheral host tissue. In these cases, surgical intervention is contraindicated, as the iris will become more sticky with additional manipulation, and even the use of viscoelastic material at this point will frequently be doomed to unsatisfactory results. It is imperative that the surgeon be sure that the wound is watertight prior to leaving the operating room; if this is the case, the patient may be treated with topical or systemic corticosteroids to quiet the inflammatory response and should be observed for several days, frequently with deepening of the chamber.

Primary Donor Failure

If, during the immediate postoperative period, the donor tissue is swollen with striae and is thickened more than 50 percent compared with normal tissue, primary donor failure must be considered. Donor failure may occur because of primary donor failure or because of considerable intraoperative trauma to the donor endothelium. An assessment must be made at that point, based on experience, as to what the chances are of recovery of the donor endothelium and how long it is likely to survive if it does recover. Occasionally there may be delayed clearing of the corneal transplant if the storage conditions are such that the donor endothelium becomes dysfunctional but cells are not lost. It is usually not possible to get an assessment of endothelial cell size in these cases, and clinical judgment is necessary. It is generally best to wait 1 week before determining whether there is primary donor failure. In phakic eyes, in which there is not a considerable amount of inflammation, the donor tissue may be replaced within 1 to 2 weeks if primary donor failure or mechanical trauma to the donor endothelium during the operative procedure results in donor failure. If the patient is aphakic and has had vitreous or extensive iris manipulation, it is best to wait 1 to 2 months prior to replacement of the donor tissue. Otherwise the iris is frequently sticky and may result in extensive anterior synechiae with a clear graft but a markedly elevated IOP due to loss of the angle.

Epithelial Defects

Every attempt should be made to heal epithelial defects during the immediate postoperative period. A persistent epithelial defect tends to result in edema of the stroma, loss of endothelial cells, poor wound healing, and a propensity to infection. Epithelial defects may be healed by frequent lubrication, patching, or the use of a therapeutic soft contact lens. Failure to recognize and heal these defects may lead to stromal melting and eventual perforation.

Endophthalmitis: Diagnosis and Treatment

This condition is similar to that after cataract surgery, except that the organism may have been transmitted from the donor. Culture results from the corneoscleral rim may be helpful in initiating therapy.

Elevated Intraocular Pressure

It is imperative that IOP be controlled prior to keratoplasty, as it may become further elevated during the immediate postoperative period and for many months thereafter. With the use of better suturing techniques, markedly elevated IOP generally does not occur unless there has been extensive manipulation of the iris or vitreous or a considerable amount of viscoelastic material has been used. With oversized donor buttons and the use of looser sutures, elevated IOP is not as frequent.[30] Pressure may be measured with an electronic applanation tonometer or a pneumotonometer. The Goldmann applanation device and the Schiøtz tonometer are not reliable.

If the IOP is elevated, medical treatment with the appropriate topical medications and carbonic anhydrase inhibitors is indicated.[31] Frequently IOP will return to preoperative levels after several weeks, and intervention is best avoided. If IOP remains excessively high during the first few days, intermittent hyperosmotic agents may be given by mouth, if tolerated. If IOP still remains elevated, further intervention may be required. Laser trabeculoplasty may be used if the angle is open and visualization possible. If not, a conventional filtering procedure may succeed or cyclocryotherapy may be used. All these procedures may endanger the graft endothelium because of the tendency for a shallower anterior chamber and the inflammatory response that may follow any of them.

Late Postoperative Problems

Glaucoma is handled as it is during the immediate postoperative period, except that surgical intervention is often required. The surgeon should be aware of the possible role of prolonged use of topical corticosteroids in elevating IOP. The possible contribution of topical steroids to the development of lens changes is also important.[32]

Immune Rejection

Immune rejection is a not-uncommon cause of graft failure, which occurs after several weeks to several years.[33] It is frequently heralded by the onset of blurred vision and a line of keratic precipitates along the endothelium, with overlying edema of the epithelium and stroma (Fig. 15-16). This may occur in any area but frequently occurs in that area closest to the limbus, especially if there is vascularization in this area and if there is iris incarceration in the wound. There is usually no antibody response to a nonrejected corneal transplant, but following recognition that the keratoplasty is for-

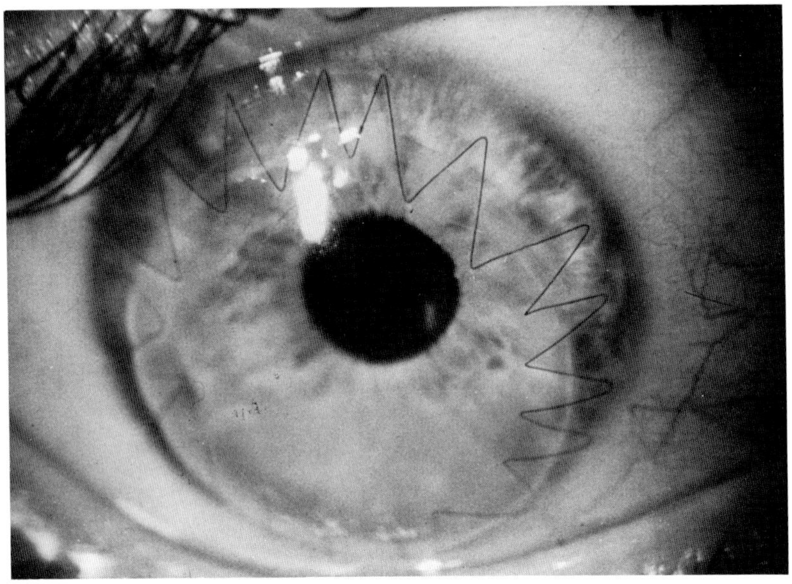

Fig. 15-16. Immune corneal graft rejection. Most of the corneal button is still clear, but edema occurs over the lower one third.

eign and the development of an immune response, a systemic response is detectable. Treatment consists of frequent topical corticosteroids, oral corticosteroids, and occasionally periocular steroids. Approximately one half of corneal transplant rejections can be reversed if they are not extensive. The patient must be warned to seek medical attention immediately should any signs of corneal rejection occur, such as a red eye or blurred vision due to corneal edema. Occasionally it is not possible to differentiate uveitis from corneal graft rejection, but the treatment for both is similar. Occasionally it is not possible to differentiate nonimmune, late endothelial failure from trauma or endothelial dropout from immune rejection. An attempt to treat with corticosteroids should be made if the IOP is not elevated and there is no contraindication.

Suture Problems

Suture problems consist of exposed sutures, which may break down the epithelium and stimulate vascularization and may lead to corneal ulcers. Once a suture has come to the surface, is loose, and there is vascularization up to it, it should be removed. If this is an interrupted suture, it poses no problem. If it is part of a running suture, and the entire suture is loose, it should be removed. If only one segment of the running suture is loose and vascularized and the rest appears to be necessary for wound support, that section of the suture may be removed and the suture knotted to itself at either end. This requires considerable manipulation at the slit-lamp or operating microscope but will frequently allow a section of vascularized cornea with loose suture to be taken care of without jeopardizing the wound strength of the remaining corneal tissue. Once a suture begins to decolorize and thin, it should be removed. Removal at this point is not difficult but, if the patient is sent away and the suture continues to decolorize and break down, multiple small breaks will occur. This may necessitate urgent care and, because of the very fragile nature of the suture at this point, its removal may be rather tedious and difficult.

Astigmatism

Most grafts heal and have a degree of astigmatism that is well tolerated by the patient. However, approximately 10 percent of grafts are left with a relatively high astigmatic error that makes corrected and uncorrected visual acuity less than ideal and spectacle and contact lens fitting difficult. If the patient sees well and comfortably with spectacles or contact lenses, no further attempt should be made to correct the astigmatism. Removing sutures along the steep meridian will frequently decrease the astigmatic error, and removing the running suture at the appropriate time will also frequently alter the astigmatic error. If the patient still retains a degree of astigmatism that is not tolerated, then relaxing incisions or corneal wedge resections may be done.[34] Thus it should be possible to provide adequate visual results in the vast majority of patients.

Retinal Complications

Retinal detachments[35] and cystoid macular edema[36] occur following penetrating keratoplasty, especially in aphakic eyes. They are treated similarly to when they occur in other aphakic eyes.

PROGNOSIS

The prognosis for penetrating keratoplasty in most cases is excellent with clear grafts in more than 80 percent of cases.[37] Several corneal and ancillary factors may contribute to reduced prognosis. Extensive vascularization may reduce the prognosis by leading to immune rejection in certain cases. These patients can frequently be treated with extensive topical and systemic corticosteroids, however, and occasionally with tissue-typed tissue. Patients with disorders of the lids and conjunctiva are the most susceptible to corneal graft failure. This problem occurs when there is extensive symblepharon, when the eye is very dry, or when there is a condition such as mucous membrane pemphigoid or Stevens-Johnson syndrome. This frequently leads to vascularization and breakdown of the epithelium with failure of the graft. Patients who have had extensive chemical burns have an extremely poor prognosis in many cases. This is due to disorganization of the lids and conjunctiva, frequently with loss of the mucoid and aqueous layer of the tear film. Furthermore, there has often been extensive damage to the ciliary body from a chemical injury with defective aqueous production of glucose, which results in graft failure.

Patients with uncontrolled IOP, whether it be too high or too low, are not ideal candidates for keratoplasty. If the glaucoma is severe, the pressure must be brought under control prior to keratoplasty. If not, the failure rate will be extremely high.

Patient compliance is extremely important in keratoplasty as opposed to many other intraocular procedures. The frequent use of topical corticosteroids to prevent corneal graft rejection and the recognition of corneal graft rejection, if it does occur after corticosteroids have been discontinued, depend heavily on patient compliance. If a patient is not compliant and is not going to use medication, keratoplasty is frequently doomed to failure from technical and immune factors. With a helpful patient and absence of other complicating factors, the success rate for keratoplasty should exceed 90 percent.

REFERENCES

1. Waltman SR: The cornea. p. 38. In Moses RA (ed): Adler's Physiology of the Eye. 7th Ed. CV Mosby, St. Louis, 1981
2. Binder PS, Wickham MG, Zavala EY, Akers PH: Corneal anatomy and wound healing. p. 1. In Borraquer I, Binder PS, Buxton J, et al (eds): Symposium on Medical and Surgical Diseases of the Cornea. Transactions of the New Orleans Academy of Ophthalmology. CV Mosby, St. Louis, 1980
3. Sugar J, Mitchelson J, Kraff M: Endothelial trauma and cell loss from intraocular lens insertion. Arch Ophthalmol 96:449, 1978
4. Paton D: The prognosis of penetrating keratoplasty. Based upon corneal morphology. Ophthalmic Surg 7(3):36, 1976
5. Abbott RL, Forster RK: Determinants of graft clarity in penetrating keratoplasty. Arch Ophthalmol 97:1071, 1979
6. West CE, Wood TD, Kaufman H: Cyclocryotherapy for glaucoma pre- or post-penetrating keratoplasty. Am J Ophthalmol 76:485, 1973
7. Eye Bank Association of America Medical Standards, 1984
8. Forster RK, Fine M: Relation of donor age to success in keratoplasty. Arch Ophthalmol 85:42, 1971
9. Duffy P, Wolf J, Collins G, et al: Possible person-to-

person transmission of Creutzfeldt-Jakob disease. N Engl J Med 290:692, 1974
10. Baer GM, Shaddock JH, Houff SA, et al: Human rabies transmitted by corneal transplant. Arch Neurol 39:103, 1982
11. Shaw EL, Aquavella JV: Pneumococcal endophthalmitis following grafting of corneal tissue from a (cadaver) kidney donor. Ann Ophthalmol 9:435, 1977
12. Stainer GA, Brightbill FS, Calkins B: A comparison of corneal storage in moist chamber and McCarey-Kaufman medium in human keratoplasty. Ophthalmology 88:46, 1981
13. McCarey BE, Meyer RF, Kaufman HE: Improved corneal storage for penetrating keratoplasties in humans. Ann Ophthalmol 8:1488, 1976
14. Waltman SR, Palmberg PF: Human penetrating keratoplasty using modified M-K medium. Ophthalmic Surg 9:48, 1978
15. Doughman DJ, Harris JE, Schmitt MK: Penetrating keratoplasty using 37°C organ cultured cornea. Trans Am Acad Ophthalmol Otolaryngol 81:778, 1976
16. Capella JA, Kaufman HE, Polack FM: Prognosis of keratoplasty in phakic and aphakic patients and the use of cryopreserved donor tissue. Trans Am Acad Ophthalmol Otolaryngol 76:1275, 1972
17. Olson RJ: The effect of scleral fixation ring placement and trephine tilting on keratoplasty wound size and donor shape. Ophthalmic Surg 12:23, 1981
18. Polack FM: Penetrating keratoplasty using MK stored corneas and Na hyaluronate (Healon). Trans Am Ophthalmol Soc 80:248, 1982
19. Stegmann R, Miller D: Protective function of sodium hyaluronate in corneal transplantation. Ocul Ther Surg 12:28, 1981
20. Davison JA, Bourne WM: Results of penetrating keratoplasty using a double running suture technique. Arch Ophthalmol 99:1591, 1981
21. McNeill JI, Kaufman HE: Early visual rehabilitation after keratoplasty. A double running suture technique. Ann Ophthalmol 10:652, 1978
22. Mackman G, Brightbill FS: Combined penetrating keratoplasty and mechanical anterior vitrectomy. Ophthalmic Surg 11:330, 1980
23. Waltman SR: Penetrating keratoplasty for pseudophakic bullous keratopathy. Visual results. Arch Ophthalmol 99:415, 1981
24. Meyer RF, Sugar A: Penetrating keratoplasty in pseudophakic bullous keratopathy. Am J Ophthalmol 90:677, 1980
25. Sugar A, Meyer RF, Heidemann D, et al: Specular microscopic follow-up of corneal grafts for pseudophakic bullous keratopathy. Ophthalmology 92:325, 1985
26. Lindstrom RL, Harris WS, Doughman DJ: Combined penetrating keratoplasty, extracapsular cataract extraction and posterior chamber lens implantation. J Am Intraocular Implant Soc J 7:130, 1981
27. Hunkeler JD, Hyde LL: The triple procedure. Combined penetrating keratoplasty, extracapsular cataract extraction and lens implantation. An expanded experience. J Am Intraocular Implant Soc J 9:20, 1983
28. Purcell JJ Jr, Krachmer JH, Doughman DJ, Bourne WM: Expulsive hemorrhage in penetrating keratoplasty. Ophthalmology 89:41, 1982
29. Urrets-Zavalia A: Fixed dilated pupil, iris atrophy and secondary glaucoma. A distinct clinical entity following keratoplasty in keratoconus. Am J Ophthalmol 56:257, 1963
30. Zimmerman T, Olson R, Waltman S, Kaufman H: Transplant size and elevated intraocular pressure. Postkeratoplasty. Arch Ophthalmol 96:2231, 1978
31. Wood TO, West C, Kaufman HE: Control of intraocular pressure in penetrating keratoplasty. Am J Ophthalmol 74:724, 1972
32. Donshik PC, Cavanagh D, Boruchoff SA, Dohlman CH: Posterior subcapsular cataract induced by topical corticosteroids following keratoplasty for keratoconus. Ann Ophthalmol 13:12, 1981
33. Stark WJ: Transplantation immunology of penetrating keratoplasty. Trans Am Ophthalmol Soc 78:1079, 1980
34. Krachmer JH, Fenzl RE: Surgical correction of high postkeratoplasty astigmatism. Relaxing incisions vs wedge resection. Arch Ophthalmol 98:1400, 1980
35. Forstot SL, Binder PS, Fitzgerald C, Kaufman HE: The incidence of retinal detachment after penetrating keratoplasty. Am J Ophthalmol 80:102, 1975
36. Kramer SG: Cystoid macular edema after aphakic penetrating keratoplasty. Ophthalmology 88:782, 1981
37. gOlson RJ, Waltman SR, Mattingly TP, Kaufman HE: Visual results after penetrating keratoplasty for aphakic bullous keratopathy and Fuchs' dystrophy. Am J Ophthalmol 88:1000, 1979

Lamellar Keratoplasty

16

Stephen R. Waltman

CLINICAL PICTURE

Lamellar keratoplasty involves replacement of the patient's diseased anterior corneal stroma and Bowman's membrane with donor material. Host endothelium, Descemet's membrane, and a part of the deep stroma are preserved. The donor corneal disc becomes repopulated with host fibroblasts, and the recipient epithelium usually covers the anterior corneal surface. This procedure is technically more difficult than penetrating keratoplasty, especially in inexperienced hands, and the visual results are not usually as good. It has the advantage of being primarily an extraocular procedure that preserves the host endothelium. The risk of rejection is therefore markedly diminished. The risks of wound leaks or flat anterior chambers associated with an intraocular procedure are eliminated. Microsurgical techniques have vastly improved the technique of lamellar keratoplasty, but they have also substantially improved the results with penetrating keratoplasty. The use of conjunctival flaps and therapeutic soft contact lenses has reduced the indications for lamellar keratoplasty.

SURGICAL ANATOMY

The surgical anatomy of the cornea is as discussed in Chapter 15. The major point to be stressed is that the lamellae of the host and recipient cornea are much more easily separated with a smooth dissector when this is done in the deeper one half of the stroma. In the deeper stroma, the corneal lamellae are arranged in much more discrete isolated lamellae with less criss-crossing of the fibrils than occurs in the anterior stroma.

The criteria for the selection of donor tissue are similar to those for penetrating keratoplasty except that the donor tissue is usually preserved as a whole globe. Furthermore, since the donor endothelium is not preserved, the tissue may be stored for a considerably longer period of time at 4°C, and donors with unacceptable endothelium because of age or time to enucleation may be suitable donors for lamellar keratoplasty. Every effort should be made so as not to transmit a disease from the donor to the host.

INDICATIONS

The indications for lamellar keratoplasty are optical, techtonic, or therapeutic. Patients whose disease lies in the anterior corneal stroma, especially the anterior one third, are thought to be ideal candidates for lamellar keratoplasty. Included are patients with anterior corneal stromal dystrophies, of which Reis-Bücklers dystrophy is a prime example.[1] Patients with Salzman's nodular dystrophy or irregular anterior stromal scars from trauma or infections are also candidates.

Lamellar keratoplasty may be done for techtonic reasons if the corneal stroma of the host is quite thinned peripherally, either circumferentially or in isolated areas. This is sometimes done as preparation for full-thickness penetrating keratoplasty. Indications include cases of Terrien's marginal dystrophy or pellucid marginal degeneration or when corneal scarring in the periphery makes this necessary prior to penetrating keratoplasty. This may occur from peripheral corneal infectious or inflammatory disease. In certain cases of keratoconus, if the periphery of the cornea is quite thin or the patient's compliance is likely to be poor, lamellar keratoplasty may be preferred to penetrating keratoplasty.[2,3] In these cases, there are both optical and techtonic considerations.

Therapeutically, lamellar keratoplasty is used in some cases of recurrent pterygium[4] with deep stromal scarring and more especially for the therapy of descemetoceles. Descemetoceles may be treated with soft contact lenses or by tissue adhesive after the disease processes are sterilized. Each procedure has its advantages and disadvantages, but the use of soft contact lenses or tissue adhesive requires daily observation for weeks to be sure the therapy continues successfully. The use of a patch lamellar keratoplasty may speed the rehabilitation period in certain cases.[5]

CONTRAINDICATIONS

Disease processes that affect the deeper stromal layers and the endothelium should not be treated by optical lamellar keratoplasty, as these layers are not replaced. Corneal edema due to endothelial dysfunction will recur, and failure to remove deeper stromal opacities will result in continued visual decrease. Corneal vascularization may regrow at deeper levels following surgery. Fungal corneal ulcers are absolute contraindications to lamellar keratoplasty, as the fungi tend to grow at the interface.

RECOMMENDED TECHNIQUE

According to this author's preferred technique, the host is prepared first so that if there is difficulty and extensive perforation, a penetrating keratoplasty may be performed if suitable donor tissue is

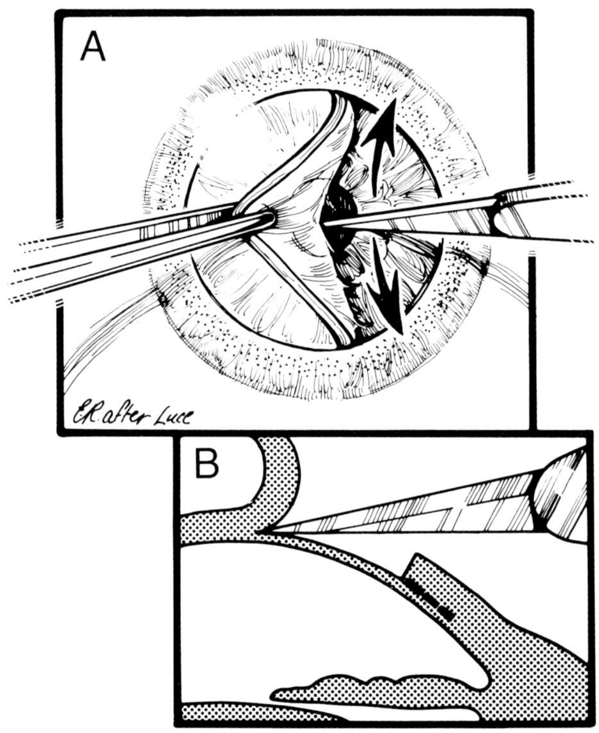

Fig. 16-1. (A) The base of the recipient bed is dissected with a back-and-forth motion of the dissector against taut stromal fiber. **(B)** The level of dissection and peripheral undermining are shown.

available. Especially in cases of therapeutic or techtonic keratoplasty, lamellar grafts of nonstandard sizes and shapes are frequently used.

The ophthalmic surgeon must prepare the host with perpendicular sharp edges to prevent override of the donor tissue. A smooth dissection of the base of the host tissue is also critical, as healing occurs along this interface. Irregularities and foreign bodies with resultant scarring at the host–donor lamellar interface may be responsible for considerable vision decrease. With optical lamellars, the trephine is set an appropriate depth of 0.2 to 0.4 mm after achieving adequate fixation of the eye. This is usually done with superior and inferior rectus bridle sutures and grasping one of the rectus muscles at its insertion. Trephine blades of 9 to 11 mm are used, and a uniform circumferential incision is made. If the incision is not of uniform depth, it may be deepened with a razorblade knife. The anterior stromal tissue is grasped with a 0.12-mm Bonn forceps and gently elevated, usually in the horizontal meridian, at approximately the 9 o'clock position on the globe. Using a razorblade knife, a constant to-and-fro or back-and-forth motion of the blade, applied against the stretched lamellae at the base of the dissection, achieves a uniform, smooth plane (Fig. 16-1). The dissecting blade should be kept perpendicular to Descemet's membrane at all times to achieve a uniform plane and reduce the danger of anterior or posterior perforation. If stromal opacity remains in the deeper tissue, the procedure may be repeated, although it is considerably easier to do it all in one dissection. Dissections down to Descemet's membrane may be carried out. After the dissection is completed and the diseased corneal tissue removed, the host bed is undermined 360 degrees for approximately 1 mm. This allows placement of the sutures deeper and ensures that the donor tissue will not override the host–donor interface. Constant irrigation and suction at the base of the dissection are done to prevent foreign body accumulation at the interface, with subsequent scarring. In patients with descemetoceles the eye is frequently soft, and the trephine can only be very gently applied for fear of rupturing the descemetocele. The trephine mark is outlined, and a very sharp razorblade knife is used to achieve a perpendicular edge. The base of the descemetocele is then dissected from peripherally to centrally 360 degrees to remove the diseased anterior stromal tissue. In this condition, a trephine blade of somewhere between 3.5 and 4.5 mm may be used to get around the area of descemetocele. If the area of descemetocele is considerably larger and the eye is not overly inflamed, consideration may be given to penetrating keratoplasty, especially if the descemetocele is central. The base of the descemetocele after dissection is frequently ir-

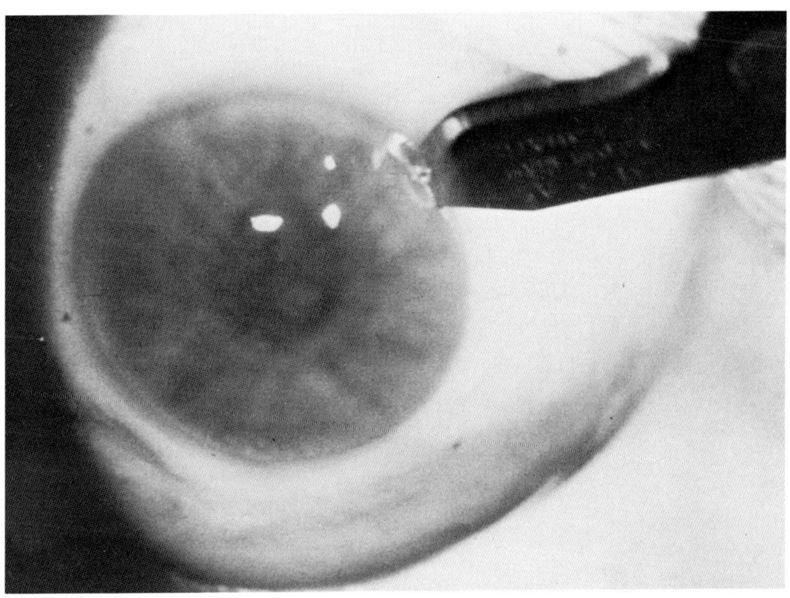

Fig. 16-2. Lamellar dissection of the donor is started with a 3- to 4-mm razorblade incision.

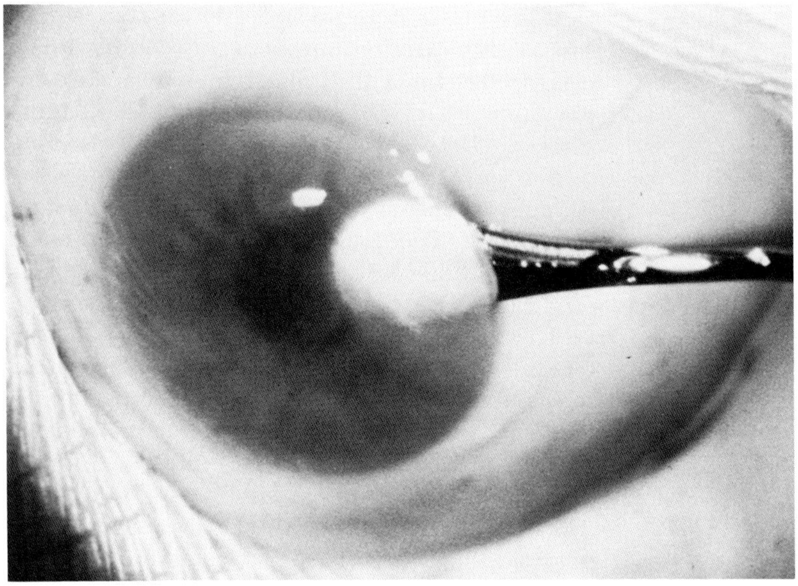

Fig. 16-3. The Martinez dissector is inserted into the intralamellar space.

regular with a considerable amount of corneal scarring; however, this is not avoidable and frequently may only lead to a slight decrease in vision if a smooth, regular anterior corneal surface can be achieved.

The donor tissue used is usually prepared as a whole globe and soaked in a broad-spectrum antibiotic. The donor epithelium is frequently irregular and edematous and is easily removed with a cotton swab and irrigation. The globe is then wrapped in a gauze sponge and held in the surgeon's nondominant hand. This facilitates control of the intraocular pressure and firmness of the globe, to keep a regular anterior corneal surface. A 3- to 4-mm incision is made at the limbus to within 0.2 mm of Descemet's membrane (Fig. 16-2). A

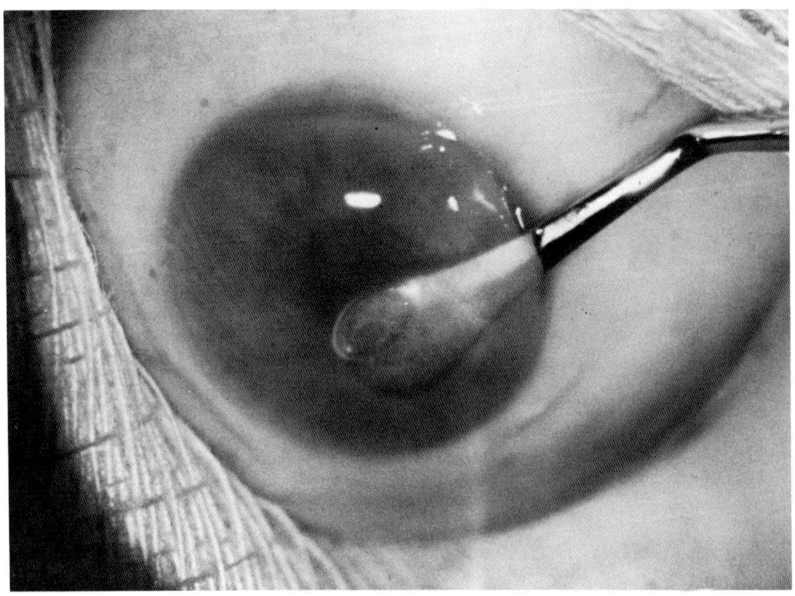

Fig. 16-4. A complete deep dissection is done with the dull end of the Martinez dissector.

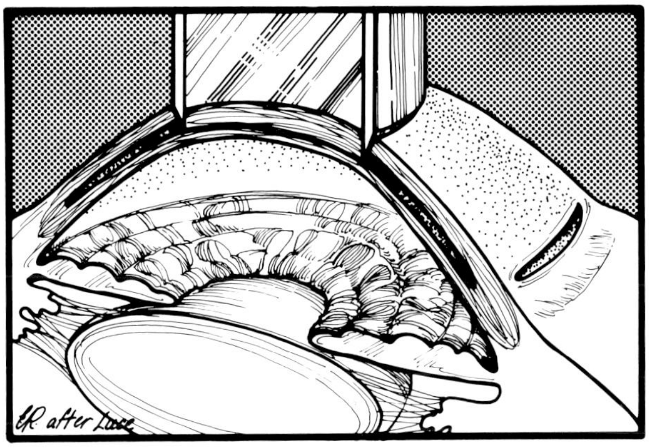

Fig. 16-5. The appropriate-size trephine is selected, and the anterior corneal button is trephined.

Martinez lamellar dissector is then used to finish the dissection. The dissector is pushed laterally and not up or down to maintain a smooth, sharp cleavage plane (Fig. 16-3). If the cleavage plane is in the posterior one half of the donor stroma, the dissection is usually easily done with a minimal amount of pressure. The curve of the dissector is kept parallel to the curve of the cornea. If the correct plane is achieved, the dissection may be performed from limbus to limbus and even extended into the adjacent sclera (Fig. 16-4). The dull end of the dissector should be used after starting the dissection with the sharp edge for 1 to 2 mm. The appropriate-size trephine with the plunger partially retracted is then applied to the donor tissue (Fig. 16-5). A round disc with a perpendicular edge and a smooth, regular base is achieved in this manner (Fig. 16-6). The deeper donor lamellae are undisturbed. A microkeratome may also be used for the dissection.

The donor tissue is placed in the recipient bed and secured with eight interrupted 10-0 nylon sutures. The sutures are placed to three quarter depth in the donor tissue and then to full depth in the undermined area of the host tissue. It is important to pull these sutures very tightly, as the donor tissue, which is initially somewhat edematous, dehydrates during the procedure, and the initial sutures may loosen. If it is difficult to secure the donor tissue in place in the host bed, a paracentesis through a separate limbal incision may facilitate suturing. The donor tissue is chosen to be 0.5 mm larger in diameter than the host tissue. After placing the interrupted sutures, a continuous nylon suture may be used for complete closure. It is imperative that the donor tissue be flush with the edge of the recipient bed, especially in the vertical meridian. Failure to achieve this will result in elevation of

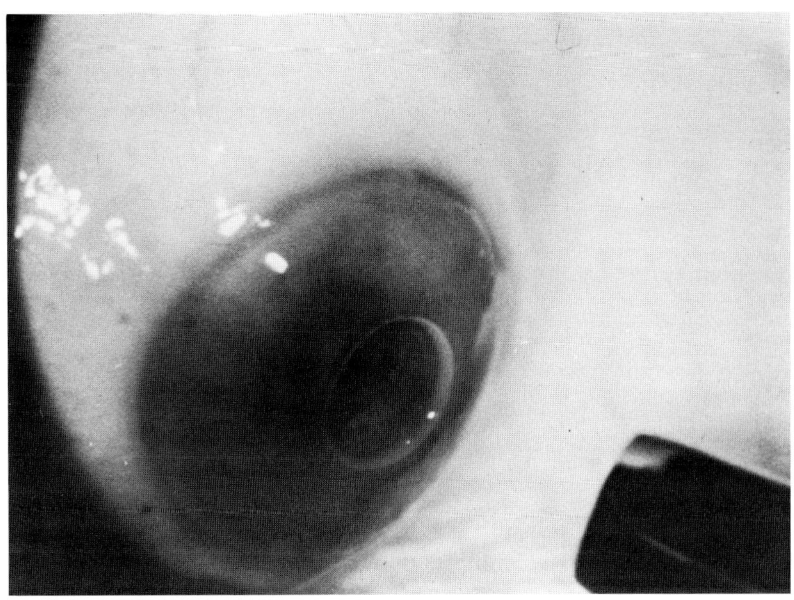

Fig. 16-6. The donor button remains in the trephine, leaving the deeper stromal tissue intact.

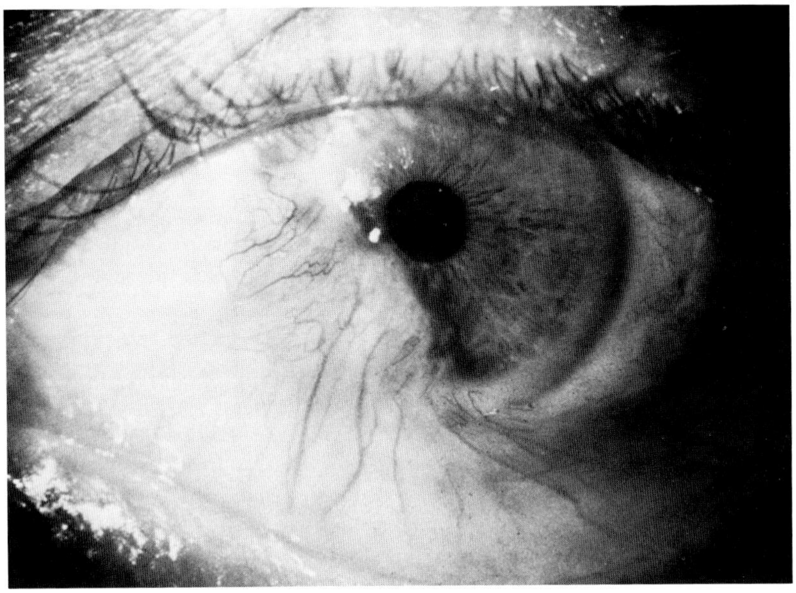

Fig. 16-7. Extensive recurrent pterygium with invasion of the anterior two thirds of the stroma.

the donor tissue by edema and by movement of the lids and may result in loss of the graft. A similar technique is used for techtonic grafts, such as those used after pterygium removal (Figs. 16-7 and 16-8). In the presence of a descemetocele, eight to ten interrupted 10-0 nylon sutures are used without a continuous suture.

COMPLICATIONS

Complications may arise when cutting the donor or the host tissue. In cutting the donor tissue, it is advantageous to practice this beforehand or to

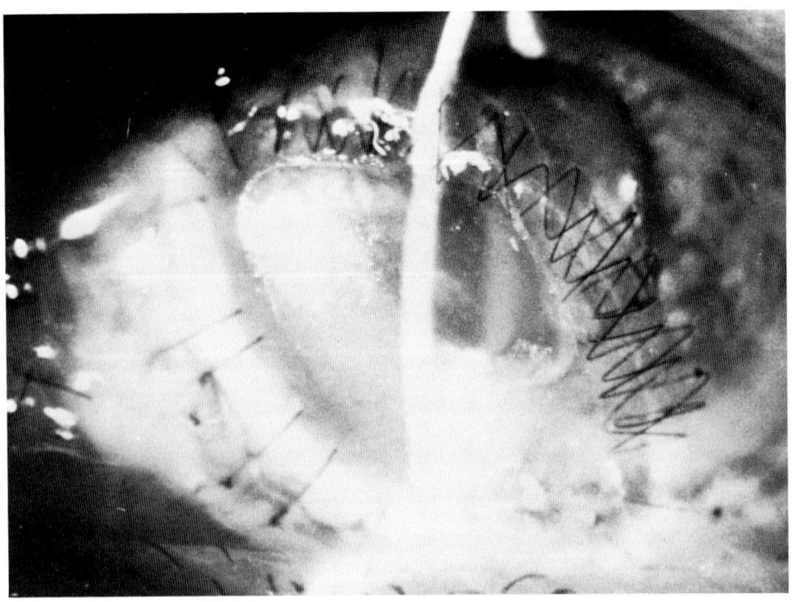

Fig. 16-8. Appearance on the second postoperative day after lamellar keratoplasty for pterygium.

have additional donor material available, as anterior or posterior perforation of the donor tissue is not unusual, especially in inexperienced hands. If the cut is very irregular, the donor tissue may not be suitable, especially for an optical lamellar. If the donor tissue is somewhat irregular, but this is primarily a techtonic or therapeutic graft, it may be employed. In cutting the host tissue, perforation of the deep lamella early on in the course of the dissection, especially if the perforation is large, may necessitate ending the procedure here, filling the anterior chamber with air and waiting for healing or converting to a penetrating keratoplasty if suitable donor tissue is available. If the perforation is small, sometimes the deeper stroma and Descemet's membrane may be sutured with a mattress-type 10-0 nylon suture and the dissection completed. If the base of the host tissue is quite irregular, it may be possible to deepen this along selected areas by further deep lamellar dissection. Great care must be taken to avoid entering the anterior chamber at this point.

One of the major difficulties with lamellar keratoplasty is the occurrence of foreign bodies at the host–donor lamellar interface with subsequent scarring. Once this has occurred, the foreign bodies can sometimes be removed intraoperatively by continuous irrigation and aspiration with copious volumes of balanced salt solution. If noticed during the postoperative period or following suturing, no therapy is available. Rejection of the donor tissue is quite uncommon because only a small amount of collagen tissue and no live fibroblasts are transplanted. Recurrences of Reis-Bücklers dystrophy in the donor tissue have been reported.[6]

If the donor tissue overrides the donor–host interface, an attempt must be made to resuture it or place a soft contact lens to allow this area to smooth out and not be traumatized by continued lid movement. If a suture breaks and there is wound separation, it should be corrected, especially if this is an optical or techtonic graft. In certain therapeutic cases, when one of the eight to ten sutures breaks, it may be possible to leave this, as long as the wound remains watertight.

PROGNOSIS

The prognosis for lamellar keratoplasty is quite good, although it is not performed as often as penetrating keratoplasty because of the less than ideal visual results that frequently result from scarring at the interface. It may be used in certain cases of keratoconus and the anterior stromal dystrophies as well as techtonically to reinforce an area of thin cornea or therapeutically for descemetoceles or after pterygium excision.

REFERENCES

1. Akiya S, Brown SI: The ultrastructure of Reis-Bücklers dystrophy. Am J Ophthalmol 72:549, 1971
2. Wood TO: Lamellar transplants in keratoconus. Am J Ophthalmol 83:543, 1977
3. Gasset AR: Lamellar keratoplasty in the treatment of keratoconus. Conectomy. Ophthalmic Surg 10:26, 1978
4. Paton D: Pterygium management based on a theory of pathogenesis. Trans Am Acad Ophthalmol Otolaryngol 79:603, 1975
5. Dohlman CH, Boruchoff SA, Sullivan GL: A technique for the repair of perforated corneal ulcers. Arch Ophthalmol 77:519, 1967
6. Olson RJ, Kaufman HE: Recurrence of Reis-Bücklers corneal dystrophy in a graft. Am J Ophthalmol 85:349, 1978

Radial Keratotomy

17

William D. Myers

EVOLUTION OF RADIAL KERATOTOMY

In 1898, Lans[1] performed radial incisions in an attempt to flatten the corneal curvature. In 1939, Sato[2] published a report on the use of nonperforating incisions starting from the epithelial and endothelial corneal surfaces. By 1953, Sato et al.[3] had extended the use of such incisions to the treatment of myopia. These workers made up to 64 incisions from both the anterior and posterior corneal surfaces with a central 6-mm diameter optical zone into which no cuts extended. Since the importance of the endothelium was not established in Sato's time, Sato had no reason to suspect that corneal edema would be a future complication of his procedure. In 1972, Fyodorov[4] noted in one of his patients a marked reduction in the patient's myopia following an injury in which multiple anterior corneal lacerations were created. Because of this clinical observation, he reasoned that anterior incisions alone could be used to reduce myopia surgically. Since by now the importance of the corneal endothelium was well known, it was obviously desirable on Fyodorov's part to avoid endothelial incisions of any type.

Fyodorov's major innovation to the radial keratotomy procedure was the concept of radial cuts of uniformly varying length to correct various degrees of myopia. In other words, he varied the optical zone according to the degree of myopia. The larger the degree of myopia, the smaller the optical zone. Fyodorov and Durnev[5] first reported on his clinical studies in the American literature in 1979. After investigating the effects of 32, 16, and 8 radial incisions in reducing the corneal curvature, they decided that 16 was the optimal number of incisions in most cases. The original Fyodorov procedure also included extending the incisions to, the sometimes through, the limbus. In 1978, Dr. Leo Bores performed the first radial keratotomy in the United States at the Kresge Eye Institute. Dr. Bores and the director of the institute, Dr. Robert Jampel, established a protocol for proper evaluation of this procedure. Those of us who perform refractive surgery are indeed indebted to these two opthalmologists, who elected to pursue an investigation that did not find widespread support among their colleagues at the time. Once a clinical investigation of radial keratotomy in the United States was initiated, several modifications to the procedure were adopted. The author noted in one case, in which a perforation occurred on the eighth incision, that the final optical result was exactly what would have been expected had the case included 16 incisions. In the subsequent clinical study, 16 patients were given 8 incisions in one eye and 16 in the other. The optical results in both eyes were quite similar.[6] This clinical conclusion found support from Schachar et al.,[7] who determined after evaluating a mathematical model of radial keratotomy that 8 incisions could come close to achieving the same degree of corneal flattening as could 16 incisions. During the early clinical investigation in the United States, some patients were noted to develop neovascularization of their incisions. These patients all had radial incisions extending to the peripheral vascular arcades and also had soft lenses applied within several weeks following the radial keratotomy procedure.[8] This problem was solved by keeping the incisions at least 1 mm short of the limbus and not applying soft lenses to the cornea of undercorrected patients until the normal postoperative corneal changes had stabilized. This meant waiting at least several weeks to several months following the radial keratotomy procedure before applying soft lenses. As the procedure evolved in the United States, surgeons not only reduced the number of incisions and their length but also changed the direction of the incisions from centripetal (as favored by the Russian surgeons) to centrifugal (as favored by the American surgeons). This change was made in order to avoid inadvertently incising into the optical zone, which can occur when incisions are made toward the visual axis. During the early 1980s, as the radial keratotomy procedure evolved from a surgical standpoint, it also changed with regard to the manner in which it was clinically investigated. As in generally the case with new surgical procedures, the initial investigations were conducted by a few individuals involved in the early clinical use of the surgical technique. These early efforts were first reported to American ophthalmologists in 1979.[9–11] These early studies were rightfully viewed in a circumspective manner by most ophthalmologists due to lack of adherence to a rigid experimental protocol.

An attempt was made by two national organizations to compile the results of many radial keratotomy surgeons.[12,13] While this approach enabled us to look at many more results than was theretofore possible, it did little to instill a higher level of confidence in the scientific validity of the data, since it simply pooled the information and failed to correct the deficiencies of the earlier reports. Specifically, there was no reliance on independent observers, no control of follow-up losses, and no standard methodology in all cases. Two early studies deserving of particular mention because they involved the use of an independent observer and had no patients lost to follow-up were the studies of Hecht and Jamara,[14] reported in 1982, and the studies of Nirankari et al.,[15] reported in 1983. The analysis of radial keratotomy (ARK) study has given a careful statistical analysis of the results of three surgeons with significant experience in radial keratotomy.[16] Since the surgeon did not follow a standard protocol and an independent observer failed to record the data, it can be criticized from a purely scientific posture. The value of this report, however, is the manner in which it reflects the results of experienced surgeons in variable clinical settings. This mimics what might be expected in the very practical world of clinical practice.

The Prospective Evaluation of Radial Keratotomy (PERK) study, a multicenter study funded by the National Eye Institute, is a study to which many ophthalmologists look for information that will be considered clinically and scientifically valid. This multicenter study funded by the National Eye Institute avoids many of the criticisms of the aforementioned approaches to the study of radial keratotomy. Specifically, it addresses the requirements of an independent examiner, safeguards against follow-up losses, and takes place within the framework of a proper experimental design.[17]

VARIATIONS IN RADIAL KERATOTOMY TECHNIQUE

Radial kertotomy has often been criticized because of the lack of a standard technique. This criticism is not peculiar to radial keratotomy, as it is obvious that there are multiple approaches to cataract extraction, muscle surgery, and many other ophthalmic surgical procedures. In addition to differences in surgical technique, differences also exist in the method of determining the patient's corneal thickness. In the United States, some surgeons have traditionally preferred optical pachometry, while others prefer ultrasonic pachometry.

Surgeons who favor the optical means of corneal thickness determination generally use a Haag-Streit pachometer I, which attaches to the Haag-Streit 900 slit lamp or its equivalent produced by other manufacturers. The pachometer is placed on the fixation post of the slit lamp after removing the applanation tonometer and locating the slit-lamp housing to the left of the microscope. The pachometer provides a split image of the corneal section by using two plano glass plates located edge to edge that divide equally and horizontally the reflected light entering the right objective of the microscope. This reflected light is seen through the 10× split-image eyepiece, which replaces a normal right ocular. When using the special pachometer lens, it is necessary to add +2.5 diopters to the normal setting.[18] In order to measure the central corneal thickness, the patient is asked to fixate the slit beam while the examiner focuses the slit lamp with the joystick until the split corneal section is seen through the right ocular. Using the measurement scale of the pachometer, the split image is adjusted until the endothelial surface of the top corneal section just touches the epithelial surface of the bottom section. The illumination of the slit lamp should be reduced to a minimal level that permits clear visualization of the corneal section. If the illumination is increased from this minimal level, it will provide a corneal section that will appear falsely thickened. Once familiar with the basic operation of the Haag-Streit pachometer, the surgeon will quickly appreciate the necessity of knowing that the slit-lamp beam is perpendicular to the corneal surface. Without a guarantee of true perpendicularity, it is possible to generate readings that are generally too thick or occasionally too thin. To avoid false optical measurements, it is important that the Mishima-Hedbys pinlight attachment be used in conjunction with the Haag-Streit optical pachometer.[19] The A-A′ measurement represents the true thickness of the central cornea (Fig. 17-1). If, however, the incidence of the slit-lamp beam is not perpendicular to the corneal surface, the measurement on the corneal pachometer will be falsely exaggerated, as shown by section B-B′. With the Mishima-Hedbys attachment, two pinlights are placed 10 mm apart in the vertical plane. The distance between the pinlights and the slit-lamp beam is equal to the distance between the slip-lamp beam and the right microscope objective (x-y in Fig. 17-2). Thus, when the optical section or slit beam is perpendicular to the cornea, the angle of incidence i will be equal to the angle of reflection r, and the pinlights will be seen on the surface of the corneal sections by the biomicroscopist (Fig. 17-3). Using this method, one will obtain the most accurate optical pachometry measurements possible. To use the Haag-Streit pachometer without the Mishima-Hedbys attachments makes such measurements difficult at best. Once the central optical pachometry is determined, the examiner measures the peripheral areas of the cornea by having the patient

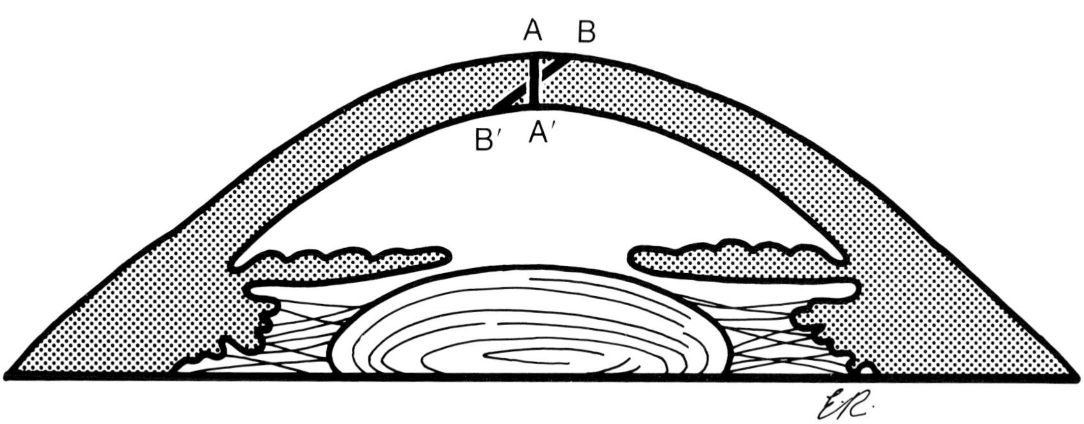

Fig. 17-1. Only an optical section that is perpendicular to the corneal surface as represented by the line A-A′ gives a true corneal thickness. Any nonperpendicular section as in the case of the line B-B′ will give a false reading.

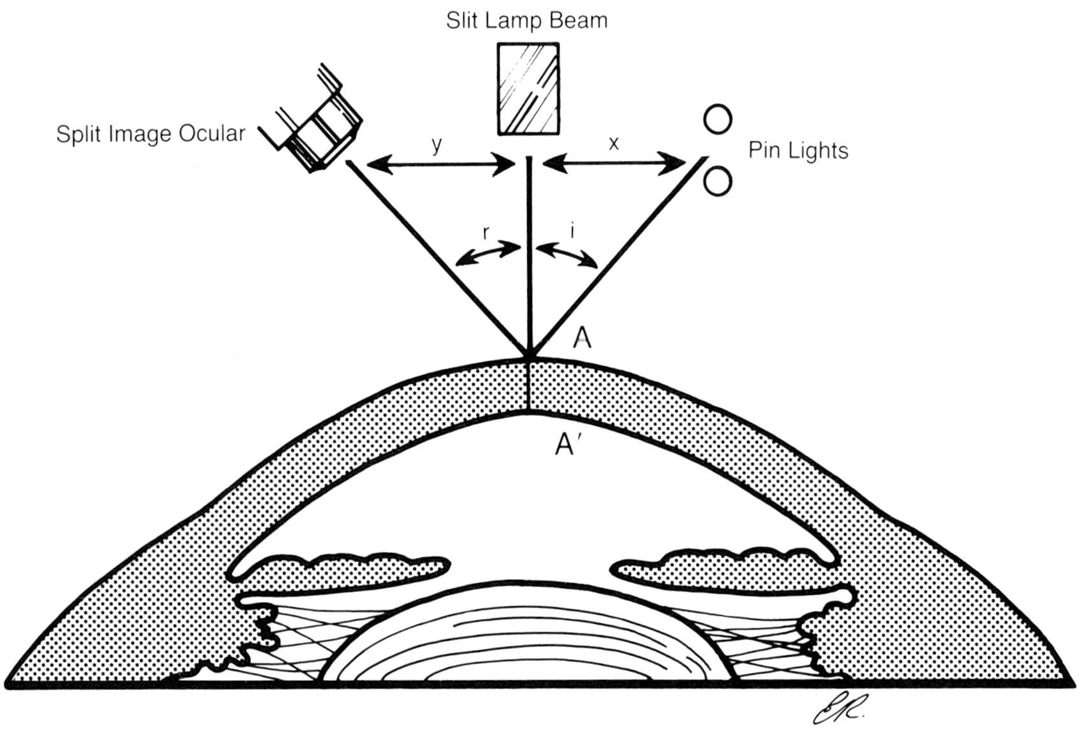

Fig. 17-2. When the beam of the slit lamp cuts the optical section A-A′, which is perpendicular to the corneal surface, the examiner will see the reflection of the Mishima-Hedbys pinlights on the surface of the cornea through the split-image ocular. Since the distance from the pinlights to the slit-lamp beam x is equal to the distance from the slit-lamp beam to the split image ocular y, the angle of incidence i will equal the angle of reflection r only when the slit beam is perpendicular to the corneal surface.

look straight ahead while the examiner swings the slit beam to the mid- and far periphery. It is in measuring the noncentral cornea that the pinlights are most vital in guaranteeing true perpendicularity of the measurement.

While some surgeons prefer to measure the corneal thickness optically, many others use ultrasonic instruments. Ultrasonic instruments have several advantages. While the optical pachometer can only measure the corneal thickness in the 180-degree meridian, the ultrasonic apparatus readily measures the corneal thickness in any given meridian. This permits contour mapping of the cornea, which is practically impossible to achieve by optical means. The ultrasonic devices can also be used intraoperatively, whereas the optical measurements cannot be. One further advantage of the ultrasonic instrument is that most surgeons find it much easier to learn that the method of optical pachometry. The major disadvantage to the ultrasound instruments is that they are extremely expensive compared with their optical counterparts.

When using the optical measurement, I take a central measurement and one peripheral reading at the optical zone radius in the 180-degree meridian (Fig. 17-4). When using the ultrasonic pachometer, I take one central reading and four peripheral readings at the optical zone radius in the 180- and 90-degree meridians (Fig. 17-5).

Variation in Surgical Methods

Once having decided on the preferred method of pachometry, the surgeon is still faced with several choices relating to the surgical approach to radial

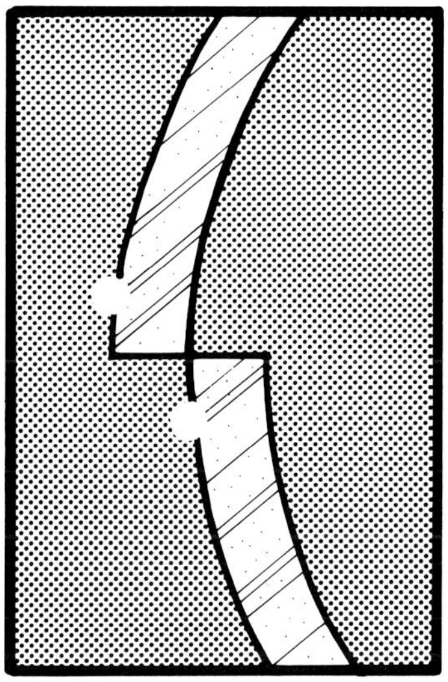

Fig. 17-3. The Haag-Streit pachometer I is adjusted so that the endothelial surface of the upper corneal section touches the epithelial surface of the lower corneal section. If the examiner can then see the reflection of the pinlights on the epithelial surfaces of both corneal sections, the perpendicularity of the measurement is ensured.

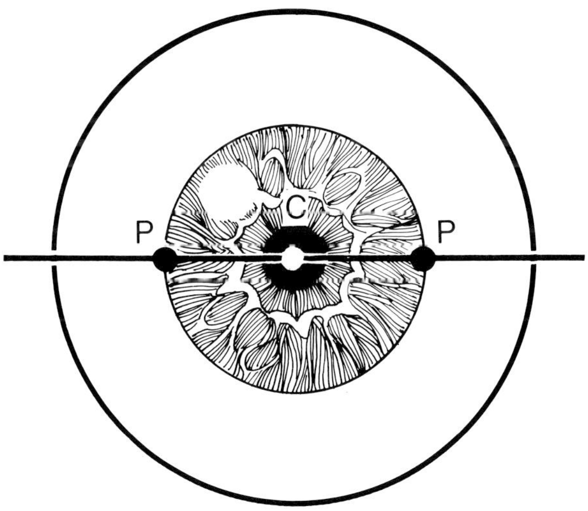

Fig. 17-4. When using the Haag-Streit pachometer I, the examiner is limited to readings in the 180-degree meridian. The central reading (C) is taken with the patient fixating the beam of the slit lamp. The peripheral reading (P) is taken with the patient looking straight ahead while the examiner swings the slit lamp so that it intersects the estimated position of the optical zone radius in the 180-degree meridian. The diamond blade is set at the mean of the central and peripheral readings.

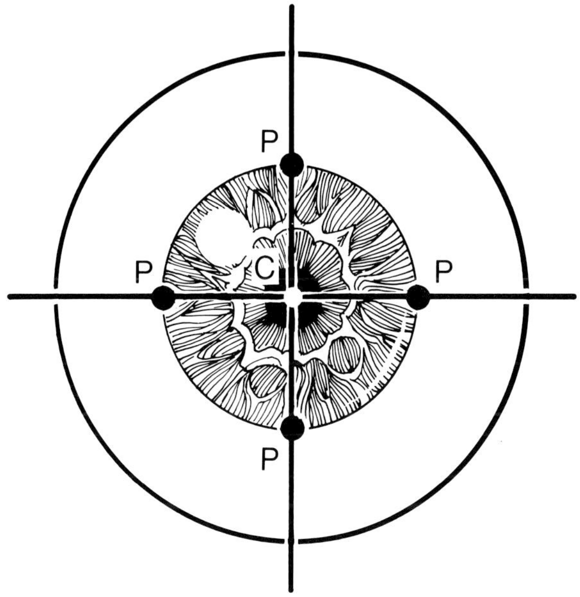

Fig. 17-5. In performing ultrasound pachometry, the Kremer Corneometer I with a sound velocity of 1,640 m/sec is used to measure the central cornea in the optical zone radius at the 90 and 180-degree meridians. The diamond blade is set at 100 percent of the thinnest optical zone radius reading.

keratotomy. The surgeon must choose between radial keratotomy knives using metal, ruby, or diamond blades. The surgeon is further confronted with tables and formulas using 16, 8, and 4 incisions, which can be made in a single surgical pass or in multiple passes to achieve redeepening. Obviously, experienced radial keratotomy surgeons are achieving excellent results using all the above variations. Each successful radial keratotomy surgeon has developed a specific way of performing pachometry, setting the blade of the micrometer knife, making the incision, and establishing personal formulas for determining the optical zone size and the depth of cut. Within a given surgeon's system, all the parts of the procedure add up to a successful outcome. Beginning radial keratotomy surgeons, however, must avoid an eclectic approach whereby various aspects of different surgeons' methods are randomly combined. As a starting point, the novice radial keratotomy surgeon should attempt to duplicate the complete technique of a single surgeon.

RECOMMENDED TECHNIQUE

Under the proper conditions, radial keratotomy can be a very brief, atraumatic, and very effective procedure. With less than optimal conditions, its potential for disaster should not be underestimated. Attention to the following details should facilitate a successful procedure. Preparation of the patient starts in the preoperative holding area with the instillation of a drop of 0.5 percent proparacaine. This eliminates the stinging that would otherwise occur when sterile 0.5 percent tetracaine is given in the operating room. In almost all cases, I prefer to avoid any type of local injection. This pertains to both retrobulbar injections and seventh nerve blocks of any type. I rely primarily on a very small dose of intravenous Valium, generally less than 5 mg, and large doses of verbal reassurance. The anesthesiologist is instructed to give only enough intravenous Valium to take the edge off the patient's anxiety, but never enough to interfere with the patient's full cooperation.

In order to perform the procedure using only 0.5 percent tetracaine, it is necessary to explain every step of the procedure to the patient. It is also crucial that the patient be made aware that certain sensations will be felt during the procedure that are quite normal. I make it a point to tell every patient that pressure will be felt on the eye during the procedure. While instructing the patient of this, I grasp the conjunctiva with forceps and press gently on the globe, so that the patient knows that this pressure sensation is normal. Without the proper mental set, the patient interprets the first tactile sensation as a pain impulse, which can create instantaneous anxiety. I find this method of using verbal reassurance far more effective than any pharmacologic approach.

Positioning the Patient and the Microscope

Next, the patient's head and neck should be positioned, so that the patient's visual axis is perpendicular to the ceiling of the operating room. It is important to make sure the eye is centered in the field of the microscope. It is also important to make sure the patient's eye is centered between the lids. The body of the microscope should be aligned in a perfectly vertical manner. Thus, the axis of the body of the microscope and the patient's visual axis form a plumb line (Fig. 17-6). The power of the microscope is adjusted so that the cornea fills the field of the microscope. This is approximately the 12X setting on the Zeiss Opmi 6-S. If the alignment should

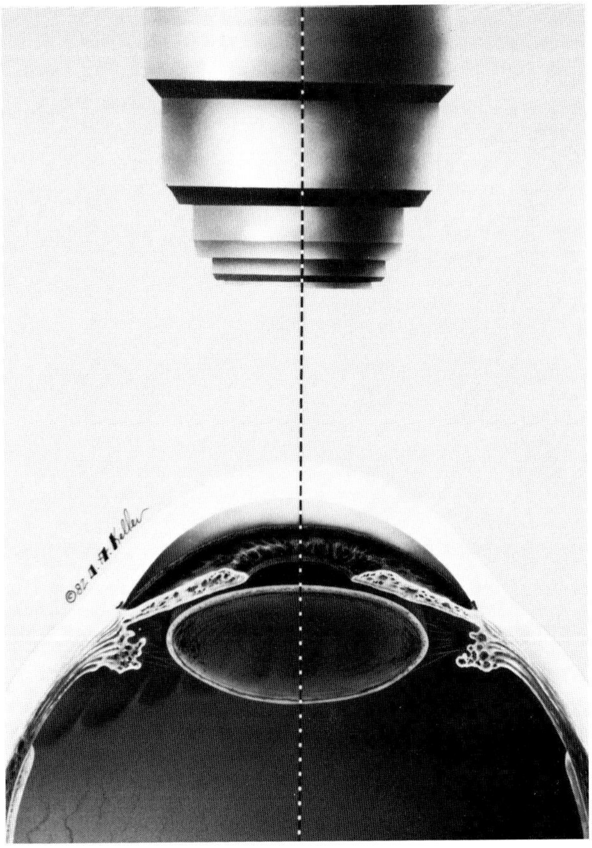

Fig. 17-6. Positioning of the microscope and patient. In radial keratotomy, the axis of the microscope body and the patient's optical (visual) axis should form a plumb line. Those of us who operate normally with a tilted microscope must adapt to this perpendicular alignment. The patient's head should be fixated, since any movement can compromise accurate measurement of the visual axis. The microscope power is adjusted so that the cornea "fills the field." Make sure that the eye is centered and that the viewing angle is perpendicular to the iris plane. (Myers WD, Keller DA: Radial keratotomy: The procedure. Ophthalmic Forum 1:46, 1982.)

change during the procedure, it is vital to recognize it and correct it. Too frequently, the beginning radial keratotomy surgeon will continue to operate, even though the patient's position is such that a proper control of the incision is no longer possible. One common misalignment problem occurs when the patient flexes the neck, in turn causing a downward slope from the head to the chin. This, in turn, causes the patient's upper lid to cover the upper portion of the cornea. This misalignment can be corrected by placing a rolled towel at the junction of the patient's neck and upper back to facilitate cervical extension.

Marking the Visual Axis

The general principles of this technique can be adapted to any microscope with a coaxial illumination system. The specifics given herein, however, relate only to the Zeiss Opmi 6-S microscope, with which the author is most familiar.

Using coaxial illumination and the green filter in the microscope, the patient is asked to look at the center of the microscope filament. The surgeon closes the left eye and makes an epithelial defect with a 26-gauge needle to mark the center of the visual axis. This mark should generally be inferior to the lower edge of the filament reflex, approximately one width of the light reflect inferior to the reflection itself. This is to compensate for prismatic displacement within the microscope system. The mark should also be slightly to the opposite side of the surgeon's fixating eye. Placement of this mark is shown in Figure 17-7. This method of marking the visual axis is generally accurate for most microscopes. If any modification of this technique is necessary, however, it can be determined in the following manner. A patient, having had radial keratotomy, is asked to fixate the light of a direct ophthalmoscope. The surgeon then observes to ensure that the reflex from the patient's cornea is centered with regard to the optical zone, as defined by determination of the cuts. If the epicenter of the optical zone, as defined by determination of the cuts, coincides with the light reflex and the ophthalmoscope (Fig. 17-8, left) the optical zone has been placed properly. However, if there is eccentricity of the optical zone with regard to the light reflex (Fig. 17-8, right) an appropriate adjustment must be made in the way the optical zone is centered operatively.

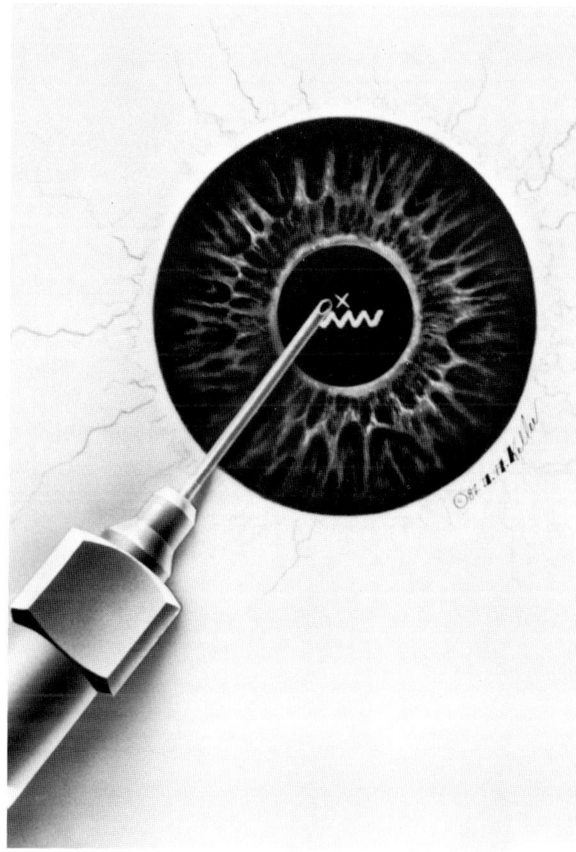

Fig. 17-7. Marking the visual axis. With coaxial illumination and the green filter in the microscope, the patient is asked to look at the center of the filament. The surgeon closes one eye and makes a small epithelial defect with a 26-gauge needle to mark the center of the visual axis (the intersection of the visual axis with the corneal surface). This mark generally should be on the lower edge of the filament reflex, one width of the light reflection inferior to the reflection itself (to compensate for the prismatic displacement of the light by the microscope), and slightly to the side opposite the surgeon's fixating eye. (Myers WD, Keller DA: Radial keratotomy: The procedure. Ophthalmic Forum 1: 46, 1982.)

Checking the Optical Center Mark

The patient is asked to look up and down and to the right and to the left, followed by looking back to the center of the reflex of the coaxial light (Fig.

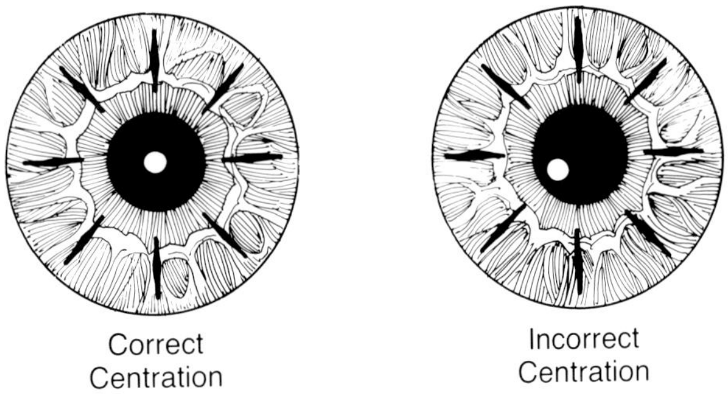

Fig. 17-8. To check the centration of the optical zone, the patient is asked to fixate the light of the direct ophthalmoscope. If the examiner sees a corneal light reflex centered with regard to the central termination of the radial incisions, the intraoperative method of optical zone centration is correct. If the corneal light reflex is not centered, the intraoperative method of centration should be modified accordingly.

17-9). The surgeon verifies that each time the patient looks at the filament, the pupil becomes miotic (indicating foveal fixation) and the filament reflex and the optical center mark are constant.

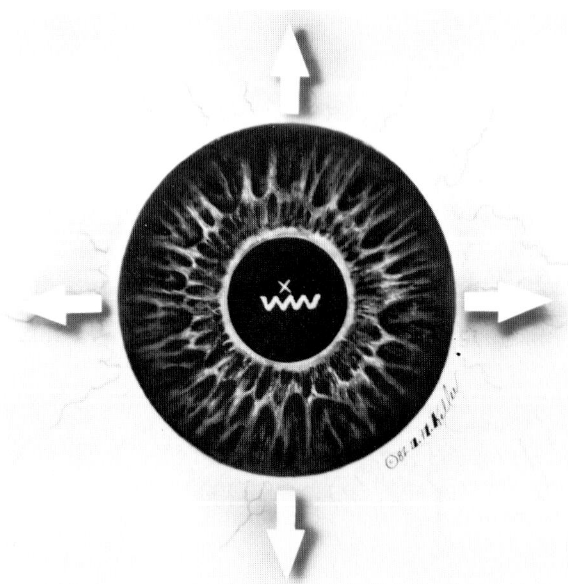

Fig. 17-9. Checking the optical center mark. The patient is asked to look up, down, left, right, and back to the center of the filament. The surgeon verifies that each time the patient looks at the filament, the pupil "snaps down," indicating foveal fixation, and that the filament reflex and the optical center mark alignment are constant.

Marking the Optical Zone

A dull circular marking trephine is placed with its cross-hairs centered over the central optical mark (Fig. 17-10). Depending on the magnitude of the angle κ, this circular mark will have varying amounts of horizontal eccentricity with regard to the pupil. The surgeon should not be concerned about this once having determined that the method of marking the optical center is proper. It is important to note when using both the needle to mark the visual axis and when using a trephine to define the optical zone, the marks should create only indentations in the epithelium, and not damage Bowman's

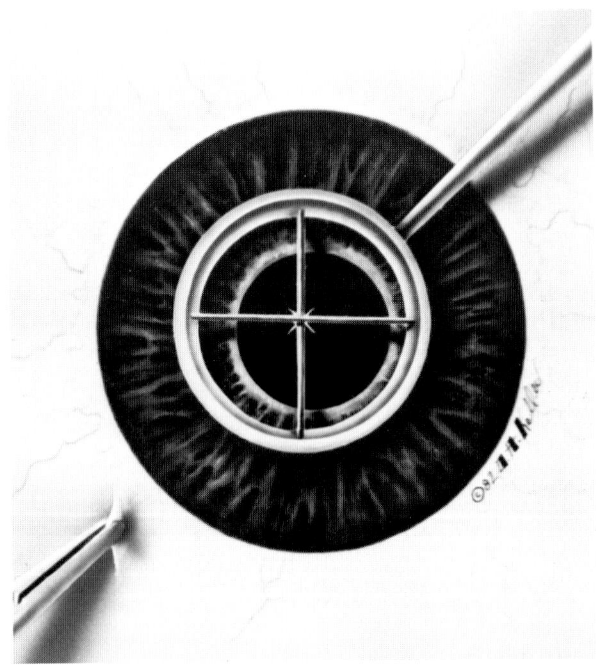

Fig. 17-10. Marking the optical zone. A dull, circular marking trephine (Hoffer) is placed with its cross-hairs centered over the central optical mark, while the eye is fixated at the limbus with forceps. If either the optical center mark or the trephine mark is not apparent, it can be visualized by drying with a Weck-cel sponge. The surgeon then measures the corneal thickness with an ultrasonic pachymeter in which the speed of sound in the cornea is set at 1,630 m/sec. After calibrating the instrument on a test block, the surgeon places the sterile probe tip perpendicular to the cornea centrally and at the 3, 6, 9, and 12 o'clock meridians, just outside the trephine mark. The length of the knife blade is set at 100 percent of the thinnest paracentral reading.

Table 17-1. Nomogram for Optical Zone Diameter for Ages 20 to 60[a]

Degree of Myopia (diopters)	Optical Zone Diameter (mm)				
	20 yr	30 yr	40 yr	50 yr	60 yr
8	3.0[b,c]	3.0[b,c]	3.0[b,c]	3.0	3.25
7	3.0[b,c]	3.0[b,c]	3.0[b]	3.24	3.50
6	3.0[b,c]	3.0[b]	3.25	3.50	3.75
5	3.0[b]	3.25	3.50	3.75	4.00
4	3.25	3.50	3.75	4.00	4.25[d]
3	3.5	3.75	4.00	4.25[d]	4.5[d]
2	3.75	4.0	4.25[d]	4.5[d]	4.75[d]

[a] The diamond blade is adjusted at 100 percent of the thinnest paracentral ultrasound pachometer measurement; alternatively, if using optical pachometry, the mean of the central and peripheral pachometer reading is used to determine the depth of blade. In the case of ultrasound, the speed of sound should be set at 1,640 m/sec.

[b] A diamond blade is advanced 0.02 on the second four incisions.

[c] Patients will probably require a second series of eight incisions after the eye heals from the first eight incisions.

[d] A series of four incisions should be considered on the first eye.

membrane. When these superficial marks are moistened with balanced salt solution or the patient's own tears, they will become barely noticeable to disappear entirely. They can be made readily visible, however, by drying the central cornea with a Weck-cel sponge. A guide to the size of the optical zone is shown in the momogram of Table 17-1.

Optical Zone Determination and the General Surgical Approach

Every experienced radial keratotomy surgeon I know believes that the optical zone size, the depth of the incisions, and the age of the patient are all important variables that affect the amount of correction possible using radial keratotomy. The nomogram shown in Figure 17-1 is one that the beginning surgeon can use as a starting point. As the surgeon gains clinical experience with the procedure, he or she will be in a position to develop a personal nomogram that eventually will provide even better clinical results. This simplistic nomogram adjusts the optical zone according to the degree of myopia and the patient's age. The resultant depth of the incision is held constant at 90 percent, and the number of incisions is held constant at eight, except as otherwise noted. Only in those cases marked with 1, 2, or 3 is any variation made in either the depth of cut or the number of incisions. It is important to remember that a surgeon's nomogram, surgical technique, and preoperative pachometry form an integrated unit. The beginning surgeon must adopt all aspects of this approach. For example, some surgeons adjust the optical zone size according to the patient's preoperative intraocular pressure (IOP).[20] Although I do not consider IOP in selecting my optical zone, I do notice that in particularly soft eyes I tend to press harder with the fixation forceps on the globe and tend to make my incisions at a slower rate. This often gives me a slightly greater depth of cut. This would increase the degree of myopic correction, as well as shrinking the optical zone according to the dictates of the nomogram. Thus, while I ignore IOP in my nomogram, I do not in fact ignore it at the time of surgery. I would furthermore advise that the inexperienced radial keratotomy surgeon not be concerned with redeepening incisions until having gained experience with the single incision technique described in this section.

Setting the Diamond Knife

I currently prefer a diamond blade to any of the metal blades I have tested. This is not to say that excellent results cannot be achieved using other materials for making radial keratotomy incisions, since the experience of many surgeons indicates excellent results with ruby and metal knives. The use of a diamond blade is such an important constant in my technique, however, that to substitute another type of blade would be incompatible with the total approach, presented herein. When setting the diamond blade, it is important to use a depth of blade gauge matched to the diamond knife. Both Pilling and Micra manufacture gauges to be used in conjunction with their diamond knives. An example of the Micra gauge and diamond knife is shown in Figure 17-11. One frequently finds with many instruments that there is a discrepancy between the setting of the micrometer adjustment of the diamond knife and the true setting as registered on the gauge block. It is always the setting of the gauge

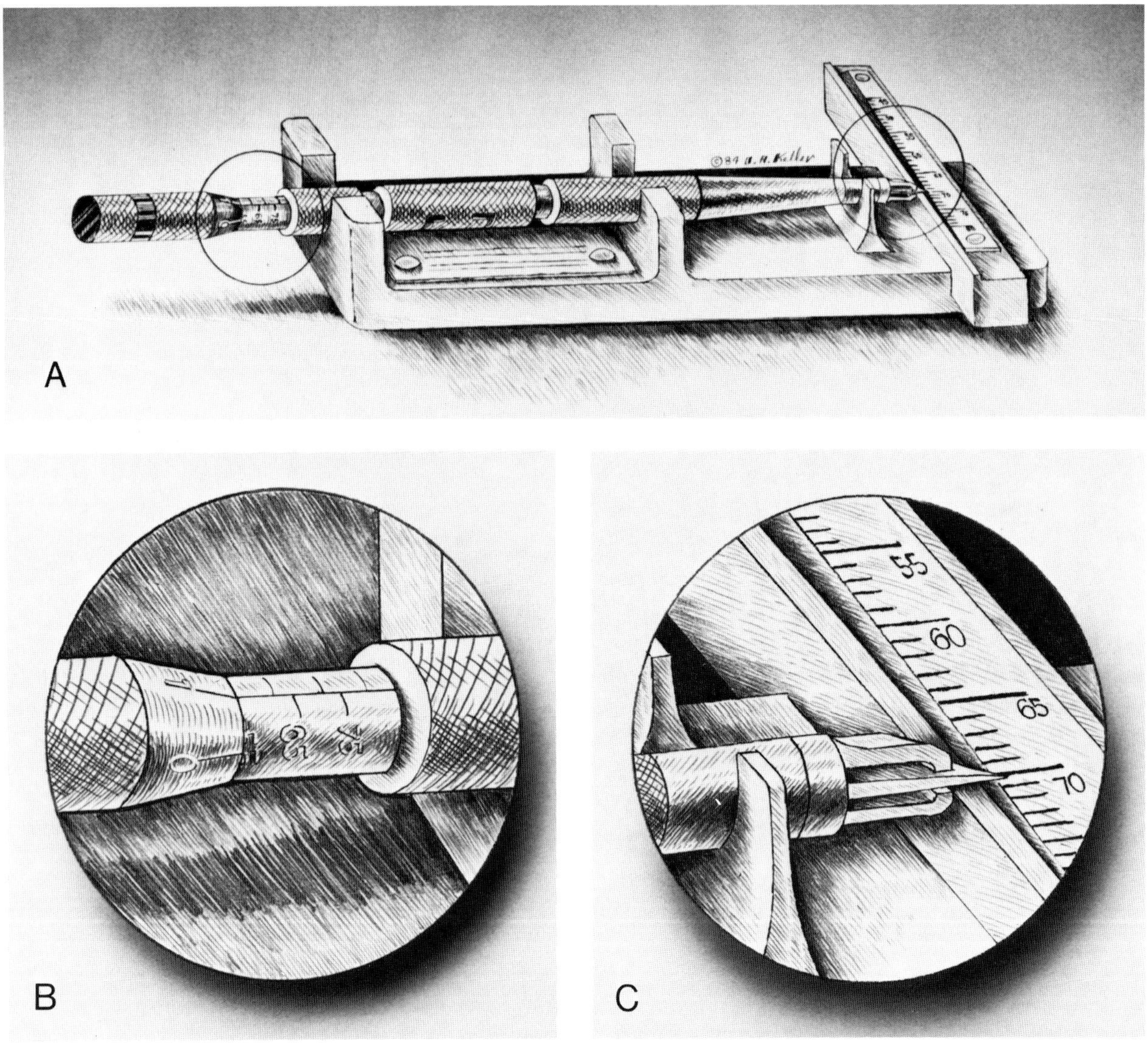

Fig. 17-11. After advancing the diamond blade the desired amount with the micrometer, the surgeon verifies its length with an appropriate measuring gauge. **(A)** The diamond knife is seen here in its holder and measuring device. The inserts show **(B)** the micrometer handle and **(C)** verification of the blade depth along the blade gauge.

block that should be used a guide to proper blade setting. The setting of the depth of the blade should be performed under the highest power possible with the microscope. It helps to use a Mayo stand or some other supportive stand when making the blade depth adjustment. The microscope illumination should be just bright enough to define the tip of the blade clearly in relationship to the gauge block. Excessive illumination will produce glare off the diamond and metal block, which will interfere with proper visualization.

Making the Radial Incisions

The surgeon grasps the conjunctiva with the fixation forceps at the 9 o'clock position (Fig. 17-12). The noncutting back edge of the diamond blade is

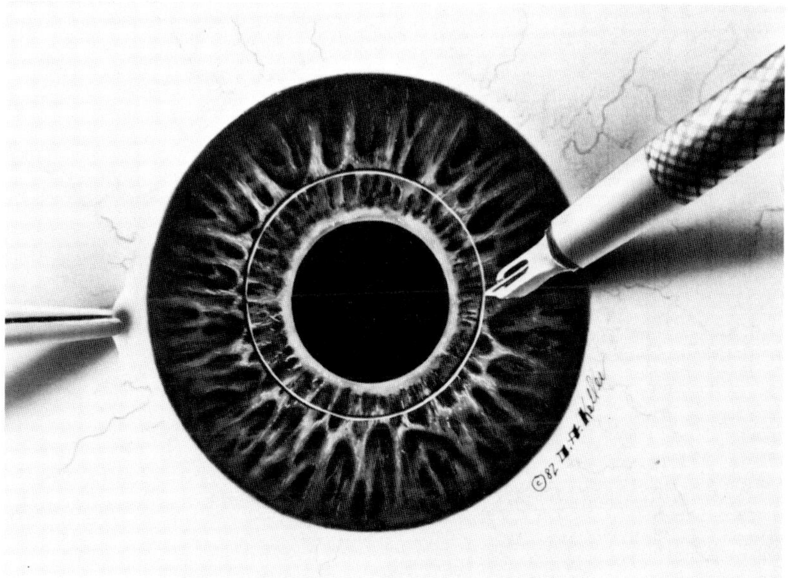

Fig. 17-12. The radial incision. The surgeon grasps the conjunctiva with fixation forceps at the 9 o'clock position. The surgeon then incises the cornea with a diamond blade, making sure that the noncutting, back edge of the blade is placed just touching the optical zone and the incision is perpendicular to the corneal surface. Before exiting 1 mm short of the limbus, the knife handle is tilted toward the optical center to create incisions with internal and external aspects equal in degree of arc.

placed just touching the optical zone and is plunged in perpendicular to the cornea. Once the blade is inserted to its fullest extent, it is held there for 2 or 3 seconds before being moved. This will ensure a full depth of incision at the start of the incision. Without this intentional delay, there is a tendency for the surgeon to move the blade away from the optical zone before achieving the maximum cutting depth. This in turn produces incisions that are not deep enough adjacent to the optical zone. As the incision is extended in a radial manner, care should be taken to be sure that the incision is perpendicular to the cornea; otherwise an oblique incision will result (Fig. 17-13).

A common error in making a radial incision frequently occurs when a patient intorts or extorts the globe while the surgeon is making the radial incision. If, for example, the cut is being made in the 180-degree meridian and the patient rotates the eye in a counterclockwise manner, a curvilinear incision will be the end result (Fig. 17-14). However, if the surgeon adjusts for any rotational movement of the patient's eye and concentrates on radiality at all times, a straight incision is guaranteed. Frequently the eye becomes softer with each succeeding incision. When this happens, the surgeon should increase IOP of the eye by pressing with the fixation forceps, and not the diamond knife itself. If an attempt is made to increase the pressure of the eye by pressing with the diamond knife, the footplate of the knife will indent the cornea, and a cut of insufficient depth may result. Specific care should be taken to move the blade in a slow and deliberate manner and to observe the tip of the diamond blade at all times. In so doing, the surgeon can immediately visualize a microperforation and stop the cut before the perforation enlarges. The radial incisions are made with both the right and left hands. One of the most common errors noted when observing the beginning radial keratotomy surgeons is a tendency not to terminate the incision until the blade has cut into a portion of the vascular arcades of the limbus. The bleeding produced by this excessively peripheral cut is quite persistent and often results in postoperative deposits in the wound. A constant effort should be made to stop the cut 1 mm away from the limbal vascular arcades. The pattern of the radial kertotomy incisions is shown in Figure 17-15.

Checking the Depth of the Incisions

A Fyodorov dipstick is placed in the incision perpendicular to the endothelium as shown in Figure 17-16. This will ensure the incision depth and uniformity. To check the incision depth, the surgeon should align the patient's visual axis away from the

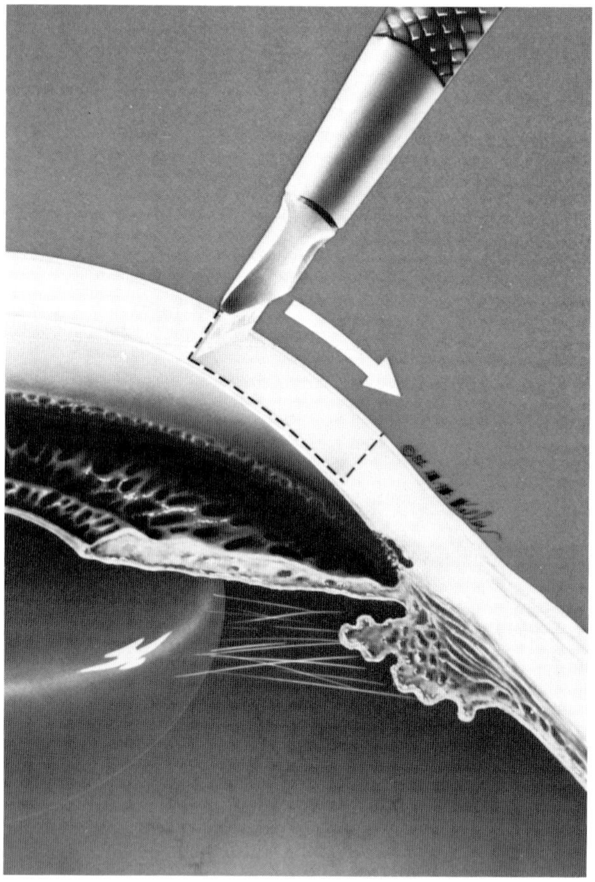

Fig. 17-13. As the incision is extended in a radial manner, care should be taken to ensure that the incision is perpendicular to the cornea, or an oblique incision will result. The surgeon makes the incisions slowly, while observing the tip of the blade so that if a perforation occurs (<1 percent of cases in the author's series), it can be limited to a microperforation (no suture required). The thickness of the microdiamond blade spreads the wound so that the tip may be visualized. (The blade used in the PERK study is not depicted. PERK uses the KOI Piling Knife, Model No. KO-100-041, manufactured by the KOI Associates, Frazer, PA 19355. The blade gauge assembly is manufactured by KOI, Model No. KO-100-032.)

perpendicular axis of the microscope, in order to be able to view the incision from the side. Such a check of the incision depth should be made immediately after the cut has been made with the diamond knife. This is because as the radial keratotomy surgery proceeds, the cornea can either swell due to irrigation with balanced salt solution, or dehydrate due to the heat from the microscope itself

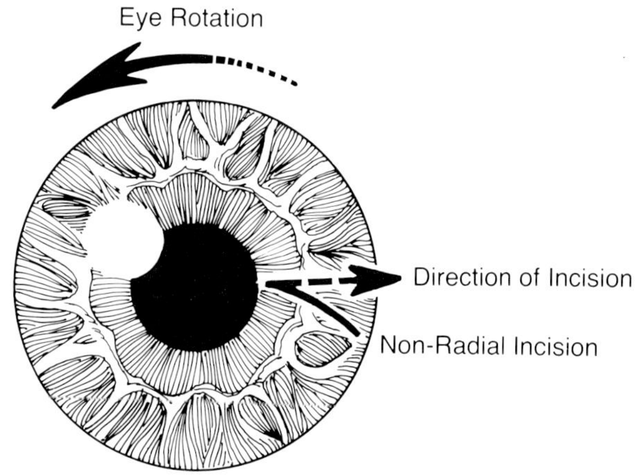

Fig. 17-14. If the patient intorts or extorts the eye, the surgeon must adjust the direction of the incision relative to the new rotational position of the eye. Otherwise, a curved, nonlinear incision will result.

and low humidity in the operating room. This change in the corneal thickness can make the wound appear too deep or too shallow when checked with a dipstick at the end of the operation. The surgeon should avoid pressing too firmly with the dipstick, which will indent the internal stroma layers and Descemet's membrane into the anterior chamber. This will make the incision appear excessively deep (Fig. 17-17). Any incision that is found to be too shallow should be recut to the proper depth. Once surgeons gain experience with the

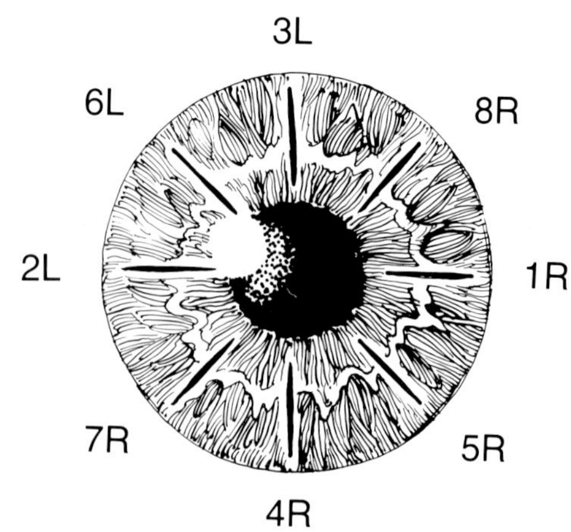

Fig. 17-15. Right-hand, left-hand order of incisions. The incisions are made in the order indicated in the diagram. Letters R & L indicate which hand the surgeon uses to make each incision.

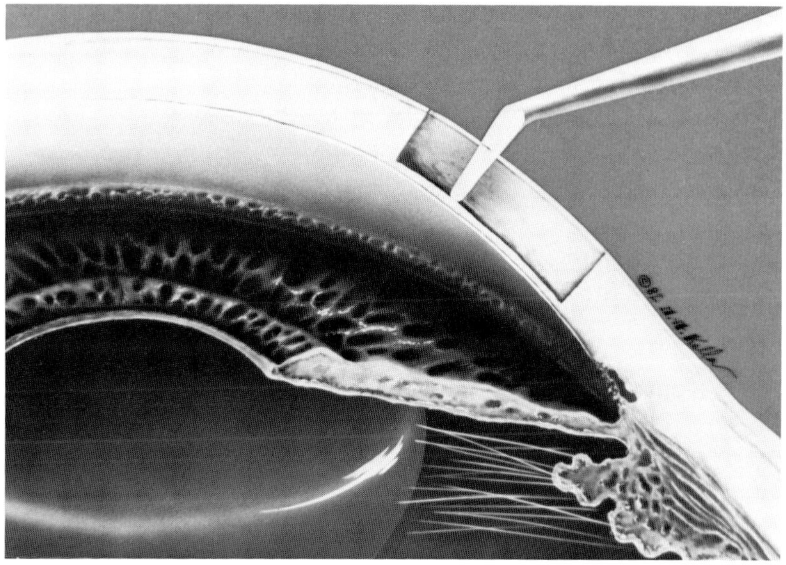

Fig. 17-16. Checking the incisions. A Fyodorov dipstick is placed in the incision perpendicular to the endothelium. To check the incision depth and uniformity, the surgeon aligns the visual axis away from that of the microscope in order to view the incision from the side.

procedure, they will routinely produce cuts of proper depth, and it will be unnecessary to check such incisions with the dipstick.

Irrigating the Incision

The surgeon should then irrigate the incisions with balanced salt solution through a small-gauge needle in order to facilitate complete removal of any debris from the radial keratotomy incisions. Weck-cel sponges are used to absorb any excess fluid, thereby removing foreign material that might otherwise reenter the incisions during the immediate postoperative period (Fig. 17-18). Tobrex drops and 1 percent Cyclogyl are instilled into the cul-de-sac at the termination of the procedure. The patient's eye is not patched, as patients are generally much more comfortable without patching.

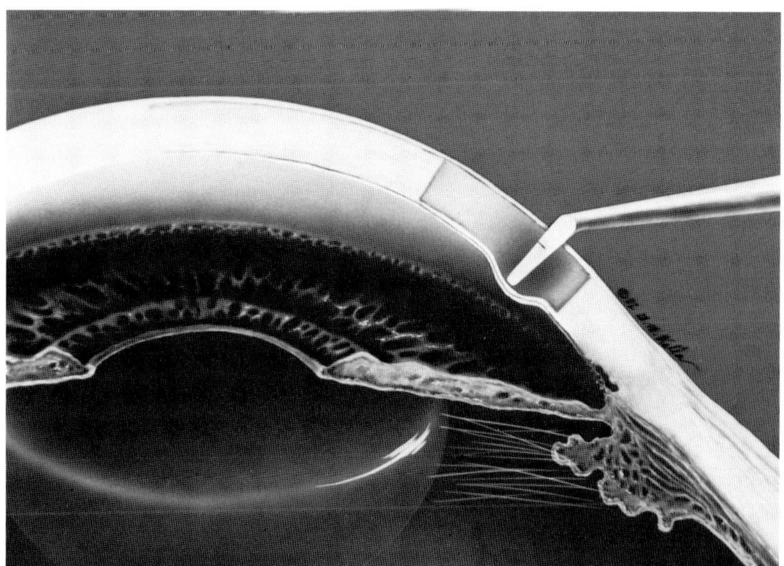

Fig. 17-17. Idention of the internal stromal fibers and Descemet's membrane into the anterior chamber should be avoided, since it magnifies the appearance of the incision depth. Any incision that is too shallow can be recut, although this usually becomes unnecessary as the surgeon gains experience in the procedure.

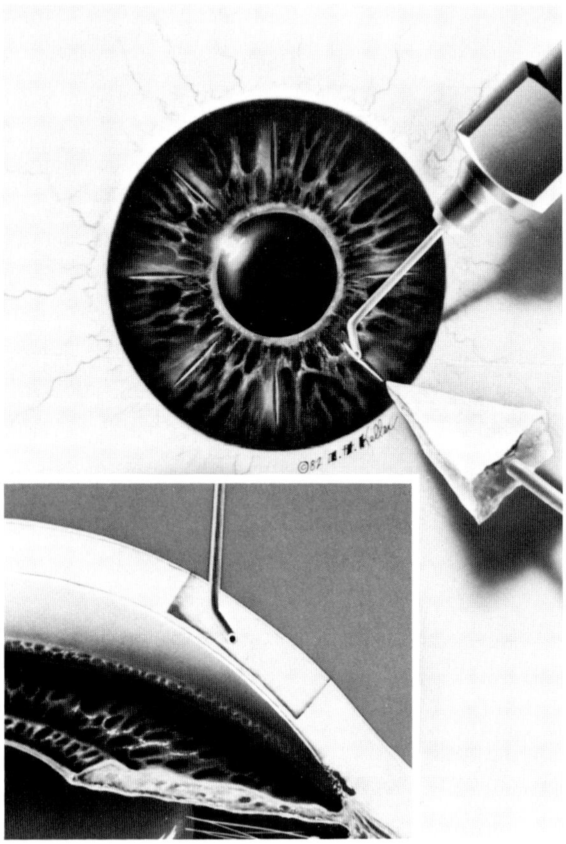

Fig. 17-18. Irrigating the incisions. The surgeon irrigates the incisions with balanced salt solution through an air-injection needle, making sure that all foreign material is removed. Weck-Cel sponges are used to absorb the excess BSS, thereby removing foreign material that might otherwise find its way back into the incisions during the immediate postoperative period. Topical 0.3 percent gentamicin and a mydriatic with cyclopegic are instilled, and the eye is patched for 24 hours.

INDICATIONS

Radial keratotomy should be considered when the following criteria have been met:

Myopia that appears stable: A review of the patient's current and past prescriptions should be your guide in this determination. Make sure patients that have had their contacts out for at least 1 to 2 weeks prior to the preoperative radial keratotomy exam. Generally patients with stable myopia will be at least in their 20s.

Freedom from any significant past or present ocular pathologic changes: This condition applies to the current status of the patient's cornea but should also apply to the total ocular and periocular structures. For example, it is possible that a patient with a significant posterior subcapsular cataract change might implicate the radial keratotomy procedure as its cause. It is also important to rule out a history of recurrent iritis or herpetic keratitis in all radial keratotomy candidates.

Fully informed patient: The patient must be fully informed about the procedure and its complications. The informed consent document must fully cover such areas as infection, glare, variable vision, and overcorrection. While it is true that most patients are not bothered by these problems once they stabilize, it is also true that a properly performed radial keratotomy can produce these problems in a given patient. It is therefore important that the patient fully understand this.

Dissatisfaction with glasses or contact lenses: It should not be assumed that just because patients have expressed a desire to have radial keratotomy they are truly dissatisfied with their current situation. It is important to document each patient's specific indications, whether they be occupational, recreational, psychological, or functional.

Patient's needs potentially met by the procedure: If the patient desires the operation for occupational reasons, it is important to know exactly what the occupational visual requirements are. If the patient desires a career in a branch of the armed services, the patient should determine whether the service has an official policy concerning radial kerototomy. The Air Force, for example, does not officially allow radial keratotomy patients to enter their flight programs. Patients desiring full surgical correction of myopia should generally be in the range of 2.0 to 8.0 diopters. Any patient falling outside the range of the nomogram shown in Figure 17-1 should be fully aware that only a partial correction is likely.

Astigmatism of less than 1.5 diopters: Since this discussion is concerned with the use of radial keratotomy to correct spherical myopia, a discussion of astigmatic correction is outside the scope of this chapter.

CONTRAINDICATIONS

Radial keratotomy is contraindicated under the following circumstances:

The myopic presbyope who wants to be totally free of glasses: Many patients in this category harbor the misconception that radial keratotomy will correct both the myopia and the presbyopia. The surgeon must stress that even if all the myopia is corrected, the patient will still be obliged to wear reading glasses. This must be covered fully in the informed consent.

The marginally successful contact lens wearer with a relatively flat cornea and a relatively high degree of myopia: If, for example, the patient has a K reading of 41.00 sphere and 9.0 diopters of myopia, it is likely that there will be a postoperative residual myopia. The patient's postoperative corneal curvature will no doubt now be too flat to be properly fit with a contact. This patient must be informed that the procedure will probably make contact lens wearing difficult or impossible. The patient who finds this unacceptable is not a candidate for radial keratotomy.

PROGNOSIS AND COMPLICATIONS

A review of the American ophthalmic literature from 1979 until 1984 shows a high degree of correlation between multiple independent surgeons with regard to their results and complications. Fyodorov[4] provided us with the first major report on radial keratotomy. In his series he reported a high degree of efficacy and a surprising lack of complications. Bores, the first American ophthalmologist to perform radial keratotomy, reported on an initial series of 303 eyes. Of these, 61 percent achieved a postoperative acuity of 20/40 or better.[11] In this series, Bores measured an endothelial cell loss of 6.3 percent and recorded no serious surgical complications. Nirankari et al.[15] conducted a well-controlled series on 58 eyes, which used an independent observer and in which no follow-up losses occurred. In those eyes with 5.0 diopters of myopia or less, an uncorrected visual acuity postoperatively of 20/40 or better was achieved in 65 percent. Hecht and Jamara[14] also used an independent observer, and all 17 of their patients were fully followed. These investigators noted that with a myopia range of −2.0 to −7.5 diopters, the postoperative correction was 20/50 or better in 94 percent of their cases. Kremer and Marks[21] reported on 105 consecutive radial keratotomy procedures. They noted that 93 percent of their patients with refractive errors of −3.0 diopters or less achieved 20/50 or better visual acuity without correction. In those patients with myopia of −6.0 diopters or less, the percentage of patients achieving 20/50 or better was 82 percent.[21] Recently, Dietz et al.[22] reported on their first 290 cases. One year postoperatively, 83 percent of patients achieved 20/40 or better without correction. It should be noted that in all the above reports no complications of a serious nature were encountered. My own initial series of 400 radial kertotomy patients, first reported in 1981, corresponds well with the early results of other surgeons. Seventy-three percent of all patients had postoperative uncorrected visual acuities of 20/40 or better. The breakdown of the postoperative visual results is shown in Table 17-2. The patients' preoperative refractive errors ranged from 1.5 to 18.0 diopters, with a mean of 5.49 diopters. There was a correlation between the degree of preoperative myopia and the resultant uncorrected postoperative visual acuities. It was found that 202 of 259 eyes (78 percent) with refractive errors of 6.0 diopters or less had postoperative uncorrected visual acuities of 20/40 or better. For cases with 5.25 diopters or less, the percentage achieving 20/40 or

Table 17-2. Postoperative Visual Acuity: First 400 Patients

Uncorrected Visual Acuity Postoperatively	No. of Patients	Percentage
20/20	56	14
20/25	56	14
20/30	88	22
20/40	92	23
		73
20/50–20/100	48	12
≥20/200	60	15
		27

better increased to 81 percent. The complications in this series (see Table 17-3) were generally caused by imperfect surgical technique or the fitting of soft contact lenses during the early postoperative phase. Since the time of this initial series of 400 cases, our ability to make uniformly deep incisions has improved due to the perfection of diamond micrometer knives and their integrated gauge blocks. A review of my last 400 cases shows how these advances in instrumentation have positively influenced the results. As shown in Table 17-4, 86 percent of patients in this latter series achieved uncorrected postoperative acuities of 20/40 or better. The only complication in the first series that occurred in the last series of 400 cases was seven eyes having a small induced cylinder (Table 17-5).

Table 17-3. Complications of First 400 Cases

Complication	*N*
Microperforations	3
Macroperforations	0
Recurrent erosions	0
Infections	0
Induced cylinder (0.5–1.0 diopters)	19
Irregular astigmatism	3
Reduction in best corrected acuity	2
Neovascularization	4

Table 17-4. Postoperative Visual Acuity: Last 400 Patients

Uncorrected Visual Acuity Postoperatively	No. of Patients	Percentage
20/20	92	48
20/25	56	14
20/30	52	13
20/40	44	11
		86
20/50–20/100	32	8
≤20/200	24	6
		14

Table 17-5. Complications of Last 400 Cases

Complication	*N*
Microperforations	0
Macroperforations	0
Recurrent erosions	0
Infections	0
Induced cylinder (0.5–1.0 diopters)	7
Irregular astigmatism	0
Reduction in best corrected acuity	0
Neovascularization	0

The most frequently reported complications following radial keratotomy include perforation, neovascularization, overcorrection and undercorrection, glare, variable vision, and iron lines of the cornea.

Perforation

The incidence of perforation varies depending on the surgeon's individual technique. In my series using the technique described, the perforation rate was 0.6 percent. When a technique of redeepening of the incisions is used, the change in the perforation percentage obviously increases. For example, Dietz et al.[22] reported a 37 percent incidence of perforation in their series. Normally a perforation carries no significant complications. However, the first reported case of endophthalmitis following radial keratotomy occurred in a case involving a perforation.[23] If a perforation causes significant softening of the globe or shallowing of the anterior chamber, the surgeon should not attempt to continue with the procedure. In the case of a significant loss of the anterior chamber that does not spontaneously resolve, a repair of the wound is indicated.

Neovascularization

Neovascularization was noted in some of the first cases performed in the United States. Neovascularization, in the experience of most surgeons, requires incisions that cut into the vascular arcades in association with the application of soft lenses in the early weeks or months following the procedure. By avoiding this combination of causative factors, this complication can be obviated.

Hyperopia

A complication reported in most series to varying degrees is that of induced hyperopia. Creating hyperopia in a previously myopic patient is optically the least desirable outcome. Patients are generally very tolerant if they are left with residual postoperative myopia; however, patients in whom hyperopia is induced are understandably disturbed by their new refractive state. Their degree of distress is directly proportional to the amount of overcorrection and the patient's age. Because patients are selected for radial keratotomy due to an inability to tolerate contact lenses, such overcorrected patients are obliged to wear hyperopic spectacles. Since overcorrections are most likely to occur in older persons with lower amounts of myopia, it is wise to use a larger than normal optical zone than indicated in Table 17-1 and to reduce the number of incisions from 8 to 4. It is always possible to perform a second radial keratotomy in the case of an undercorrection. It is obviously far better to achieve emmetropia with two surgical procedures than hyperopia in one.

Undercorrection

Undercorrections tend to occur with a frequency generally in the range of 10 to 20 percent, depending on the series reviewed. Most patients in this group are younger and have higher degrees of preoperative myopia. Along with patient selection, the depth of incisions is closely related to the problem of undercorrection. If the incision is less than 90 percent of the total corneal thickness, the possibility of an undercorrection increases.

Glare

Almost all radial keratotomy patients experience glare in the early postoperative phase. In almost all these patients it is not bothersome after several months. Glare can be caused by incisions that occur too close to the visual axis. This can result from a surgical error in the marking of the optical zone center or in the making of an individual cut. When selecting patients initially for radial keratotomy, it is prudent to select patients who require a large optical zone. Once these patients have been checked postoperatively and the optical zone is found to be properly centered, the surgeon can safely move on to patients requiring smaller optical zones. The problem of individual cuts that migrate close to the visual axis can be avoided by cutting from the optical zone to the periphery, and not in the reverse direction. Since some patients will notice postoperative glare even following a perfectly performed radial keratotomy procedure, it is imperative that glare be mentioned as a possible complication on the informed consent form. It should be noted that some patients with residual myopia or physiologic myopia at night will complain of glare, when it is really simply the uncorrected refractive error that they notice. Glasses are the solution in such cases. Pilocarpine 0.5 percent used at night can be helpful in those patients experiencing postoperative glare and who have larger than normal pupils.

Variable Vision

Fluctuating vision, like glare, is present in all cases during the initial postoperative stage. It is gone after several months in the vast majority of patients. In those patients in whom the fluctuating vision is bothersome, glasses for night driving are generally required.

Recurrent Erosion

Some radial keratotomy patients describe symptoms compatible with small recurrent erosions. This diagnosis is frequently made by history, since generally at the time of the examination the patient's epithelial surface appears totally intact. Generally these patients will be in the older age group. The use of Lacri-Lube HS is effective treatment in these cases.

Iron Deposits

Careful biomicroscopy following radial keratotomy frequently demonstrates iron lines in approximately 20 percent of all radial keratotomy patients. Surface irregularities during the postoperative period are probably responsible for this finding.

REFERENCES

1. Lans LJ: Experimentelle untersuchung uber die entstellung von astigmatismus durch nicht-perforirende corneawunden. Albrecht von Graefes. Arch Ophthamol 45:117, 1898
2. Sato T: Treatment of conical cornea. Nippon Ganka Gakkai Xasshi 43:541, 1939
3. Sato T, Aklyama K, Shibata H: A new surgical approach to myopia. Am J Ophthamol 36:823, 1953
4. Fyodorov SN: Surgical correction of myopia and astigmatism. p. 103. In Schachar RA, Levy NS, Schachar L (eds): Keratorefraction. LAL, Denison, 1980
5. Fyodorov SN, Durnev V: Operation of dosage dissection of corneal circular ligament in cases of myopia of mild degree. Ann Ophthalmol 11:1855, 1979
6. Myers WD: 400 cases of radial keratotomy. p. 101. In Schachar RA, Levy NS, Schachar L (ed): Refractive Heratoplasty. LAL, Denison, 1983
7. Schachar R, Black T, Huang T: A physicist's view of radial keratotomy with practical surgical implications. p. 195. In Schachar RA, Levy NS, Schachar L (eds): Keratorefraction. LAL, Denison, 1980
8. Bores LD, Myers WD, Cowden J: Radial keratotomy: An Analysis of the American experience. Ann Ophthalmol 13:941, 1981
9. Fyodorov, SN: Surgical correction of myopia and astigmatism. p. 141. In Schachar RA, Levy NS, Schachar L (eds): Keratorefraction. LAL, Denison, 1980
10. Myers WD: Initial experience with radial keratotomy. p. 173. In Schachar RA, Levy NS, Schachar L (eds): Keratorefraction. LAL, Denison, 1980
11. Bores LD: American experience with myopia, procedure of Fyodorov. p. 175. In Schachar RA, Levy NS, Schachar L (eds): Keratorefraction. LAL, Denison, 1980
12. Bores LD: Purpose, protocol and goals of the National Radial Keratotomy Study Group. p. 21. In Schachar RA, Levy NS, Schachar L (eds): Radial Keratotomy. LAL, Denison 1980
13. Farkas TG: Role of the Keratorefractive Society in evaluation of radial keratotomy. p. 25. In Schachar RA, Levy NS, Schachar L (eds): Radial Keratotomy. LAL, Denison, 1980
14. Hecht SD, Jamara RJ: Prospective evaluation of radial keratotomy using the Fyodorov formula: Preliminary report. Ann Ophthalmol 14:139, 1982
15. Nirankari VS, Katzen LS, Karesh JW, et al: Ongoing prospective clinical study of radial keratotomy. Ophthalmology 90:637, 1983
16. Arrowsmith PN, Deitz MR, Marks RG, et al: In Sanders DR (ed): Radial Keratotomy. Slack, Thorofare, 1984
17. Waring GO, Moffitt SD, Gelender H, et al: Rationale for and design of the National Eye Institute prospective evaluation of radial keratotomy (PERK) study. Ophthalmology 90:40, 1983
18. Haag-Streit Pachometer Manual.
19. Mishima S, Hedbys B: Measurement of corneal thickness with the Haag-Streit pachometer. Arch Ophthalmol 80:710, 1968
20. Dietz RM: Determination of operative parameters. p. 45. In Sanders DR (ed): Radial Keratotomy. Slack, Thorofare, 1984
21. Kremer F, Marks R: Radial keratotomy: Prospective evaluation of safety and efficacy. Ophthalmic Surg 14:925, 1983
22. Dietz MR, Sanders DR, Marks RG: Radial keratotomy: An overview of the Kansas City study. Ophthalmology 91:467, 1984
23. Gelender H, Flynn HW: Bacterial endophthalmitis resulting from radial keratotomy. Am J Ophthalmol 93:323, 1982

Epikeratophakia for Aphakia, Myopia, and Keratoconus

18

Marguerite B. McDonald
Herbert E. Kaufman

We believe that refractive surgery will become a progressively more important part of ophthalmic surgery and that, in fact, insertion of intraocular lenses is a kind of refractive surgery. Spectacles are no longer uniformly accepted and satisfactory, and some patients cannot see even with them. For some, refractive surgery represents the only alternative to a functionally blind eye. For others, the expectation of reducing dependency on artificial visual aids has made refractive surgery increasingly attractive and worth some slight surgical risk.

Among the procedures currently available in the United States, including the Barraquer procedures and radial keratotomy, only epikeratophakia is truly reversible, making it relatively safe; only epikeratophakia offers the potential for such a wide range of correction, from at least 27 diopters of hyperopia to unlimited amounts of myopia. Epikeratophakia is technically simple, requires no complex or unusual instrumentation, and can be learned quickly and easily, with minimal risk, even to early or infrequent patients. The epikeratophakia lens and surgical procedure can also be used to treat keratoconus and to reinforce corneas with pterygia or perforations.

EARLY LAMELLAR REFRACTIVE PROCEDURES

Keratophakia and Keratomileusis

Methods for profoundly altering the shape of the cornea were first devised by Dr. Jose Barraquer of Bogotá, Colombia.[1] Twenty years ago, before intraocular lenses were available, Barraquer sought a means to provide a permanent aphakic correction for the large numbers of people in his country who were unable to afford cataract spectacles or handle the early, primitive hard contact lenses. Barraquer developed a number of specialized instruments, such as the microkeratome and the cryolathe, and used these to perform his first refractive procedure, which he called keratophakia.

This procedure involves removal of a lamellar section of the cornea with the microkeratome. A tissue lenticule shaped on the cryolathe is then placed in the stromal bed and the lamella replaced (Fig. 18-1). The increase in corneal thickness provides increased dioptric power, replacing the function of the natural lens.

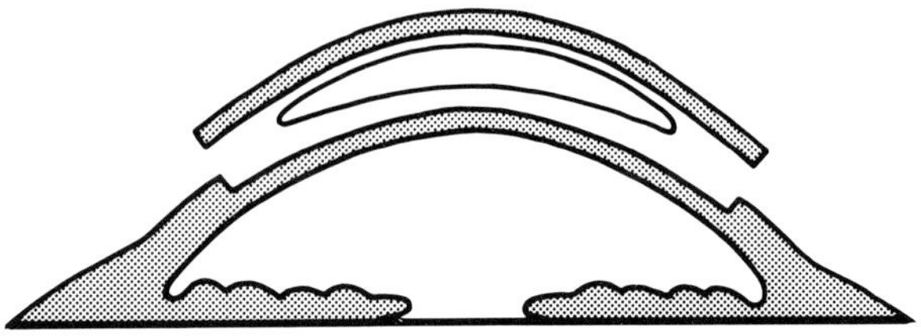

Fig. 18-1. Keratophakia. The donor tissue lenticule is sandwiched between the stromal bed and the anterior lamella. Keratophakia can correct aphakia, but not myopia.

The second procedure, keratomileusis, was developed because there was a chronic and severe shortage of donor tissue in Colombia, limiting the number of keratophakias that could be performed. In the classic keratomileusis procedure, the corneal lamella is removed, frozen, and shaped on the cryolathe and replaced in the stromal bed, all in the course of a single operation (Fig. 18-2). Keratomileusis today is also performed with shaped donor tissue placed in the stromal bed, particularly when the patient's lamella is inadequate.

Both refractive procedures can effectively correct aphakic vision and, with changes in the shaping procedures, keratomileusis can also be used to correct myopia. However, there were problems with the accuracy of the correction, and the various surgical and technical skills as well as the instrumentation needed to lathe the lenticule and perform the surgery were many and complex. The microkeratome, which is essential to both keratophakia and keratomileusis, is a difficult instrument to use, requiring the selection of multiple rings, the raising of the intraocular pressure (IOP) to 65 mmHg, and dissection of the patient's central optical axis. These procedures are not reversible, and the risk of perforation and high astigmatism remains. Over the past few years, both procedures have been improved, and both are currently being performed in the United States by a small number of surgeons.

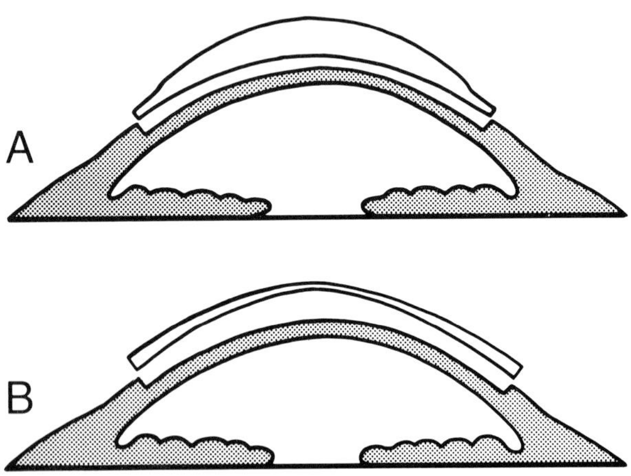

Fig. 18-2. Keratomileusis. The patient's cornea is sectioned with the microkeratome, and the lamella is frozen and shaped on the cryolathe and replaced in the stromal bed. In a variation of this procedure, donor tissue can be used to shape the lenticule; this is called homoplastic keratomileusis. **(A)** Keratomileusis for aphakia. **(B)** Keratomileusis for myopia.

EPIKERATOPHAKIA FOR THE CORRECTION OF REFRACTIVE ERROR

Aphakia

Epikeratophakia for the correction of aphakia (Fig. 18-3) evolved from the Barraquer procedures, with modifications to eliminate the microkeratome, simplify the surgery, and reduce the risk to the patient.[2–9] Once it became clear that freezing and shaping the lenses on the cryolathe left no living cells,[10] and studies confirmed that living cells in the stroma are unnecessary for the clarity of the lenses, the next step was to preserve the shaped

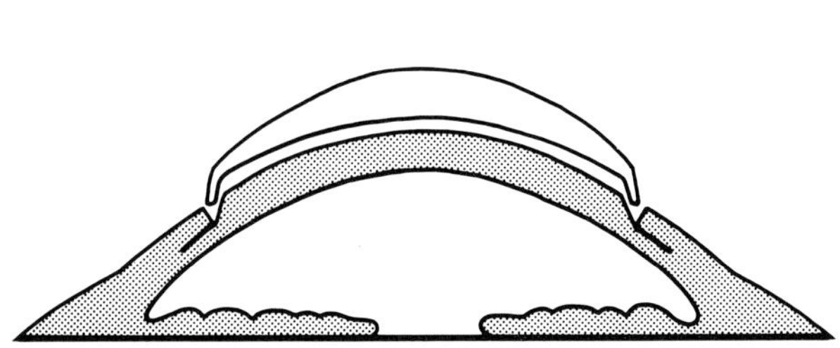

Fig. 18-3. Epikeratophakia for aphakia. The donor tissue lens is shaped and preserved by lyophilization until surgery, then rehydrated in balanced salt solution with antibiotics. The wing (edge) of the tissue lens is sutured into a peripheral keratectomy in the cornea.

tissue so that it could be stored safely and easily. In this way, mass production of tissue lenses with the necessary dioptric correction was made possible, and the lenticule could be ordered by the surgeon from a central source, dispensing with the cryolathe, computer programs, and complex calculations. Putting the donor lens on the anterior surface of the cornea achieved the refractive goal and, at the same time, eliminated the use of the microkeratome. These changes, coupled with refinements in tissue handling,[11,12] have resulted in a procedure that is relatively simple to perform, that carries a low risk of damage to the patient's cornea, and that is reversible, if necessary.[13-15]

Clinical Picture and Indications

Adult Epikeratophakia. The patient for whom epikeratophakia was originally designed is unilaterally aphakic, unable or unwilling to wear a contact lens, and is not a candidate for secondary intraocular lens implantation. Because these patients are unable to resolve the image disparity produced by monocular aphakic spectacles, without refractive surgery they may have a functionally blind eye after cataract extraction.

As the epikeratophakia procedure has been developed and refined, its application has been extended to patients who are bilaterally aphakic. In some cases, epikeratophakia has been performed in preference to an invasive secondary procedure in an eye that may be at risk of endothelial damage and corneal decompensation or in an eye with a disorganized anterior chamber that cannot support a secondary implant. Other patients who are not eligible for, or who do not want, intraocular lenses simply prefer a permanent, maintenance-free correction and are willing to undergo a relatively safe and reversible surgical procedure to achieve this end. Occupational situations may also dictate a preference for refractive correction: dusty and dirty environments make contact lenses impractical, and some patients must pass minimum vision screening without correction.

As the frequency of combined cataract extraction and intraocular lens implantation has increased, the pool of aphakic or potentially aphakic candidates for epikeratophakia has diminished. However, there are still some patients for whom this type of refractive surgery may be a safer route to visual rehabilitation. These include aphakic adults without an intact posterior capsule, as well as those with traumatic cataracts, recurrent uveitis, glaucoma, marginal endothelial cell counts, cornea guttata, vitreous in the anterior chamber, or poorly controlled diabetes. In addition, patients likely to need panretinal photocoagulation or vitrectomy may be candidates for epikeratophakia.

Pediatric Epikeratophakia. Another problem group for whom epikeratophakia may provide a solution is that of children with cataracts.[16-20] Although it has been shown that congenital cataract extraction in neonates, coupled with contact lens correction and vigorous amblyopia therapy, may produce good visual results, the effort required to maintain a contact lens in the eye of a young child over long periods of time is overwhelming, and the cost is not insignificant. An epikeratophakia lens permanently corrects most of the refractive error and leaves the parents free to concentrate on the occlusion schedule.

Children with traumatic cataracts are excellent candidates for epikeratophakia as a combined procedure with cataract extraction.[21] Because we find that the epikeratophakia lenses clear quickly in children, the sutures can usually be removed 2 to 3 weeks after surgery, and amblyopia therapy is begun a week later. An alternative is to remove the congenital cataract and fit the neonate with contact lenses. When children are small, they tolerate contact lenses well, but, when contact lens intolerance develops (usually within 1 or 2 years), an epikeratophakia can be done at a time when the eye is not changing and the final correction may be easier to predict. For children with traumatic cataracts and corneal lacerations, epikeratophakia may prevent a penetrating keratoplasty because it reduces regular and irregular astigmatism while correcting the aphakia. Neither the corneal lacerations nor preoperative astigmatism appear to interfere with vision after successful epikeratophakia surgery; in fact, preoperative astigmatism due to scarring appears to be reduced 10 to 20 percent by a sort of splinting effect provided by the epikeratophakia lens. The epikeratophakia lens also supports the injured cornea and permits rapid removal of the sutures from the corneal laceration repair, before vascularization occurs.[22] More rapid visual rehabilitation also reduces the potential for the development of dense amblyopia and visual loss.

Contraindications

Adult Epikeratophakia. Lagophthalmos, blepharitis, and/or dry eyes are relative contraindications to epikeratophakia. Patients with moderate blepharitis and dry eyes are told that treatment (e.g., lid scrubs, antibiotics, artificial tears) must be continued faithfully after the refractive procedure to ensure the survival of the epikeratophakia lens. In many cases, the surgeon must make a judgment as to the reliability of the patient in following through on this chronic regimen. Because dry eyes are also a contraindication to contact lens wear, people with this condition are more likely to seek refractive surgery, but caution is necessary. Although the epikeratophakia lens can withstand somewhat more severe corneal conditions than can contact lenses, uncontrolled dry eyes and/or blepharitis predispose this surgery to failure. Vascular ingrowth from previous contact lens wear does not appear to affect the success of epikeratophakia lenses. Lagophthalmos, if severe, must be treated surgically to restore the normal anatomical function of the lid prior to epikeratophakia surgery.

Pediatric Epikeratophakia. Retrospective evaluation of visual results in pediatric epikeratophakia demonstrated that in children under 1 year of age, undercorrection was the rule rather than the exception, while the reverse was true for older children. The very short eyes and steep corneas of aphakic neonates do not seem amenable to a sufficient increase in corneal curvature for reasons that we do not yet understand. As a result, however, we suggest that epikeratophakia not be used in neonates.[23] In most neonates and infants, when cataractous lenses are removed, contact lenses can be used successfully at first; later, when contact lens correction becomes difficult because of lack of cooperation, refractive surgery may be employed. Epikeratophakia has been used successfully as a primary procedure in older children with acquired cataracts and with bilateral cataracts, and this form of correction is also better than no correction at all in a very young child who proves intolerant of contact lenses or spectacles.

Alternative Methods of Treatment

Adults. In the overwhelming majority of adults, cataract extraction is combined with intraocular lens implantation. For unilaterally aphakic patients, daily wear or extended-wear contact lenses are an alternative. The bilaterally aphakic adult can also be corrected with ahakic spectacles. Refractive procedures for the correction of aphakia include keratophakia, keratomileusis, and epikeratophakia.

Children. Contact lenses specially fabricated for very steep corneas are used in neonates; the use of contact lenses in young eyes requires constant vigilance on the part of an adult to be sure that the lens has not been decentered or lost. Spectacles can be used by older children who are bilaterally aphakic, although damage, breakage, and loss are problems. Although intraocular lens implantation has been performed in a few series of young patients, we do not recommend this form of correction because of the long-term risks of chronic uveitis and corneal endothelial damage. Invasive refractive procedures, such as keratophakia and keratomileusis, which require the microkeratome sectioning of the often small and steep cornea, carry a greater risk, compared with epikeratophakia, which is extraocular, relatively safe, and reversible.

Surgical Technique

Adult Epikeratophakia. Before surgery, each patient undergoes a complete ophthalmologic examination. Corneal curvature is measured, and the average keratometry reading is combined with the spherical equivalent of the spectacle correction corrected to the corneal plane, in order to calculate the dioptric power required in the epikeratophakia lens. The epikeratophakia lens (Keratolens) is ordered ahead of time, to the proper specifications. The tissue lens is obtained in the lyophilized (freeze-dried) state, under vacuum, and is rehydrated in BSS containing antibiotics for 20 minutes in the operating room while the patient is being prepared and draped.

At surgery, before being anesthetized, the patient is asked to fixate on the filament of the Zeiss operating microscope, while the surgeon makes a defect in the epithelium with a 27-gauge needle to mark the visual axis. After the general or local anesthesia is administered, a speculum is placed and superior and inferior 4-0 silk bridle sutures are used to stabilize the globe.

The epithelium is removed from the mid-peripheral cornea. A blunt cut cellulose sponge soaked in a 4 percent cocaine solution is used to create an epithelial defect peripheral to the visual axis mark. The epithelium is removed from the cornea by means of a Paton spatula, sparing only a central island containing the visual axis mark and a 0.5-mm cuff at the limbus (Fig. 18-4). Care is taken to push the loosened epithelium centrally, rather than outward, to prevent debris from collecting in the fornices. Copious and repeated irrigation and aspiration ensure the removal of all epithelial tissue, to prevent the later development of interface opacities between the host cornea and the epikeratophakia lens.

The cornea is incised to a depth of 0.3 mm by means of the Hessburg-Barron suction trephine (Fig. 18-5). The cut is centered over the visual axis mark (Fig. 18-6). For a hyperopic epikeratophakia lens, a 7.0-mm trephine is used. The central patch of epithelium with the visual axis mark is removed. The circular cut, which penetrates Bowman's layer, becomes the outer wall of the annular keratectomy, which is created by dissecting away the inner wall to form a wedge-shaped trough 0.5 mm across at the corneal surface (Fig. 18-7). A 0.12-mm forceps or Colibri forceps is used to hold the tissue while the wedge of Bowman's layer and anterior stroma is dissected.

The Suarez spreader, a blunt dissecting instrument that has been slightly sharpened, is employed to make a 1-mm lamellar split in the stroma for 360 degrees at the base of the annular keratectomy, in the limbal direction (Fig. 18-8). This provides a "pocket" into which the edge of the lens can be tucked, anchoring the lens more securely, and preventing any part of the edge from escaping to rise above the surface of the keratectomy and cause astigmatism as the lens heals.

Irrigation and aspiration of both the lens and the corneal bed are repeated at this point, just before the lens is placed on the eye. The lens, which is 8.5 mm in diameter, is draped over the cornea, centered over the keratectomy, in direct apposition to the bare Bowman's layer. A Polack forceps is used to hold the lens while the first suture is placed (Fig. 18-9). The 10-0 nylon suture enters the wing 0.75 mm from the edge, from the anterior surface,

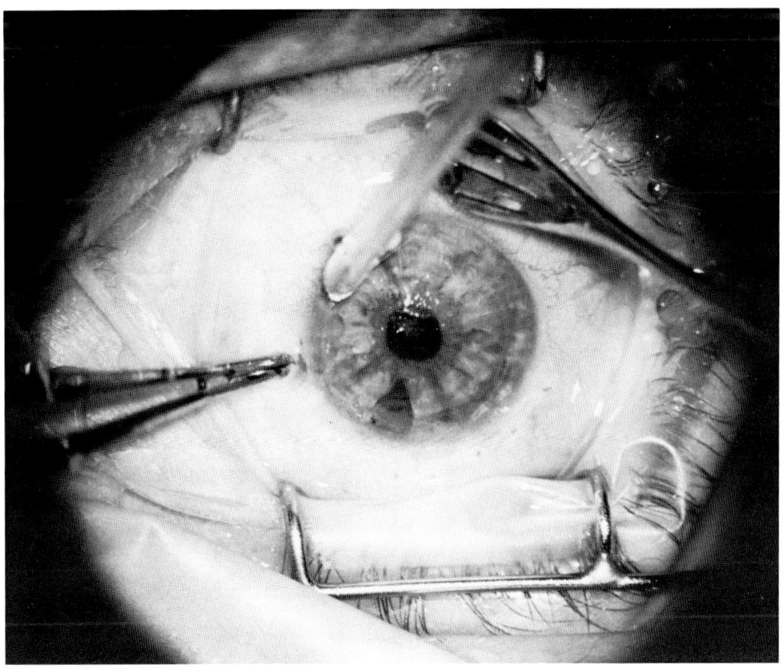

Fig. 18-4. At surgery, after the visual axis is marked, a Paton spatula and 4 percent cocaine are used to remove the epithelium from the patient's cornea, except for a 0.5-mm cuff at the limbus and a small island containing the visual axis mark.

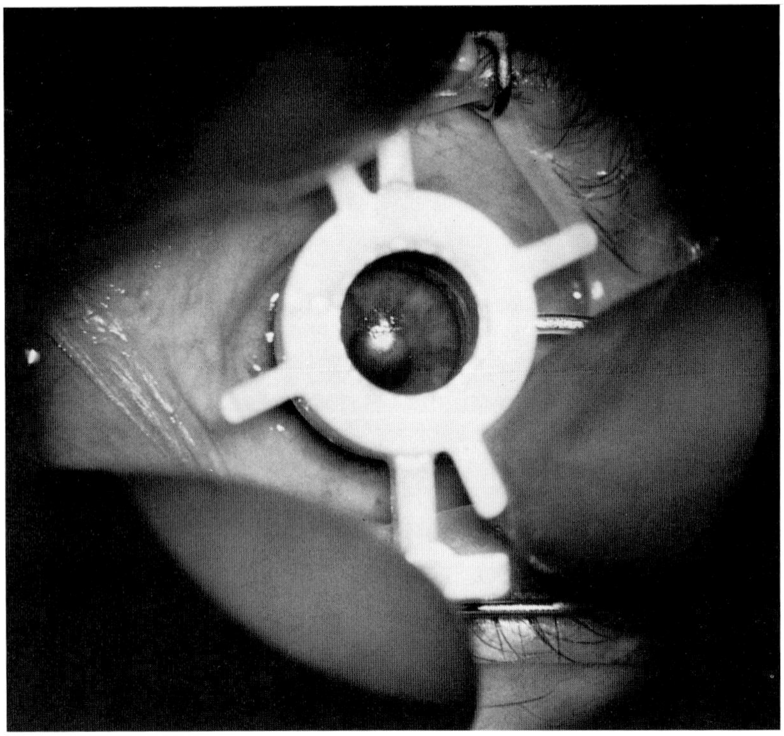

Fig. 18-5. A circular trephine cut, 0.3 mm in depth, is made with a Hessburg-Barron suction trephine.

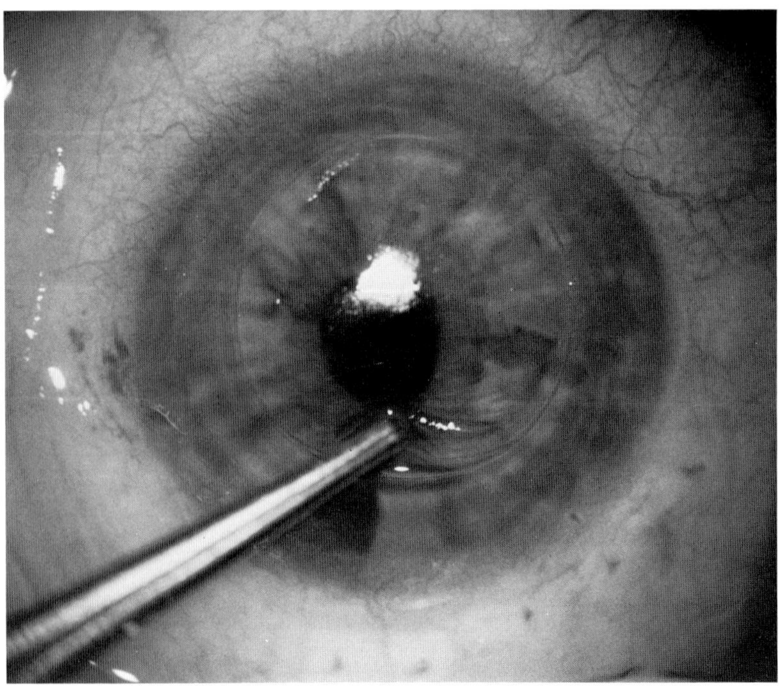

Fig. 18-6. The annular keratotomy is well out of the visual axis.

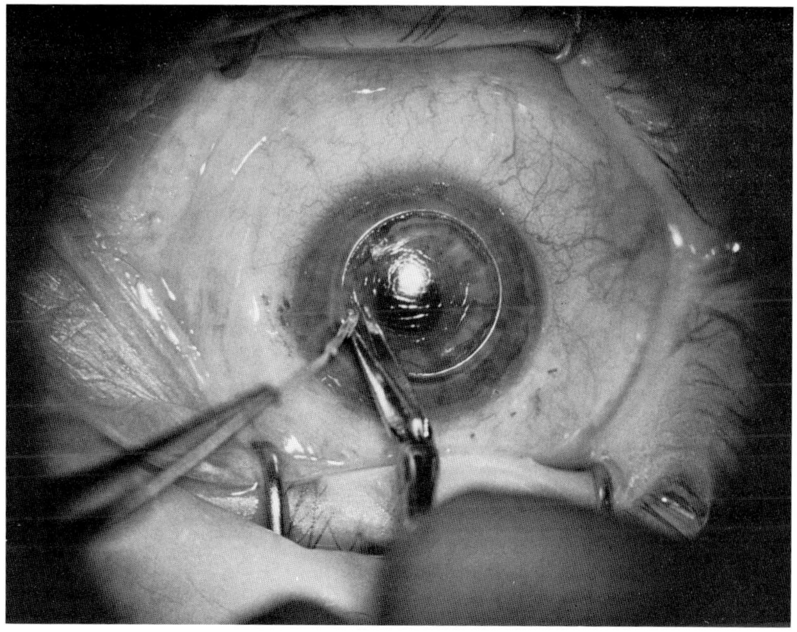

Fig. 18-7. The inner wall of trephine cut is dissected at an angle with a Vannas scissors to form the annular keratectomy, into which the wing of the tissue lens will be sutured.

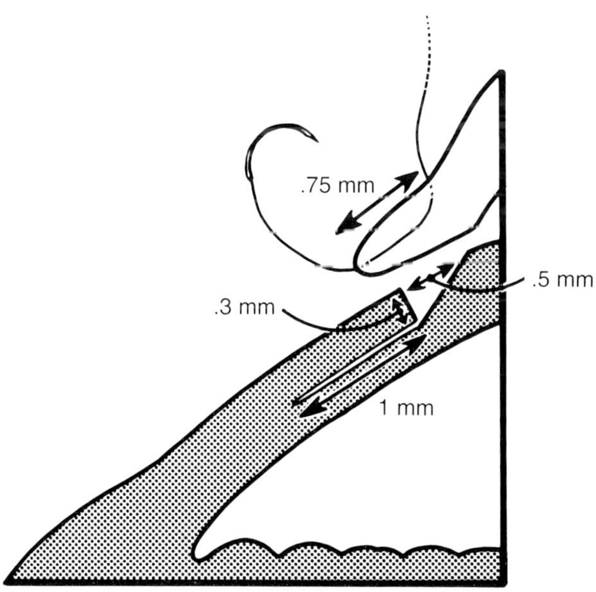

Fig. 18-8. Spreading technique. Side view of annular keratectomy with peripheral lamellar dissection at the base extending 1 mm toward the limbus. The suture is placed to split the wing of the tissue lens 0.75 mm from the peripheral edge.

passing horizontally to split the wing, rather than emerging posteriorly. The Polack forceps is removed, and the recipient lip is held with Colibri forceps or with the cross-action Maumenee forceps. The bite in the recipient cornea is 1 mm long and deep enough to pass through the pocket formed by the Suarez spreader. The suture is tied with three knots. The next seven sutures are placed in this manner, evenly spaced around the lens. The wing of the lens between the sutures is tucked into the annular keratectomy with the Barraquer iris spatula. The last eight sutures are placed blindly, evenly divided among the spaces between the first eight sutures (Fig. 18-10). No attempt is made to separate the lens and bed to inspect the precise location of these last eight sutures. Finally, the knots are rotated first through the surface of the lens and then into the stromal bed, such that the ends stream behind the knot, forming an arrow pointing toward the corneal surface (Fig. 18-11). This permits the removal of the sutures through the recipient cornea without rotating the knots through the tissue lens, possibly disrupting the healing edge.

At the conclusion of surgery, a bandage soft contact lens that covers the lens and extends out over the edge of the remaining cuff of epithelium is

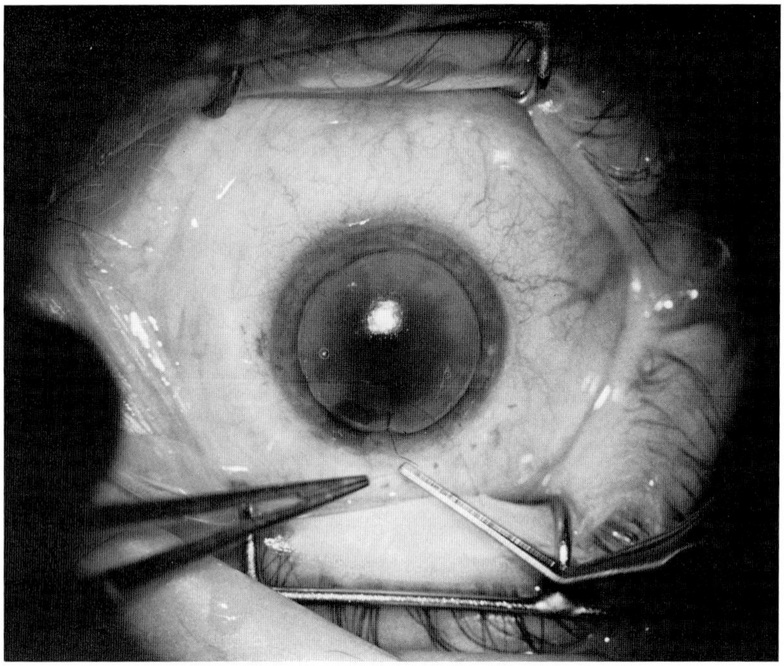

Fig. 18-9. The tissue lens is draped over the cornea, and the first suture is placed.

placed on the eye. SubTenon's gentamicin sulfate and methylprednisolone acetate are injected and gentamicin and homatropine 5 percent drops instilled. The eye is closed with a cotton patch and covered with a Fox shield. The following day, the patch is removed. The bandage lens remains on the eye until the surface of the lens is reepithelialized, usually 4 to 7 days. The metal shield is worn at night

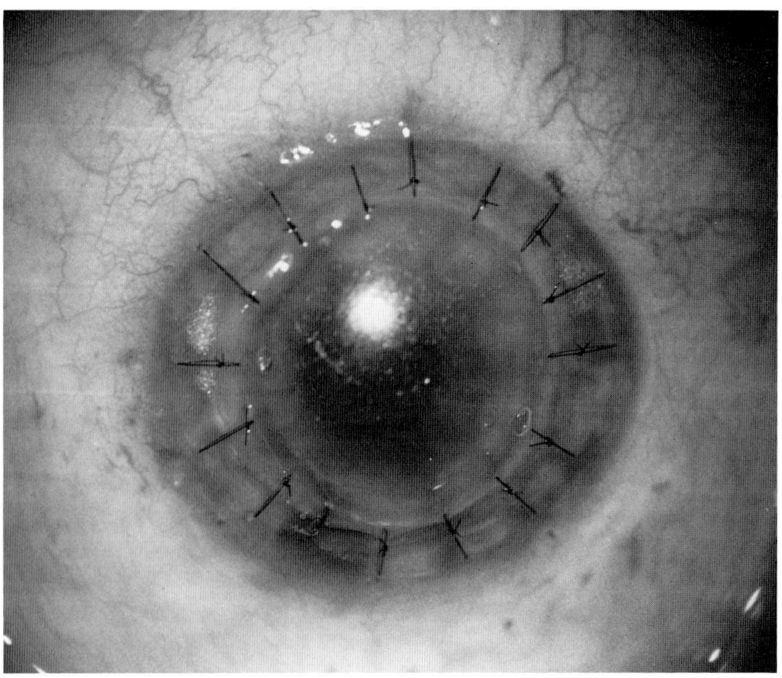

Fig. 18-10. Epikeratophakia graft in place with 16 interrupted sutures. A soft contact lens is placed over the graft to aid in epithelialization. Small air bubbles that may form under the contact lens usually disappear within 24 hours.

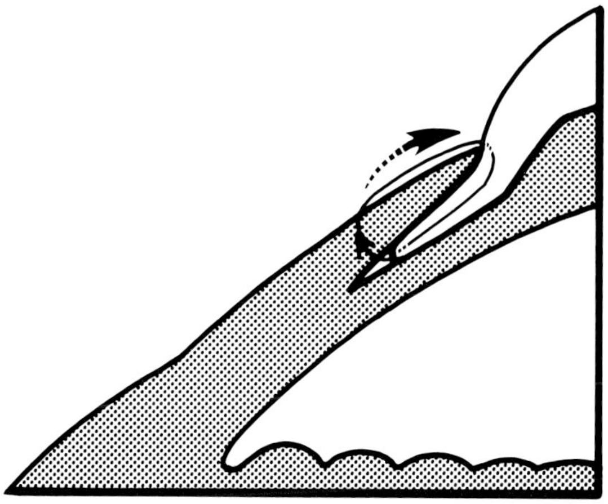

Fig. 18-11. The wing of the tissue lens is inserted into the annular keratectomy and lamellar dissection, with the suture exiting through the recipient cornea. The suture is tied with a triple throw, and the knot is rotated through the wing and into the recipient cornea, with the ends of the sutures streaming behind for ease of later removal with minimal disruption to the wing–stroma interface.

for a period of 4 weeks. After the epithelial cover is complete, the bandage lens is removed, the drops are discontinued, and a bland but protective ointment (usually Sulamyd, if there is no allergy to sulfa) is applied three or four times a day, more for the protective effect than for the antibiotic activity.

In adult aphakic patients, the sutures are removed 8 weeks after surgery (Fig. 18-12). Individual sutures may be removed earlier if vascularization appears to be a problem in a particular area, or if loosened sutures begin to collect mucus.

Pediatric Epikeratophakia. In children scheduled for a combined cataract extraction and epikeratophakia, keratometry readings and A-scan ultrasonography for axial length are used to calculate the required power of the lens. Few of our pediatric patients are old enough or cooperative enough to participate in the marking of the visual axis, so that part of the adult procedure is omitted entirely. The surgery for aphakic children is otherwise similar to that of adults. In the combined procedure, the cataract is generally removed from a limbal approach, after the trephine cut is made, and before the annular keratectomy is dissected.

After the keratectomy and Suarez spreader pocket are made, the lens is draped over the cornea and sutured as described for the adult procedure, except that a total of 20 to 24 10-0 nylon sutures are placed.

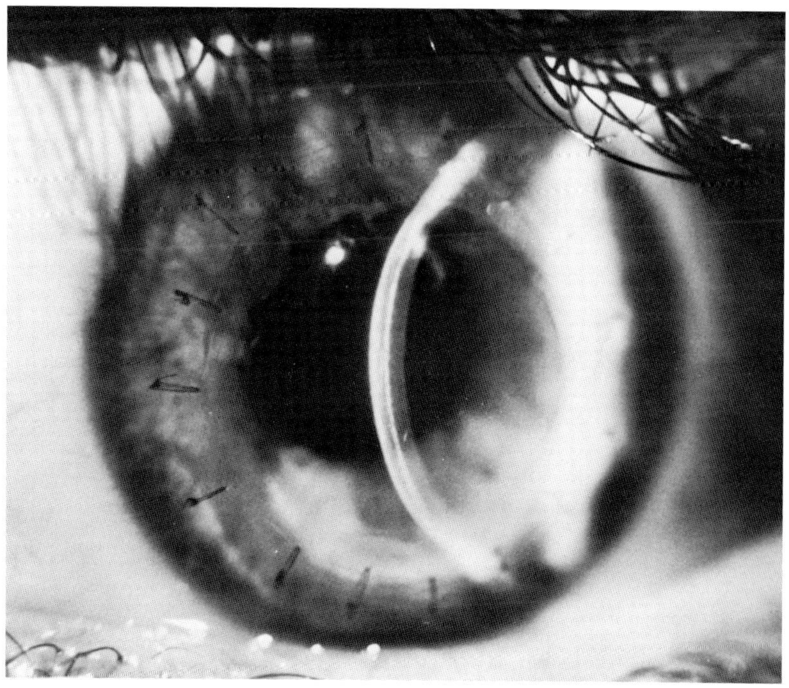

Fig. 18-12. Slit-lamp photograph of aphakic epikeratophakia tissue lens 2 months after surgery, just prior to suture removal.

Pediatric patients are given oral antibiotics (amoxicillin), as well as topical gentamicin and atropine, and the eye is covered 24 hours a day by means of a bandage soft contact lens and a plastic shield with holes through which ointments can be applied, until the sutures are removed. The sutures are usually removed 2 to 3 weeks after surgery, during the course of an evaluation under anesthesia. Topical antibiotic and atropine are instilled once a day until the eye is no longer red, after which an artificial tear (such as Duratears) is used at night for 6 months. Occlusion therapy is begun 1 week after the sutures are removed.

Prognosis

Adult Epikeratophakia. Patients who are aphakic but who can demonstrate a potential for 20/20 vision before surgery usually progress to a visual acuity of 20/50 by 3 to 6 weeks after surgery and of 20/20 to 20/25 by the third or fourth month. The final correction is generally within 1 diopter of the predicted correction. In a nationwide study of epikeratophakia, early results show that 3 to 4 months after surgery, of 42 patients with an average preoperative acuity of 20/30 − 2, 29 percent had 20/50 or better visual acuity without correction, 58 percent had 20/100 or better, and only 14 percent had less than 20/400 uncorrected vision. These were the first visual acuities obtained after suture removal and, as such, would be expected to improve with further follow-up. In terms of spherical equivalent, 34 percent were corrected to within 1 diopter of emmetropia and 59 percent to within 2 diopters of emmetropia.

Average final corrected acuity is about one Snellen chart line less than preoperative spectacle acuity. Patients are usually quite satisfied with their vision and very willing to trade one line of spectacle acuity for unaided vision in a previously functionally blind eye. The one-line loss is thought to be the result of irregular astigmatism, possibly caused by irregularities in the hand-cut keratectomy. This is a problem we hope to eliminate with the development of the new trephine.

Pediatric Epikeratophakia. Children with traumatic cataracts have shown a good response to epikeratophakia as a means of correcting aphakic vision. In our most recent series, 13 children under the age of 6, whose average age at the time of refractive surgery was 3.5 years, had been visually deprived in the affected eye for an average of 8.4 months. Three of these children developed final visual acuities of 20/100 or worse, seven achieved between 20/80 and 20/50, and three have acuities better than 20/50.

Children with congenital cataracts have shown more variable results. Individual patients have done very well, however, showing that good to excellent visual outcomes are possible. Two patients operated on before their first birthday have achieved 20/60 visual acuity; one has achieved 20/100, and one 20/200. Many patients in this category are not yet able to cooperate verbally in the measurement of acuity. Furtheremore, visual outcome is heavily dependent on the willingness and ability of the parents to maintain the occlusion schedule, and we have had a number of cases in which the epikeratophakia lens was successful and in which the potential for vision seemed excellent, but conscientious maintenance of the patching schedule was not possible, and poor vision due to amblyopia was the result.

In the nationwide study of pediatric patients receiving epikeratophakia tissue lenses for the correction of aphakia, data obtained 3 to 4 months after surgery showed that 65 percent of 27 cases were within 1 diopter of emmetropia, and 97 percent were within 3 diopters of emmetropia. Mean spherical equivalent was reduced from 14 diopters (range: 7.1 to 25 diopters) preoperatively to 0.7 diopters (range: −1.9 to +3.4 diopters).

Complications

A potential surgical complication is perforation of the cornea with the Hessburg-Barron trephine. The 0.3-mm trephine cut is made with $3\frac{1}{2}$ quarter-turns of the plunger after the blade has been leveled to the plano position (3 up, $6\frac{1}{2}$ down). Confusing complete revolutions with quarter-turns will lead to perforation, as will leveling the notch in the trephine with the outer wall of the suction ring instead of the inner wall. To prevent serious damage to the eye, the Hessburg-Barron suction trephine should be used on a relatively dry cornea. Under these circumstances, if aqueous suddenly appears, it is immediately apparent that perforation has occurred. Conversely, if the eye is wet, it is more difficult to identify escaping aqueous humor immediately, and the trephine can penetrate the iris or, in the worst possible case, hit the lens. At the first sign of perforation, the surgical assistant should break the suction, either by pushing in the plunger or by cutting through the connecting tubing.

In the event of a perforation, the damage is repaired as follows: the eye must be closed with 10-0 nylon sutures, the incision observed carefully to ensure it is watertight, and the knots rotated beneath the surface of the eye to minimize irritation. A Troutman or Keeler keratometer can be used to ensure that the eye is closed and that suturing the perforation has not created an astigmatic cornea.

In a phakic eye, damage is likely to be minimal, and often the repair can be followed by completion of the epikeratophakia procedure. In an aphakic eye, however, the problem is more serious, and the refractive procedure generally must be abandoned for the time being. In these cases, it is very likely that vitreous will be entrapped on the endothelial side of the perforation, which can lead to the development of cystoid macular edema or retinal detachment, or both. It is advisable to examine the anterior chamber for vitreous strands in the operating room. If the operating microscope is not equipped with a slit-lamp attachment, a disposable hand-held slit lamp can be used successfully. Introduction of an air bubble can also be helpful in showing strands of vitreous in a corneal wound. To clear the vitreous, a limbal stab with a No. 75 Beaver blade is made parallel to the iris, and a Barraquer sweep is passed through the anterior chamber. If none of these maneuvers is successful, the eye must be opened from the site of the Beaver blade incision and an Ocutome vitrectomy performed. Most adult candidates for epikeratophakia for aphakia are selected for this surgery because they have vitreous in the anterior chamber, making secondary intraocular lens implantation difficult and dangerous. For this reason, perforation of the anterior chamber during the epikeratophakia procedure in an aphakic eye should invariably be followed by procedures designed to locate and clear the vitreous, lest the first indication of this problem become apparent on slit-lamp examination on the first postoperative day. Epikeratophakia can be rescheduled at a later date, when the eye is quiet.

A disposable modified Hessburg-Barron trephine is available, which has a special device to break suction at a depth of 0.3 mm in the cornea and which makes two circular parallel incisions 0.5 mm apart. With this trephine, the surgeon need only lift the median strip between the incisions and sever it with the Vannas scissors at its base. For the future, we are in the process of designing a permanent knife that will make the outer perpendicular cut and the inner angled cut with diamond or ruby blades, with a fixation device at the limbus that does not depend on suction. This trephine will create the entire keratectomy and the peripheral lamellar pocket simultaneously and reduce the potential for perforation of the anterior chamber virtually to zero.

During the early phases of development of the epikeratophakia procedure, the most common postoperative complication in all aphakic patients, adult and pediatric, was undercorrection. New tissue processing and selection methods have largely eliminated this problem in the adult population and in children over the age of 1 year. At this time, the reason for undercorrection in the youngest patients is unclear. Successful correction in sporadic individual cases of neonatal congenital cataracts demonstrates that the epikeratophakia lens has the potential to meet the dioptric requirements of these eyes and that the upper limit of total corneal curvature achievable with this kind of lens, if there is an upper limit, certainly exceeds the curvature actually necessary to correct vision in these babies.[24]

Another optical complication has been postoperative astigmatism, most frequently seen when the edge of the lens escapes from the annular keratectomy and protrudes above the surface of the cornea. The use of the Suarez spreader to make a peripheral annular pocket in the stroma at the base of the keratectomy has eliminated this problem by providing a larger space and more secure fastening for the edge of the lens.

The most common factors leading to lens failure are chronic epithelial defects and scarring due to uncontrolled dry eyes and blepharitis. In the event of a chronic epithelial defect that does not change shape for two or more postoperative visits, the bandage lens is removed and a pressure patch applied. If the patient was unable to wear a bandage lens, and the eye was already patched, a tarsorrhaphy is performed. Three double-armed 5-0 Dermalon sutures are tied very tightly with long ends and no bolsters; the sutures can then be untied, the cornea examined, and the sutures retied every 7 days for 3 weeks. Should the defect persist throughout this treatment, the epikeratophakia tissue lens is removed. The graft can be replaced immediately if the eye is quiet, but generally several weeks or months of healing may be needed before a new graft is attempted.

Other problems include traumatic dehiscence of the scar during the early healing period, neovascularization resulting from delayed suture removal, epithelial rests at the lens–cornea interface, infiltrates, and infection. The incidence of infection in the pediatric patients was, at first, markedly higher than in the adult patients, probably because children are more likely to put their hands in their eyes, and their hands are less likely to be clean. Covering the eye with the plastic shield and eliminating parental handling of the eye during the early postoperative period, coupled with the administration of prophylactic antibiotics, has reduced the incidence of infection nearly to zero; in addition, pediatric patients are seen at least every 3 days after surgery until the sutures are removed, so that any incipient infection can be treated promptly.

Experience has shown that the epikeratophakia lens attaches to the cornea by healing in the area of the annular keratectomy; no permanent scar is formed across the visual axis. In cases in which epithelial ingrowth between the lens and the cornea approaches the optical zone, the healing edge of the lens can be opened for several clock hours, the extraneous material scraped with a dull curette, such as the Barraquer iris spatula, and the interface rinsed thoroughly, after which the edge of the lens is resutured, as in the original operation.

Any or all of these optical, mechanical, or medical complications can lead to the removal of the epikeratophakia tissue lens. The ultimate indication for removal of the lens is the judgment of the surgeon that no form of therapeutic intervention will result in satisfactory visual correction. At that point, depending on the healing status, either the sutures are removed or the peripheral scar is opened, and the lens is peeled off the cornea; this can easily be accomplished with topical anesthesia during an office visit. It has been our experience that the patient's cornea is re-epithelialized within 4 to 7 days after the tissue lens is removed, regardless of the length of time the lens has been in place.

In general, the epikeratophakia tissue lens can be replaced immediately in a quiet eye; an eye that is irritated or inflamed must be permitted to recover before a second procedure is performed. That is, a tissue lens removed during the early postoperative period because of neovascularization or infection can probably not be replaced for several weeks or months, while a graft fully healed into place but inadequate because of undercorrection or overcorrection, glare, or other optical problems can sometimes be removed and replaced in one surgical procedure.

Specific indications for replacing an epikeratophakia tissue lens include undercorrection or overcorrection, a substantial change in dioptic requirements, such as a myopic patient who becomes increasingly myopic some time after surgery because of the extension or enlargement of a posterior staphyloma, or failure to epithelialize the graft in spite of good compliance, appropriate follow-up, and absence of underlying ocular disease. In this last circumstance, the problem may be considered intrinsic to the graft, albeit unexplainable, and this sort of failure can usually be converted to success by repeating the graft. The occasional patient with late trauma or infection can also be successfully regrafted, as in one case of a teenager who partially dislodged his tissue lens 1 month after surgery in a motorcycle accident. The first graft was removed and replaced, and the second graft healed uneventfully with excellent resulting vision.

Contraindications to a repeat epikeratophakia are essentially similar to those for a first graft: noncompliant patients, patients who do not follow medication schedules, patients who do not return for follow-up visits, and patients with uncontrolled dry eyes, blepharitis, or lagophthalmos.

Myopia

Clinical Picture and Indications

In general, patients with 6 or more diopters of myopia, which has been stable for at least 1 year, are eligible for myopic epikeratophakia lenses.[25,26]

At Louisiana State University (LSU), the lower limit has been extended to 4 diopters of myopia, on a trial basis. Exceptions to the requirement for stable myopia are made for unilaterally highly myopic children in whom anisometropic amblyopia is developing. Patients with more than 2 diopters of astigmatism require a modified surgical protocol involving a controlled postoperative wound dehiscence in the steepest quadrant. Toric epikeratophakia tissue lenses are being tested at LSU for correction of more than 2 diopters of astigmatism; less than 2 diopters of astigmatism is generally masked by the ordinary spherical epikeratophakia tissue lens alone.

Patients seeking refractive surgery for myopia are expected to be unable or unwilling to use spectacles or contact lenses for visual correction; in particular, patients who have not tried contact lenses for several years are informed about the many advances in contact lens materials and designs over the past few years and are given the opportunity to try contact lens correction again before undergoing refractive surgery.

Contraindications

The contraindications are the same as for aphakic epikeratophakia, in terms of lagophthalmos, uncontrolled dry eyes, and/or blepharitis. Patients with less than 4 diopters of myopia who require refractive surgery can probably be managed by radial keratotomy. Astigmatism of greater than 2.5 diopters may preclude successful correction by a spherical myopic epikeratophakia lens. Preexisting conditions that may reduce the chances for a good visual outcome in myopic patients include posterior staphylomas, myopic macular degeneration, and rhegmatogenous retinal detachments.

Alternative Methods of Treatment

Myopia can be corrected by means of spectacles or contact lenses. Some surgeons have advocated the removal of the crystalline lens, with the implantation of a low plus- or minus-power intraocular lens, if necessary. However, this type of surgery in an eye at risk of retinal detachment, vitreous loss, and cystoid macular edema is generally considered extremely risky and is not often done in the United States.

Refractive procedures for the correction of myopia include keratomileusis, radial keratotomy, and epikeratophakia. The upper limit of effective correction obtained by radial keratotomy is about 6 to 8 diopters; the limit for myopic keratomileusis is about 15 diopters, and for homoplastic keratomileusis somewhat higher. There is no theoretical limit to the degree of myopia that can be corrected with an epikeratophakia lens. For many severely myopic patients, no combination of optical aids can provide adequate correction. One of our earliest myopia patients was using a combination of spectacles and contact lenses and achieving a best corrected visual acuity of only 20/200. With the epikeratophakia lens, his vision was 20/50 − 3 with spectacle overcorrection of −1.00 + 1.00 × 140 degrees about 1 year after surgery.

Surgical Technique

The surgical procedure for myopic epikeratophakia (Fig. 18-13) is similar to that of aphakic epikeratophakia. Sutures are removed 8 weeks after surgery (Fig. 18-14).

Prognosis

Because myopic lenses are thin, they clear faster than do aphakic lenses. These patients generally have usable vision 2 or 3 weeks postoperatively, while the sutures are still in place. By 3 weeks, most patients with the potential for 20/40 corrected acuity have achieved 20/50 and continue to improve thereafter. Uncorrected vision averages about 20/100 + 2, which is a considerable change for highly myopic (greater than 8 diopters of myopia, generally) patients who have undergone this procedure to date. By 3 to 4 months, uncorrected

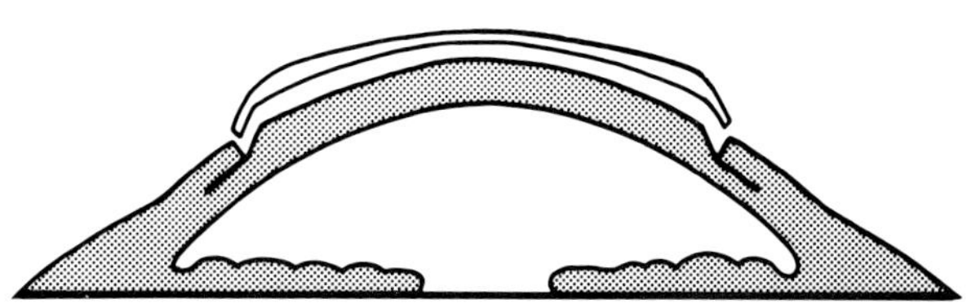

Fig. 18-13. Epikeratophakia for myopia. The tissue lens is thinner centrally and thicker peripherally, where the lens and wing meet, resulting in a net flattening of the anterior curvature of the cornea.

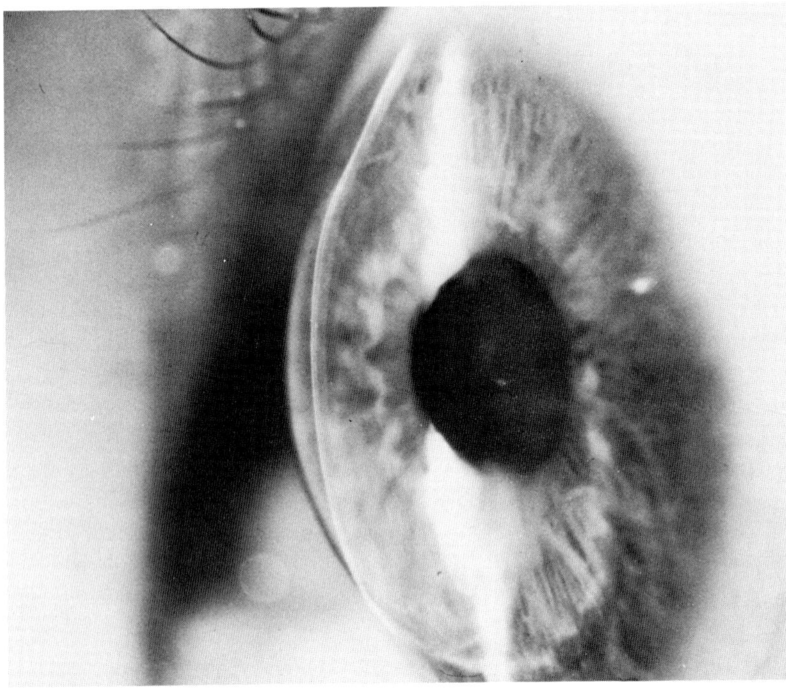

Fig. 18-14. Slit-lamp photograph of myopic epikeratophakia tissue lens 3 months after surgery. The sutures have been removed.

vision averages 20/80, and acuities continue to improve for 2 to 6 months. Of 13 patients receiving epikeratophakia tissue lenses for myopia in the nationwide study, with 3 to 4 months follow-up, one third were corrected to within 1 diopter of emmetropia, and two thirds to within 2 diopters of emmetropia. A number of LSU patients have achieved a final corrected acuity better than the best corrected preoperative spectacle acuity, probably as a result of the enlargement of the image on the retina.

Complications

Complications of myopic epikeratophakia are largely similar to those of aphakic epikeratophakia: astigmatism, undercorrection or overcorrection, traumatic separation of the healing lens, epithelial rests in the lens–cornea interface, infiltrates, persistent epithelial defects, and infection. Most of the complications represent fewer than 2 percent of cases, and most are seen during the first 2 postoperative months.

A number of the early patients who received myopic epikeratophakia tissue lenses experienced postoperative glare, often to the extent that the grafts were removed. It appeared that the tissue lenses, 1.5 mm larger in diameter than the trephine bed, were thrown into folds centrally, when the hydration of the graft stabilized. To remedy this, the tissue lens was redesigned to be only 0.5 mm larger than the trephined bed, and these grafts have been successful in patients with relatively normal K readings. We have also observed, however, that patients with very high corrections and somewhat steep corneas still suffer undercorrection and glare, probably because of the disparity between the arc and cord length. It has also, been noted that because of suture compression, patients were approximately 3 to 4 diopters undercorrected while their sutures were in place. Recently, we have modified the procedure such that an 8.5-mm graft is placed in a 7.0-mm trephined bed, with the addition of the peripheral lamellar dissection to take up the excess wing tissue and allow the graft to drape over the cornea. A loose suturing technique eliminates the problem of suture compression and prevents postoperative astigmatism. We now also use a qualitative keratometer, such as the Troutman or the Keeler keratometer, to look for distortions caused by uneven suturing. The ring of lights highlights any irregularities and permits the surgeon to adjust the tension on the sutures until the circle is perfect. A hand-held portable slit beam is also used in the darkened operating room at the end of the procedure to check the four quadrants of the graft for folds in the recipient cornea. The eye is compressed somewhat during surgery and becomes hypotonic, so that some folds will be present in virtually all cases. However, multiple folds directed toward a particular suture indicate compression and the potential for postoperative astigmatism, which can be averted by replacing that suture.

Epikeratophakia (Onlay Lamellar Keratoplasty) for Keratoconus

Clinical Picture and Indications

The indications for epikeratophakia for keratoconus[27,28] are mild to moderate keratoconus with no central scarring. Eligible patients are unable to wear contact lenses for optical correction but can demonstrate 20/40 or better best corrected visual acuity with a hard lens worn for diagnostic purposes.

The epikeratophakia lens used in this procedure is 0.3 mm thick, and plano (i.e., of equal thickness throughout), with a small peripheral wing 0.75 mm wide and 0.13 mm thick. The lens has no intrinsic optical power but serves a tectonic function, flattening and reinforcing the thinned and protruding cornea. One advantage to epikeratophakia is that the onlay lenses do not appear to elicit an immune reaction, and no cases of immunologic rejection have been seen among these patients.

Contraindications

Central scarring interferes with vision; preexisting corneal scars must be 1 mm or more from the visual axis, as flattening the cone may move paracentral scarring into the optical zone. Patients with severe scarring or less than 20/40 best corrected visual acuity with a hard lens require penetrating keratoplasty.

Surgical Technique

For keratoconus (Fig. 18-15), the lens is plano and 9.0 mm in diameter. The trephine cut is 8.5 mm in diameter. The lens is sutured tightly across the cornea. If the cone is very large and thin, as in keratoglobus, four reefing sutures may be placed at 90 degrees around the cornea and tightened to reduce the protrusion, after the annular keratectomy is made and before the lens is attached. The reefing sutures create folds in the peripheral cornea, much like those in a reefed sail, and smooth out the central cornea (Fig. 18-16). When the epikeratophakia lens is in place, additional folds form under the central area, but these generally smooth out within 6 weeks after surgery and do not interfere with vision. Paracentesis is generally unnecessary. Reefing sutures are re-

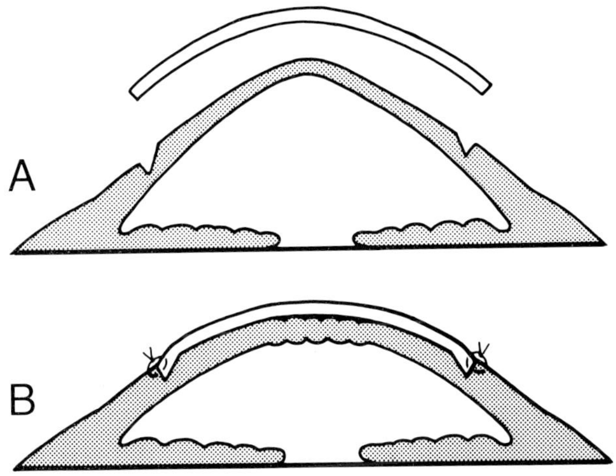

Fig. 18-15. **(A)** For keratoconus, a plano onlay lamellar graft is used to flatten and reinforce the thinned ectatic cornea. **(B)** The folds that form in the recipient cornea immediately after surgery resolve within 3 months after surgery.

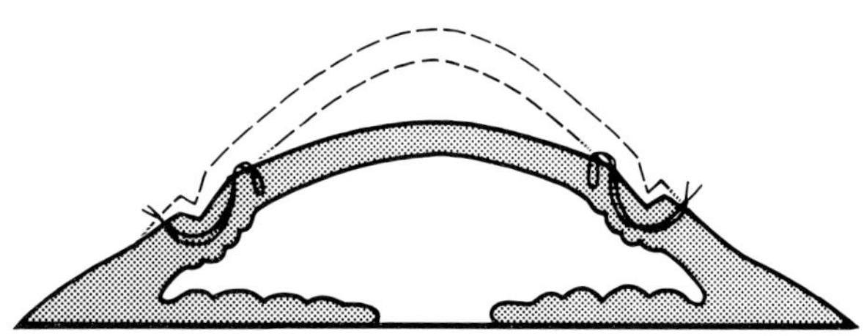

Fig. 18-16. Reefing sutures can be used to reduce the size of the cone before the epikeratophakia graft is placed. Four sutures are positioned at 90 degrees from one another and tightened, creating folds in the peripheral cornea and reducing the amount of corneal folding that will occur under the graft.

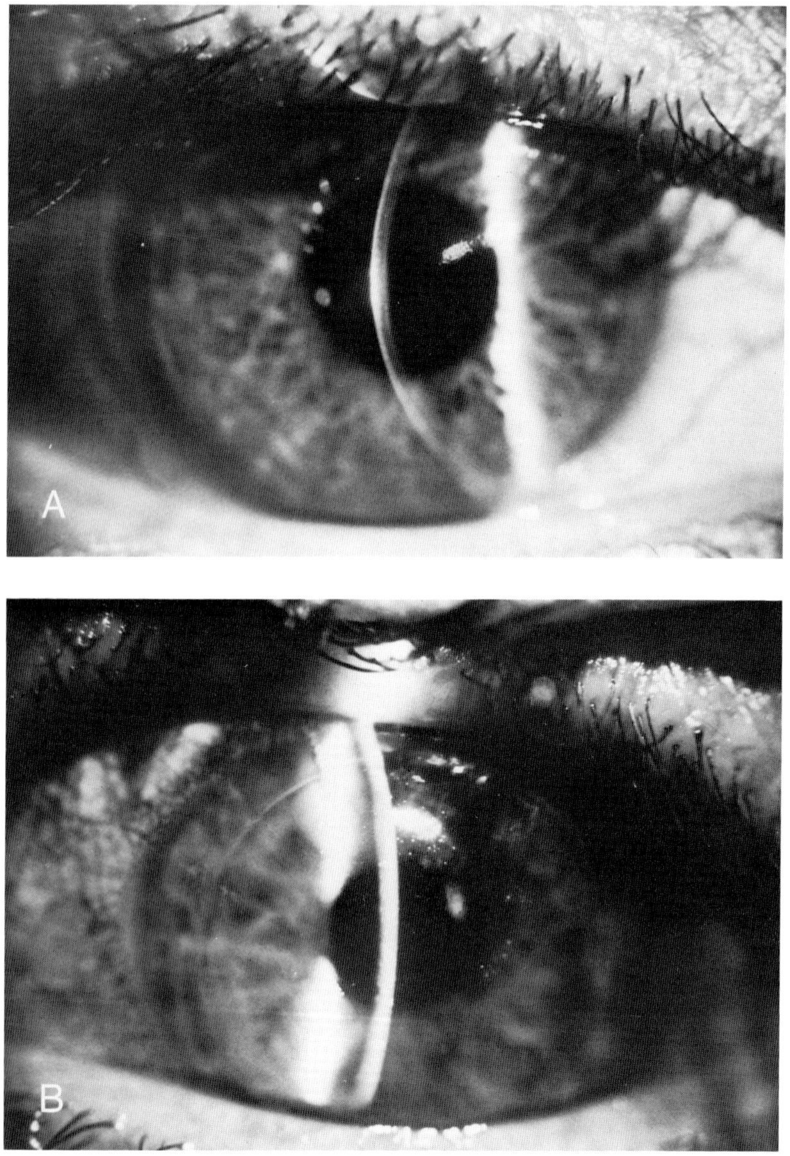

Fig. 18-17. (A) Preoperative slit-lamp view of cornea with keratoconus. **(B)** Slit-lamp view of epikeratophakia graft for keratoconus 2 months after surgery, with sutures still in place.

moved at 3 weeks. The graft sutures are removed 3 months after surgery (Fig. 18-17).

Prognosis

Although the lens has no optical properties, the corneal compression decreases myopia by 5 to 8 diopters. Regular astigmatism also decreases by about 4 diopters. By 4 months postsurgery, most of these patients have resumed full-time daily contact lens wear and have visual acuities equal to, or nearly equal to, their best corrected preoperative acuities.

Complications

Complications are largely the same as those for aphakic and myopic epikeratophakia. There is the possibility that a paracentral scar will move centrally with corneal compression and interfere with vision. Also, a large proportion of keratoconus patients, particularly young ones, react adversely to the 10-0 nylon sutures, with injection, ciliary flush, and sterile microabscesses developing around each suture. In cases in which the epithelium is intact, the use of dilation and corticosteroids, four times a day for 1 week, then tapered over 3 days and discontinued, generally resolves the problem quickly.

EPIKERATOPHAKIA PATCH FOR CORNEAL REPAIR

Pterygium

Clinical Picture and Indications

In cases of multiple recurrences of pterygium, for which adequate excision has been performed numerous times, an inlay lamellar graft cut from a plano epikeratophakia tissue lens can be used to provide tectonic support for the thinned cornea.

Surgical Technique

The pterygium and the inflamed conjunctiva to which it is attached are resected, with the leading edge conforming to a straight vertical line from limbus to limbus. A circular plano epikeratophakia lens is cut on a cord corresponding to the length of the leading edge of the dissection. The half-moon–shaped graft is sutured into place with interrupted sutures. The peripheral area of bare sclera is covered with a conjunctival flap. A strip of bare sclera is left uncovered between the inlay lens and the flap, to maintain the continuity of the tear film and minimize the formation of dellen, as well as to prevent limitations in the motion of the eye (Fig. 18-18).

Prognosis and Complications

The bed in which the inlay lamellar graft is placed must be absolutely clear of any debris. Bare stroma provides an extremely sticky surface, one that is much more difficult to irrigate and keep clean than Bowman's layer. However, any small piece of foreign material, such as sponge or suture, will be extremely difficult to remove; it will be trapped beneath the graft and will result in the invasion of numerous blood vessels, which can lead to recurrence of the pterygium.

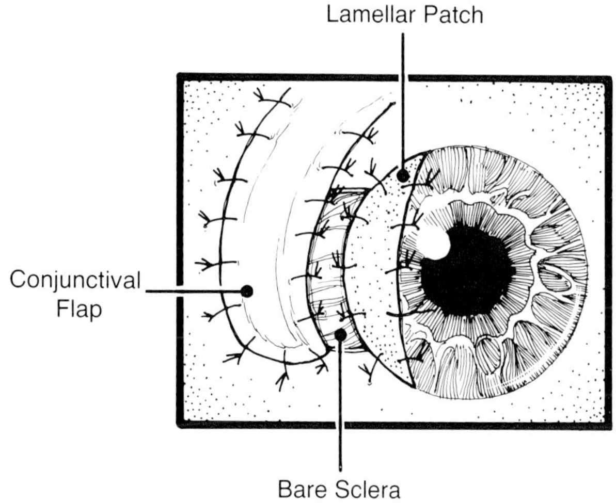

Fig. 18-18. Inlay graft for pterygium. A circular lyophilized plano tissue patch is cut to a half-moon shape, rehydrated, and sutured to the cornea to reinforce the thinned area from which the head of the pterygium has been removed. A conjunctival flap is performed to cover the bare limbal area. An area of bare sclera is left to inhibit regrowth of the pterygium.

The limbal sutures must be watched carefully and removed early, sometimes as soon as 2 weeks after surgery, to prevent vascularization. The central sutures are left in place for 3 to 6 weeks. Most patients require a new spectacle overcorrection, but vision is good. The surgery does not interfere with contact lens fitting. No cases of high induced corneal cylinder have been seen at LSU.

Perforation

Clinical Picture and Indications

An onlay tissue graft that is actually a kind of miniepikeratophakia can be used in cases of small peripheral descemetocele, corneal perforation, or deep ulcer. In very inflamed eyes, perforated ulcers that are too large to glue can be repaired with these tissue grafts, permitting medical treatment that may obviate the need for penetrating keratoplasty, or at least maximize the potential for the success of the penetrating graft by delaying surgery long enough for treatment with antibiotics, antiviral agents, or corticosteroids.

Surgical Technique

The surgeon should remove as much necrotic tissue as possible, as the situation warrants. A trephine is selected with a diameter sufficient to encompass the thinned area, such that the circular trephine cut is located in healthy tissue. A 0.3-mm–deep cut is made, and the inner wall of the cut dissected to the 0.3 mm depth plane. A thin piece of tissue is punched from the plano tissue lens to the same diameter as the trephine cut and sutured into place. For grafts 3.0 mm or more in diameter, the diameter of the patch is 0.5 mm larger than the trephine cut. The patch restores the integrity of the eye and supports the thinned area of the cornea (Fig. 18-19).

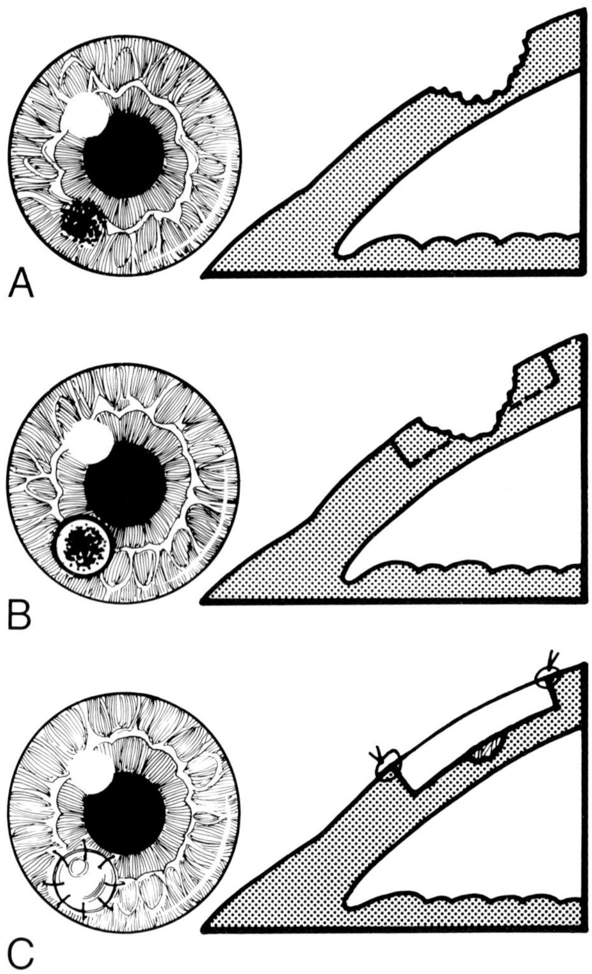

Fig. 18-19. Onlay graft for perforation. **(A)** Necrotic debris is removed from the perforation. **(B)** A trephine cut is created in healthy tissue outside the area of the perforation, and a bed is prepared for the graft tissue. **(C)** A circular patch is cut from a lyophilized plano tissue lens and rehydrated. The patch is sutured into the prepared bed to fill the wound and reinforce the cornea.

ACKNOWLEDGMENTS

This work was supported in part by U.S. Public Health Service grants EY03635, EY02580, and EY02377 from the National Eye Institute, National Institutes of Health, Bethesda, MD and by an unrestricted grant from Research to Prevent Blindness, Inc., New York City.

REFERENCES

1. Barraquer JI: Keratomileusis and keratophakia. p. 409. In Rycroft PV (ed): Corneoplastic Surgery: Proceedings of the Second International Corneoplastic Conference. Pergamon Press, New York, 1969
2. Kaufman HE: The correction of aphakia. Am J Ophthalmol 89:1, 1980
3. Werblin TP, Klyce SD: Epikeratophakia: The surgical correction of aphakia. I. Lathing of corneal tissue. Curr Eye Res 1(3):123, 1981
4. Werblin TP, Kaufman HE: Epikeratophakia: The surgical correction of aphakia. II. Preliminary studies in a non-human primate model. Curr Eye Res 1(3):131, 1981
5. Werblin TP, Kaufman HE, Friedlander MH, Granet N: Epikeratophakia: The surgical correction of aphakia. III. Preliminary results of a prospective clinical trial. Arch Ophthalmol 99:1957, 1981
6 Werblin TP, Kaufman HE, Friedlander MH, et al: A prospective study of the use of hyperopic epikeratophakia grafts for the correction of aphakia in adults. Ophthalmology 88:1137, 1981

7. Werblin TP, Kaufman HE, Friedlander MH, et al: Epikeratophakia: The surgical correction of aphakia. Update: 1981. Ophthalmology 89:916, 1982
8. Asbell PA, Werblin TP, Loupe DN, et al: Secondary surgical procedures after epikeratophakia. Ophthalmic Surg 13:555, 1982
9. McDonald MB, Koenig SB, Safir A, et al: Epikeratophakia: The surgical correction of aphakia. Update: 1982. Ophthalmology 90:668, 1983
10. Rich LF, Friedlander MH, Kaufman HE, Granet N: Keratocyte survival in keratophakia lenticules. Arch Ophthalmol 99:677, 1981
11. Safir A, McDonald MB, Klyce SD, et al: The cornea press: Restoring donor corneas to normal dimensions and hydration before cryolathing. Ophthalmic Surg 14:327, 1983
12. Safir A, McDonald MB, Friedlander MH, et al: Compensating for thermally caused dimensional changes in the cryolathe. Ophthalmic Surg 15:306, 1984
13. McDonald MB, Kaufman HE: Refractive keratoplasty. p. 276. In Steele ADMcG, and Drews RC (eds): Cataract Surgery. Butterworths International Medical Reviews: Ophthalmology 2. Butterworths, London, 1984
14. McDonald MB, Kaufman HE: Refractive Corneal Surgery. Module 11: Focal Points, 1984. Clinical Modules for Ophthalmologists. American Academy of Ophthalmology, San Francisco, 1984
15. McDonald MB, Kaufman HE: Refractive surgery for visual rehabilitation of aphakia. p. 622. In Ginsberg SP (ed): Cataract and Intraocular Lens Surgery: A Compendium of Modern Theories and Techniques. Vol. 2. Aesculapius, Birmingham, Al, 1984
16. Morgan KS, Werblin TP, Asbell PA, et al: The use of epikeratophakia grafts in pediatric monocular aphakia. J Pediatr Ophthalmol Strabismus 18(6):23, 1981
17. Morgan KS, Werblin TP, Friedlander MH, Kaufman HE: Epikeratophakia in the pediatric patient: A case report. J Ocul Ther Surg 1:198, 1982
18. Morgan KS, Asbell PA, McDonald MB, et al: Preliminary visual results of pediatric epikeratophakia. Arch Ophthalmol 101:1540, 1983
19. Morgan KS, Asbell PA, May JG, et al: Pediatric epikeratophakia. p. 937. In Reinecke RD (eds): Strabismus II: Proceedings of the Fourth Meeting of the International Strabismological Association, Asilomar CA, October 25–29. Grune & Stratton, Orlando, 1984
20. Morgan KS, Stephenson GS, McDonald MB, Kaufman HE: Epikeratophakia in children. Ophthalmology 91:780, 1984
21. Morgan KS, Marvelli TL, Ellis GS Jr, Arffa RC: Epikeratophakia in children with traumatic cataracts. J Pediatr Ophthalmol Strabismus 23:108, 1986
22. Morgan KS, Stephenson GS: Epikeratophakia in children with corneal lacerations. J Pediatr Ophthalmol Strabismus 22(3):105, 1985
23. Arffa RC, Marvelli TL, Morgan KS, et al: Keratometric and refractive results of pediatric epikeratophakia: Effect of patient age. Invest Ophthalmol Vis Sci 26(suppl):204, 1985 (Abst.)
24. Arffa RC, Marvelli TL, Morgan KS: Keratometric and refractive results of pediatric epikeratophakia. Arch Ophthalmol 103:1656, 1985
25. Werblin TP, Klyce SD: Epikeratophakia: The surgical correction of myopia. I. Lathing of corneal tissue. Curr Eye Res 1(10):591, 1981/1982
26. McDonald MB, Klyce SD, Suarez H, et al: Epikeratophakia for myopia correction. Ophthalmology 92:1417, 1985
27. Kaufman HE, Werblin TP: Epikeratophakia for the treatment of keratoconus. Am J Ophthalmol 93:342, 1982
28. McDonald MB, Koenig SB, Safir A, Kaufman HE: Onlay lamellar keratoplasty for the treatment of keratoconus. Br J Ophthalmol 67:615, 1983

Conjunctival Flaps and Pterygium 19

William M. Townsend

CONJUNCTIVAL FLAPS

The conjunctival flap has been in use for the treatment of corneal disease since the 1800s.[1] In the ensuing years, much was made of the technique used to fashion the flap, as if a racquet-shaped design offered true advantages over a bridge or other designs.[2] In reality, Gundersen's contribution of popularizing the use of conjunctiva only and leaving Tenon's capsule behind was a truly significant advance.[3] This innovation, dating from 1958, marked the beginning of the modern era in the use of the flap. In more recent years, however, the deserved popularity of the procedure waned considerably with the arrival of bandage contact lenses and the increased availability of donor corneal tissue. Some, for all practical purposes, have declared the procedure worthless,[4] thereby erasing an important modality of treatment from the repertoire of the newer generations of eye surgeons. Nevertheless, like all worthwhile things, the conjunctival flap will survive as an easily performed, highly effective solution for many vexing corneal problems.

Indications

Elimination of Resistant Active Infection

Keratomycoses. A recent major textbook states that a rationale is lacking for the use of conjunctival flaps if there is active fungal disease.[4] A corollary of this concept is that keratoplasty is a better method of eliminating a recalcitrant mycotic keratitis. The truth is quite the opposite: the best possible rationale for the use of flaps in these cases exists, in that the procedure works. Table 19-1 lists the results of treatment with this modality. A comparison with the results achieved using "a chaud" therapeutic keratoplasty in similar cases[5,6] demonstrates the greater efficacy of the flap. This empirical finding has a readily available explanation. The corneal stroma does contain immunoglobulins, elements of a humoral mediated immune system. The body defenses against fungi depend on the cell-mediated immune system, however, which is absent from the cornea.[7] As such, the tissue lacks defenses against fungi, and even saprophytic types multiply unscathed. By contrast, the conjunctival flap is rich in

Table 19-1. Conjunctival Flaps vs. Therapeutic Grafts in the Treatment of Recalcitrant Mycotic Ulcers

		Infection Cured		Good Vision Potential	
	N	*N*	%	*N*	%
Conjunctival flap	21	15	71	12	57
Therapeutic PKP	8	4	50	2	25

(Cavalcanti R, Townsend WM: unpublished data.)

vascular and lymphatic channels that provide a direct route for the local delivery of T lymphocytes. It must be emphasized that the flap is preferable to the therapeutic penetrating graft: not only is it more effective in eliminating active infection, but it also leaves the anterior segment in much better condition. Histologic examination of enucleated eyes with keratomycosis[8] shows that the hyphae select the deep layers for colonization, accumulating not only in the posterior corneal stroma but encroaching on the trabecular meshwork over the iris surface as well and even reaching the posterior chamber. The inflammatory reaction attracted to these deep sites promotes the severe complications that befall keratoplasty and render the eye useless, even if it does eliminate the actual infection: pupillary block and extensive anterior synechiae with intractable glaucoma.[9]

The actual timing of the decision to perform the conjunctival flap is crucial to the success of the operation. If the patient comes for treatment early, there is time to treat medically and observe for a beneficial response over the ensuing 5 to 7 days. Lack of response or definite progression (Fig. 19-1) is the signal for immediate surgery (Fig. 19-2). Waiting longer or allowing the process to deepen and form corneal or anterior chamber abscesses (Fig. 19-3) usually dooms the eye, and the flap is commonly eroded (Fig. 19-4). No one will dispute that a medical cure is the goal in the keratomycoses. The unfortunate fact remains that a therapeutic response with recovery of useful vision is rarely achieved with current antifungal agents. Until better agents appear on the market, the conjunctival flap is really the only effective barrier against progression of fungal infection. Bacterial ulcers, on the other hand, rarely fail to respond to aggressive treatment with the vast therapeutic armamentarium available today.

Herpes Simplex Ulceration. Among the various forms of herpetic ulceration, several produce recurrent or chronic longstanding inflammation that is unresponsive to antiviral medication. Such prolonged morbidity is common with chronic superficial keratitis and with the deep stromal ulcerative form so susceptible to necrosis and even perforation. Lamellar therapeutic keratoplasty, advocated by some as a means to eliminate active disease, has given poor results. Pfister et al.,[10] as well as Rice and Jones,[11] reported failure rates in the vicinity of 90 percent, most due to herpetic recurrence at the donor–recipient interface. Experience with therapeutic penetrating keratoplasty has also been discouraging. Polack and Kaufman[12] noted a high failure rate (almost 50 percent) in 20 eyes grafted with active disease, in contrast to the high success rate (80 percent) recorded when the procedure was performed in the inactive stage. Similar results have been reported in more recent studies.[13,14] By contrast, the conjunctival flap has been very effective in eliminating active inflammation. Paton and Milauskas[15] cited 36 cases of chronic stromal disease in which only four persisted with active inflammation after application of the flap.

Replacement of Damaged Corneal Epithelium by Conjunctiva

Whether damaged intrinsically (healing defects, chronic edema, trophic ulcers, neuroparalytic keratitis) or surrounded by a hostile environment (keratitis sicca, exposure keratitis, melting disorders), the defective corneal epithelium can be replaced by conjunctiva with beneficial results. The conjunctiva is highly resistant, bearing as it does its own vasculature as a source of nourishment, anabolic metabolites, and body defenses against infection. The other side of the coin is that the corneal area will lack transparency, interfering with good vision if the area lies within the visual axis. When the patient has a visual need for the affected eye, some method other than the flap should be considered. The same conclusion holds true if the surface disturbance is only temporary or self-limited (recurrent erosions, transient seventh nerve palsy). Even if the lesion is central but there is no visual need, however, or if the lesion occupies a peripheral position, the benefits and drawbacks

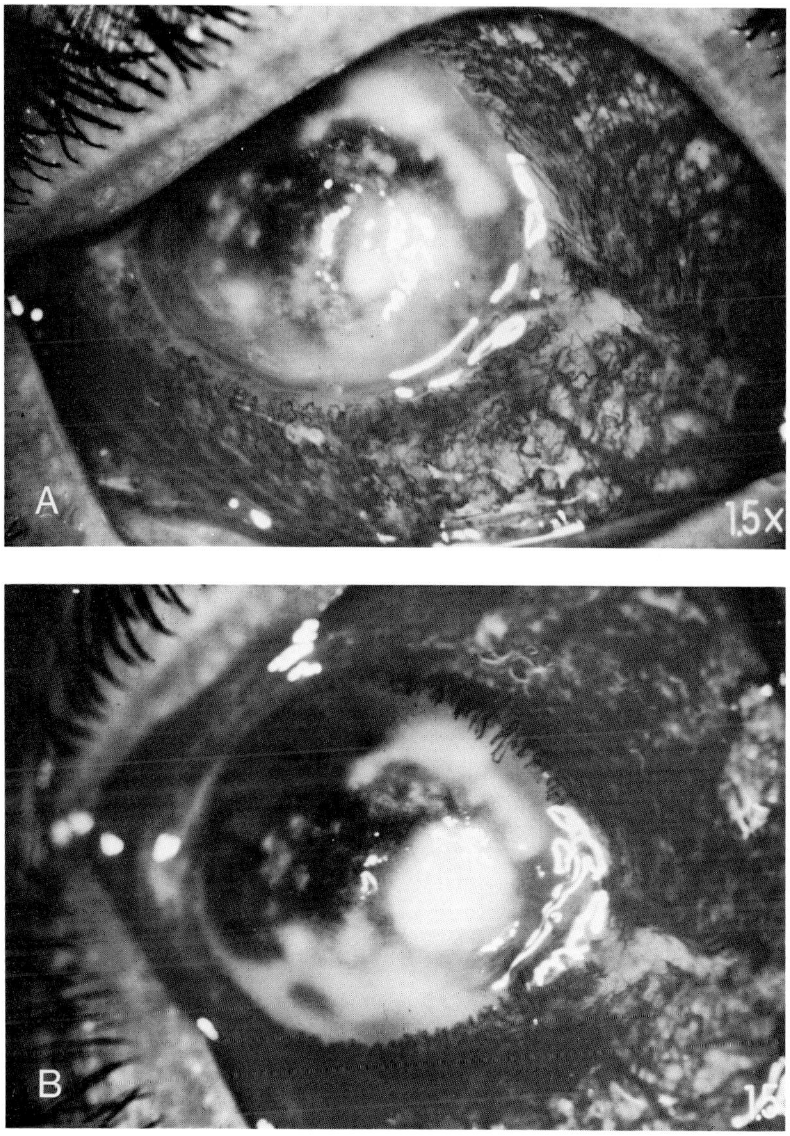

Fig. 19-1. (A) Pulularia mycotic ulcer. Note severity of involvement with deep plaques. **(B)** Three weeks later, 0.3 percent topical amphotericin B has not prevented worsening of case. Stromal abscess has formed.

of the thin conjunctival flap must be weighed against those of the therapeutic soft lens: Can the patient return every 4 to 6 weeks for observation? Can the patient wear the lens without rapid buildup of deposits? Will the patient retain the lens without losing it every 2 to 3 months? Is infection likely?

The conjunctival flap is especially suited for the treatment of bullous keratopathy in elderly patients with no visual need in the affected eye.[16] Similarly, in patients with melting disorders and severe corneal thinning, the corneal tissue used for tectonic reconstruction may suffer the same fate as the original host's cornea unless further protected with a conjunctival flap.

Tectonic Support

A taut, carefully sutured thin flap may be used to seal a perforated cornea if corneal donor tissue is not available. Although better than nothing, a flap will help the anterior chamber re-form, but previously formed anterior synechiae remain and some aqueous leakage is common during the early

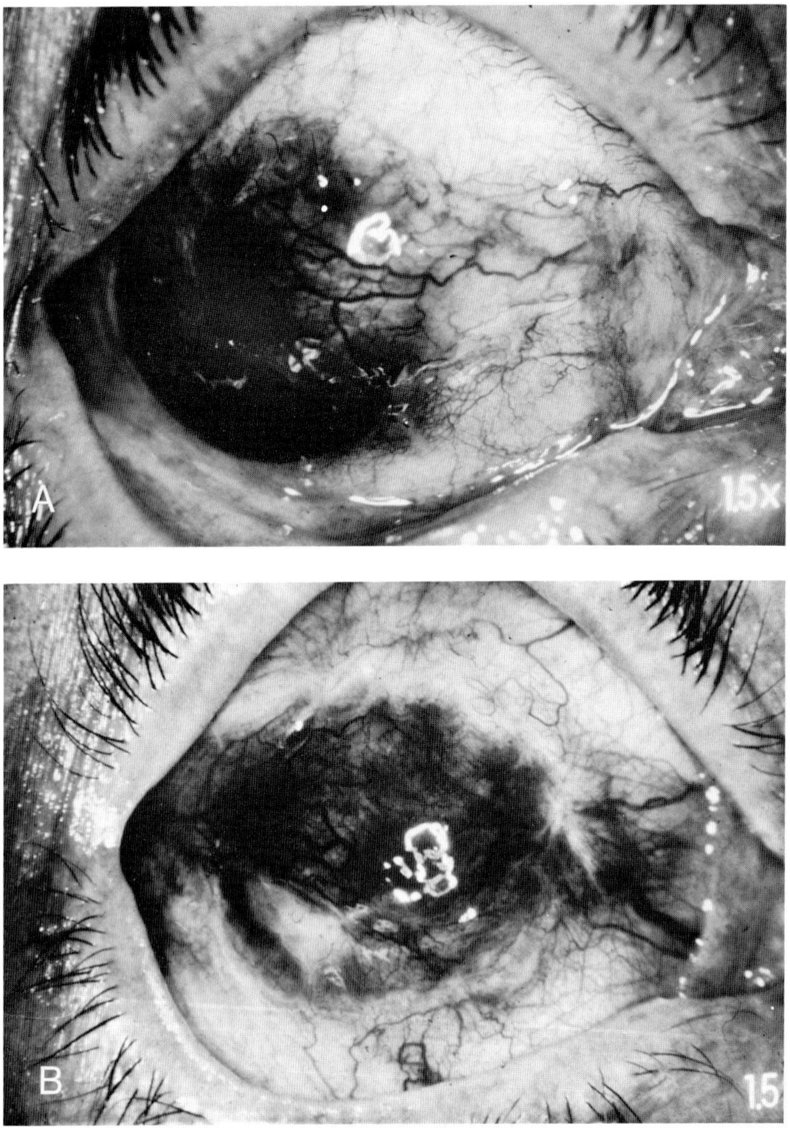

Fig. 19-2. **(A)** Less than 1 week after Gundersen flap, there is little scleral reaction as the stromal abscess has resolved. **(B)** Six months after Gundersen flap, the eye is quiet and free of infection.

postoperative period. Another tectonic application for the thin conjunctival flap relates to phthisical eyes. In preparation for the use of a cosmetic shell, the flap provides a strong lining that is less likely to be subject to erosions than the corneal epithelium.

Surgical Technique (After Gundersen)

General anesthesia is preferable for congested eyes associated with mycotic ulcers and active herpetic disease. In quiet eyes, topical anesthesia reinforced with 2 percent lidocaine infiltration under the bulbar conjunctiva is usually sufficient. A retrobulbar injection of 2 percent lidocaine is sometimes necessary, especially in the presence of mild to moderate ciliary congestion. After the speculum is applied, Gundersen[16] calls for a limbal traction at the 12 o'clock position so as to tort the globe downward. A useful variation is to place a 4-0 silk suture under the superior rectus instead. The suture serves not only to provide traction but also to indicate the superior limit of the conjunctival incision (to be made later) if significant degrees of sym-

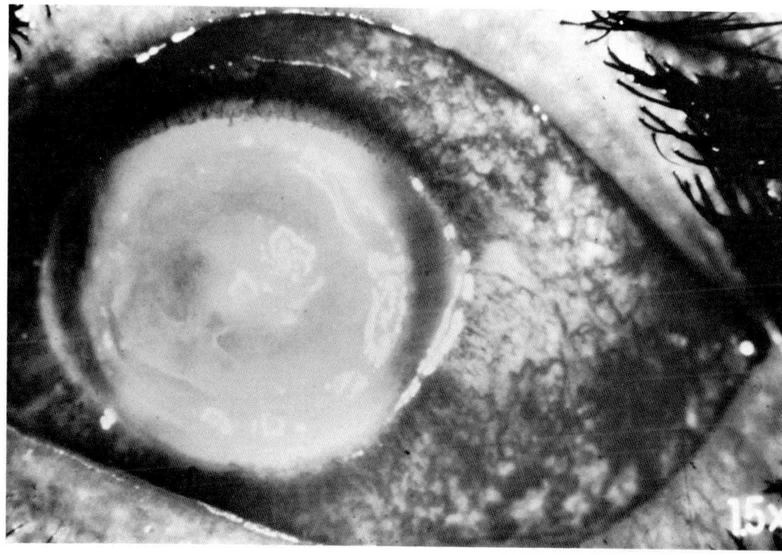

Fig. 19-3. Severe necrosis of stroma with abscess in the anterior chamber.

blepharon formation are to be avoided. One to 2 ml of lidocaine with 1 : 50,000 epinephrine is used to balloon the superior bulbar conjunctiva, which will be used for the flap. The needle is inserted, beveled side up, over the horizontal meridian, taking care not to puncture the conjunctiva to be included in the flap. The infiltration is done external to Tenon's capsule; it should balloon the conjunctival layer only, reaching from canthus to canthus (Fig. 19-5). The intention is to aid both in securing hemostasis and in separating the two layers. With fine-toothed forceps and Wescott scissors, the conjunctival incision is begun just inferior to the superior rectus suture and continued nasally and temporally, taking care to maintain the same distance parallel to the superior limbus (Fig. 19-6). Dissection of the flap now proceeds as in the preparation of a huge limbal-based flap (Fig. 19-7). In fashioning the flap, the desired thickness is obtained by placing the tip of the scissors blade on the conjunctival undersurface, but before cutting, observing the over surface to make sure that a buttonhole will not result. Dis-

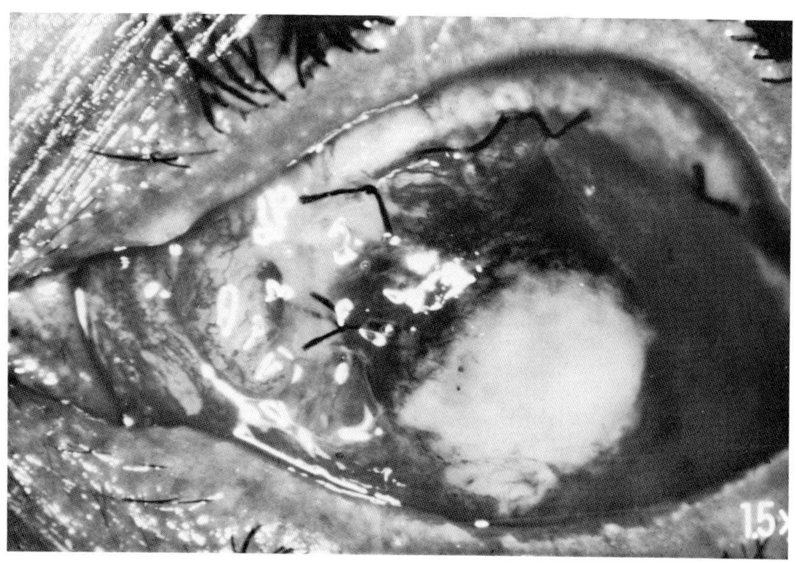

Fig. 19-4. Perforation of flap with growth of abscess. Flap applied too late.

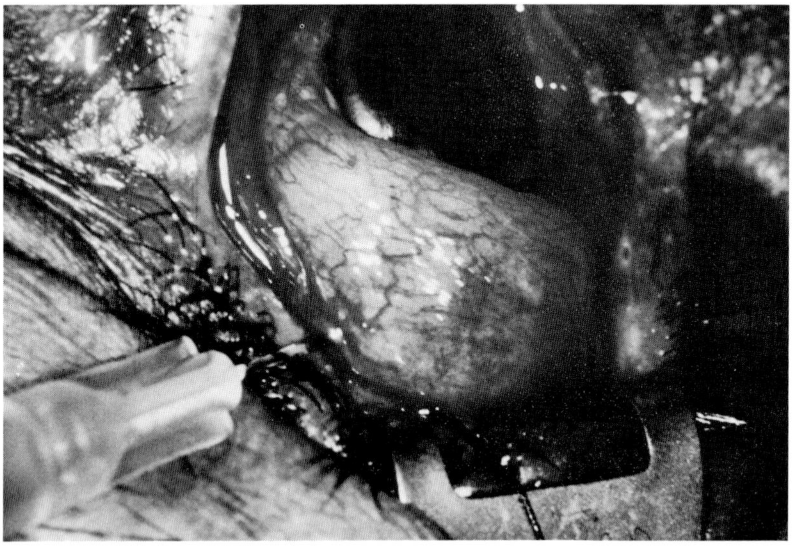

Fig. 19-5. Ballooning of conjunctiva with 1.5 ml lidocaine containing 1:10,000 epinephrine.

section is facilitated if an assistant can use a forceps to tent up the subconjunctival tissues, which is then easily cut safely between the two forceps, one holding the latter tissue and the other, held by the surgeon, grasping the conjunctiva itself. Dissection continues until the limbus is reached all around between the 9 and 3 o'clock positions. A sharp blade is then used to make a buttonhole at the limbal attached end. Through it, the Wescott scissors can be introduced, and a 360-degree peritomy is made (Fig. 19-8), thus freeing completely the bridge flap from the superior bulbar surface.

To ensure proper adhesion to the corneal surface, Gundersen advocated a superficial keratectomy. Actually, removal of the epithelium only is adequate. The flap is now slid down to cover the bared corneal surface, making sure that the conjunctival surface is not inverted. After spreading the thin flap smoothly, it is sutured both above and below to the limbal cornea or episclera using a 10, 0 nylon running suture. If the lower suture is applied first (Fig. 19-9) then upper one can be used to give the proper tension: the fit should be snug but stretching the conjunctiva is undesirable. If the

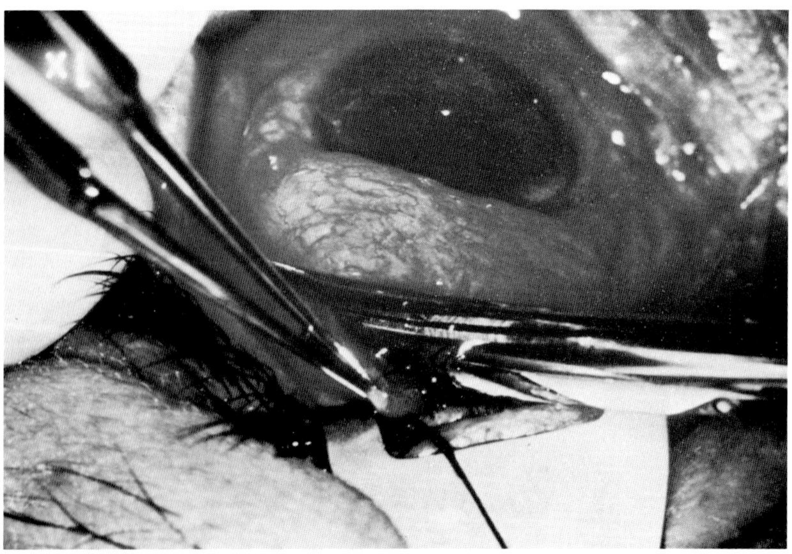

Fig. 19-6. Incision of conjunctiva continued parallel to limbus.

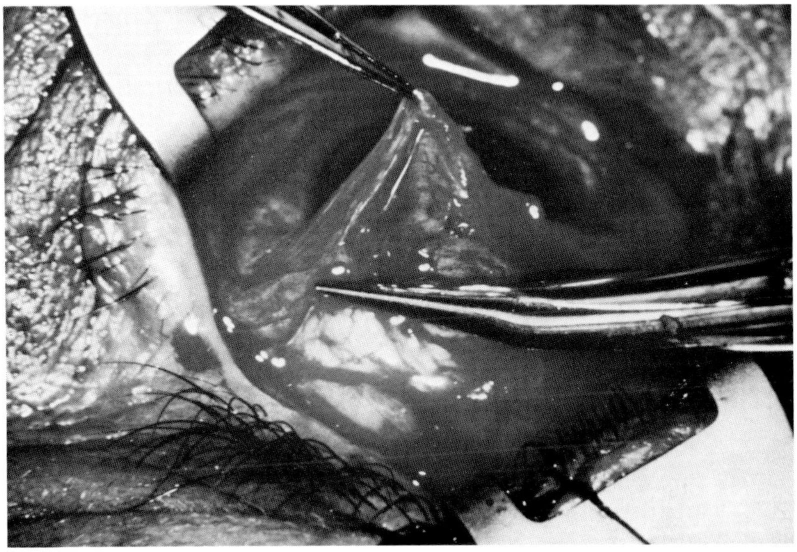

Fig. 19-7. Dissection of flap toward the limbus.

thickness obtained is the proper one, the underlying corneal surface is easily seen under the flap. The surface bared of conjunctiva is left uncovered, as a new conjunctiva re-forms rapidly.

Postoperative Care

The primary goal of postoperative care is to avoid damage to the flap. A protective patch is kept on for 48 hours, after which a mild topical antibiotic solution is used for 1 week. It is important to avoid both antimycotic and antiviral agents during this period for they only serve to irritate the fragile tissue. Sutures are removed after 1 month.

Complications

During the surgical procedure, buttonholing of the flap may be managed by placement of a suture if small. Large buttonholes require that a new flap be made. The lower bulbar conjunctiva is the second site of choice as the lateral bulbar conjunctiva is

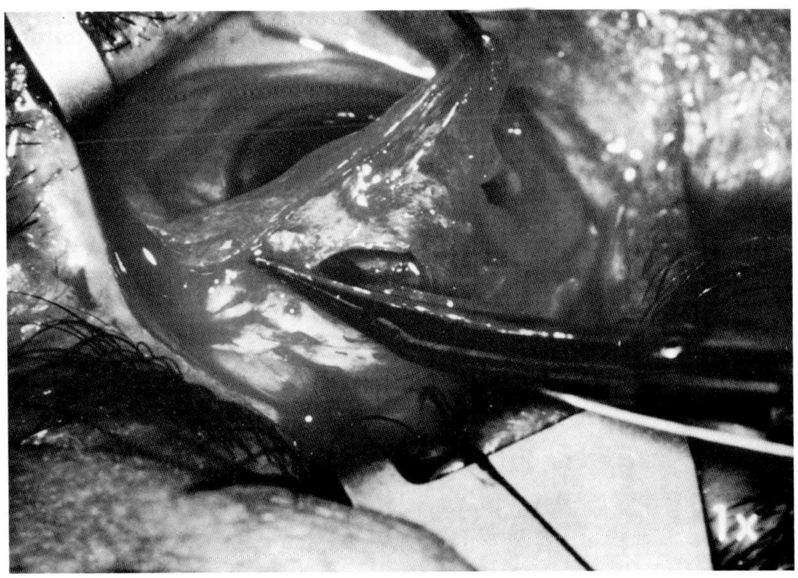

Fig. 19-8. Limbal peritomy, including not only area of flap but the entire circumference as well.

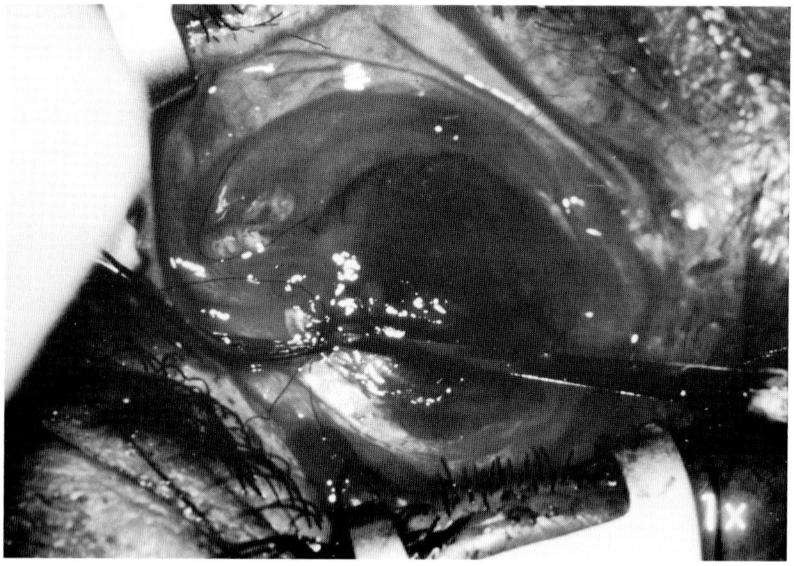

Fig. 19-9. The flap is placed over the de-epithelialized corneal surface taking care to maintain the epithelial side up. It is sutured with running 10-0 nylon both above and below.

surprisingly small in area and is of little value as a potential source of tissue. Not infrequently, the conjunctival flap dissected is seen to be insufficient to cover the entire corneal surface. Rather than force the situation by stretching the tissue, it is preferable to decrease the area of coverage and thus avoid tension.

Upward retraction of the flap is the most common significant complication during the early postoperative period. It is serious because the supply of available conjunctiva is limited and there may not be enough for a second attempt. Every possible step should therefore be taken at surgery to avoid this complication. The following principles are helpful:

1. To avoid vertical tension, do not stretch the flap.
2. Do not make flap too thin.
3. Take wide bites on the flap side when suturing its inferior edge to the limbus as the sutures tend to erode through.
4. With ocular movement, there is tugging of the flap communicated by its attachments to the normal conjunctival surface. To avoid this tension, it is logical to isolate the flap as much as possible from the contiguous conjunctiva. The bridge flap of Gundersen, sutured above and below is certainly more isolated than a partial flap, often used for peripheral lesions (Fig. 19-10).

Some degree of ptosis, usually minimal and cosmetically insignificant is noted in most patients with a flap. Severe cases require removal of scar tissue and plastic repair. Other complications include the formation of granulomas and inclusion cysts, both readily managed by simple excision.

PTERYGIUM

What is a pterygium? Most textbooks evade this question, offering a mere description of the lesion instead of a true definition. Since the days of Susruta, thousands of years before Christ, it has been known as a triangular sheet of fibrovascular tissue that appears on the epibulbar conjunctiva, disturbing both the victim for its unsightly appearance and the surgeon for its tenacious tendency to recur. A definitive classification of the lesion still eludes us. Is it a degeneration or an inflammation? There is also uncertainty regarding its etiology and pathogenesis, for the pterygium, to borrow from Amsler's comment about keratoconus, is a condition that resembles only itself.[17] Nevertheless, we can characterize the lesion as accurately as possible and point out the best available methods for its successful surgical removal.

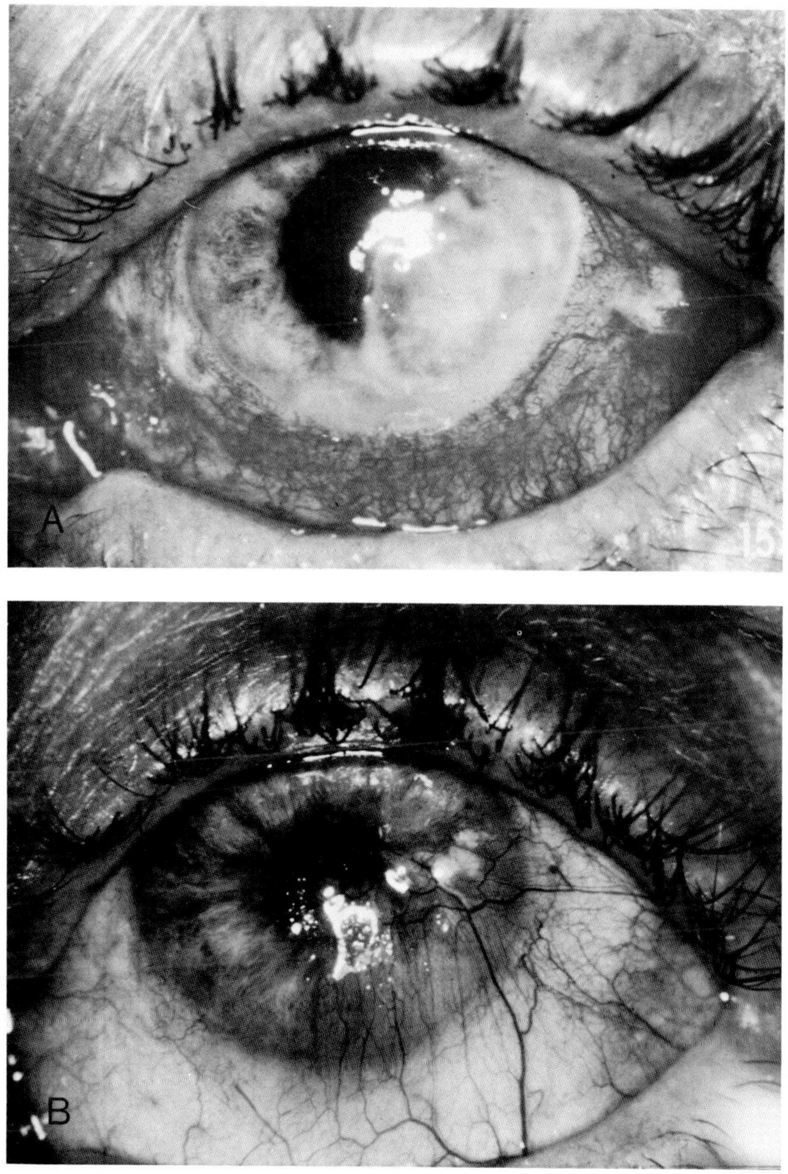

Fig. 19-10. (A) Peripheral mycotic ulcer (Fusarium). **(B)** Healed lesion after partial flap.

Clinical Picture

More often than not, the pterygium is already fully formed by the time the patient first seeks help. The history usually indicates that the tissue grew very rapidly over a period not exceeding "two or three months." At times, it will be acknowledged that prior to the burst of rapid growth the lesion had been a very small mound, present for many months or even years. In rare instances, the full evolution of the condition can be witnessed. In these cases, the initial lesion is indistinguishable from a pinguecula, which suddenly has attracted prominent vessels (old and new) from both conjunctiva and episclera (Fig. 19-11). The yellowish mound elongates, assuming the shape of an hourglass. In the following weeks or months, the prominent new vessels continue to appear nasal to the mound, while on the corneal side many delicate vascular twigs project from its base and point in the direction of the segmentally engorged limbal plexus (Fig. 19-12). Now the body of the ptery-

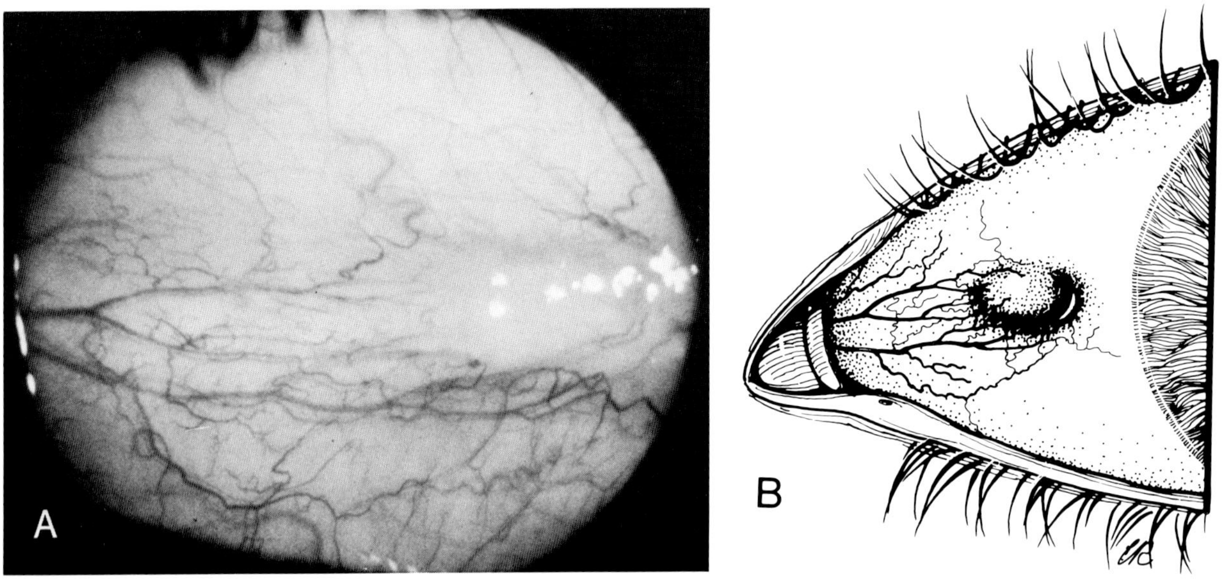

Fig. 19-11. Pinguecula. **(A)** Clinical photograph. **(B)** The initial pterygium lesion is indistinguishable from a pinguecula, which has suddenly attracted prominent vessels (old and new) from both conjunctiva and episclera.

gium becomes defined as a substantial band with the appearance of the upper and lower folds.

The entire lesion becomes a true pterygium when the yellowish mound, now the head, encroaches upon the limbal cornea (Fig. 19-13). Actual penetration is signaled by the appearance of a halolike subepithelial cap inside the cornea. In contrast to this relatively rapid formation, the march of the pterygium across the cornea is very slow, usually requiring several years to reach the

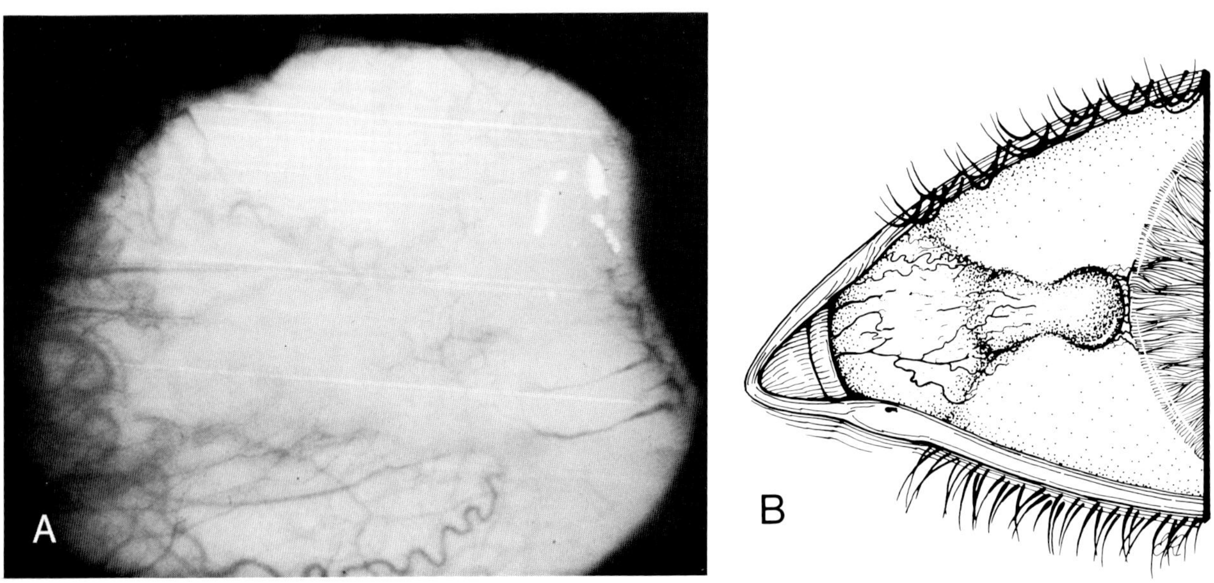

Fig. 19-12. **(A)** Elongation of pinguecula and appearance of neovascularization on its canthal end as well as over its corneal end. Note also congestion of the limbal plexus. **(B)** Drawing shows the hour-glass shape formed as the pinguecula elongates.

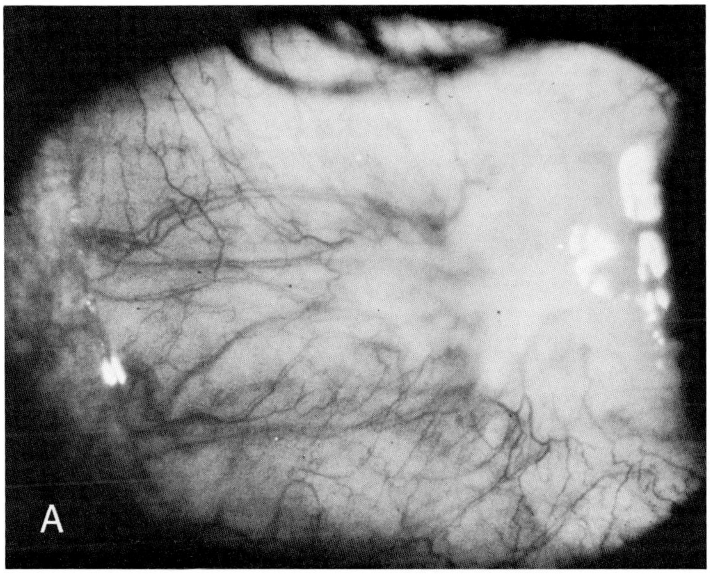

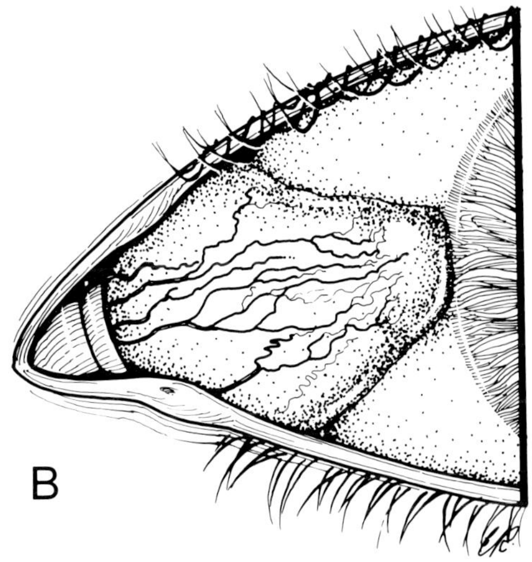

Fig. 19-13. (A) Consolidation of pinguecula into pterygium head at limbus and definition of its body. **(B)** Drawing shows well-defined pterygium.

pupillary axis. Often, however, there is a curiously abrupt cessation of growth at some point. This inactivation is characterized by the cessation of episodic congestion, disappearance of punctate staining over the body, and shrinkage of the halolike cap.

The lesion just sits there, remaining stationary for years. Symptoms produced by a pterygium relate mostly to those intermittent episodes of congestion when it becomes hyperemic, provoking severe photophobia, tearing, and foreign body sensation. The cosmetic blemish is always there. Amsler recorded up to 1.5 diopters of against-the-rule astigmatism.[17] In severe cases, the patient may complain of diplopia due to symblepharon formation and limitation of ocular rotation.

Eventually, involutionary changes set in. The head thins and flattens progressively, producing a scar of macular density that blends inperceptibly with the adjacent cornea, while the body withers into a veil-like membrane traversed by only a few delicate blood vessels (Fig. 19-14). Actively growing pterygia occur typically in the younger age group (20 to 30 years), the period of greatest incidence. The most exuberant ones, extremely fleshy masses with large corneal extension, are seen in persons exposed to the elements, such as farmers and construction workers. Primary pterygia can then be placed into one of five groups:

1. Actively growing pterygia
2. Fleshy or malignant pterygia
3. Slow-growing pterygia
4. Stationary pterygia
5. Atrophic pterygia

The successful removal of a pterygium is not only dependent on the surgical technique used, but also on the type of lesion encountered. Those falling into groups 3, 4, and 5 can be removed by just about any expedient technique, with little risk of recurrence. If the same technique is then used to remove lesions that fall into groups 1 and 2, recurrence is likely.

Surgical Pathology

Three basic elements give substance to the histologic appearance of pterygium (Fig. 19-15). An epithelial covering composed of atrophic conjunctiva reaches beyond its normal anatomic confines onto the cornea. It overlies the second important element: a bulky mass of thickened, hypertro-

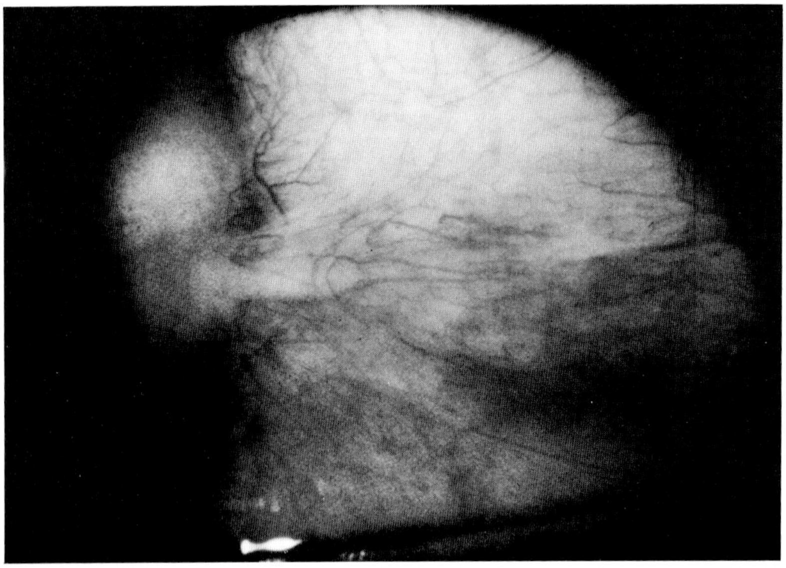

Fig. 19-14. Atrophic pterygium. Note flattening of head and veil-like thinning of body.

phied, and degenerated connective tissue. Its collagen component assumes a coiled, fibrilated pattern reminiscent of elastic tissue. Indeed, the abnormal collagen shows basophilia and affinity for elastic tissue stains but is not digested by elastase,[18] thereby falling into a category of elastoid or elasticlike degeneration. Similar changes are seen in the dermis of actinic keratosis lesions. The third important element is vascular. New blood vessels, usually congested, are dispersed between the hypertrophied collagen fibers. In addition, the episcleral bed under the pterygium shows hyperemia, thus participating in the inflammatory reaction. Figure 19-16 illustrates the limbal relationships of pterygia. Because Tenon's capsule is absent at the limbus, the subepithelial connective tissue at this site lies directly over the episclera. A short distance toward the canthus, however, Tenon's capsule

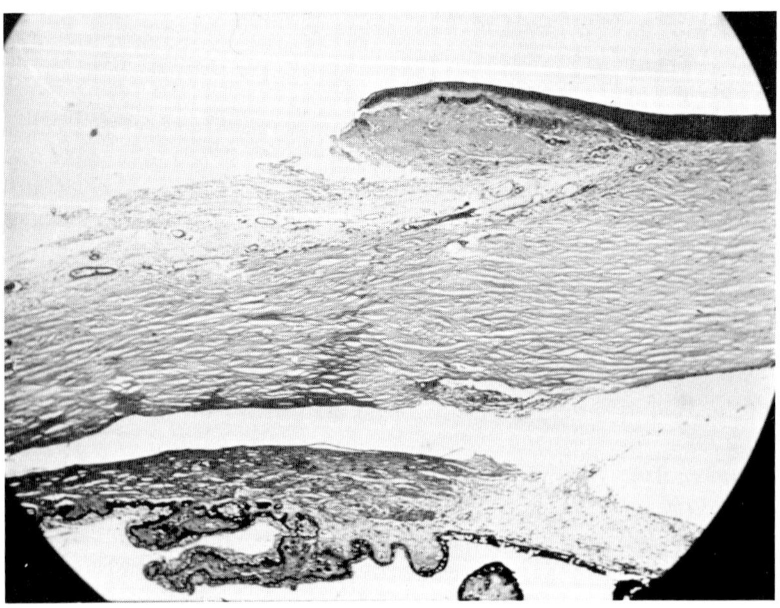

Fig. 19-15. Histologic appearance of pterygium.

makes its appearance; in this location, the same connective tissue will lie not over episclera, but over the thicker parietal layer of Tenon's tissue. This layer is probably incorporated into the pterygium body, contributing to its vasculature and bulk. Because Tenon's space is interposed between it and the episclera, the pterygium body is loose and nonadherent, thus able to slide forward across the epibulbar surface and into the cornea. On the corneal side just in front of the head, an advancing row of fibroblasts can be seen penetrating the cornea in single file, wedged between Bowman's and the basement membrane of the overlying corneal epithelium (Fig. 19-16B). These account for the gray zone or cap observed with the slit lamp and prepare a path for the head to enter the cornea. As it does, Bowman's membrane is pushed downward and eventually fragmented (Fig. 19-16C). The fibrovascular tissue of the pterygium head becomes firmly adherent to the superficial stroma over these sites of focal interruption in Bowman's membrane.

Methods of Treatment

Pterygium would certainly arouse less interest were it not for its stubborn tendency to recur despite all the techniques designed through the years to avoid just that. The earliest technique used, that of evulsion, was practiced by the Greeks and still has its devotees.[19] The method that followed, simple excision, has suffered from the same high recurrence rate obtained by evulsion, 23 to 75 percent.[20] This complication spurred the development of alternative methods for handling the pterygium once its head was dissected off the cornea.

Desmarres (1855)[21] initiated the concept that shifting the dissected pterygium head to a new position away from the cornea would lead to atrophy of the lesion by virtue of eliminating its stimulus for growth into the transparent tissue. McReynolds (1902)[22] modified the technique by burying the tissue under the conjunctiva.

Many variations have been described.[23] For example, Knapp (1868) favored splitting the pterygium before suturing it to the conjunctiva. Blaskovics (1931) folded the head under the body. Neher, Stocker, Doherty, Busacca, Miller, and others have favored other minor modifications. Pari passu to the establishment of the technique of transplantation, the excision technique itself was evolving. Some considered it essential to cover the entire exposed raw epibulbar defect with normal conjunctiva as far as the limbus. Arlt (1872), Terson (1911), Campodonico (1922), Arruga (1937), and Bangerter (1943) designed various rotating flaps to achieve this objective.

Others[24] recommended the use of a free graft to cover the scleral defect, introducing the barrier concept. In this view, the grafted tissue acts as a barrier against the passage of new vessels from the conjunctiva into the cornea, thereby helping avoid recurrence. Elsching (1926), Majoros (1930), Gómez-Marquez (1931), and others favored the use of conjunctiva obtained from bulbar surface of the same eye or from the opposite eye. Various other tissues were suggested as sources of graft. Svoboda (1946) favored buccal mucous membrane, Gifford (1909) advocated the use of skin, and Castroviejo (1950) recommended cornea. Later, the barrier concept was extended to the sclera itself. D'Ombrain (1948), McGavic (1949), Sugar (1949), and King (1961) were proponents of this modification. The barrier effect of conjunctiva is limited in value because the plane followed by the new vessels that foster recurrence is deeper, over the episclera itself. The scleral plane is the correct one. Indeed, those who introduced the bare sclera concept emphasized the importance of excising the subconjunctival connective tissue present under the body of the pterygium in deterring recurrence. Picó (1964)[25] agreed with Alger (1964)[26] that the source of recurrence is the formation of granulation tissue in the raw corneal and scleral surface. The all-important principle then becomes the prevention of new vessel formation in the bared episcleral surface with the use of such methods as cauterization and β-irradiation. The former eliminates existing blood vessels, while the latter has a delayed effect, lasting several weeks, which is particularly effective in arresting the formation of new capillary endothelium. Rapid epithelialization also helps diminish the formation of granulation tissue. A smooth surface promotes rapid ingrowth of the adjacent epithelium; the use of a burr to polish the raw limbal surface has been advocated (Paton D, personal communication, 1972). Covering the raw episcleral surface with a

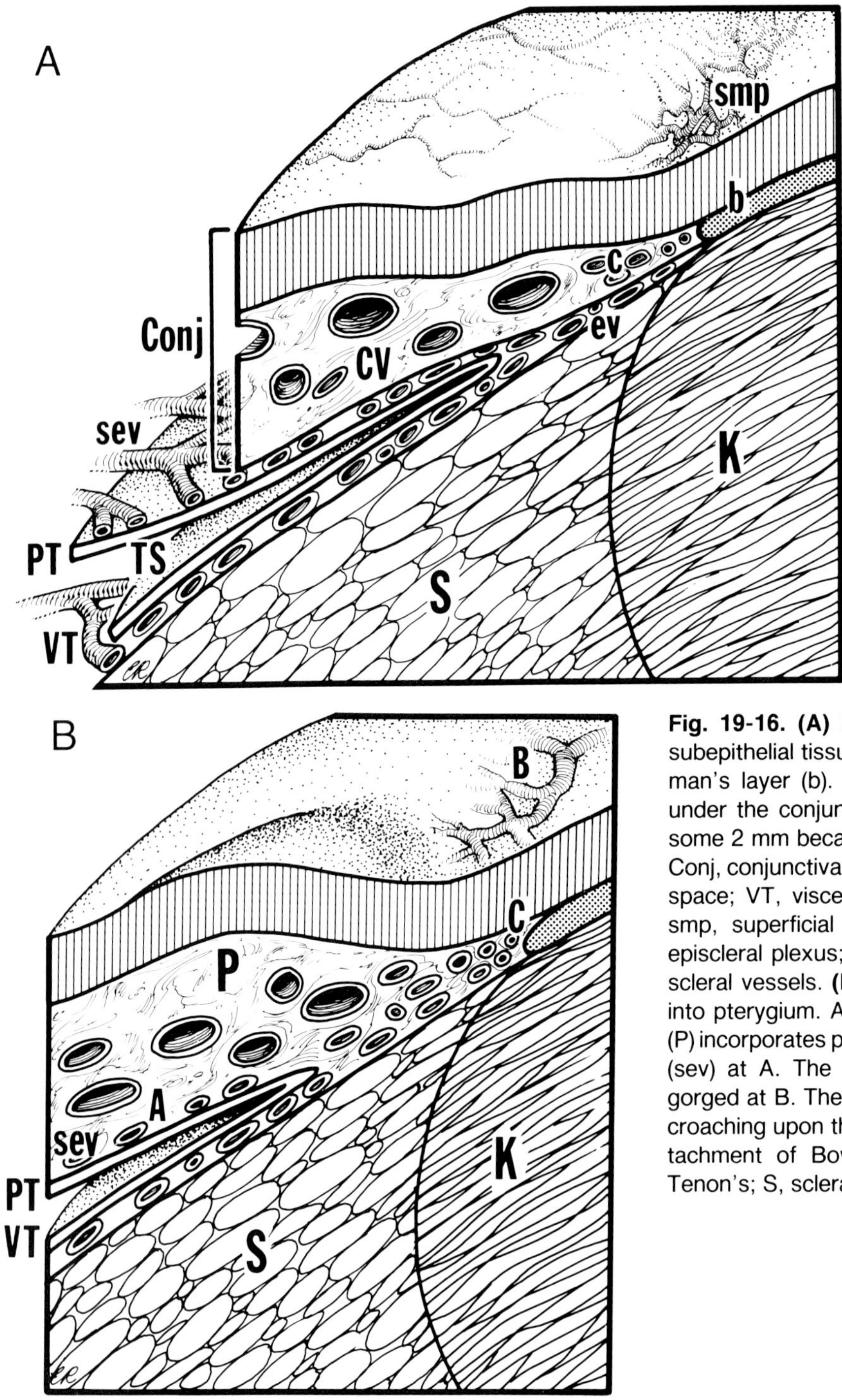

Fig. 19-16. (A) Limbal anatomy. The conjunctival subepithelial tissue (c) is in the same plane as Bowman's layer (b). The episcleral vessels lie directly under the conjunctival subepithelial tissue for only some 2 mm because Tenon's is interposed distally. Conj, conjunctiva; PT, parietal Tenon's; TS, Tenon's space; VT, visceral Tenon's; S, sclera; K, cornea; smp, superficial marginal plexus; sev, superficial episcleral plexus; CV, conjunctival vessels; ev, episcleral vessels. **(B)** Development of the pinguecula into pterygium. Abnormal connective tissue mound (P) incorporates parietal Tenon's (PT) with its vessels (sev) at A. The superficial marginal plexus is engorged at B. The abnormal connective tissue is encroaching upon the cornea (K) and there is early detachment of Bowman's layer at C. VT, visceral Tenon's; S, sclera. *(Figure continues.)*

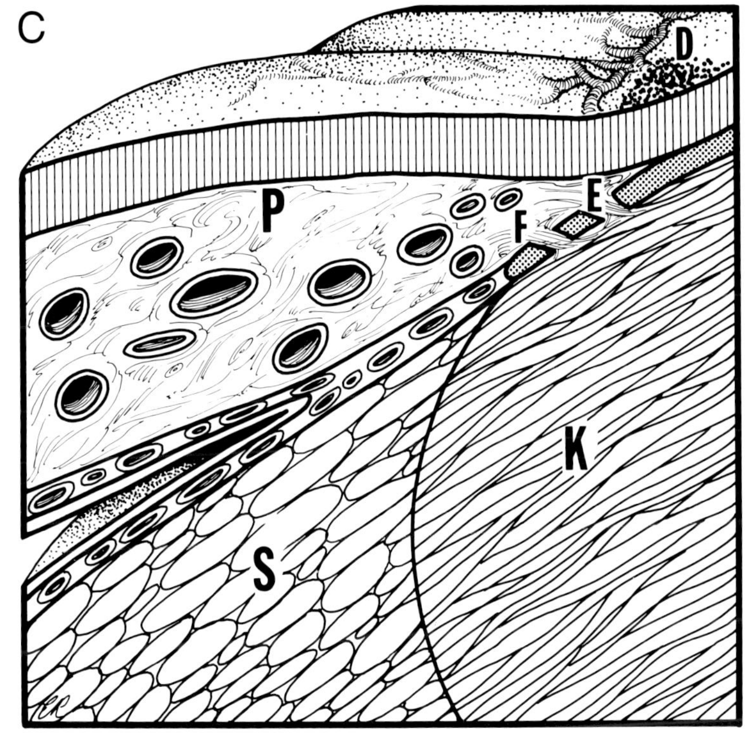

Fig. 19-16 *(Continued)*. **(C)** Formed pterygium. The pterygium head is preceded by fibroblasts between Bowman's and the epithelium, giving rise to the clinically apparent gray zone (D). The following vascularized connective tissue is seen detaching Bowman's layer (E). This tissue is penetrating the stroma through dehiscences in Bowman's itself. **(F)** These are the only sites of adhesion of pterygium to the globe because the bare episclera, and more distally, the Tenon's space, are not invaded. P, pterygium mound; S, sclera; K, cornea.

flap of healthy conjunctiva is another means of achieving this end.

The truth of the matter is that most cases with either the stationary or the atrophic form of pterygia will do well even with a simple excision or evulsion, never even hinting at recurrence. But if the same expedient technique is then used for an active or fleshy lesion, a prompt recurrence is bound to occur.

Recommended Technique

The technique recommended makes every possible maneuver to prevent recurrence. The results are gratifying in that observed rates are as low as 3 percent, a far cry from those cited by other investigators. The procedure has been used for many years by Picó[25] with some modifications from the method described by Castroviejo.

Anesthesia

Following the application of a topical anesthetic, 1.5 ml 2 percent lidocaine (Xylocaine) with epinephrine (1 : 10,000) is injected under the body of the pterygium, using a short 26-gauge needle (Fig. 19-17). The body of the pterygium and the surrounding conjunctiva are readily ballooned by the solution. Very fleshy, extensive, or recurrent pterygia may require retrobulbar anesthesia. Van Lint akinesia is also recommended for these cases.

Partial Superficial Keratectomy

A sharp blade is used to make incisions into clear cornea some 0.75 mm in front of and parallel to the edges of the head (Fig. 19-18). The depth of penetration is just beneath Bowman's membrane. Some cases require deeper penetration before a bed clean of pterygium tissue is reached. A scleral dissector is important for fashioning a smooth and even keratectomy, while a fine-toothed forceps (0.12 Castroviejo) is essential for adequately grasping the keratectomized tissue.

Transition to Limbus

The approach of the dissection to the limbal plane is signaled by a shift of the bed's transparent quality to a more opaque one and frequently by bleeding (Fig. 19-19). In order to avoid continuing the dissection along a deeper level than desired,

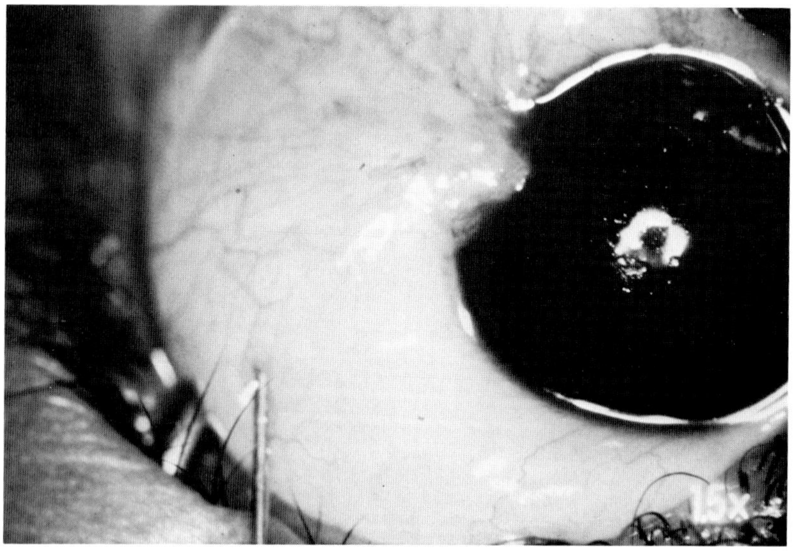

Fig. 19-17. Anesthesia. After topical anesthesia, 1.5 ml 2 percent lidocaine (Xylocaine) with epinephrine (1 : 10,000) is injected under the body of the pterygium.

into the episclera itself, it is important to shift to Wescott scissors and to step up with the tip of the blades directed upward, thereby piercing the undersurface of pterygium. Alternatively, Wescott scissors may be introduced at right angles over one of the limbal ends and the neck cut in this manner (Fig. 19-19). When the entire width of the pterygium neck is thus severed from the limbus, the head and body become loose and freely movable.

Excision of the Pterygium

Horizontal incisions above and below the body of the pterygium are continued in angular fashion toward the semilunar fold, where they converge. The pterygium is then excised en bloc (Fig. 19-20). The remaining bed should reveal a clean episcleral surface adjacent to the limbus; more laterally, the rectus insertion is visible under a covering of fascia.

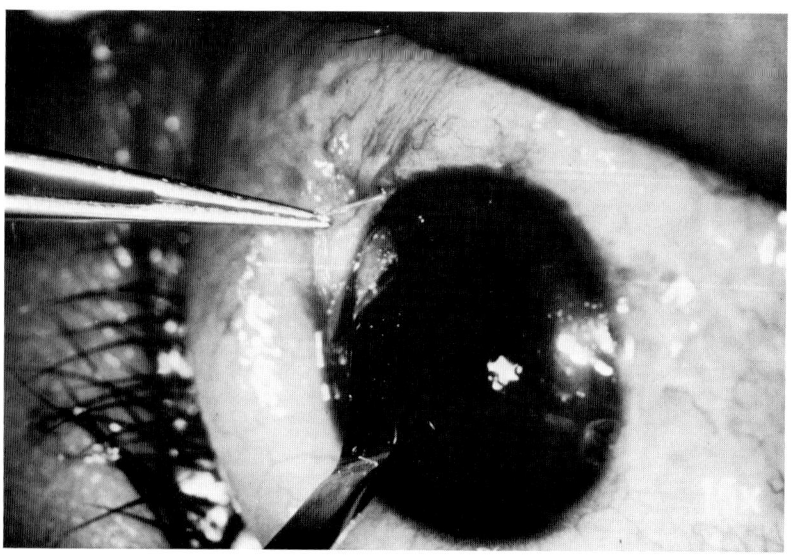

Fig. 19-18. Partial superficial keratectomy. Dissection is deeper than Bowman's layer and should include all blood vessels.

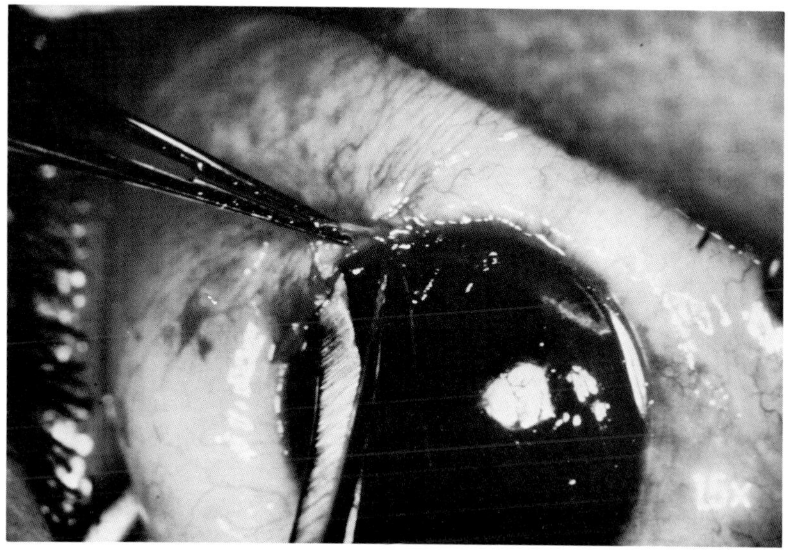

Fig. 19-19. Transition to limbus, stepping up to limbus with scissors to avoid sclera. The pterygium is now free, since its body is not adherent to the sclera.

The subepithelial connective tissue excised with the pterygium will have included the limbal portion of Tenon's capsule (parietal layer). The remaining cut edges are seen to be smooth, pale, and uninvolved.

Scraping and Cauterization of the Bare Area

A rectangular area 3 mm wide adjacent to the limbus is cleaned of tissue tags by scraping the episcleral surface with the flat side of the blade (Fig. 19-21). Light cautery is then applied to close all vessels in the area.

Sliding Conjunctival Flap

The superior horizontal free edge of conjunctiva is lifted with a fine-toothed forceps and, with the help of Wescott scissors, separated from the underlying Tenon's capsule (Fig. 19-22). The thinned conjunctiva is now incised vertically about 3 mm from the limbus. The incision is continued superiorly until the superior fornix is approached. The

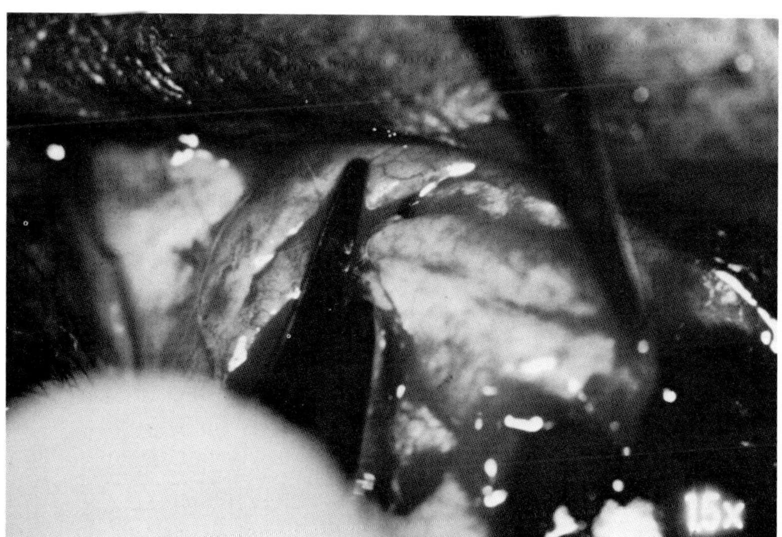

Fig. 19-20. Excision of pterygium. The body is excised. Rectangular incisions above and below converge to meet at the plica semilunaris.

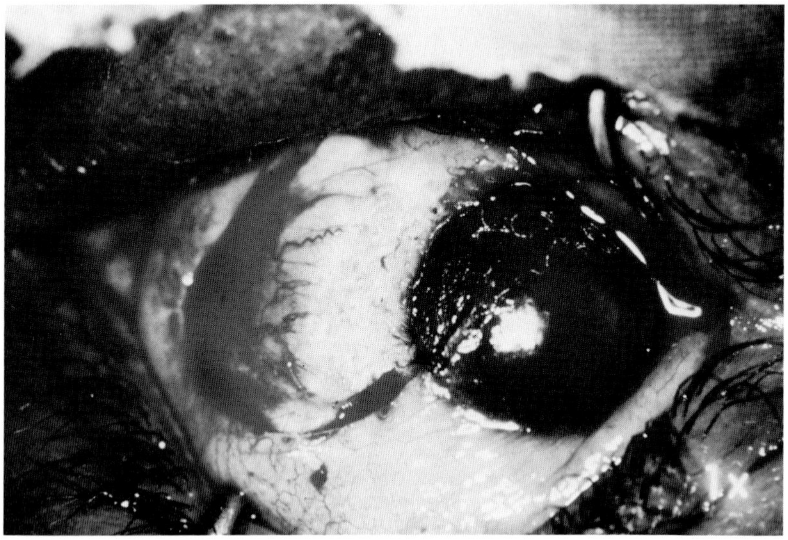

Fig. 19-21. Scraping and cauterization of bare area. Rectangular area 3 mm wide adjacent to the limbus is scraped; light cautery is applied, leaving the zone clean and smooth.

distal or canthal segment of conjunctiva thus formed is brought down and sutured both to the episclera and to the overlying inferior horizontal conjunctiva near its free edge. The slid flap now covers the raw epibulbar surface, leaving, however, a 3-mm bare sclera adjacent to the limbus. Additional sutures may be necessary to close horizontal or vertical gaps between the flap and the adjacent conjunctiva; 8-0 silk is recommended.

Application of β-Radiation

The bare area is subjected to the application of 2,000 REP of β-radiation with a ^{90}Sr applicator. This procedure is performed before the patient leaves the operating room (Fig. 19-23).

The radiation is applied with the intention of preventing the formation of new episcleral capillaries that might act as a source of granulation tissue and recurrence. At the same time, it provides a scleral barrier, an avascular zone that hinders the forward growth of episcleral vessels into the limbus and cornea. The effectiveness of β-radiation becomes readily apparent when different series, with and without radiation, are compared. Picó[25] observed a recurrence rate of 3 percent with and 8 percent without. In Hilger's[27] series, it was 8 percent with and 23 percent without, while Cameron[28] cited higher rates, 16 percent with and more than 50 percent without. Like x-rays and γ-rays, β-rays are emissions of high-speed electrons that induce ionizing radiation, leading to tissue damage. The penetration of β-rays is very limited, however, with only 20 percent of the surface dose penetrating a distance of 3 mm.[29] Furthermore, β-rays are highly selective in the type of tissue affected, with collagen showing little change while vascular walls and young, actively dividing endothelium displaying exquisite sensitivity.[30] The tissue effect appears within a very short latency period (hours) but persists for several weeks. The long duration of action and the conveniency of working with the anesthetized eye make the operative moment ideal for application.

Postoperative Care

The overriding principle in postoperative care is prevention of vascularization. The pressure bandage is removed after 48 hours. If, as usually happens, the corneal and conjunctival epithelium have re-formed, the patch is discarded and topical steroids are applied frequently, with the intention of arresting the inflammatory process as much as possible. Steroids are continued for a period of 4 to 6 weeks, the usual time required for all inflammation to subside. All sutures are removed 5 days after surgery.

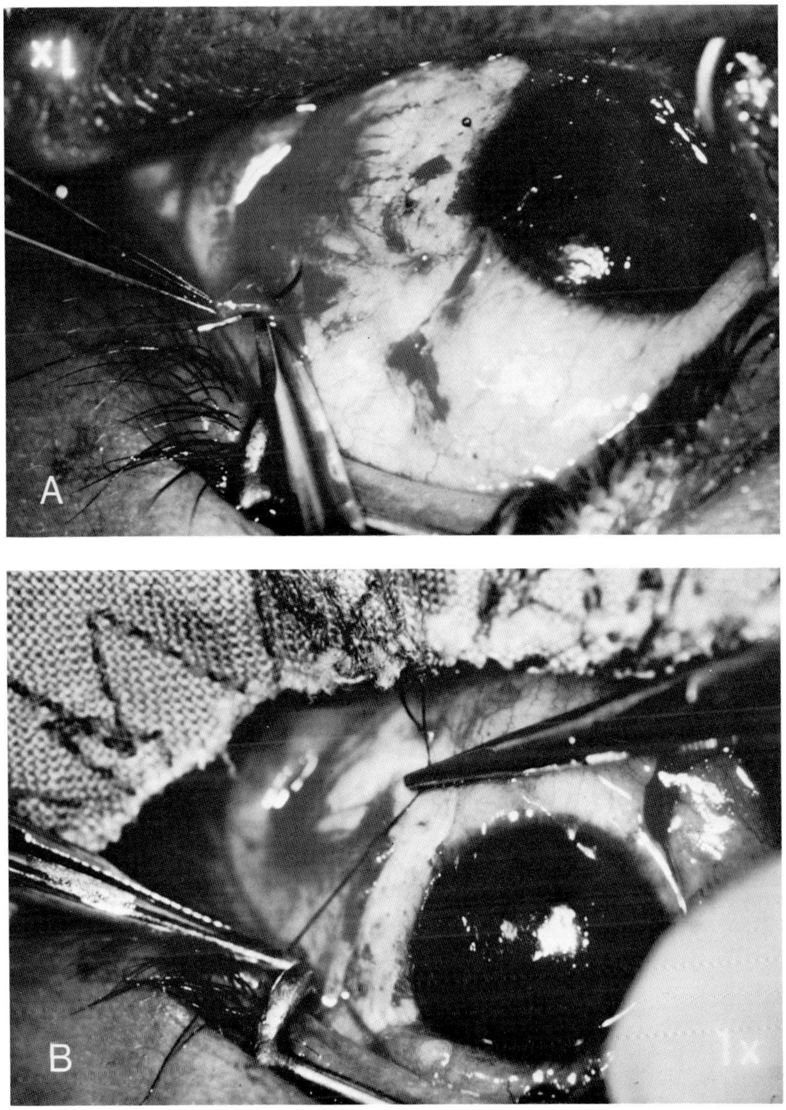

Fig. 19-22. (A,B) Sliding conjunctival flap.

Complications

All the complications that may occur at surgery can be avoided with proper care. Perforation of the cornea during the keratectomy is nearly impossible with microscopic visualization and maintenance of a superficial plane of dissection. If it does occur, the dissected tissue should be sutured back when donor tissue is not available. Perforation or dissection into the sclera is avoidable by taking care to observe the limbal junction and then shifting to a more superficial plane. Damage to the horizontal muscles is prevented by careful separation of the subconjunctival scar tissue and identification of the tendon prior to excising the former, especially in recurrent lesions.

Postoperative complications include infection, usually of the scleral bed, granuloma and dellen formation, as well as the appearance of amputation neuromata.[31] Some degree of scarring is inevitable at the keratectomy site. Usually of mild degree, it does not interfere with vision unless the pupillary axis is encroached upon. Minor degrees of astigmatism may occur with excision of lesions with consid-

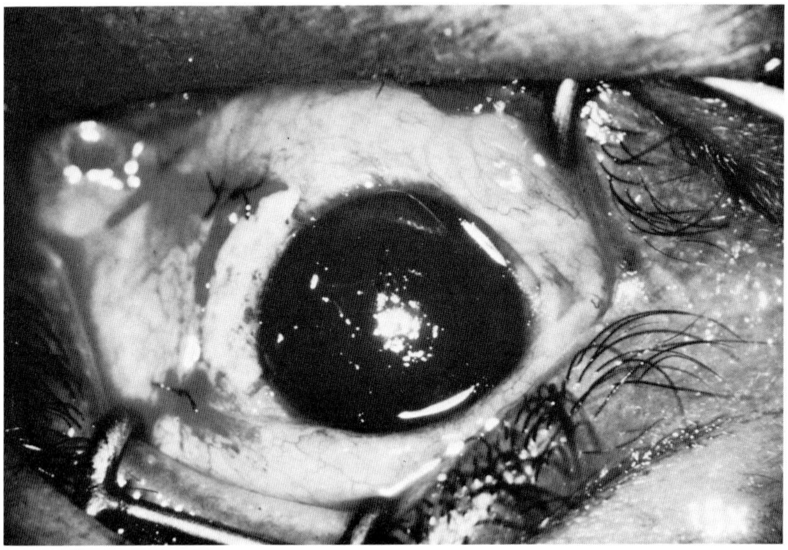

Fig. 19-23. Appearance after application of β-radiation.

erable corneal involvement. Complications may also result from the application of β-radiation. Telangectasia of the episcleral and conjunctival vasculature, conjunctivitis, and episcleritis have occurred rarely[32] in large series. Cataract formation has been described frequently, but usually when total surface dosage considerably exceeded the ceiling level of 4,000 REP.[33]

Recurrence

Within 2 or 3 weeks of surgery, fine capillaries may be seen in some cases. Appearing to arise from the episcleral surface under the flap, many parallel vessels race forward toward the bare area in brushlike fashion. If left alone, they often cross the bare area and extend into the cornea with surprising speed. Within a matter of weeks, the vascularized region becomes covered by fibrous tissue similar in appearance to the original pterygium body, leaving the patient with a lesion as unsightly as the original one. Whether this lesion constitutes a true recurrence or not is academic. From the patient's viewpoint, the pterygium has surely grown back. Therefore, prompt action is required as soon as the brushlike vessels are detected. They should be scraped and cauterized under local anesthesia, and an additional 1,000 REP of β-radiation should be applied to the area.

Once the recurrence is fully developed, further surgery is inevitable, but the surgeon should regard the lesion as one considerably different from the original one. The subconjunctival fibrous tissue element is more abundant and tightly bound to the underlying sclera. As such, Xylocaine infiltration will be impossible, as the liquid will no longer reach the adherent areas. This factor as well as the sharp dissection that will be required to free the sclera require the use of retrobulbar or even general anesthesia. The involved sector of cornea may be too thin, due to previous keratectomies, or the planned procedure may require a deep lamellar resection if deep-lying vessels are present. In either circumstance, a peripheral lamellar keratoplasty is indicated.[34]

Aside from these considerations, which may apply in general to any recurrent lesion, the surgeon must take into account the amount of conjunctiva remaining as well as the possible presence of symblepharon, with limitation of ocular rotation (Fig. 19-24). This latter complication is readily evident upon inspection of the involved eye, but judging the adequacy of conjunctival supply must wait until surgery. At this time, in contrast to the primary procedure, the conjunctiva covering the pterygium body is saved until after its separation from the subconjunctival scar tissue. Often it is found to be shrunken and actually smaller than anticipated.

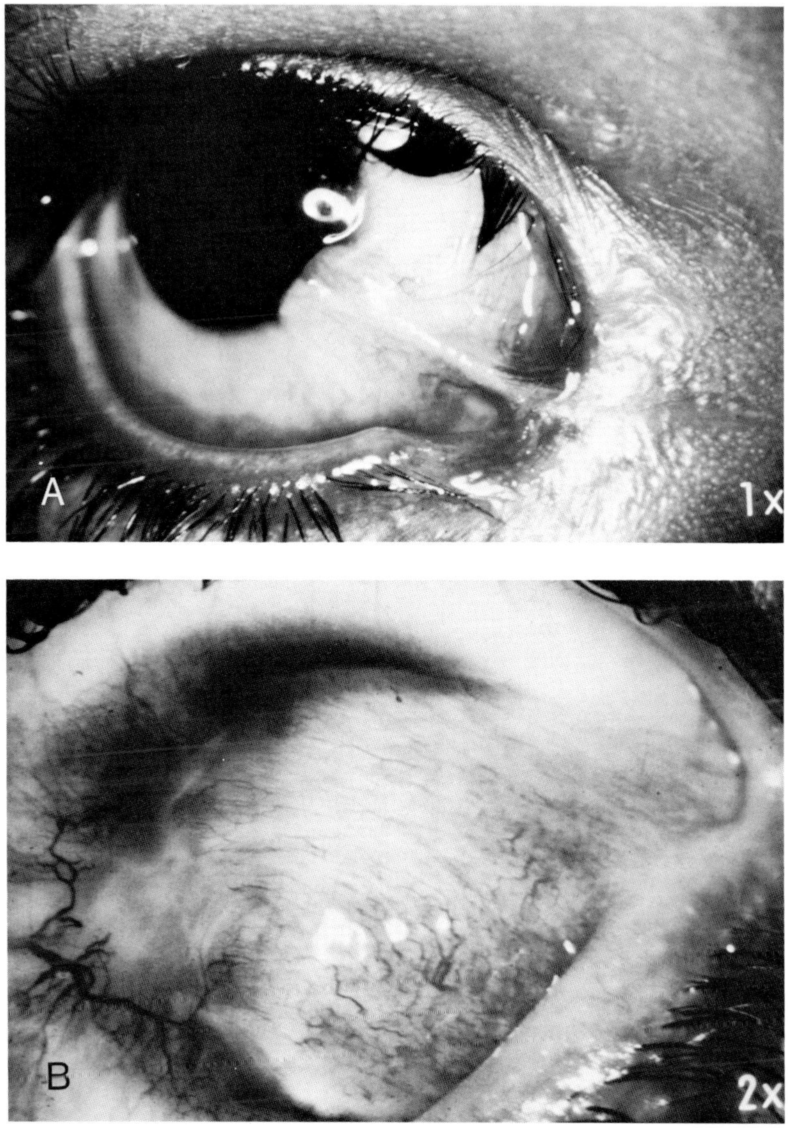

Fig. 19-24. (A) Symblepharon without limitation of ocular rotation. **(B)** Symblepharon with severe limitation of ocular rotation.

Picó[35] clearly outlined the course of action to be followed. When symblepharon formation is absent and conjunctiva is found to be plentiful, the situation is equivalent to the original one and the steps of the primary procedure are repeated. If the amount of conjunctiva remaining after excision of the fibrous tissue element is insufficient, only the head is excised, and the mucosa covering the body is used to clothe the denuded epibulbar area. It is tacked to the episclera some 3 mm from the limbus using interrupted 8-0 silk sutures. When symblepharon is present, this same recession maneuver is employed if there is enough mucosa to cover the raw epibulbar area and to correct the symblepharon. By contrast, severe degrees of symblepharon with restricted ocular movement are usually associated with the presence of insufficient amounts of conjunctiva. In these cases, it becomes necessary to use a graft of buccal mucosa or autologous conjunctiva to cover the large expanse of bare sclera. Failure to cover the raw area is promptly followed by reappearance of the symblepharon. All recurrences should receive additional application of β-radiation at the end of the procedure.

REFERENCES

1. Kuhnt H: Uber Die Verwertbarkeit Der Bindehaut in Der Praktischen Und Operativen Heilkünde. Bergmann. Weisbaden, 1898
2. Haik GM: A fornix conjunctival flap as a substitute for the dissected conjunctival flap: A clinical and experimental study. Trans Am Ophthalmol Soc 52:497, 1954
3. Gundersen T: Conjunctival flaps in the treatment of corneal disease with reference to a new technique of application. Arch Ophthalmol 60:880, 1958
4. Forster RK: Fungal diseases. p.176. In Smolin Q, Thoft RA (eds): The Cornea. Little, Brown, Boston, 1983
5. Polack FM, Kaufman HE, Newmark E: Keratomycosis, medical and surgical treatment. Arch Ophthalmol 85:410, 1971
6. Sanders N: Penetrating keratoplasty in the treatment of fungus keratitis. Am J Ophthalmol 70:24, 1970
7. Williams DM, Weiner, MH, Drutz DJ: Inmunologic studies of disseminated infection with *Aspergillus fumigatus* in the mouse. I. Infect Dis 143:726, 1981
8. Naumann G, Green NR, Zimmerman LE: Mycotic keratitis. A histopathologic study of 73 cases. Am J Ophthalmol 64:668, 1967
9. Jones BR: Principles in the management of oculomycosis. Trans Am Acad Ophthalmol Otolaryngol 79:15, 1975
10. Pfister RR, Richards JSF, Dohlman CH: Recurrence of herpetic keratitis in corneal grafts. Am J Ophthalmol 73:192, 1972
11. Rice NSC, Jones BR: Problems of corneal grafting in herpetic keratitis. In Ciba Foundation Symposium on Corneal Graft Failure. Association Scientific Publ. 15:221, 1973
12. Polack FM, Kaufman HE: Penetrating keratoplasty in herpetic keratitis. Am J Ophthalmol 73:908, 1972
13. Langston RHS, Pavan-Langston D, Dohlman CH: Penetrating keratoplasty for herpetic keratitis. Prognostic and therapeutic determinants. Am Acad Ophthalmol Otolaryngol 79:577, 1975
14. Cobos LM, Coster DJ, Rice NS, Jones BR: Corneal transplants in herpetic keratitis. Arch Ophthalmol 98:1755, 1980
15. Paton D, Milauskas AT: Indications, surgical technique and results of thin conjunctival flaps on the cornea. p.329. In Bronson NR, Paton RT (eds): Advances in Keratoplasty. International Ophthalmology Clinics 10:329, 1970
16. Gundersen T: Surgical treatment of bullous keratopathy. Arch Ophthalmol 64:260, 1960
17. Amsler M: Zur Frage des Pterygiumbedingten Astigmatismus. Ophthalmologica (Basel) 126:52, 1953
18. Cogan DG, Kuwabara T, Howard J: The nonelastic nature of pingueculas. AMA Arch. Ophthalmol 61:388, 1959
19. Tower P: Corrugated silver wire for severing pterygium from the cornea. Am J Ophthalmol 33:1439, 1950
20. Gibson JBG: Brisbane survey of pterygium. Trans Ophthalmol Soc Aust 16:125, 1956
21. Desmarres LA: Traité Théorique et Practique des Maladies des Yeux. Vol. 2. Baillière, Paris, 1855
22. McReynolds JO: The nature and treatment of pterygia. JAMA 39:296, 1902
23. Berens C, King TH: Atlas of Ophthalmic Surgery. JB Lippincott, Philadelphia, 1961
24. Rosenthal TW: Chronology of pterygium therapy. Am J Ophthalmol 36:1601, 1953
25. Picó G: Pterygium. Current concept of etiology and management. p.280. In King JH, McTigue JW (eds.): The Cornea World Congress. Butterworths, Washington, DC, 1965
26. Alger LH: Etiology of pterygium recurrence. Am J Ophthalmol 57:450, 1964
27. Hilgers JHC: Pterygium on the Island of Aruba. Klein Offset Drukkerij Poortpers NV, Amsterdam, 1959
28. Cameron ME: Pterygium Throughout the World. Charles C Thomas, Springfield, IL 1965
29. McDonald JE, Wilson FM: Ocular therapy with beta particles. Trans Am Acad Ophthalmol Otolaryngol 63:468, 1959
30. Blum HF: Histopathology of Irradiation. McGraw-Hill, New York, 1948
31. Johnson R, Preston R, Newton JC: Amputation neuroma following pterygium excision. Am J Ophthalmol 62:569, 1966
32. Hughes WF: Beta radiation sources, uses and dangers in treatment of the eye. JAMA 170:2096, 1959
33. Haik GM, Lyda W, Waugh RL Jr, Ellis G: Cataract formation following beta-ray radium therapy. Am J Ophthalmol 38:465, 1954
34. King JH Jr: The pterygium. AMA Arch Ophthalmol 44:854, 1950
35. Picó G: Tratamiento de las Complicaciones de la Cirugía del Pterigion.p.83. In Eighth Congreso Panamericano de Oftalmología, Mar del Plata, Argentina, Vol. I, 1968

Surgical Correction of Astigmatism

20

Richard C. Troutman
Casimir A. Swinger

PREVENTION

According to Troutman,[1] a principal cause of excessively high postoperative astigmatism is defective surgical technique. Although this is better controlled, other causes of excessive residual astigmatism are more difficult to eliminate, especially those arising from either variable anatomic and physiologic characteristics of the recipient or donor tissue, or both.

Perhaps one of the best methods with which to develop awareness of surgical technique is the use of the surgical keratometer, first introduced and long advocated by Troutman et al.[2] Whether one employs a qualitative or a quantitative instrument, the keratometer rapidly improves the surgeon's wound-closure technique and results. For uniformity, only elastic monofilament nylon sutures should be used for optical wound closure.

In cataract surgery, faulty incision and wound closure are the major sources of postoperative astigmatism, such errors being produced by sutures placed too superficially, too loosely, too tightly, or a combination, and by malposition of (or defective) wound margins. Poor closure technique is readily detected during surgery by observing the reflex of the keratometer, enabling the surgeon to make any necessary corrections intraoperatively. Working with a keratometer, the surgeon develops increased awareness of the optical significance of a given procedure. When used in conjunction with preoperative and postoperative office keratometry, the surgeon begins to think "optically" and enters the domain of refractive surgery, thereby increasing his or her ability to provide the patient not only with a good anatomic result, but with the best optical result possible as well. It is important that surgeons continuously evaluate their technique and modify it as necessary to obtain the best final optical results.

In keratoplasty the situation is even more complex. Here the surgeon works with a donor as well as with the patient's cornea. We use tissue-culture–preserved corneas in all cases and cut the buttons from their endothelial surface with a vertically directed pistonlike punch. This technique provides a round vertical-sided button. A good cut is more apt to be ensured if the edge of the disposable trephine blade is carefully examined for sharpness under magnification prior to use.

Most surgeons attribute the greater percentage of high astigmatism following keratoplasty to the recipient cornea, either from irregularities of the trephine incision and casting or from preoperative pathology, such as in keratoconus. First, the surgeon must ensure that there is even, vertically directed pressure on the cornea at trephination to avoid distortion of the globe and a defective recipient cut. Distorting forces can also arise from the lids, the speculum, a superior rectus suture, or a too tightly sutured scleral expander or ring. An obturator should not be used on steep or keratoconic corneas, as it may distort the cornea during the cut should it come into contact with the steep central cornea. We use a universal trephine handle and disposable blade without an obturator to cut the recipient opening.

During completion of the excision, poor technique with the corneal scissors can produce irregular wound margins and resultant postoperative astigmatism. A vertical edge matching that of the punched donor button should be obtained.

After placing the graft in the bed, it is rotated, while the reflex of the keratometer is being observed, until the position of least astigmatism (approximately round reflex) is found, as confirmed by the surgical keratometer. When suturing, regardless of the suture pattern used, one must strive to place the sutures radially, deep, and with the loops under equal tension, such that the graft is not shifted from this ideal position. Finally, while observing the reflex, the suture tension is adjusted to complete the closure with minimal astigmatism.

Despite meticulous surgical technique, high astigmatism will still occur in a number of eyes following the removal of all sutures. The various techniques for surgical correction of this residual astigmatism are the subject of this chapter.

CLINICAL PICTURE

Patients selected for surgical correction of astigmatism vary widely. Candidates include patients with congenital astigmatism and those with excessive astigmatism induced from a cataract incision or following keratoplasty. Until recently, refractive surgery for astigmatism was limited to patients whose visual problem could not be corrected by spectacles or contact lenses. With increased experience and improved accuracy of results, correction of less debilitating astigmatism is more frequently achieved.

Spectacles should always be tried before surgical treatment is considered. Patients will tolerate high cylindrical corrections of 10 diopters or more in some instances.

The astigmatic error of corneal astigmatism will be demonstrated on refraction, keratometry, or photokeratoscopy. It is unusual for such data to be inconsistent with respect to axis. There can be a significant difference in the magnitude, depending on the spherical equivalent accepted at refraction. For example, a patient with a high hyperopic correction accepts less cylinder by manifest refraction than measured objectively by keratometry, due to the efficiency of the correcting lens. The opposite is the case for a high myope.

The presenting clinical signs depend on the etiology of the astigmatism. For example, in congenital astigmatism the only findings are the refractive cylinder and, as observed by Barraquer,[3] a sometimes more oval shape to the limbal ring. In astigmatism following cataract surgery, sector or meridional suture compression may be observed; conversely, a poorly apposed or dehisced wound may be present. Following keratoplasty, excessive suture tension, scarring, or vascularization in a sector can result in steepening in that meridian. A poorly formed scar, override, or dehiscence of the graft edge results in flattening of the incident meridian.

SURGICAL ANATOMY

Correction of astigmatism is best accomplished within the cornea, except in the case of an ectatic cataract wound at the limbus. When an astigmatism is regular, the corneal surface is toric in shape; there is an axis of greatest curvature (steep) and, approximately 90 degrees away, a corresponding axis of least curvature (flat) (Fig. 20-1). When an irregular astigmatism is present, the axes are more or less than 90 degrees apart, and asymmetric sur-

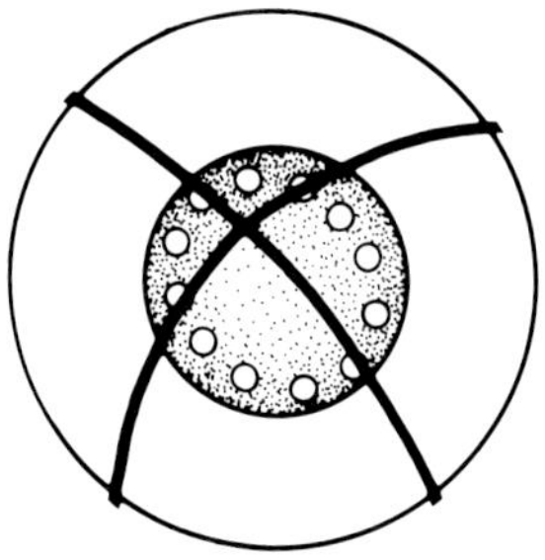

Fig. 20-1. Keratometric reflex on astigmatic cornea demonstrates typical ellipse with a major axis (flat) of least refractive power and a minor axis (steep) of greatest refractive power.

face irregularities may be detected with a photokeratoscope or keratometer.

In the normal cornea, the thickness varies from approximately 0.52 mm centrally to a peripheral value of 0.65 mm or more.[4] Optical or ultrasonic pachymetry should be used to determine corneal thickness before refractive surgical procedure is attempted.

INDICATIONS

Indications for the surgical correction of astigmatism vary not only with its cause and degree but also with the needs of the individual patient. A high degree of astigmatism satisfactorily compensated for with spectacles or contact lenses should not be surgically corrected unless the patient's concerns or needs change. An operation should not be performed simply because an astigmatism exists, in the absence of symptoms.

The principal indications for the surgical correction of an astigmatism are as follows:

1. Patients who, following surgery, are symptomatic or whose astigmatism cannot be fully corrected with their astigmatic spectacle correction or who cannot tolerate hard contact lenses
2. Patients requiring good uncorrected visual acuity for professional reasons, which can include cosmesis, when the astigmatism is the primary cause of the decreased acuity or as an adjunct to surgery for a spherical error
3. All patients unable to tolerate hard contact lenses or who, because of corneal astigmatism, are unable to wear cosmetic soft contact lenses, especially patients requiring a contact lens for significant anisometropia

There are no defined limits as to the minimal or maximal degree of astigmatism for which to operate. A vision-compromising residual astigmatism following cataract/IOL may be operated on for a cylinder as low as 2 or 3 diopters. Following otherwise successful keratoplasty or in a wound slippage following cataract surgery, the cylinder operated may be as high as 15 to 20 diopters. Again, it is the need of the patient as well as the magnitude and etiology of the astigmatism that determine whether surgery should be performed and the best procedure to employ.

CONTRAINDICATIONS

The major contraindications to the surgical correction of astigmatism are as follows:

1. Irregular astigmatism, which cannot be regularized by corneal refractive surgery—although in high degrees it sometimes proves beneficial
2. When vascularization of the cornea may be increased if radial incisions are made in a vascularized cornea, causing vessels to grow toward the visual axis, decreasing vision, or, in the case of a graft, precipitating a homograft reaction
3. In a cornea with numerically or morphologically deficient endothelium, for which surgery may induce corneal decompensation (specular microscopy should be performed before refractive surgery when an endothelial deficit is suspected)
4. When astigmatism is combined with other, more severe, pathology from which visual improvement cannot be demonstrated preopera tively by other means of correction or a potential acuity meter

METHODS OF TREATMENT

Theory

The goal of any corrective surgery for astigmatism is a spherical cornea. This is accomplished either by steepening the flat corneal meridian or by flattening the steep corneal meridian (see Fig. 20-1). Of a number of techniques proposed or attempted, only the following are in a widespread use at this time:

- Techniques that steepen the flatter corneal meridian
  - Corneal wedge resection (Troutman)
  - Wound revision or block resection and resuture
- Techniques that flatten the steeper corneal meridian
  - Selective suture removal
  - Sector circumferential relaxing incisions (Troutman)
  - Trapezoidal keratotomy (Ruiz)
  - Sector radial incisions with or without perpendicular flag or T incisions (Fyodorov)

Since we have not found radial incisions effective for the correction of higher degrees of astigmatism, and because the flat and T incisions are used primarily for correction of small degrees of astigmatism in combination with surgery for myopia, these are not discussed in this chapter.

Techniques

The following is a brief description of the techniques used to reduce residual astigmatism, after all sutures are removed, following cataract or keratoplasty.

Corneal Wedge Resection

In the corneal wedge resection, a crescentic shaped, wedge-profiled area of tissue is resected from the healed keratoplasty incision centered across the axis of the flat corneal meridian (Fig. 20-2).[5] The resection extends along approximately 90 degrees of arc length, the crescent being widest at the axis of the flat meridian and tapering gradually to either end. The two curvilinear incisions outlining the crescent are deepened to meet at the level of Descemet's membrane.

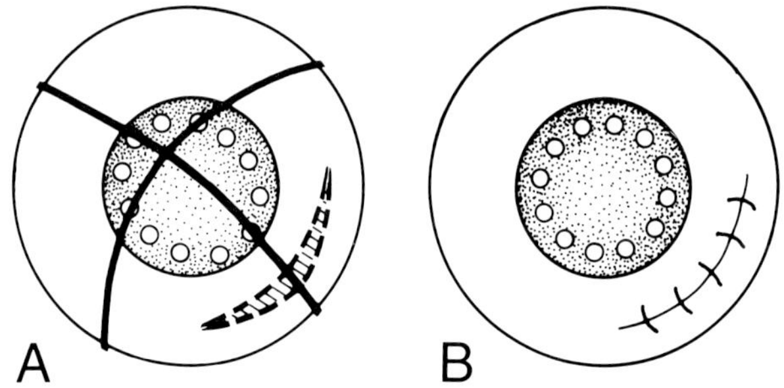

Fig. 20-2. Corneal wedge resection. **(A)** Crescent of tissue is resected across flattest corneal meridian. **(B)** After sutures have been placed, keratometric reflex indicates an overcorrection.

The amount of correction obtained is related to the width of the resection at the middle of the crescent. The first 0.5 mm of resection results in about 5 to 8 diopters of astigmatic correction. Each 0.05 mm of resection width above the initial 0.5 mm gives approximately 1 diopter of further correction.[5] In practice, less than a 0.5-mm resection is ineffective and rarely will more than 1.0 mm be required.

Steepening the flat corneal meridian by a corneal wedge resection induces a compensatory flattening of the perpendicular, or previously steep, corneal meridian. These changes are additive and serve to bring the meridional refractive powers closer in value. Approximately 0.5 diopter of flattening at the steep meridian is obtained for each 1 diopter of steepening obtained at the operative or flat meridian.

Wound Revision by Block Resection and Resuture

This technique is used primarily for the repair of ectatic superior limbal cataract wounds that induce high degrees of against-the-rule astigmatism. Here the cataract wound is exposed. Thinned, misaligned tissue is removed by block resection and the new wound resutured in its full thickness with elastic monofilament nylon suture.

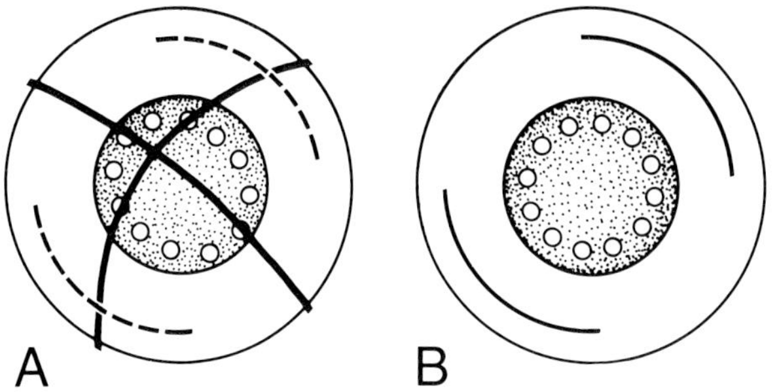

Fig. 20-3. Circumferential relaxing incision. **(A)** Bipolar arcuate incisions are made in the graft wound at opposite poles of the steep corneal meridian. **(B)** After healing, the astigmatic cornea is now spherical, as indicated by keratometric reflex.

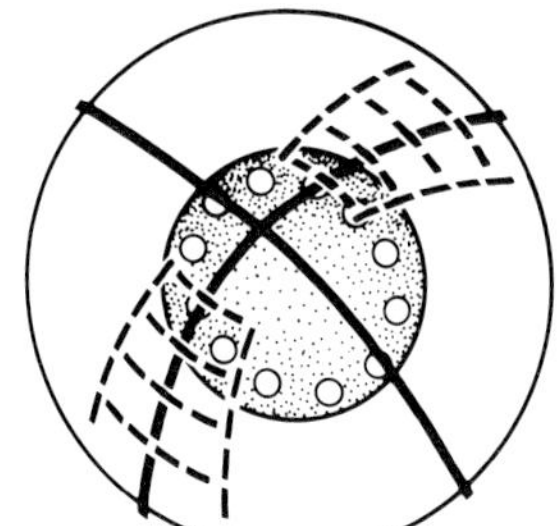

Fig. 20-4. Trapezoidal keratotomy. A series of transverse and semiradial incisions are made across the steep corneal meridian.

This technique is used in high astigmatism, for which relaxing incisions or trapezoidal keratotomy would be ineffective. Corrections of up to 18 diopters have been reported.[6]

Circumferential Relaxing Incision

In this technique, one incises in a healed keratoplasty or cataract wound producing a wound gape that flattens a too steep corneal meridian (Fig. 20-3).[7] When performed for correction of astigmatism after cataract surgery, a single incision is made in the cataract incision across the axis of the steep corneal meridian. In postkeratoplasty astigmatism, two incisions are made in the incision at opposite poles of the steep corneal meridian.

Each relaxing incision is made deep into the graft recipient cicatrix and is centered on the axis of the steep corneal meridian. In postkeratoplasty astigmatism, two compression sutures are placed across the graft scar at 90 degrees to the steep meridian. The suture loops are tightened to induce a temporary overcorrection by gaping the relaxing incision wounds to prevent early apposition, adding to the final effect.

Although circumferential relaxing incisions have corrected up to 16 diopters of astigmatism, they are most useful in astigmatic errors of less than 10 diopters.

Trapezoidal Keratotomy

In this technique, two series of four transverse incisions are made perpendicular to and centered on opposing poles of the steep corneal meridian[8] (Fig. 20-4). Two radial incisions are made to each side of each set of transverse incisions, but not intersecting them. The two groups of incisions are separated by a clear central optical zone of varying diameter. An optical zone of less than 3 mm is not advisable because of induced glare and irregular astigmatism.

Shorter transverse incisions (1.5 to 2.0 mm in length) produce significant flattening of the steep meridian while having minimal effect at the opposite meridian, unlike the corneal wedge resection and the circumferential relaxing incisions, wherein the wounds extend further laterally and have more influence on the opposite meridian. This greater control over the effects at the opposite meridian improves the accuracy. Also, by increasing the length of the transverse incisions to as long as 5 mm, the spherical equivalent corneal power can be variably corrected. Since the trapezoidal keratotomy produces flattening of the steep corneal meridian and compensatory steepening of the flat meridian, a hyperopic spherical equivalent may be decreased by making the transverse incisions longer to induce more myopia at the opposite meridian. By contrast, if the spherical equivalent is emmetropia or myopia, the incisions are usually made shorter to reduce the myopic spherical equivalent.

Table 20-1 is a rough guideline to estimate the amount of astigmatic correction that may be obtained with various optical zone diameters, when the depths of the incisions are constant at 80 percent or more of corneal thickness. As with circumferential relaxing incisions, trapezoidal keratotomy is capable of correcting up to 11 diopters of astigmatism.[9] However, excessive glare and irregu-

Table 20-1. Astigmatic Correction Obtained with Trapezoidal Keratotomies of Various Optical Zone Diameters

Diameter of Optical Zone (mm)	Astigmatic Correction (diopters)
3.0	7.0–11.0
3.5	5.0– 7.0
4.0	4.0– 5.0
4.5	3.0– 4.0
5.0	1.0– 3.0

(Data derived a from computer program developed by Dr. Luis Ruiz of Bogotá, Colombia.)

lar astigmatism can result from the small optical zones necessary for high corrections; a corneal wedge resection or relaxing incisions at the graft scar are preferred techniques when less than a 3.5-mm optical zone is required to obtain the correction.

The correction obtainable may well depend on the etiology of the astigmatism. It is not yet known whether comparable results will be obtained for a given optical zone diameter when the technique is performed for congenital astigmatism in a patient who previously has had cataract surgery, or in patients who have astigmatism following keratoplasty. The current technique is similar for all three types of patients.

Surgical Approach

The following summarizes our approach to the correction of various astigmatic errors.

Postkeratoplasty Astigmatism

Selective removal of interrupted sutures over a period of months may be used in an attempt to alter wound healing and to produce a cornea with minimal astigmatism. If high astigmatism still exists after final suture removal, we perform circumferential relaxing incisions for cylinders up to 10 diopters. We recently investigated the trapezoidal keratotomy for cylinders up to this value. The latter has the advantage of not disrupting the graft–host interface and of being more quantifiable. However, it does involve considerably more surgery than the circumferential relaxing incisions and can cause endothelial damage and glare. Complications such as perforation, necessitating suturing, as well as graft rejection, have been reported. For cylinders above 10 diopters, a corneal wedge resection is the procedure of choice.

Postcataract Astigmatism

With-the-Rule Astigmatism. This can be reduced by removing sutures selectively. If there remains a significant astigmatism, a single circumferential relaxing incision is preferred, for errors up to 3 diopters, if the cataract incision was corneal. The trapezoidal keratotomy may be used for errors up to 10 diopters, again with the precaution of an optical zone not less than 3.0 mm.

Against-the-Rule Astigmatism. We perform a trapezoidal keratotomy for cylinders up to 8 to 10 diopters and a wound revision for errors greater than 8 to 10 diopters.

Congenital Astigmatism

It is unusual to see eyes with exceptionally high degrees of congenital astigmatism. Almost all such cases can be corrected with trapezoidal keratotomy.

RECOMMENDED TECHNIQUE

Postkeratoplasty Astigmatism

Suture Modulation

When a continuous or double-continuous suture is used to close the wound, suture modulation obviously cannot be practiced during the early postoperative period. However, we find that the double-continuous suture does have the advantage of decreasing postoperative myopia in keratoconic patients.[10] With continuous sutures, one is committed to final suture removal to determine the final astigmatic result. In our experience, however, when sutures are properly tensioned under keratometric control, the "sutures-in" astigmatism will rarely exceed 5 diopters. Modification of residual astigmatic error following suture removal can be achieved by surgery.

If multiple interrupted sutures are used, whether alone or in conjunction with a running suture, modification of the "sutures-in" postoperative astigmatism can be attempted by selective suture removal. Nevertheless, when all sutures are removed, significant astigmatism may persist or recur, requiring surgical correction.

We follow all graft patients with refraction, keratometry, and photokeratoscopy. In cases in which interrupted sutures were used, if regular or irregular astigmatism of any significant degree is noted at 8 weeks follow-up, selective interrupted suture removal is performed, removing the suture(s) tensioning the steep meridian — these sutures are easily identified by their compressive effects on keratometry and photokeratoscopy. This often results in a significant decrease in excessive "sutures-in" astigmatism. Additional interrupted sutures may be removed, as necessary, to regularize the rings of the photokeratoscope and to reduce the postoperative cylinder.

Such suture modulation has two obvious advantages. First, it reduces regular and irregular astigmatism during the early postoperative period, which may allow for more rapid optical rehabilitation of the patient. Second, it has been suggested that it reduces the surgically induced or final astigmatic error. However, when suture modulation has been completed and a minimal astigmatic error has been achieved, the remaining sutures must be left in place for about 15 months before removal. Only then will the final result be known.

Corneal Wedge Resection

The corneal wedge resection may be performed in either of two ways.[5] A double-blade knife may be used and both superficial incisions made simultaneously, or the incisions may be made sequentially with a single blade. In either case, the basic concept is to remove a section of the cicatrix across the flat corneal meridian.

Surgery begins by observing the reflex of the surgical keratometer and identifying the steep and flat meridians. These should confirm the preoperative keratometric and refractive values.

If sequential incisions are made, we make the first incision either inside or outside the cicatrix in order to produce the inner or outer curve of the tissue crescent to be resected. The second incision is then made to the opposite side of the cicatrix. The location of the first incision relative to the cicatrix depends on the etiology of the astigmatism. If we believe that the etiology is an irregularly cut or oval graft (i.e., the astigmatism results from the shape of the donor button), we make the initial incision more within the graft and the second just peripheral to or at the cicatrix, with most of the wedge coming from the donor. However, if we believe that the astigmatism arises from an abnormal or thinned recipient zone, as in keratoconus, we then make the initial incision more in the recipient, outside the cicatrix, and the second just inside or at the scar to remove more tissue from the recipient.

Initially, both incisions are made to the calculated resection width, approximately 90 degrees in arc length, and at about one half of the corneal thickness (Figs. 20-5 and 20-6). The primary incisions, which are perpendicular to the corneal surface, can be made with a thin diamond or metal blade. The initial incisions are deepened gradually

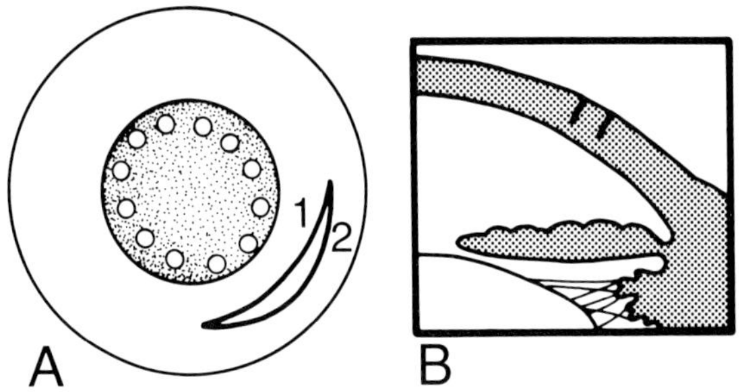

Fig. 20-5. Corneal wedge resection. **(A)** Initial incisions (1, 2) are made to mid-stromal depth **(B).**

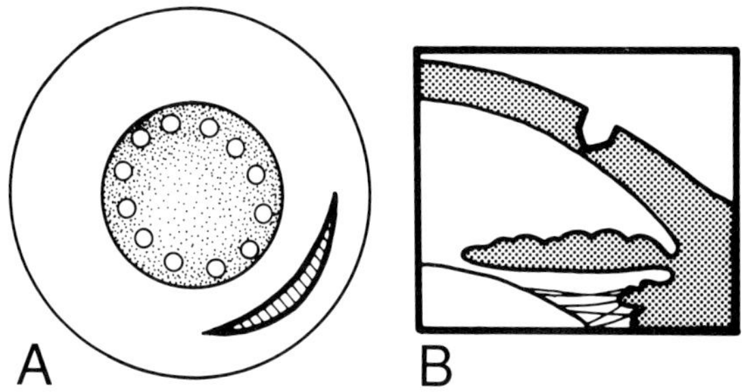

Fig. 20-6. Corneal wedge resection. **(A)** Initial incisions are deepened to meet Descemet's membrane, and **(B)** the wedge is excised.

with a single-blade knife and extended obliquely so that they meet at the level of Descemet's membrane, to effect the wedge-shaped excision.

Incisions performed simultaneously with the double-blade knife are made parallel for a greater distance into the corneal stroma than two successive incisions. This produces a different excision profile than that of sequential incisions and results in somewhat more correction for a given width of anterior resection (Fig. 20-7). For this reason, the width of the excision is reduced by 20 percent.

When the outline of the excised area has been completed, the wedge of tissue is excised at depth with the diamond blade or a Vannas scissors. The curved cuts should be smooth and regular for good wound coaptation and healing.

After the wedge has been excised, a small paracentesis is made in the depth of the wound to facilitate approximation of the wound margins during suturing (Fig. 20-8). The wound is closed with five interrupted through-and-through 10-0 nylon suture loops beginning at each end of the resection, where the gape is more easily approximated, and progressing centrally to close the deep aspect of the wound. Four additional interrupted sutures are placed at mid-stromal depth between the deep bites in order to better approximate the anterior corneal surface (Fig. 20-9).

Sutures are tied first with double slip knots to allow for optimal adjustment of suture loop tension, as determined with the surgical keratometer. The double slip knot is formed by combining two single slip knot ties and locked with a square knot. The suture loops should be tensioned so the flat meridian becomes the steep corneal meridian with

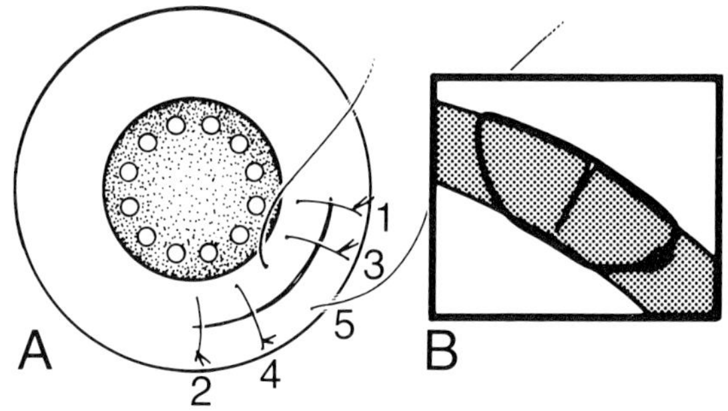

Fig. 20-8. Corneal wedge resection. **(A)** Initial wound closure obtained with multiple interrupted sutures beginning in the periphery, as indicated by the numbers typifying the sequence of placement. **(B)** Sutures are placed deep or through and through.

an overcorrection of 30 to 50 percent, as indicated by the surgical keratometer. Otherwise, when some of the initial correction is lost with decreased wound edema, undercorrection will result. Finally, the slip knots are locked down successively with square knots to produce even compression of the wound. They are buried in the donor cornea.

To compensate for the overcorrection, two interrupted through-and-through suture loops are placed across the graft scar approximately 60 degrees from either end of the closed resection (Fig. 20-10). They are tensioned to round out the keratometric reflex, thereby decreasing the astigmatism induced by the wedge sutures and providing improved optical rehabilitation with sutures in. They also support the wound opposite to the wedge, preventing wound stretch or dehiscence.

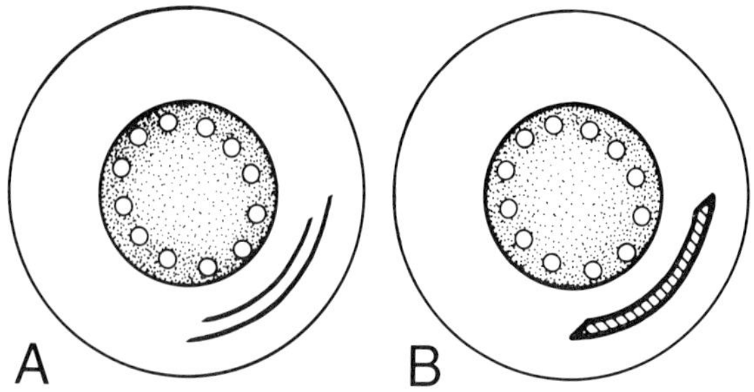

Fig. 20-7. Corneal wedge resection. **(A)** Double-bladed knife performs both incisions simultaneously. **(B)** Incisions are joined at their terminations by linear incisions.

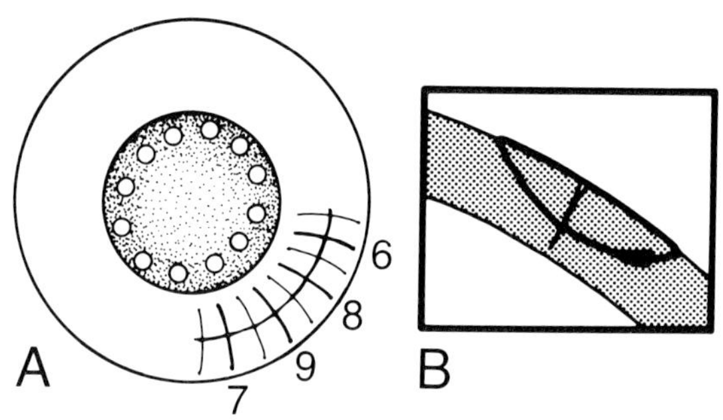

Fig. 20-9. Corneal wedge resection. **(A)** Additional sutures are placed to give temporary overcorrection as indicated by keratometric reflex. **(B)** Second series of sutures (6–9) are placed at mid-stromal depth to achieve closure of the anterior corneal surface.

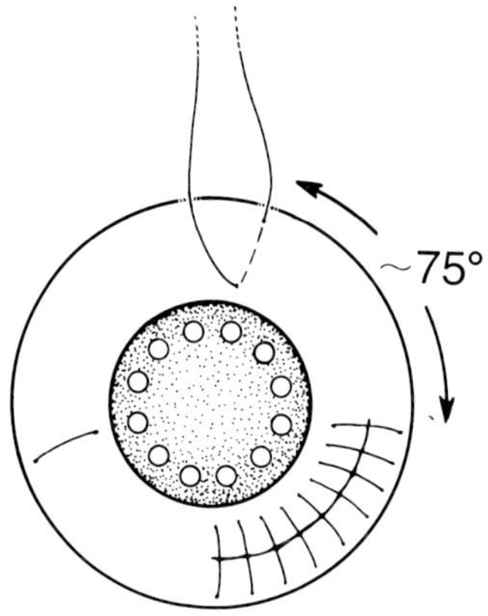

Fig. 20-10. Corneal wedge resection. Following closure of wedge, compression sutures are placed approximately 75 degrees away from termination of both sides of the wound.

At the conclusion of surgery, a subconjunctival injection of antibiotic is given and the eye patched. All knots must be buried.

Postoperatively, a steroid and an antibiotic drop are used for 1 to 2 weeks. There is usually minimal or no iritis, and cycloplegics are rarely used.

The keratometry will stabilize sufficiently after several weeks to permit temporary spectacle correction. Sutures are removed sequentially, but not before the third month. The compression sutures are typically the first to be removed, followed by any wedge sutures that are loose or excessively tight. If an overcorrection persists, additional suture loops are removed. If sphericity or a slight undercorrection is obtained, either before sutures are removed or after the removal of some sutures, the remaining sutures are left in situ indefinitely. If an overcorrection persists after removal of the remaining sutures, relaxing incisions or trapezoidal keratotomies are performed to correct the residual astigmatism.

Circumferential Relaxing Incisions

Technically this procedure is more simple than corneal wedge resection. Although initially this technique was performed at the slit lamp, it is now performed in the ambulatory surgery unit under the microscope to allow use of the surgical keratometer and to place compression sutures.

The steep corneal meridian is identified, and the epithelium is abraded to mark its axis. Initially, a relaxing incision was performed across only one pole of the steep corneal meridian. Now it is almost always done paired, as a bipolar procedure.

A suction ring may be used to fixate the globe during the incisions, but this can be precarious if the eye is entered. A double-pronged fixation forceps, such as used for radial keratotomy, is preferred. A steel or diamond blade may be used to make the incisions under direct visualization with gradual deepening, or a preset micrometer knife may be preferred. Intraoperative pachymetry is used to determine the blade length, which is set typically at 80 percent of corneal thickness in the area of the incision. Because the graft wound may be irregular in thickness, the surgeon must evaluate the wound biomicroscopically to avoid areas of posterior gape. If the depth of the wound is too irregular, a modified trapezoidal keratotomy or wedge resection should be done.

The incision is made directly into the cicatrix to maximum depth (Fig. 20-11). As a curvilinear incision is somewhat more difficult to make than a linear incision, an unguarded incision should be deepened gradually. As a variation, one may use the double-blade diamond knife to make paired parallel incisions, 0.5 mm apart, to enhance the effect of the relaxing incision. The incisions, however made, are duplicated at the opposite pole of the steep corneal meridian.

After completing the relaxing incisions, interrupted compression sutures are placed across the graft scar at opposite poles of the perpendicular meridian (at 90 degrees). These induce gaping of the relaxing incisions, delaying healing and enhancing the final optical effect (Fig. 20-12). The

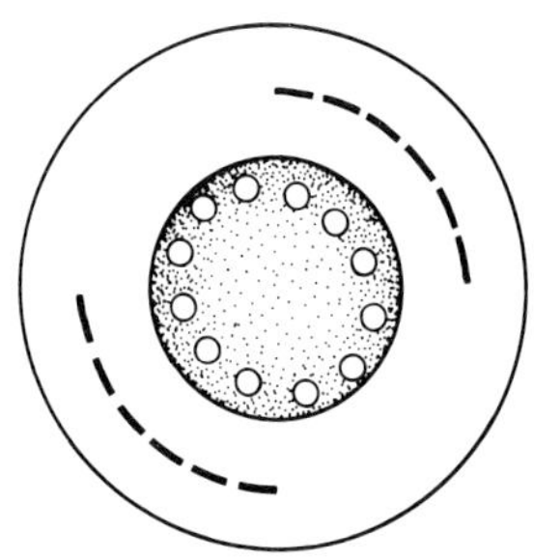

Fig. 20-11. Circumferential relaxing incision. Deep arcuate incisions are made within the graft cicatrix at both poles of the steep corneal meridian.

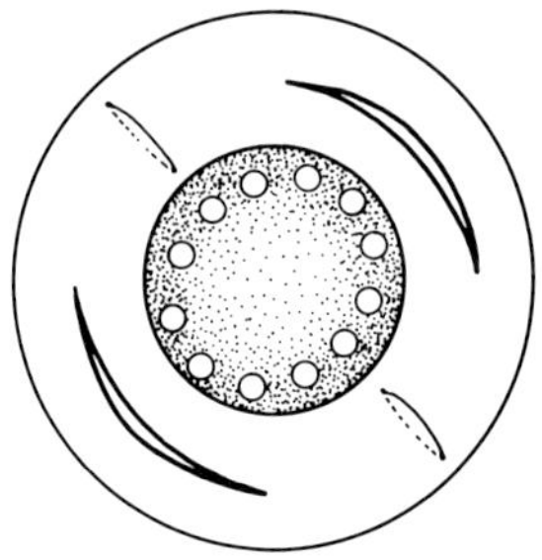

Fig. 20-12. Placement of compression sutures at the previously flat meridian produces a gaping of relaxing incisions and temporary overcorrection.

compression sutures produce corneal steepening and temporary overcorrection in their meridian. They are left in place approximately 6 weeks, unless the postoperative result is a spherical cornea or an undercorrection, in which case they are left in place indefinitely. At the conclusion of the procedure, an injection of antibiotic is given, and the eye is patched. A steroid and an antibiotic are administered for 1 to 2 weeks. As there is usually minimal discomfort from circumferential relaxing incisions, a bandage lens is unnecessary.

The final optical result is often manifested variably. For example, there may be little initial effect followed by a gradual improvement over several weeks. By contrast, initially, an overcorrection may be obtained, followed by a decay to a spherical cornea or an undercorrection, especially when the compression sutures are removed.

Trapezoidal Keratotomy

This technique is also performed on an ambulatory basis, usually under topical anesthesia (ophthaine or tetracaine), adding a retrobulbar when the patient is highly sensitive. If necessary, 4 to 10 percent cocaine, applied with a cotton swab, can be used to anesthetize the limbus.

The steep and flat axes are identified with the surgical keratometer and a small peripheral reference mark is made in the epithelium. The diameter of the optical zone is calculated with a computer program or is estimated from Table 20-1 (data in this table have not been verified clinically, and each surgeon must adjust the surgical variables according to personal technique). The optical center is identified while the patient fixates on the coaxial light of the operating microscope. Rather than mark the light reflex directly, which may cause an opacity at the visual axis, the marking trephine should be centered over the light reflex on the visual axis with a slight inferior displacement (to account for the fact that the microscope light is not truly coaxial). The displacement is approximately one half the light reflex in width.

After the optical zone is delimited, a caliper is used to mark the lengths of the transverse incisions (determined by the effect desired on the spherical equivalent) by placing radial delimiting marks in the epithelium to either side of the meridian to be incised.

If one does not have a computer program (especially since the accuracies of computer programs for incisional refractive surgery are yet to be demonstrated), one can estimate the lengths of the transverse incisions as follows. First, the refraction is written in plus cylinder form. If emmetropia is desired, and the spherical component is minus or plano, a short incision of about 1.5 mm is made. If the spherical component is hyperopic, the lengths of the incisions depend on the values of the refractive sphere and keratometric cylinder. The value of the plus sphere is divided by the value of the plus cylinder to find the ratio of the two. The estimates in Table 20-2 are examined to determine the incisional length that corresponds most closely to the ratio calculated. For example, a refraction of $+1.00 +5.00 \times 90$ gives a ratio of 0.20. An incisional length of 3 mm would be selected (see Table

Table 20-2. Estimates of Lengths of Transverse Incisions for Trapezoidal Keratotomy for Various Ratios of Sphere/Cylinder

Sphere/(+)Cylinder Ratio	Length of Transverse Incisions (mm)
Negative	1.5
Zero	1.5
0.08	1.5
0.10	2.0
0.16	2.5
0.20	3.0
0.23	3.5
0.25	4.0
0.30	4.5
⩾0.33	5.0

(Data derived from a computer program developed by Dr. Luis Ruiz of Bogatá, Colombia.)

2). It must be remembered that these are crude estimates, and neither the effects of various optical zone diameters nor the lengths of transverse incisions have been adequately evaluated in experimental or clinical studies.

The incisions are made with the micrometer-adjusted diamond blade used for radial keratotomy. The blade is set at 100 percent of the sonic pachymetric reading obtained at the optical zone delimiting mark as it intersects the axis to be incised. A bipolar forceps fixates the globe. A transverse incision of the "calculated" length is made across both poles of the steep corneal meridian at the optical zone intersection. Each of these incisions is followed in turn by three additional transverse incisions of equal length, equally spaced, with the fourth, outermost incisions, lying close to the limbus. The diamond knife is extended by 0.02 mm for each corresponding pair of incisions as one moves outward. This approach permits a more constant percentage depth, as normal corneal thickness increases peripherally.

When the paired transverse incisions have been completed, the diamond knife is then reset for the optical zone reading, and paired radial incisions are made to either side of the transverse incisions. The radial incisions must not join or cross any transverse incisions, but each should begin near the optical zone just beyond their termination, diverging slightly and ending just short of the limbus.

Recently, we had a case of a perforation at the graft scar after trapezoidal keratotomy following penetrating keratoplasty. A persistent shallow chamber necessitated suturing. We are now evaluating a modification of trapezoidal keratotomy for astigmatism following keratoplasty, where the radial incisions do not cross the graft scar but end and begin just adjacent to it. This approach should prevent accidental perforation but might affect the correction obtained.

Upon completion of all incisions, each is inspected for appropriate depth. They are then copiously irrigated with filtered BSS to remove epithelium, blood clots, and debris.

Subconjunctival antibiotics are injected, and the eye is patched for 1 to several days. Typically, pooling or staining is noted in the incisions for several days following surgery. Topical antibiotics are used until no further staining is noted.

A small overcorrection should be induced at 1 to 2 weeks, if a final more spherical result is to be obtained. If an undercorrection persists, topical steroids, such as 1 percent prednisilone acetate qid, are given for up to 6 weeks in order to slow wound healing and reduce the decay in the correction. On the other hand, if after 2 weeks a significant overcorrection has been obtained, timolol, 0.5 percent bid, may be used to lower the IOP and perhaps decrease the overcorrection. This use of medication to alter wound healing and the final astigmatic error is based on empirical evidence only.

Postcataract Astigmatism

Astigmatism following cataract extraction is usually regular, involving the vertical meridian. Typically, it is either with the rule or against the rule. With-the-rule astigmatism indicates an excessively tight or compressive situation in the wound near the axis of the plus cylinder, as it passes through the arc of the wound. Against-the-rule astigmatism indicates a weak or ectatic wound with stretching or slippage.

Suture Cutting or Removal

If a compression-induced with-the-rule astigmatism is noted, the simplest method for reducing postoperative astigmatism is to cut or remove excessively tight suture loops. When nylon sutures have been used and the compressive effect is observed with the photokeratoscope, some reduction in cylinder will usually be obtained regardless of the length of time that has elapsed since surgery. If no compressive effect is recorded, little or no change in cylinder may be anticipated. Although suture cutting or removal may reduce with-the-rule astigmatism, if used too early an opposite error may be induced.

Usually, the offending suture loop lies at the axis of the plus refractive cylinder and at the axis of greatest dioptric power as determined with the clinical keratometer. When astigmatism is the result of multiple vectors of force, the steep axis may lie in a meridian between the tight suture loops.

For cataract wounds at or posterior to the limbus, corrective suture removal can begin as early as 8 weeks postsurgery. If a corneal incision has been used, it is best to wait at least 12 weeks.

If against-the-rule astigmatism is present, it is best to leave all sutures in place to support the wound for as long as possible, as suture removal will almost always increase the error.

Wound Revision

High against-the-rule astigmatism is usually associated with silk or absorbable sutures, poorly sutured wounds, or too early removal of nylon sutures. It occurs more often in a wound placed close to the cornea than more posteriorly, as in a scleral flap. Surgical correction begins by raising a conjunctival flap over the wound area, so as to better observe the ectatic tissue to be excised. The area can be delimited with a double-blade knife or by sequential curvilinear incisions, as for the wedge resection. The block of tissue is resected, and the wound is closed with interrupted, through-and-through nylon sutures. Vitreous at or near the wound should be displaced with Healon or air; if necessary, a vitrectomy should be performed.

The superficial wound is also coapted by sutures placed more superficially. A reversal of the astigmatism to a minimal, with-the-rule astigmatism should be obtained (as at the conclusion of cataract surgery). As astigmatism decays following a decrease in wound edema, a more spherical cornea is obtained. Here, too, compensating compression sutures may be used to reduce sutures-in astigmatism.

At the conclusion of the procedure, the patient is given an antibiotic injection. Postoperative care is similar to that for the routine cataract patient.

Trapezoidal Keratotomy

See under Trapezoidal Keratotomy, above, for a description of this technique.

Congenital Astigmatism

For the correction of congenital astigmatism, in which there is no cicatrix to be excised or released, either a corneal wedge resection, a semilunar incision, or a trapezoidal keratotomy may be employed. In almost all cases, however, congenital astigmatism is best corrected by trapezoidal keratotomy, as exceptionally high cylinders are rarely seen on a congenital basis.

PROGNOSIS AND COMPLICATIONS

Although current procedures for the correction of astigmatism are not readily quantifiable, except for some recent attempts to do so with the trapezoidal keratotomy, results are good. In a high percentage of cases, the cylinder can be reduced to a level at which spectacles can be tolerated.[11] In addition, many patients can have their astigmatism reduced to a level at which even a soft contact lens can be fit. This is especially the case following trapezoidal keratotomy for the correction of mild congenital astigmatism. Obviously, the higher the astigmatic error, the lower the chances of producing a spherical cornea.

Few complications have been reported following procedures for astigmatism. The major complications common to all techniques for astigmatism are undercorrection or overcorrection. In one case, angle-closure glaucoma following corneal wedge resection resulted after a large correction was attempted in a patient with an abnormally small, shallow anterior segment. It was successfully treated with miotics.

The complications reported following the circumferential relaxing incisions include several inadvertent perforations into the anterior chamber, causing shallowing and requiring suturing, as well as a vitreous wick following a relaxing incision in an aphakic eye in which the incision was made too deeply into the cornea.[12,13] Recently, Healon has been of value in keeping back the vitreous face in such eyes.

Thus far, few complications have been reported following trapezoidal keratotomy. The major complication appears to be optical, in the form of glare, which increases as the optical zone is decreased. Trapezoidal keratotomy can produce more glare than can a radial keratotomy of comparable optical zone diameter. This is probably because of the more numerous transverse incisions, the first of which is tangential to the optical zone. In addition, we have seen one case of a graft rejection that developed within 10 days following a trapezoidal keratotomy, there was also a case of shallowing of the anterior chamber, requiring suturing, in which a microperforation occurred at the intersection of the graft wound and a radial incision.

REFERENCES

1. Troutman RC: Surgical correction of high corneal astigmatic errors after successful keratoplasty—A preliminary report. Adv Ophthalmol 27:170, 1972
2. Troutman RC, Kelly S, Kaye D, Clahane AC: The use and preliminary results of the Troutman surgical keratometer in cataract and corneal surgery. Trans Am Acad Ophthalmol Otolaryngol 83:232, 1977
3. Barraquer J: Results of the crescentic resection for the correction of congenital astigmatism and astigmatism following penetrating keratoplasty. Arch Soc Am Oftal Optom 16:211, 1982
4. Mishima S: Corneal thickness. Surv Ophthalmol 13:57, 1968
5. Troutman RC: Improved techniques in refractive surgery for astigmatism. Cornea 1:57, 1982
6. Cravy TV: Secondary astigmatism control without wedge resection. p. 244. In Current Concepts in Cataract Surgery. CV Mosby, St. Louis, 1980
7. Troutman RC, Swinger C: Relaxing incision for control of postoperative astigmatism following keratoplasty. Ophthalmic Surg 11:117, 1980
8. Nordan LT: Current Status of Refractive Surgery. CL Printing, San Diego, 1985
9. Lavery GW, Lindstrom R: Ruiz keratotomy corrects high astigmatism. Ocul Surg News 2:1, 1985
10. Troutman RC, Meltzer M: Astigmatism and myopia in keratoconus. Trans Am Ophthalmol Soc 70:265, 1972
11. Troutman RC: Corneal wedge resections and relaxing incisions for postkeratoplasty astigmatism. p. 161. In Binder PS (ed): International Ophthalmology Clinics. Refractive Corneal Surgery: The Correction of Astigmatism. Little, Brown, Boston, 1983; #4, 23:161–168.
12. Stainer GA, Binder PS: Vitreous wick syndrome following a corneal relaxing incision. Ophthalmic Surg 12:567, 1981
13. Sugar J, Kirk AK: Relaxing keratotomy for postkeratoplasty high astigmatism. Ophthalmic Surg 14:156, 1983

Keratoprosthesis

21

Frank M. Polack

Replacement of opaque corneas with glass or plastic materials has been performed experimentally with varying degrees of success. Corneal implants require the insertion of an optical cylinder held in place by a flange or supporting material. The optical device has almost always been made of methyl methacrylate, but the retaining device has been composed of a variety of materials, such as plastic, gold, and bone.[1–8] Visual results depend on the condition of the retina. Initially they have been satisfactory because in most cases in which a corneal implant is used, the disease affects exclusively the anterior segment of the eye. For this same reason, the long-term results are not very good because retention of the implant is complicated by lack of bonding between the implant and the soft tissues with subsequent extrusion, infection, and/or retinal detachment. A ceramic keratoprosthesis has been made following the design of Cardona's adjustable through-and-through prosthesis. Improved adherence of soft tissue to the ceramic material has been observed,[9] and in a 3-year study we obtained good results in implantations through the cornea and conjunctiva but unsatisfactory results when exteriorized through the lid.[10] We consider this an unsolved mechanical problem, to be avoided whenever possible. However, in many cases (i.e., pemphigoid), it is the only method of implantation possible. The surgical procedure is described in detail in this chapter; the prostheses used are those of the author and of Cardona et al.[3]

INDICATIONS

Keratoprosthesis is indicated in patients with advanced stages of corneal disease when keratoplasty offers no possibility of success, such as in cases of repeated graft failure, chemical injuries when corneal transplants have failed, or when keratoplasty is not indicated; in thin and vascularized corneas, in ocular pemphigoid or end-stage dry eye syndrome, in cases of reconstruction of the anterior segment with no feasibility of corneal grafting, and in exceptional cases of corneal scarring due to disease or absence of the eyelids. The operation presupposes an adequately functioning retina and optic nerve. Since most of these corneas are scarred and irregular, determination of the intraocular pressure (IOP) is made with an electronic tonometer or an air tonometer. Visual requirements should consist of a degree of light perception and projection, as well as color discrimination. Ultrasound examination is essential to determine the anatomic status of the posterior pole of the eye.

CONTRAINDICATIONS

The procedure is not indicated in patients who have traveling vision in one eye, severe diabetes, or longstanding glaucoma.

MATERIALS AND INSTRUMENTS

The corneal prosthesis used is made of aluminum oxide ceramic. The retaining disk is an opaque 8.5-mm ring made of Frialit or corundum, slightly rough with a central threaded perforation 3.5 mm in diameter and with 12 perforations for sutures. The thickness is 1.2 mm centrally, tapering down to 0.2 mm in the edges. The optical cylinder is made of a single corundum crystal ($N = 1.767$). It is 10 mm in length and 3.5 mm in diameter with a thread to fit the retaining ring and optical surfaces, providing 60 diopters of power (Fig. 21-1).*

Instruments

Most instruments used in blepharoplasty and keratoplasty will be required. The techniques of implantation necessitate the use of periosteum or fascia lata. Fascia lata can be obtained by the direct approach from the side of the quadriceps and periosteum is acquired from the upper third of the tibial surface. Instruments required for this procedure include a scalpel, Stevens scissors, skin retractors, Freie periosteal elevator, 4-0 catgut, and 5-0 nylon.

The technique for periosteal removal is as follows: about 5 ml of 1 or 2 percent lidocaine (Xylocaine) with epinephrine is infiltrated along the anterior crest of the tibia in its upper third. The skin is then prepped and draped. An incision is made in the skin over the crest of the tibia, deep to the bone, for an extension of about 15 cm. The skin is then retracted; blunt dissection with scissors separates the subcutaneous fat from the surface of the periosteum. About 2 × 2 inches (5 × 5 cm) of per-

* This prothesis is available from Dr. G. Heimke, Zinkgrafstr 62, D-6940 Weinheim, West Germany.

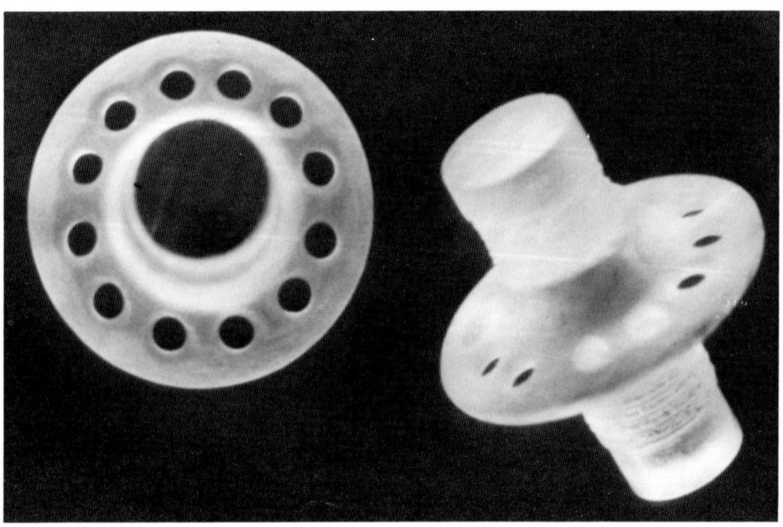

Fig. 21-1. The ceramic keratoprosthesis is made of aluminum oxide or corundum. The optical cylinder is 10 mm long and 3.5 mm in diameter with a thread to fit the retaining ring. This ring is 8.5 mm in diameter and has 12 perforations for sutures.

iosteal tissue is then isolated from the fat and connective tissue. The periosteum is elevated from the bony surface with the periosteal elevator and removed with scissors. The subcutaneous tissue is approximated with 4-0 catgut suture and the skin is closed with interrupted or continuous 5-0 nylon sutures. A compressive dressing is then applied to the leg.

Extremely thin corneas will require a full-thickness total corneal graft. A cryounit for cataract extraction will be required and a vitrectomy instrument should be available. Fine hemorrhages are controlled with a solution of 0.002 percent epinephrine.

Trephines

Ten- or-11 mm trephines are used in cases where the corneas must be replaced. A 3.5-mm trephine is needed for the optical portion of the keratoprosthesis.

Sutures

For keratoplasty, 8-0 black silk sutures are used; 6-0 black silk (Ethicon TG140-8) sutures secure a Flieringa ring, and 5-0 catgut fixes the periosteal donor tissue. When required, 5-0 nylon sutures are used for skin closure. The footplate of the keratoprosthesis is sutured to the cornea with a special-order Ethicon 8-0 prolene on a TG140-8 needle or a similar suture up to 5-0 size.

OPERATIVE TECHNIQUES

Technique I: Transcorneal Implantation

The surgical techniques, with minor modifications, are those of Castroviejo et al.[3] The typical indication for transcleral implantation is that of a chemical burn of the cornea and several failed grafts. Patients with scarred conjunctiva have required previous conjunctivoplasty or buccal mucosa graft. The prosthesis should be applied to the cornea only if it is of normal thickness. This can be determined with an ultrasonic pachymeter. Plans should be made to remove the lens if the patient is phakic. A generous vitrectomy is also required and resection of the iris should be done. After insertion of a lid speculum or traction sutures to the lid borders, a 360-degree peritomy of conjunctiva and Tenon's capsule with dissection toward the fornices is done (Fig. 21-2).

Bleeding is controlled with diluted epinephrine (1 : 20,000) and cautery. A single Flieringa ring, 18 or 20 mm, is sutured to the sclera immediately in front of the recti muscles with 6-0 silk sutures. The corneal limbus or corneal center may need to be identified and should be marked for future reference (Fig. 21-3). A corneal transplant is done at this point, if it is required. In this case, the 3.5-mm trephination is done before the graft is sutured in place. Lens extraction and total iris excision are done before vitrectomy. Since the plate of the prosthesis is 8.5 mm in diameter, the graft must be 10.5 or 11 mm. It is sutured with 8-0 silk material. It is

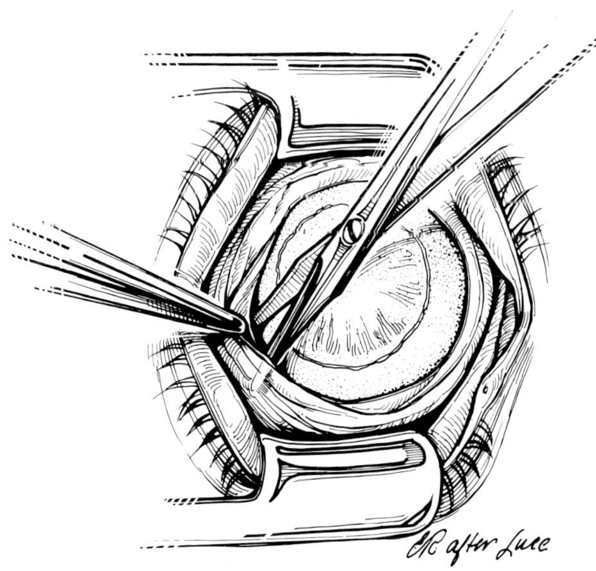

Fig. 21-2. A 360-degree peritomy is performed. The dissection is carried up to the fornices trying not to destroy usable conjunctiva. In cases of ocular pemphigoid, or scarred conjunctiva, this tissue must be removed completely in preparation for placing the prosthesis through the lid.

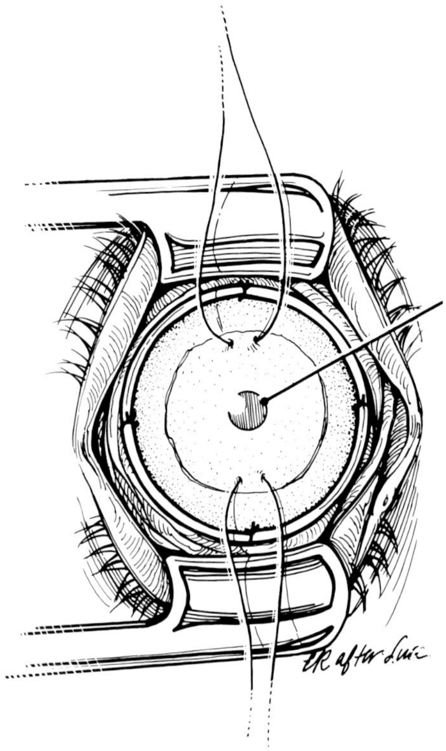

Fig. 21-3. A large Flieringa ring is secured to the sclera and the corneal center is identified. A 3.5-mm trephination is performed and preplaced sutures may be placed through the cornea about 4 to 5 mm from the center. If a cataract extraction is required, it is done before the steps here described.

convenient to perforate the exact center of the cornea partially with a 3.5-mm trephine, since this procedure is more difficult to perform after keratoplasty and vitrectomy. If the eye is aphakic, a large, wide basal iridectomy is done through a limbal incision. Vitrectomy can be performed through this incision or through the 3.5-mm opening. The plate of the keratoprosthesis is placed over the cornea aligning the central opening with the 3.5-mm trephination marking; two or three preplaced 8-0 prolene sutures are then passed through the cornea and perforations in the prosthesis. The sutures can be left alone without passing through the prosthesis, as long as they are in the correct position, thereby facilitating the start of fixation of the prosthesis. At this time, the 3.5-mm perforation is completed with a razorblade knife and Vannas scissors. The optical portion of the prosthesis is inserted into the eye (Fig. 21-4A), leaving about 4 mm of the optical portion to protrude out of the retaining plate. The preplaced sutures are tied and additional sutures are applied (Fig. 21-4B).

Balanced salt solution (BSS) is injected into the globe to provide normal eye pressure. Fluorescein may be used to check for leaks in cases with corneal grafts.

The periosteum, preserved in a Petri dish with BSS, is placed over the prosthesis; a small slit is made in its central portion so that the optical cylinder can be pushed through it; the periosteum is then sutured to the sclera with 5-0 catgut or 7-0 Vicryl. The conjunctiva and Tenon's are sutured over the prosthesis with 8-0 silk (Fig. 21-5). Sliding flaps may be required in order to place healthy and thick conjunctiva over the implant. Sutures will be removed within 2 to 3 weeks, at which time a slit is made in the conjunctiva over the optical portion (Fig. 21-6).

Technique II: Implantation through the Lid

This technique is used for eyes with severe scarring of the conjunctiva and dry eyes. As in the previous method, keratoplasty may be indicated if the cornea shows evidence of necrosis or thinning. Lensectomy, iridectomy, and vitrectomy are required in almost all cases.

An injectable anesthetic with epinephrine is injected through the lid borders and the symblepharon to reduce the amount of bleeding. The lid is separated from the adhesions to the globe with a #11 Beaver blade, while traction is made on the lid borders with 4-0 silk sutures. The dissection is continued with curved Westcott scissors and all remnants of diseased conjunctiva are removed (Fig. 21-2). The corneal limbus is identified and marked before a large Flieringa ring is sutured to the sclera (Fig. 21-3).

Keratoplasty, iris removal, lensectomy and vitrectomy are then performed. Suturing of the prosthesis and periosteal coverage is done as previously described after the ring is removed (Fig. 21-5A). The lateral and medial recti are severed to reduce eye movements. The lid borders are then removed (Fig. 21-7) and an incision made; the skin is sepa-

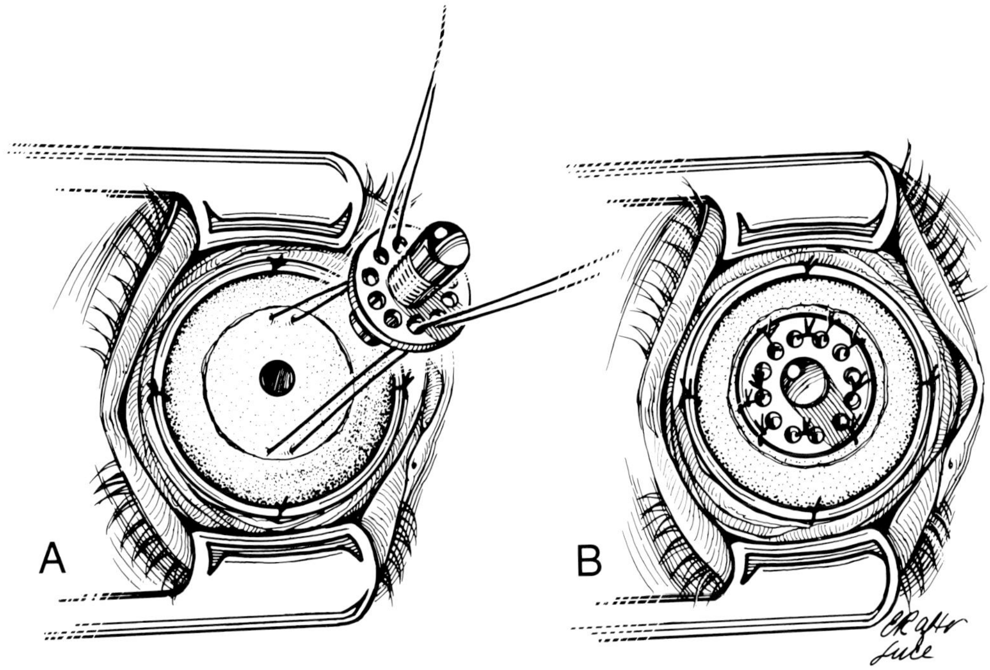

Fig. 21-4. (A) The central perforation is completed and a vitrectomy is performed through the opening. **(B)** The corneal prosthesis is then inserted through the opening and secured with the preplaced sutures.

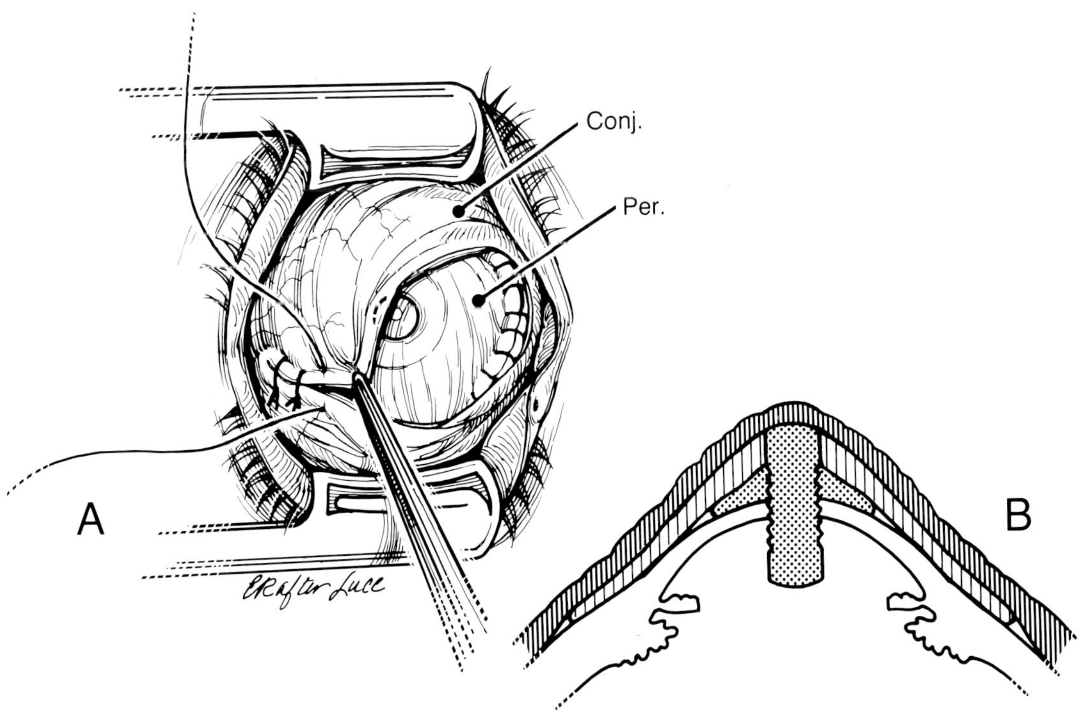

Fig. 21-5. (A) Once the prosthesis is secured in place with 8-0 prolene sutures, the Flieringa ring is removed and the area is covered with periosteum. **(B)** If the implant is to be covered with conjunctiva, the surface of the optical cylinder should be flush with the periosteum. If the prosthesis should be covered with skin of the eyelids, it should protrude 3 to 4 mm above the periosteum.

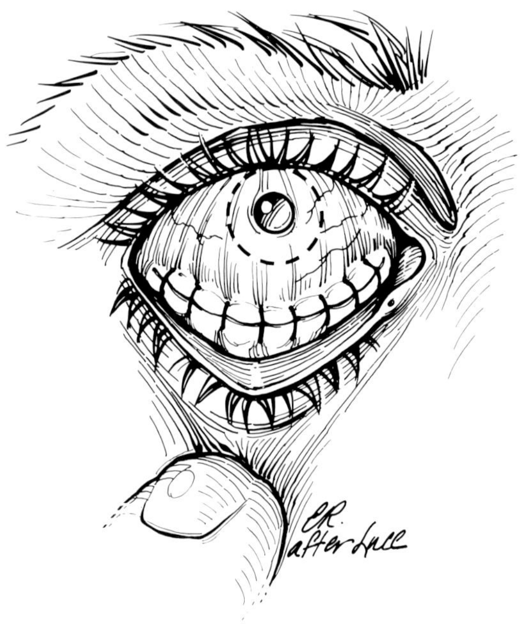

Fig. 21-6. Illustration showing the final result of a kerato-prosthesis placed through the conjunctiva.

rated by dissection from the orbicularis muscle, the levator, and the tarsus. These structures, including remnants of the conjunctiva, are removed with scissors, first from the lower lid, followed by the upper lid. Bleeders are tied or cauterized; the skin is closed over the prosthesis, which should protrude no more than 5 mm from the plate surface (Fig. 21-7). A perforation is made on the skin of the upper lid to pass the optical cylinder; this perforation can be done 2 weeks later, however, when the skin has adhered to the periosteum.

POSTOPERATIVE CARE

A firm bandage is applied to the eye for 24 hours and changed daily until the lid swelling disappears. Systemic antibiotics are used for 7 to 10 days. Strong analgesics are administered during the first 2 or 3 postoperative days.

The leg should be dressed with an elastic bandage and kept elevated for 48 hours. With the first method, the conjunctiva may be opened after 2 weeks. With the second method, the skin sutures on the lids are removed after 10 days and the leg sutures after 5 days.

The surface of the prosthesis is cleaned in a clockwise direction with saline solution. Antibiotic steroid drops as well as artificial tear solutions are applied frequently in the first technique. In the second technique, the skin of the lid is cleaned daily with baby liquid soap and tap water. The opti-

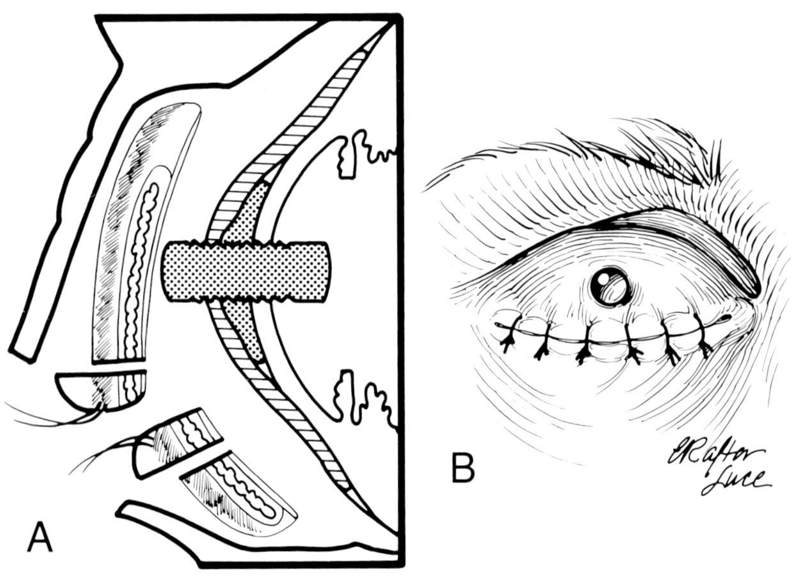

Fig. 21-7. (A) Insert shows a kerato-prosthesis in place covered with periosteum and about to be covered with skin of the eyelids. The lid borders, tarsus, and conjunctiva, will be removed. **(B)** The optical portion of the prosthesis is then exteriorized through the upper lid.

cal surface of the prosthesis can be cleaned daily with a contact lens-wetting solution.

If vision appears cloudy or if the fundus view through the prosthesis is cloudy, we use systemic steroids for a period of 1 week. Acetazolamide is given to patients with a history of glaucoma or when IOP elevation is suspected.

OPERATIVE AND POSTOPERATIVE COMPLICATIONS

The most serious complications during the surgical procedure are persistent bleeding from the ocular surface and intraocular hemorrhage. The first complication is mostly an annoyance that can be controlled with wet-field cautery and diluted epinephrine solution.

I caution against opening the eye until all bleeders have been controlled, to prevent blood from running into the vitreous cavity. Another problem occurs at the time the iris is excised. This procedure usually causes minimal bleeding, but at times it may bleed severely and blood may fill the vitreous if the eye is aphakic. If the lens is in situ, it is important to wait until the hemorrhage has subsided before removing it. Severe staining of the vitreous with blood may require a subtotal vitrectomy through a limbal port after suturing a corneal graft or via pars plana.

Since adopting the procedure of the lid scalping with removal of the tarsal plate, no infections of the tarsorraphy borders have occurred in any of our patients. Cloudiness of the vitreous has been observed during the first 2 postoperative weeks; this has been interpreted as vitritis by some authorities. Systemic steroids usually improve this problem.

Protrusion of the optical cylinder over the conjunctiva or lid occurs with both surgical techniques. Turning is required using two cellulose sponges or cotton-tipped applicators in a wrench-like fashion.

Prostheses through the skin have two frequent complications during the late postoperative period: retraction of the skin and periosteum around the implant, and partial dislocation or tilting of the prosthesis. The first complication can be repaired by opening the skin on either side of the prosthesis, dissecting it from the periosteal tissue. This layer is sutured with catgut and brought close to the optical cylinder. The skin borders are revived and closed around the prosthesis with nylon sutures. Partial dislocation of the prosthesis indicates that the plate has separated from its attachment to the cornea because of either suture rupture or corneal rupture by the prolene suture. This is frequently accompanied by a retrocorneal membrane. Excessive movement of the prosthesis requires resuturing. This implies the need for an almost complete procedure, and the surgeon must be ready to replace the prosthesis and to do a corneal graft if necessary. Retrocorneal membranes are not frequently seen with this material and if vitrectomy has been performed. Surgical division is almost impossible, but Nd:YAG laser discision has been done in one case with the Cardona prosthesis.[11]

Separation of the conjunctiva around the prosthesis in the first procedure, transcorneal implantation, occurs frequently. Repair is easy to perform and usually works wells for a period of several months.

Endophthalmitis has occurred in several cases following loosening of the prosthesis, persisting leakage, and poor patient compliance with medication or follow-up. If diagnosed early and treated vigorously, some vision can be spared. Unfortunately, in most cases this problem occurs insidiously and the patient is unaware of the severely compromised vision until it is too late.

Glaucoma is another well-known complication. Finger tension is about the only way to determine increased pressure of the eye, in addition to pain, increased cupping, and decreased field of vision. However, with a 3.5-mm opening the latter is impossible to evaluate adequately.

REFERENCES

1. Alamillo M, Alamillo R: Implantation of an artificial cornea. Am J Ophthalmol 56:937, 1963
2. Barraquer J: Inclusion de protesis opticas corneanas,

corneas acrilicas o queratoprotesis. Ann Inst. Barraquer 1:243, 1960
3. Castroviejo R, Cardona H, DeVoe AG: Present status of prosthokeratoplasty. Am J Ophthalmol 69:613, 1969
4. Choyce DP: The treatment of bullous keratopathy with acrylic inlays: Experience with Choyce two-piece acrylic keratoprosthesis. p. 399. In Rycroft PV (ed): Corneo-Plastic Surgery. Proceedings of the Second International Corneo-Plastic Conference. Pergamon, London, 1967
5. Girard LJ, Moore CD, Soper JW, O'Bannon W: Prosthetosclerokeratoplasty—Implantation of a keratoprosthesis using full-thickness onlay sclera and sliding conjunctival flap. Trans Am Adad Ophthalmol 73:936, 1969
6. Hoffman F, Harnisch JP, Strunz V, et al: Osteo-Keramo-Keratoprothese. Eine Modifikation der Osteo-Odonto-Keratoprothese nach Strampelli. Klin Mbl Augenheilkd 173:747, 1978
7. Strampelli, B: Osteo-odontocheratoprotesi. p. 1039. Ospedali Riuniti di Roma, Report Oculistico, Ospedale di S. Giovanni, 1963
8. Polack FM, Heimke G: Ceramic keratoprosthesis. Ophthalmology 87:693, 1980
9. Heimke G, Polack FM: Keramische Keratoprothesen. p. 28. In Proceedings of the German Congress in Ophthalmology, Heidelberg. Bergmann, Munich, 1977
10. Polack FM: Clinical results with a ceramic keratoprosthesis. Cornea 2:185, 1983
11. Bath P, McCord RC, Cox KC: Nd:YAG Laser dicision of retroprosthetic membrane: A preliminary report. Cornea 2:229, 1983

Section IV

GLAUCOMA

Jonathan Herschler

Section Editor

22 Clinical Presentation

Jonathan Herschler

Glaucoma is not a single disease entity but a category of diseases, all of which have in common the problem that the intraocular pressure (IOP) is too high for the health of the optic nerve. In other words, glaucoma is a pressure-induced optic neuropathy.

In certain instances, IOP is so high that, if it were allowed to remain so, damage to the trabecular drainage apparatus, and ultimately the optic nerve, would be expected shortly. Such cases require a surgical approach that is often directed to restoration of function of the patient's own outflow system, that is, peripheral iridectomy, goniotomy, trabeculodialysis, or trabeculotomy. In other glaucoma types, the pressure elevation is low grade and chronic. Medical therapy is usually effective. When progressive damage occurs in spite of maximal medical treatment, however, surgery is mandated.

If a specific defect can be found in the outflow structures, a surgical procedure to correct that defect is most appropriate. If no specific defect can be found, and when maximal medical therapy fails, an operation to create new outflow by bypassing the impaired drainage structures is in order.

If multiple attempts at bypassing the drainage structures fail, attempts to decrease aqueous production become the next line of defense. However, the secret to the successful choice of an operation is the proper diagnosis of the glaucoma type, the correct and maximal use of medical therapy, and, only when medical treatment fails, the appropriate choice of a surgical procedure.

The following is a guide through the glaucoma puzzle that may serve as an aid in selecting the proper procedure once an appropriate diagnosis has been made (Table 22-1).

Congenital glaucoma (glaucoma in infancy) should be handled as surgical disease. The procedures of choice are goniotomy and trabeculotomy (see Chapter 26). Filtration procedures (Chapter 27) are used only if multiple goniotomies and trabeculotomies have failed.

Primary angle-closure glaucoma caused by relative pupillary block also should be considered solely as a surgical problem, with medication used only to treat the acute attack. Peripheral iridectomy is the procedure of choice, whether performed with the laser in the office or in the operating room with a scalpel (see Chapter 24).

For other glaucoma types, maximal medical therapy — which will differ depending on patient and glaucoma variety — is indicated prior to surgical intervention.

Table 22-1. Glaucoma Road Map

Diagnosis	Procedure	Chapter Ref.
Congenital glaucoma	Goniotomy	26
	↓ if fails	
	Trabeculotomy	26
	↓ if fails	
	Trabeculectomy	27
Primary angle closure (relative or complete pupil block)	Laser or surgical iridectomy	24
Primary open angle Pseudoexfoliation Pigmentary Traumatic	Laser trabeculoplasty	25
	↓ if fails	
	Filtration	27
ICE syndrome Neovascular	Filtration	27
	↓ if fails	
	Filtration with seton	29
	↓ if fails	
	Cyclodestructive	30
Aphakic open-angle glaucoma	Laser trabeculoplasty	25
	↓ if fails	
	Filtration	
	↓ if fails	
	Cyclodialysis	31
	↓ if fails	
	Filtration with seton	29
	↓ if fails	
	Cyclodestructive	30
Inflammatory	Trabeculodialysis	26
	↓ if fails	
	Filtration	27
	↓ if fails	
	Filtration with seton	29
Cataract and primary open-angle glaucoma	Filtration	27
	⇅	
	Cataract extraction	
	Combined	28

Anatomy in Glaucoma-Related Surgery

23

Donald S. Minckler

This discussion of ocular anatomy is limited to features of the eye that are relevant to glaucoma surgery; detailed discussions of ocular anatomy and histology are available in several current texts.[1–3] Because the area of interest to the glaucoma surgeon is usually the anterior segment of the eye, especially the superior portion, it is essential that he or she be intimately familiar with major external and internal anatomic features and surgical landmarks. This is particularly true in procedures for congenital or secondary glaucomas, where the disease and previous surgery may have distorted the normal anatomic features of the anterior segment.

During the preoperative evaluation of any patient in whom filtration surgery is contemplated, an examination of the eyelids, conjunctival fornices, and lacrimal apparatus should be conducted. Infections, inflammations, or anomalies of these structures, including lacrimal drainage difficulties, may predispose to postoperative infection or failure of the filtration surgery; disease of the lacrimal system should be treated and, ideally, resolved prior to surgery. Preoperative treatment or chronic treatment with topical antibiotics may be indicated if persisting inflammation is infectious in origin. Inadequacies of basal tear secretion or diseases affecting the mucous membrane function, such as ocular pemphigoid, may be serious obstacles to sucessful filtration surgery, and such eyes are probably at significantly greater risk of immediate or delayed postoperative infection. Chronic inflammation associated with external disease probably also increases the risk of failure of filtration surgery.

Primary filtration surgery is almost always performed in the superior portions of the anterior segment. Since most types of filtration surgery use approximately one quadrant of the limbal circumference, it is highly desirable to place the initial incision in the middle of one or the other superior quadrants, thereby preserving the opposite quadrant for future use if necessary. Placement of the initial incision at the 12 o'clock position should be avoided.

In preoperative evaluation of previously operated eyes, the surgeon should be particularly interested in the mobility of the conjunctiva and the extent of scarring in episcleral tissues with regard to the likelihood of excessive scarring postoperatively. Avoiding previously operated areas leads to a greater chance of success for the subsequent procedure. The most difficult and least desirable area in which to perform standard filtration surgery is certainly the inferior nasal quadrant since one must operate across the nose, making visualization and tissue manipulation extremely awkward.

CORNEA

The adult human cornea appears horizontally elliptical when viewed externally, but is in fact round at Schwalbe's line when viewed posteriorly. The apparent contraction in the vertical meridian externally is created by fibrovascular ingrowth at the level of Bowman's membrane superiorly. Normal corneal measurements are listed in Table 23-1.

Eyes with buphthalmia secondary to congenital glaucoma undergo marked stretching of the eye wall, especially in the region between the rectus muscle insertions and the cornea. Eyes with corneal diameters of 14 mm or more will demonstrate marked distortion of limbal anatomy, making procedures requiring anatomic precision, such as trabeculotomy, difficult to perform. Buphthalmos is often also associated with marked thinning of the sclera, making the dissection of lamellar scleral flaps exceedingly difficult. Such eyes are prone to develop staphylomata in sites where dissection further weakens the sclera.

Table 23-1. General Ocular Dimensions (Adult)

Anterior–posterior diameter	24 mm (21–26-mm range)
Vertical/horizontal diameter at equator	23–25 mm
Weight	7.5 g
Volume	6.5 ml
Anterior chamber volume	0.25 ml
Posterior chamber volume	0.06 ml
Vitreous volume	3.9 ml
Anterior chamber depth (age-dependent)	3.6 mm (males) 3.4 mm (females)
Central corneal thickness	0.52 mm
Corneal thickness at limbus	0.67 mm
Scleral thickness at limbus	0.67 mm
Scleral thickness at equator	0.4 mm
Peripapillary scleral thickness	1.0 mm
Optic nerve diameter (including dura)	4.5 mm
Corneal diameter	
Horizontal	11.75 mm
Vertical	10.6 mm

Rectus Muscle Insertions	Width (mm)	Distance from Limbus (mm)
Medial	10.6	5.5
Inferior	10.0	6.5
Lateral	9.4	6.9
Superior	10.8	7.7

Every effort should be made to avoid injury to the corneal epithelium during glaucoma surgery, especially in eyes with epithelial disease such as chronic herpes keratitis. In such cases, when surgery is necessary, it may be preferable to use limbal-based conjunctival flaps to reduce the chances of epithelial injury, delayed wound healing, and postoperative aqueous leaks.

CONJUNCTIVA

The conjunctival epithelium blends with the corneal epithelium at the end of Bowman's membrane. The corneal and bulbar conjunctival epithelium are nonkeratinizing and stratified squamous in type. The conjunctival epithelium contains goblet cells, normally absent in the corneal epithelium. The epithelium of the bulbar conjunctiva and its scanty stroma fuse with Tenon's capsule for 2 to 4 mm posterior to the end of Bowman's membrane. Subconjunctival hemorrhages will often dissect to the edge of clear cornea. Retrobulbar hemorrhages will usually dissect anteriorly only to the line of fusion between Tenon's capsule and episcleral connective tissues, leaving a ring of blood-free space posterior to the margin of clear cornea. While normally transparent and moderately mobile, the conjunctiva rapidly becomes thickened and semitransparent during the trauma associated with surgery. If torn, the conjunctiva can usually be easily repaired at the conclusion of filtration surgery. During the preparation of a fornix-based conjunctival flap, the fused portions of Tenon's capsule and conjunctiva can be separated as a single layer near the end of Bowman's membrane.

Lymphatic channels, which may play an important role in removal of aqueous from the subconjunctival spaces following glaucoma surgery, are present in the substantia propria of the conjunctiva.[2] An incomplete pericorneal lymphatic network has been described, including collector channels running circumferentially as far posterior as 7 or 8 mm from the limbal area.[2]

Bleeding from limbal arcades invariably accompanies separation of the conjunctiva and Tenon's capsule from the edge of the cornea. Bleeding often continues, from severed vessels on the corneal side of the incision. Light cautery may be safely applied to the corneal side of the wound, but is inadvisable along the anterior edge of the conjunctiva because of concern about increasing the likelihood of postoperative wound leak. Cautery of the conjunctival wound posteriorly during dissection of a limbal based flap is seldom necessary. Bleeding will almost always occur from episcleral vessels during dissection of conjunctival flaps, regardless of whether they are limbal or fornix-based.

TENON'S CAPSULE

Tenon's capsule (fascia bulbi) surrounds the globe, extending from the corneal–scleral junction anteriorly to the optic nerve posteriorly. This

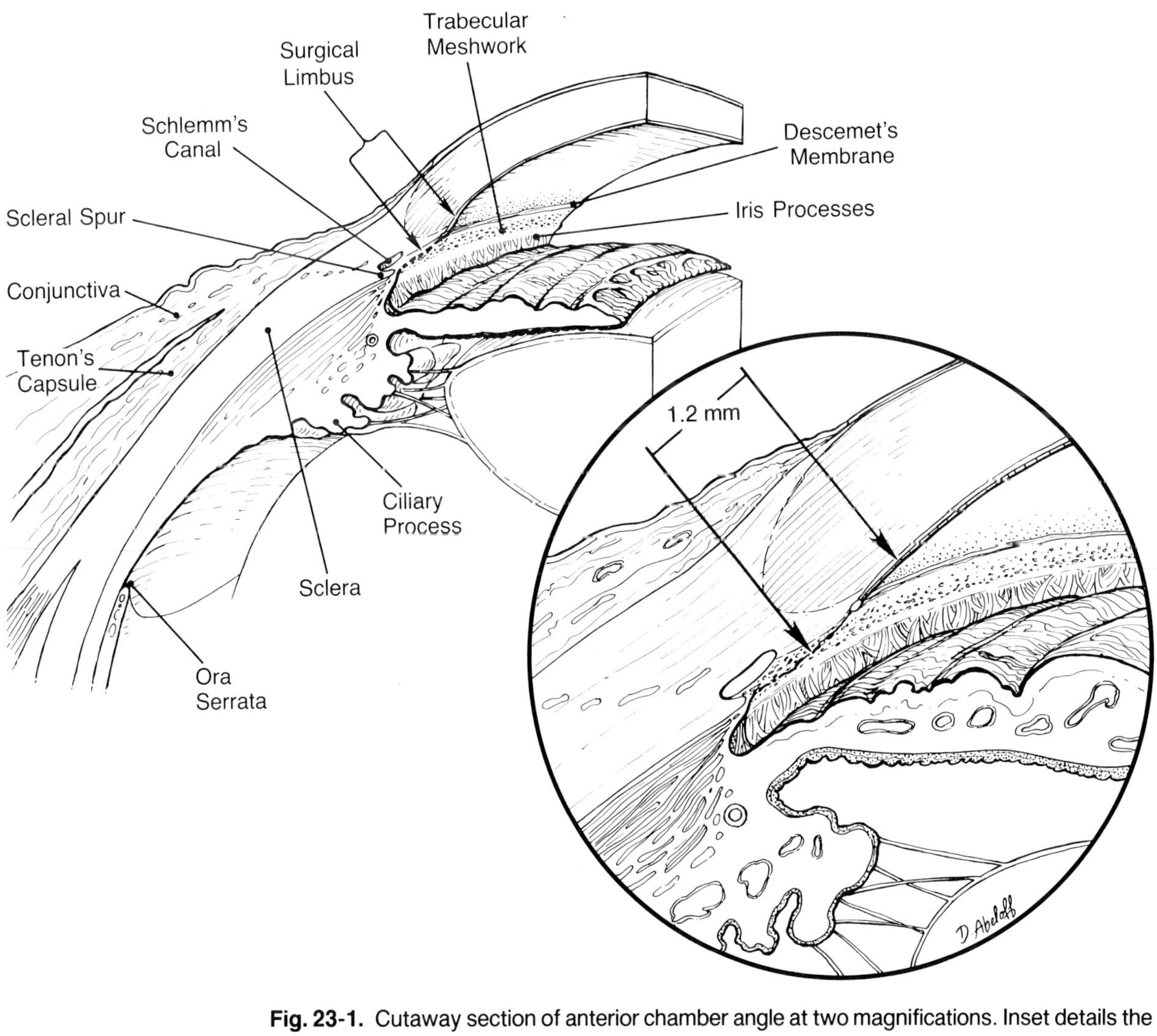

Fig. 23-1. Cutaway section of anterior chamber angle at two magnifications. Inset details the 1.2-mm surgical limbus.

connective tissue layer is probably a major site of fibroblastic activity during wound healing. Anteriorly Tenon's capsule fuses with the conjunctiva and episclera for 2 to 4 mm posterior to the cornea (Fig. 23-1). The more posterior portions are thicker, except adjacent to the optic nerve. Tenon's capsule is thickest between the insertions of the external rectus muscles and is often identifiable as a distinct layer during filtration surgery while dissecting a limbal-based flap. Tenon's capsule is attached to connective tissue between lobules of retrobulbar fat and fuses inferiorly with the suspensory ligament of Lockwood. The rectus muscles are completely ensheathed by extensions of Tenon's capsule. Extensions of Tenon's capsule also compartmentalize the orbital tissues into a peripheral space and a central space. The central space, containing the optic nerve, is the compartment into which local anesthetics are most often injected for ocular surgery. Tenon's capsule is generally more prominent in the young than in the aged, and it may be more substantial in heavily pigmented than in lightly pigmented individuals.

It remains controversial whether or not Tenon's capsule should be removed during filtration surgery, since its role in subsequent function of filtering blebs is not clear. Certainly Tenon's capsule should not be left exposed or protruding through conjunctival wounds, since it may act as a wick for infection of subconjunctival spaces or produce a formidable granulation tissue response (pyogenic granuloma). During enucleation, in order to obtain a significant length of optic nerve with the globe, it is helpful to break through Tenon's capsule around the nerve that joins the episcleral space with the central space and to slide the enucleation scissors posteriorly along the nerve. The episcleral space can be greatly expanded by fluid accumulations; and it would be the ideal space into which local anesthetics might diffuse to secure complete anesthesia of the globe, since all sensory branches of the fifth nerve from the eye must cross this space.

Scar formation as a result of previous injury or surgery involving Tenon's capsule may restrict rectus muscle function or lead to fusion of muscles and episcleral tissues. Tenon's capsule usually persists as a distinct layer over scar tissues formed around retinal buckle elements or glaucoma drainage implants.

SURGICAL LIMBUS

The limbus can be defined histologically as the junction between cornea and sclera. For practical purposes, the surgical limbus is defined as the region bounded medially by a line between the termination of Bowman's and Descemet's membranes, posteriorly by the trabecular meshwork and scleral spur, laterally by a line perpendicular to the surface of the conjunctiva intersecting the lateral wall of the iris recess, and anteriorly by the junction between corneal and conjunctival epithelium. Within this region lie structures of utmost concern to the glaucoma surgeon, including the trabecular meshwork, Schlemm's canal, and major portions of the deep and superficial aqueous drainage channels (Fig. 23-1). The surgical limbus comprises a zone measuring approximately 1.2 mm in width along the conjunctival surface superiorly.[1]

The most consistent and surgically useful landmark of this region when viewed from the subconjunctival space is the posterior border of the so-

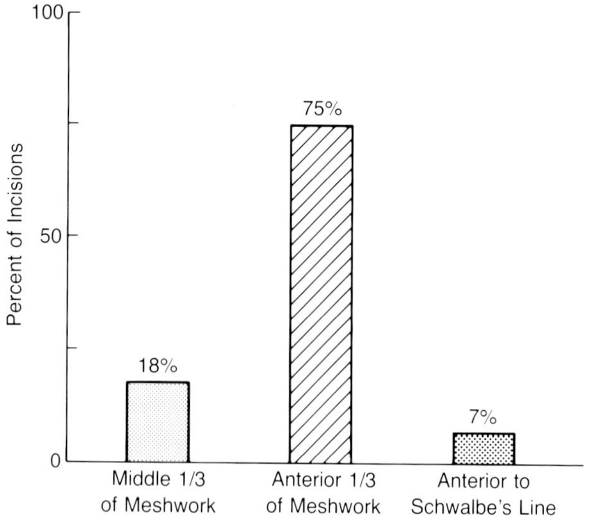

Fig. 23-2. A histologic study of 69 normal autopsy eyes demonstrated that a superior scleral incision perpendicular to the posterior margin of the blue limbus entered the middle third of meshwork in 18 percent of the cases, the anterior third in 75 percent, and anterior to Schwalbe's line in 7 percent.

called blue limbus (Fig. 23-1). The blue limbus, adjacent to the cornea, varies in clarity in different eyes and is apparently created by scatter of light by pericorneal scleral tissues. In our own histologic study of 69 normal autopsy eyes, a superior scleral incision perpendicular to the posterior margin of the blue limbus entered the eye in the middle of the trabecular meshwork 18 percent of the time, in the anterior one third of the trabecular meshwork 75 percent of the time, and anterior to Schwalbe's line 7 percent of the time (Fig. 23-2). Similar experiments involving incisions corresponding to 3, 6, and 9 o'clock positions around the circumference of the blue limbus demonstrated the same general relationships. A line perpendicular to the surface at the posterior border of the blue limbus will generally intersect the inner eye wall in the middle or more anterior meshwork. The glaucoma surgeon, when faced with the need to rotate his incisions into the inferior quadrants, can thus use the blue limbus as a reliable anatomic marker denoting his relative position with regard to the internal structures of the angle. The blue limbus is widest at 12 o'clock, least wide at 3 and 9 o'clock, and intermediate in width at the 6 o'clock position (Fig. 23-3).

As long as the deep incision is at or anterior to a perpendicular drawn from the posterior edge of the blue limbus externally, the surgeon will avoid the increased vascularity of the more posterior limbal region, the ciliary body, and the iris root. Since

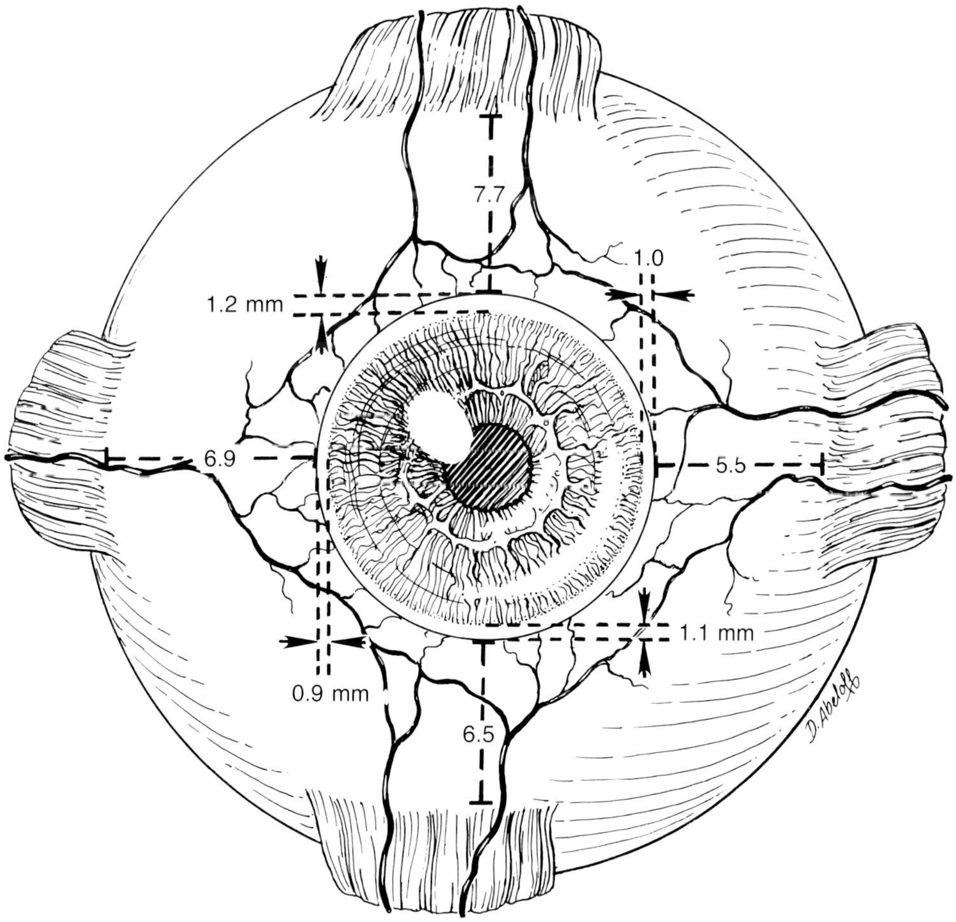

Fig. 23-3. Anterior view of the globe. Width of blue limbus is widest at 12 o'clock, and most narrow at 9 o'clock. The differing widths result in a good anatomic marker denoting the relative position with regard to internal structures of the anterior chamber angle.

the posterior margins of the blue limbus will move posteriorly during dissection of scleral flaps as the sclera is thinned over the scleral sulcus, the surgeon should be anatomically oriented before beginning the dissection.

In summary, the posterior margin of the surgical limbus is anatomically marked externally by the posterior edge of the blue limbus and internally bears a reasonably consistent relationship to the end of Descemet's membrane. The anterior margin of the surgical limbus externally varies by quadrant with the location of the end of Bowman's membrane. The zone between clear cornea externally and the end of Descemet's membrane internally is widest superiorly.

ANTERIOR CHAMBER

The relative depth of the anterior chamber angle is of obvious concern to the glaucoma surgeon during filtration procedures. The deeper the angle, the less likely the surgeon is to encounter iris vessels or iris prolapse during filtration surgery. Anterior chamber depth, while averaging approximately 3.5 mm centrally in adults, varies markedly peripherally. Eyes anatomically predisposed to angle closure typically have extremely narrow anterior chamber angles. If angle closure has occurred and peripheral anterior synechiae are present, the angle may be obliterated, making a clean anterior chamber entrance impossible. The likelihood of prolapse of iris root and ciliary processes into filtration fistulas is increased in eyes with relatively small, crowded anterior segments. Anterior chamber depth generally is dependent on multiple variables, including refractive error, age, and sex.[1]

The major gonioscopic landmarks of anterior chamber angle anatomy include Schwalbe's line anteriorly, the trabecular meshwork, the scleral spur, the angle recess, and the iris surface (Fig. 23-4). By far the most important landmark for purposes of internal angle surgery, including laser trabeculoplasty, is the scleral spur, which represents a horizontally arranged bundle of collagenous tissues and increases in prominence with age (Figs. 23-1, 23-4). Pigmentation of the trabecular meshwork varies markedly from eye to eye, but when present is a valuable aid to anatomic orientation. Pigment anterior to or at Schwalbe's line (Sampaolesi's line) can be confused gonioscopically with pigment in the meshwork. Pigmentation of the meshwork in normal eyes occurs in maximal

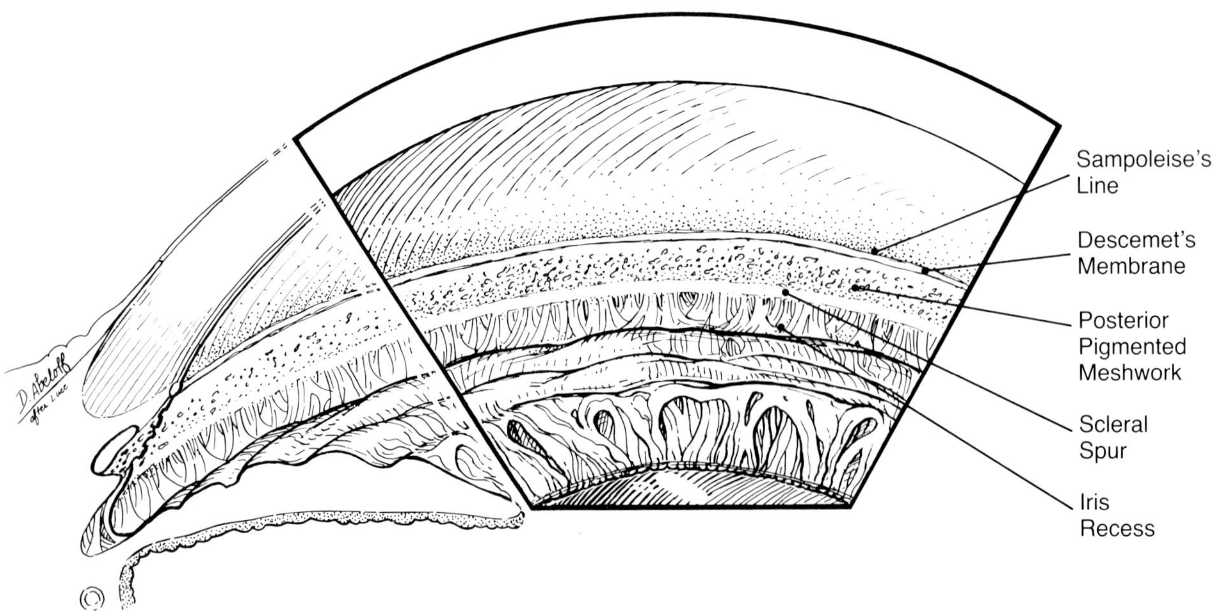

Fig. 23-4. Anatomic and gonioscopic view of the anterior chamber angle.

amounts inferiorly, and is progressively less prominent nasally, temporally, and superiorly. Pigment in the filtering meshwork may mark the location of major aqueous collector channels.[4] The trabecular meshwork is approximately 0.8 to 1 mm in meridonal width. Schlemm's canal, not ordinarily visible gonioscopically except when filled with blood, is approximately 30 to 45 μm in meridonal width. The anterior border of Schlemm's canal is usually close to a perpendicular line from the posterior margin of the blue limbus, approximately 1.5 mm posterior to the edge of Bowman's membrane externally. Schlemm's canal can usually be found by making a small radial incision into the base of a lamellar dissection and carefully examining the incision edges between 1 and 2 mm posterior to the edge of Bowman's membrane externally (Fig. 23-5). The inner surface of Schlemm's canal will often appear mucoid in texture. During trabeculotomy, it is wise to place the searching incision so that it may be converted to one arm of a trabecular excision (trabeculectomy) if the canal is not clearly identified (Fig. 23-5).

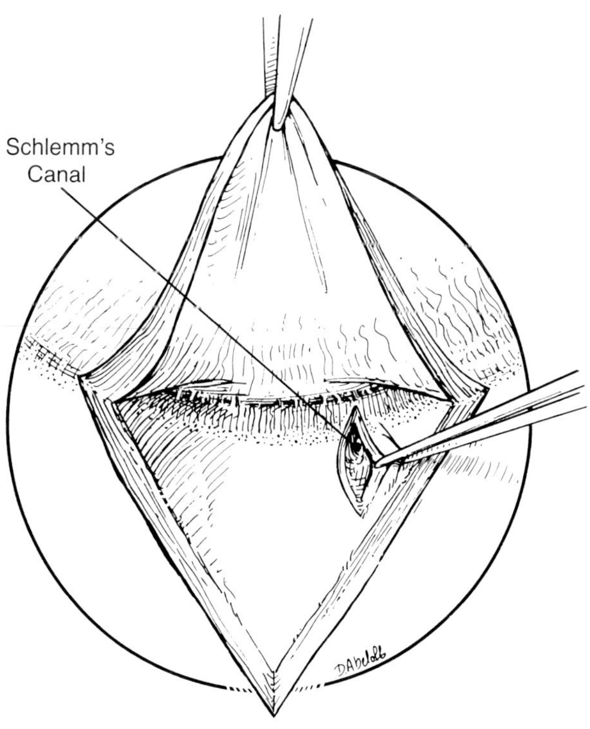

Fig. 23-5. Schlemm's canal can usually be found by making a small radial incision into the base of a lamellar dissection and carefully examining the incision edges between 1 and 2 mm posterior to the edge of Bowman's membrane externally.

During trabeculectomy the trabecular meshwork can often be clearly identified by pigment if the surgeon first completes the anterior three limbs of the excision and folds the flap externally with direct visualization of the inner surface prior to removal. This technique has the added advantage of ensuring clearance of ciliary processes.

SCLERA

The sclera varies in thickness from 0.67 mm at the limbus to 0.4 mm at the equator, thickening to approximately 1 mm adjacent to the optic nerve. The sclera is thinnest and most easily ruptured just posterior to the rectus muscle insertions, and is increased in thickness at the tendinous insertions of rectus muscles (Fig. 23-1). In contrast to the cornea, which has a highly organized collagenous structure, the sclera is composed of more randomly arranged collagen fibrils apparently coated with less intervening ground substance than in the cornea.[2] Spatula needles (side cutting) should be used exclusively when placing sutures into sclera to avoid perforation of the choroid and laceration of the retina. Anteriorly, as viewed in a coronal section, sclera blends with cornea in a curvilinear line marking the outer edge of the scleral sulcus, in which the trabecular meshwork is embedded. This histologic boundary cannot be clearly identified surgically. The disparity in light scatter created by this boundary probably accounts for the abovementioned blue limbus. During the course of a lamellar flap dissection, the blue limbus recedes posteriorly, corresponding to the curve of the scleral sulcus. During the dissection of lamellar flaps hinged at the cornea, the surgeon will usually notice the change in organization from compact to more loosely arranged collagen lamellae near clear cornea. Often aqueous or mixtures of aqueous and blood will leak from severed collector channels near the cornea. Cautery causes marked shrinkage of sclera and must be used with caution, especially along the edges of scleral flaps.

CILIARY BODY

The ciliary body extends peripherally from the ora serrata to the root of the iris, where the longitudinal ciliary muscle inserts into the scleral spur (Fig. 23-1). The supraciliaris comprises a loose, fibrillar elastic tissue joining the sclera to the ciliary portion of the uveal tract. Ciliary muscles are embedded in a connective tissue stroma, which along with a vasculature, forms the main substance of the ciliary process. The pigmented (external) and nonpigmented (internal) ciliary epithelium, continuous with the iris epithelium anteriorly, line the inner aspect of the ciliary body, forming the boundary between ciliary body and posterior chamber. Approximately 70 to 80 prominent folds (ciliary processes) arranged meridionally comprise the pars plicata. Ciliary processes measure approximately 2 mm in length and 0.5 mm in width.[1] The anterior edges of the ciliary processes are immediately posterior to the plane of the iris insertion. Ciliary processes are frequently exposed during basal iridectomies. In eyes with crowded anterior segments (hyperopic eyes) prone to angle closure, ciliary processes have considerable proclivity to rotate anteriorly and herniate into glaucoma fistulas. Bleeding from the posterior edge of the deep scleral excision during trabeculectomy may be from ciliary body vessels or damaged ciliary processes.

IRIS

The iris is normally thinnest, often consisting of only two layers of pigment epithelium including dilator muscles and minimal stroma, at its insertion into the ciliary body. The mobility of the peripheral iris varies markedly depending upon preexisting disease and will be minimal with peripheral anterior synechiae or rubeosis iridis. Posterior synechiae between iris and lens may also greatly limit iris mobility during iridectomy. Significant bleeding from the iris during iridectomy is infrequent. Care must be taken during iridectomy to ensure that both layers of the pigment epithelium are removed and that sufficient iris is excised to preclude its herniation into the glaucoma fistula. The edges of the iridectomy should lie beyond the edges of the internal fistula. Care should be taken to not inadvertently produce a cyclodialysis cleft or iris disinsertion during iridectomy. Ciliary processes may lie in close apposition to the posterior iris surface and are at hazard during iridectomy.

LENS

The adult human lens has an average equatorial diameter of approximately 9 to 10 mm and a thickness of 4 to 5 mm. The anterior surface of the lens contacts the pupillary margin of the iris, most often the site of pupillary block. The more curved posterior lens surface rests in the hyaloid fossa of the vitreous body. The lens is mobile, remarkably flexible, and may herniate without rupture into a wound, including a glaucoma fistula. Approximately 140 zonular fiber bundles have been defined comprising the lens suspensory ligaments that surround the lens equator in a 1.5-mm zone anteriorly and a 1-mm zone posteriorly. The zonules extend to adjacent ciliary processes and into ciliary valleys to the region of the ora serrata. Zonular fibers attach to the vitreous base over the pars plana. The glaucoma surgeon must use caution during manipulations of angle structures to avoid injury to the lens. The lens is at risk during cauterization of the posterior edge of trabeculectomy wounds.

NEUROVASCULAR STRUCTURES

Vessels sufficiently consistent in location to warrant attention for surgical considerations include the long posterior ciliary arteries, the anterior cili-

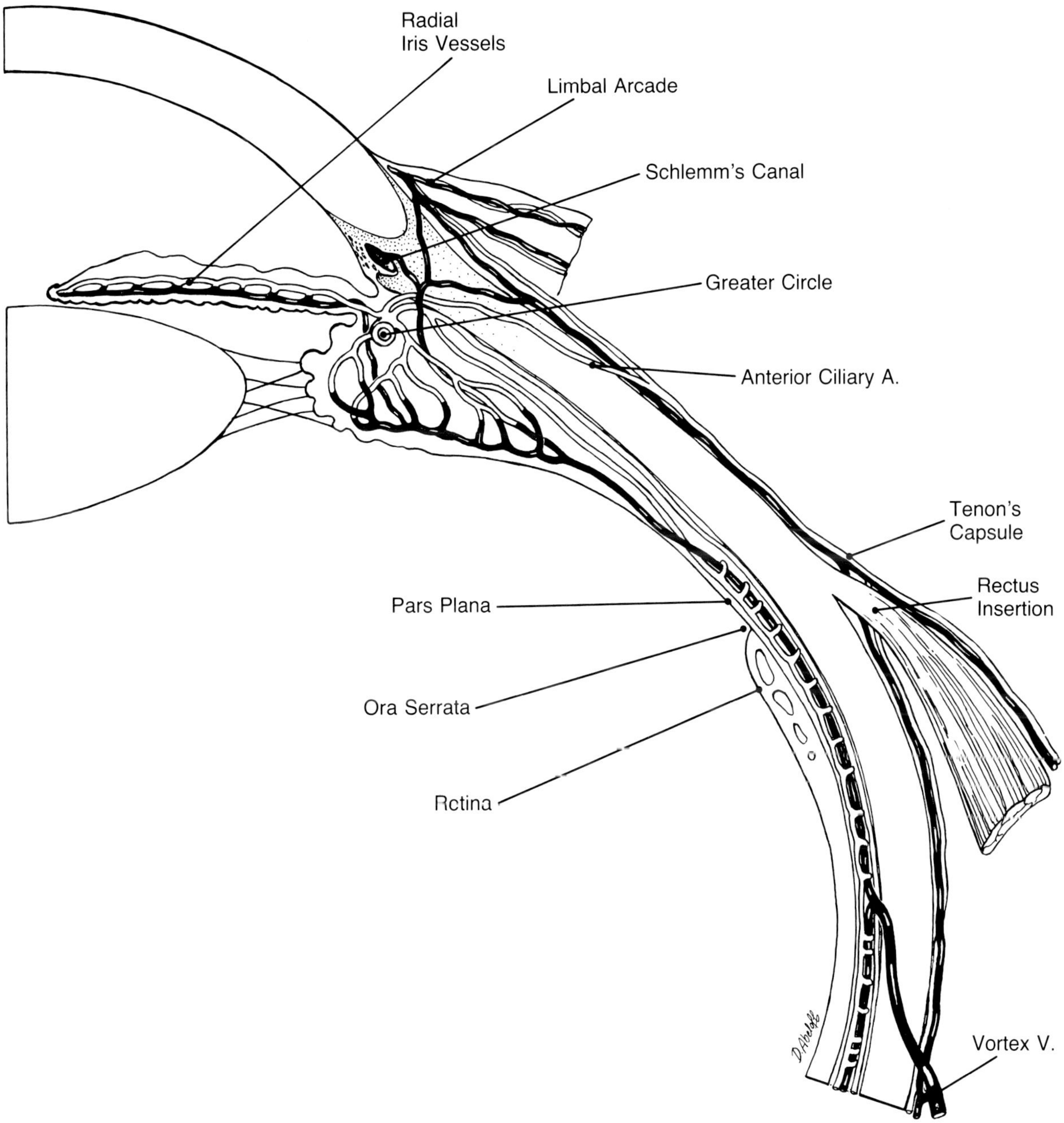

Fig. 23-6. Sagittal view of the main arterial and venous channels pertinent to glaucoma surgery.

ary arteries, the major circle of the iris, and vortex veins (Fig. 23-6).

The two long posterior ciliary arteries enter the globe in the horizontal meridian posteriorly on each side and superior to the optic nerve. These relatively large vessels run anteriorly within the sclera and choroid in the company of the long ciliary nerves to break into branches at the ora serrata and anastomose with the anterior ciliary circulation. The medial long posterior ciliary artery and nerve are often accompanied by significant pigment along their course through the sclera and are usually easily identified externally.

The anterior ciliary arteries enter the eye wall through the insertions of the rectus muscles, two for each muscle, except the lateral rectus, which typically has only one. After entering the sclera, they branch and join the major circle of the iris lying in the anterior aspect of the ciliary body. Branches of the anterior ciliary vessels extend posteriorly to anastomose with branches of the long posterior ciliary arteries. Radial branches of the greater circle extend forward into the iris.

Vortex veins, normally one per quadrant, exit the sclera approximately 3 mm posterior to the equator. The vortex veins drain virtually the entire choroid, posterior to the ora serrata. Veins accompanying the anterior ciliary arteries anastomose with veins in the anterior uveal tract and iris via the limbal region, in addition to draining the limbal arcades.

The glaucoma surgeon will encounter various degrees of bleeding, depending primarily on preexisting disease or chronic medications. Recently operated eyes tend to be extremely congested and areas of scar formation from previous injury or surgery may harbor large vessels. Marked variation in the size and arborization of anterior ciliary vessels around rectus muscle insertions will be encountered. Lowering intraocular pressure (IOP) during surgery may be accompanied by an increase in bleeding.

The long posterior ciliary nerves, carrying primarily afferent branches of the fifth cranial nerve, run in association with the long posterior ciliary artery through the sclera and choroid. The long posterior ciliary nerves branch extensively in the region of the ciliary body.

Nerve loops of Axenfeld, most common nasally, may occur as small pigmented nodules 3 to 4 mm posterior to the limbus. They are typically heavily pigmented, especially in darkly pigmented individuals, and may be painful if touched. These structures, which mark the junction of the pars plicata and pars plana internally, represent externalized loops of ciliary nerves and are often accompanied by small blood vessels and occasionally smooth muscle.

CHOROID

The choroid, representing the pigmented and richly vascular posterior extension of uveal tissues, ensheaths the globe between sclera and retina posterior to the ciliary body. Histologically, the choroid includes several layers of venous channels decreasing in size as they progress internally toward the choriocapillaris. The choriocapillaris receives arterial blood directly via perpendicularly oriented arterioles that branch into capillary lobules. Venous return from the choroid is largely dependent on the vortex vein system, which includes multiple inner ampulles concentrating into at least four vortex veins externally, at least one in each quadrant. Relatively rapid decrease of intraocular pressure, such as during glaucoma surgery, may trigger choroidal effusion and occasionally choroidal hemorrhage, apparently by constriction of vortex vein outflow. Maintenance of intraocular pressure within relatively normal ranges may be necessary to protect vortex vein outflow since vortex veins may be constricted by the sclera when intraocular pressure falls. Shearing forces generated by low intraocular pressure and globe collapse may also contribute to rupture of small arteries, especially in atherosclerotic individuals. The glaucoma surgeon should make every effort during surgical procedures to minimize hypotony and avoid undue distortion of the globe.

Choroidal effusion and choroidal hemorrhage typically initially expand the suprachoroid, the space between the sclera and the outer portions of the choroid. With massive hemorrhage, blood may infiltrate virtually all layers of the choroid in addition to rupturing internally into the subretinal and vitreous spaces.

VITREOUS

The vitreous in the average adult eye is relatively syneretic posteriorly. Formed vitreous tends to collapse anteriorly and almost always persists as relatively firm gel in the region of the vitreous base lining the junction between retina and pars plana. The formed vitreous base can easily participate in closure of glaucoma drainage fistulas when it is incarcerated or sufficiently mobile to enter the internal opening. Vitrectomy performed through glaucoma fistulas must be sufficient to clear the immediate area of formed vitreous. Aphakic eyes, following intracapsular cataract extraction, are at high risk for vitreous loss during glaucoma-filtering procedures. Filtering surgery on pseudophakic eyes following extracapsular cataract surgery will usually not involve vitreous loss, unless zonular damage or vitreous loss were encountered during cataract extraction. The use of a Flieringa ring or anterior segment support system and provision for infusion should vitrectomy be necessary, are advisable modifications of surgical technique in many aphakic eyes, especially following intracapsular cataract extraction. Compression of vitreous gel anteriorly probably plays a role in blocking aqueous flow into the anterior segment in "malignent glaucoma." In this syndrome misdirected aqueous apparently accumulates behind the posterior hyaloid.

RETINA

Fortunately, the retina is infrequently encountered by the glaucoma surgeon! He must remember, however, that any vascularized "membrane" suddenly appearing during surgery, may represent a detached retina or evidence of an expanding choroid. Previously operated or traumatized eyes may harbor traction detachments of the retina, including anterior displacement of retina with adhesion to ciliary body, iris, or lens remnants. A preoperative ultrasound evaluation is wise in any situation in which a clear appraisal of intraocular tissues cannot be accomplished by other means.

OPTIC NERVE

The optic nerve, while ostensibly the main benefactor of glaucoma surgery, may suffer indirect damage during filtration procedures. The central retinal artery and vein are both at some risk during marked fluctuations of IOP. Especially in eyes with badly damaged nerves, the surgeon must be careful not to inadvertently raise IOP during surgical manipulations prior to entering the eye and he should strive to keep changes in IOP during surgery as gradual as possible. Postoperative retinal or optic disc hemorrhages may occur following glaucoma surgery, probably secondary to large changes in IOP over short periods of time. Aggravation of preexisting disease such as cellophane retinopathy or creation of cystoid macular edema may be complications of manipulation or inflammation following glaucoma surgery. Collapse of the globe during glaucoma surgery may aggravate detachment of a recently buckled retina.

RECTUS MUSCLES

The insertions of the rectus muscles correspond externally to the ora serrata internally (Fig. 23-1). This anatomic relationship provides a reliable guide to the width of the pars plana and access to the suprachoroidal space or anterior vitreous during glaucoma surgery. The distances between the edge of the cornea and the rectus muscles are illustrated in Figure 23-1 and Table 23-1. In the phakic eye, a site 4 mm posterior to the limbus regardless of the quadrant should provide a safe port for drainage of choroidal effusion or placement of instruments into the anterior vitreous, avoiding the lens anteriorly and the retina posteriorly. In aphakic eyes, many surgeons routinely choose a site 3 mm posterior to the limbus to further decrease risk of damage to the peripheral retina. The glaucoma surgeon can use muscle insertions, identified by muscle hook, as a guide to placement of filtration fistulas. Muscle insertions vary in width and in location, and it is advisable to always identify the two adjacent muscles before proceeding with placement of a fistula. Disorientation is easily created by inadvertent torsion of the eye during surgical manipulation.

REFERENCES

1. Hogan MJ, Alvarado JA, Weddell JE: Histology of the Human Eye: An Atlas and Textbook. WB Saunders, Philadelphia, 1971
2. Jakobiec FA: Ocular Anatomy Embryology and Teratology. Harper & Row, Philadelphia, 1982
3. Duke-Elder S, Wybar KS: The anatomy of the visual system. In Duke-Elder S (ed): System of Ophthalmology. Vol. 2. CV Mosby, St. Louis, 1961
4. Tanchel NA, Aiken DG, Woods WD, et al: Correlation of segments of trabecular meshwork pigmentation and collector channels. Invest Ophthalmol Vis Sci, suppl., 25:122, 1984

Iridectomy

24

Jacob Wilensky

HISTORY

In 1856, von Graefe[1] first introduced iridectomy, the first effective surgical treatment for acute glaucoma. It was not until 1938, when Barkan[2] published his differentiation of glaucoma into open angle and angle-closure forms and elucidated the relative pupillary block mechanism as the cause of the angle closure that the rationale for iridectomy became apparent. It was realized then that this allowed aqueous in the posterior chamber to flow freely into the anterior chamber, by passing any resistance caused by apposition of the iris against the lens. This eliminated the previously higher pressure in the posterior chamber that could bow the peripheral iris forward and push it against the trabecular meshwork. Because of its high success rate and low incidence of complications, iridectomy was reputed to be the epitome of ophthalmic surgery. However, even this method could be improved. Laser iridectomy was introduced during the 1970s[3,4] and, after a slow beginning, it has largely replaced standard surgical iridectomy.

INDICATIONS

Pupillary Block Glaucoma

Iridectomy is the definitive treatment for all forms of pupillary block glaucoma. This includes both the primary forms such as acute, subacute, and chronic angle-closure glaucoma as well as secondary forms of pupillary block angle-closure glaucoma. This latter group comprises conditions such as vitreous block in aphakia and following trauma, phakomorphic pupillary block, eyes with retrolental fibroplasia, and some cases of uveitis in which pupillary block is present. Iridectomy is also indicated for the treatment of narrow angles in the fellow eyes of patients with primary angle-closure glaucoma, because of the well-known risks of subsequent closure in these eyes.[5] It may also be indicated in some patients with open-angle glaucoma but anatomically narrow angles, as some medications used to treat the open-angle component have led to closure of the angle in these eyes.

Inadequate Pupillary Opening

Iridectomy is also indicated as a means of creating an optical opening in eyes with opacities (particularly of the cornea or lens) in which more definitive treatment is impossible or has to be postponed. Optical iridectomies are probably much less common since the development of microsurgical techniques for the removal of cataracts in infants and children and similar progress in corneal transplantation surgery. Specific indications for optical iridectomy may include (1) polar or zonular congenital or infantile cataracts when the rest of the lens is clear and a good retinal image can be seen through a dilated pupil; (2) eyes with severely updrawn pupils, which may be associated with overlying corneal opacities following trauma; and (3) eyes with small localized opacities of the cornea overlying the pupil but that still offer a good view of the retina when the pupil is dilated.

Miscellaneous

Other indications for iridectomy include the completion of an imperforate surgical iridectomy performed during cataract extraction (Fig. 24-1). Since only the pigment epithelium is intact, these partial iridectomies can and should be completed with the laser. A second indication is plateau iris syndrome. The extent of pupillary block present in eyes with plateau iris syndrome is uncertain. The general consensus, however, seems to advocate iridectomy as part of the treatment for this condition.[6]

CONTRAINDICATIONS

There are no specific contraindications to the performance of an iridectomy, per se. There are, however, specific contraindications to certain techniques for iridectomy.[7] Laser iridectomy cannot be performed when the cornea is cloudy, when there is considerable anterior chamber reaction, when the anterior chamber is extremely shallow, or when the patient is unable to hold still and sit at the slit lamp. Surgical iridectomy may be contraindicated in patients who are unable to lie flat on the

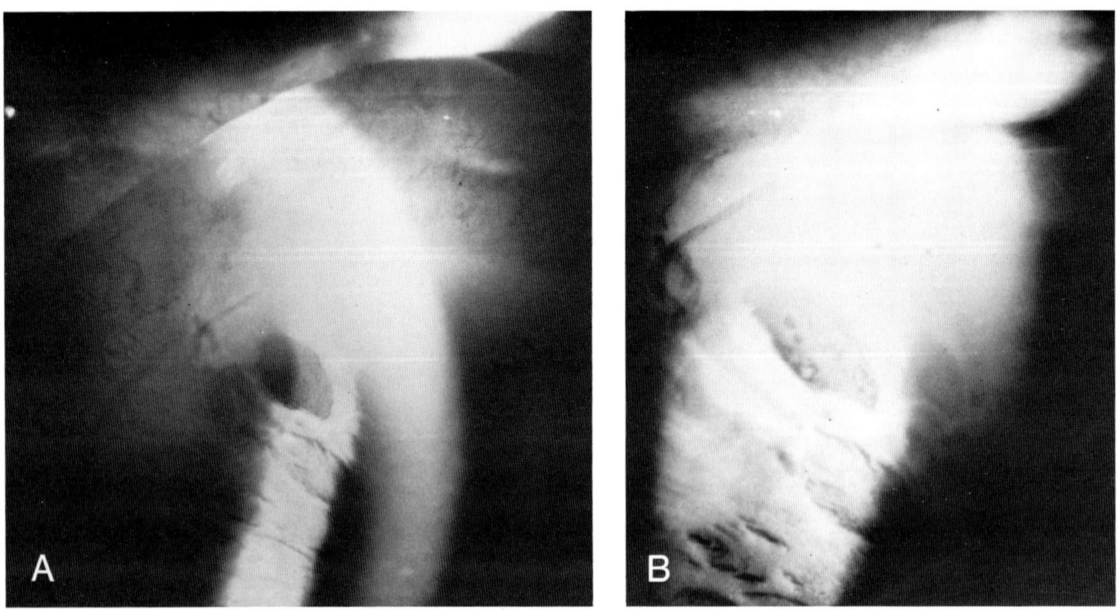

Fig. 24-1. (A) Slit-lamp photograph of an iridectomy. Note the intact pigment epithelium bowing forward. **(B)** Slit-lamp photograph of the same eye after laser iridotomy. Note the small holes in the pigment epithelium, which is no longer bowing forward.

operating table or hold still and in those who cannot tolerate general anesthesia. Surgical iridectomy may also be relatively contraindicated in patients in whom malignant glaucoma has developed following an iridectomy in the fellow eye. In this last situation, a noninvasive laser iridectomy might be preferable.

METHODS OF TREATMENT

Invasive (Surgical) Iridectomy

For many years, the standard procedure for iridectomy involved a surgical technique in which an incision was made into the eye and a piece of iris was excised.[8] The size and location of the hole in the iris depend on the indications for the procedure and the status of the patient's eye. Either a small hole was made in the iris in the form of a peripheral iridotomy (making a hole in the iris without excising tissue) or iridectomy, or a considerably larger hole was made in the form of a radial iridotomy (keyhole pupil) or sector iridectomy. In general, eyes in need of an optical opening would require a large hole. Similarly, a large opening would be needed in eyes with bounddown miotic pupils or with known retinal disease, and in patients with diabetes mellitus, to facilitate visualization of the posterior pole.

A surgical iridectomy could be performed via two approaches. The first involved making a conjunctival flap and then incising the sclera at the limbus. This incision was subsequently covered by the conjunctival flap. The second approach involved incising the eye through clear cornea. This approach did not involve the conjunctiva. Advocates of the limbal approach believed that the more posterior incision facilitated spontaneous prolapse of the iris into the iridectomy wound and that the conjunctival flap helped protect against wound leaks. Proponents of the corneal approach favored its relative simplicity and the fact that the conjunctiva was not manipulated, thereby preserving this area for later use in filtering surgery, if necessary.

Noninvasive (Laser) Iridectomy

Over the past decade the use of laser energy to create a hole in the iris has very rapidly supplanted the invasive technique as the standard method for producing iridectomies. Two basic types of lasers can be used.[9] The first is a relatively low-energy laser (e.g., argon lasers) that uses continuous-wave energy for relatively long periods of time (usually about 0.1 second). With this type of laser, light energy is converted into heat, which burns a hole through the iris tissue. Other types of lasers emit ultrashort-duration (10^{-9} to 10^{-12} seconds) bursts of ultrahigh-laser energy. With this type of pulsed laser, the light energy is so intense that it actually strips electrons off atoms, causing a small explosion in the tissue that in turn produces a shock wave, which mechanically disrupts the tissues.

Continuous-wave lasers have some advantages over pulsed lasers. They are more available, ophthalmologists are more familiar with them, and they allow somewhat greater ability to shape and enlarge holes in the iris. Continuous-wave lasers also coagulate the blood vessels, creating a hole by burning through the tissue. Pulsed lasers that disrupt tissue do not coagulate the blood vessels and thus tend to cause bleeding, which can be a particular problem in eyes with neovascularization. There is also a potential risk of rupture of the lens capsule. Continuous-wave lasers probably carry a slightly greater risk of burning the lens, producing a small, localized nonprogressive cataract. There are several advantages to pulsed lasers: (1) only one or two bursts of energy are required to create an iridectomy, (2) iris color or thickness is less of a factor in the success of treatment, and (3) there appears to be a much lower incidence of subsequent proliferation of pigment epithelium that can cause late closure of the iridectomy.

RECOMMENDED TECHNIQUES

Invasive Technique

When performing a surgical iridectomy, I prefer to use the corneal incision. The procedure is usually performed with the patient under local anesthesia, achieved by a retrobulbar injection of 2 percent lidocaine (Xylocaine). The procedure can be performed with only a two-quadrant block with infiltration of the anesthetic along the bellies of the two adjacent rectus muscles, but this is more difficult and less desirable. A bridle suture is passed through the superior rectus muscle to stabilize the globe and expose the limbus. The globe is grasped near the limbus with a 0.20-mm Castroviejo forceps. A beveled incision is made into the clear cornea in the superotemporal quadrant with a 64 Beaver blade (Fig. 24-2). The incision is started at the front edge of the limbal vascular arcade and is made relatively flat. The width of the incision is not much greater than that of the Beaver blade. A 9-0 or 10-0 nylon suture is then passed across this wound and looped out. The assistant grasps the two loops and gapes the wound open. A more vertical incision is then made through the base of this incision into the anterior chamber with either a razorblade fragment or a Super blade. In an attempt to get the iris to prolapse, this incision is made as wide at its base as it is at the top.

Once the chamber is entered, slight pressure is placed over the scleral edge of the wound. The iris will then prolapse spontaneously into the wound at this point. If it does not, slight counterpressure near the limbus at 6 o'clock may help induce it. The prolapsed iris is then grasped with a forceps, and the iridectomy is performed with DeWecker scissors. If the iris does not prolapse into an adequately wide (2- to 3-mm) wound, it is necessary to enter the anterior chamber with a Pierce-Hoskins forceps (which has no teeth), grasp the iris, and bring it out of the wound for excision. Note that when performing an optical iridectomy, two forceps are used, and the iris is grasped a second time more anteriorly, so that the sphincter is brought out of the wound. In this way, a sector iridectomy is performed rather than a peripheral one. The wound is irrigated gently with balanced salt solution (BSS); if necessary, the iris is massaged gently through the closed cornea to ensure that it is completely reposited and totally free of the incision. The pupil should be checked for a rounded-up appearance, and the iridectomy should be clearly visible. The preplaced nylon suture is then pulled and tied. The wound is tested for adequate closure; if necessary, a second 10-0 suture can be placed. If the procedure has been done properly, the anterior chamber will have remained formed, eliminating the need for re-formation with BBS. In most cases, no instrument other than the tip of the knife will have entered the anterior chamber throughout the procedure. I do not dilate the pupil at the end of the procedure. At the first dressing change, I instill 1 percent cyclopentolate eyedrops. The corneal sutures may be removed after 3 to 4 weeks, if they are causing irritation or astigmatism; if not, they may be left in place.

Noninvasive Technique

Two separate laser techniques for performing an iridectomy are described. Although Nd:YAG lasers are used to perform an iridectomy on many occasions, they are still not widely available to many ophthalmologists. They are clearly the instruments of choice for performing an iridectomy on certain occasions. Nevertheless, the argon technique is still preferable for eyes with neovascularization. I currently use both techniques on a regular basis.

Argon Technique

When performing an iridectomy, laser energy should be focused on the iris as sharply as possible. Any manipulations that reduce the clarity of the corneal epithelium (e.g., gonioscopy) should therefore be avoided. A drop of pilocarpine should be instilled to maximize pupillary block. The oculars of the laser slit lamp are adjusted to ensure that the instrument is in focus for the surgeon. The magnification is set in the range of 16 to 25×. The eye is anesthetized with a drop of proparacaine hydrochloride. An Abraham iridotomy lens is placed on the eye (Fig. 24-3).

The power settings for the procedure vary according to the pigmentation of the iris. In a light blue or gray iris, I begin with approximately 750 mW for a 0.2-second burn (Table 24-1). For a light brown iris, I use only 0.1-second burns and perhaps reduce the power to 650 mW. In a very heavily pigmented iris (Oriental or black patient), I reduce the power to 500 mW and occasionally may decrease the duration of the burn to 0.05 second. In all cases I use a 50-cm spot size treat between either the 10 and 11 o'clock position or the 1 and 2

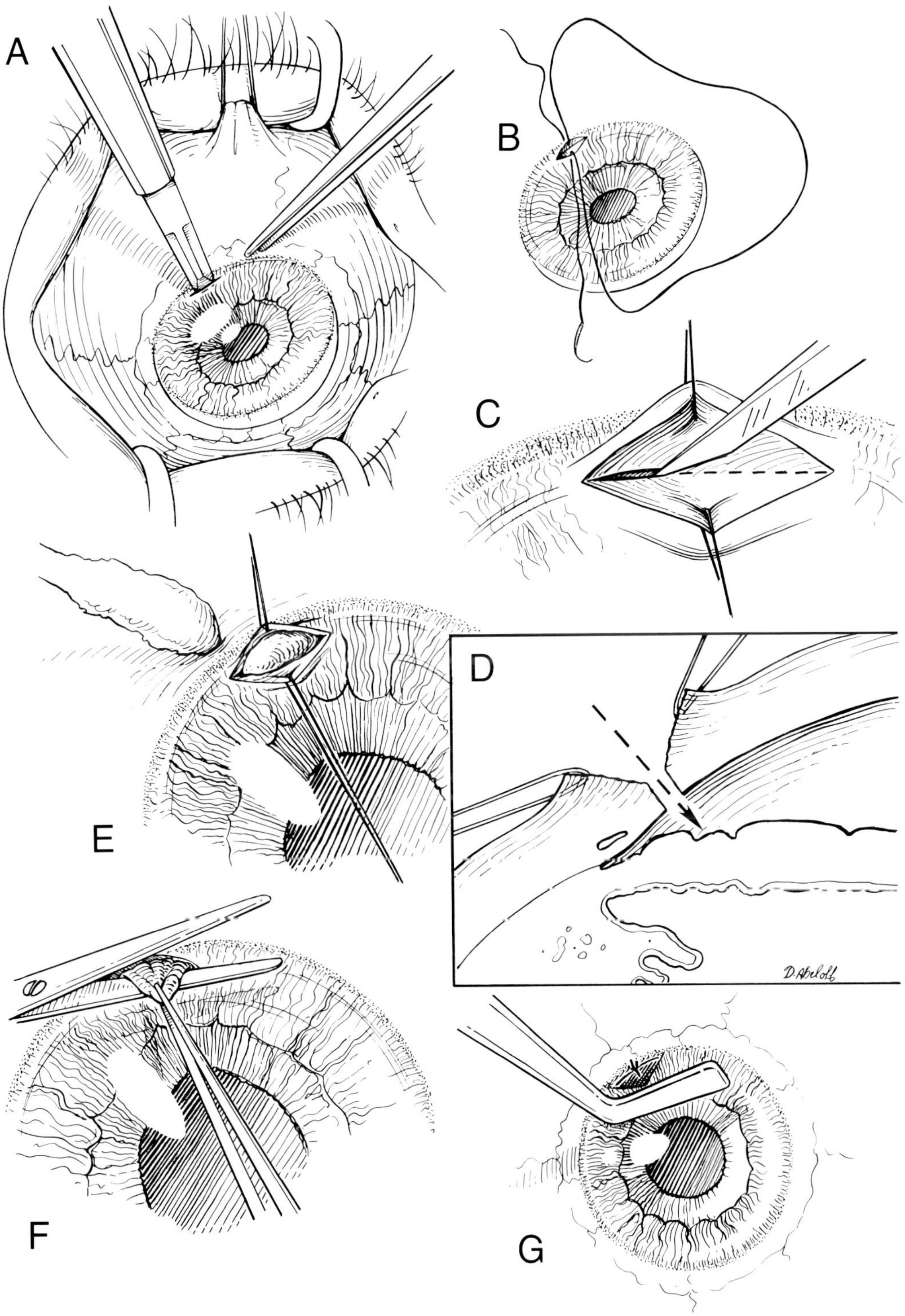

Fig. 24-2. Illustration of technique recommended for clear corneal surgical iridectomy. See text for details.

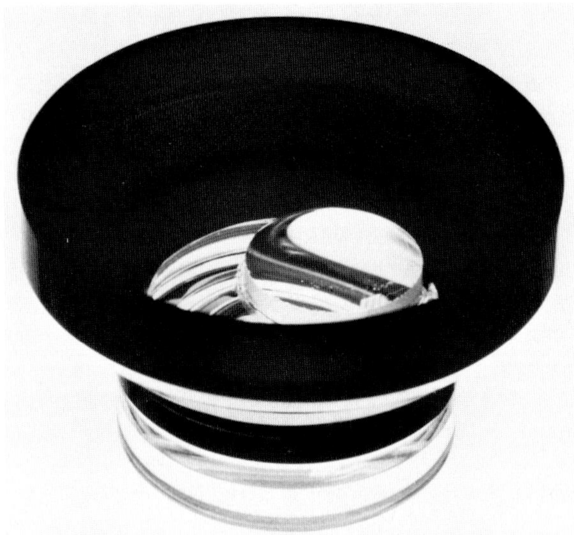

Fig. 24-3. Abraham iridotomy lens.

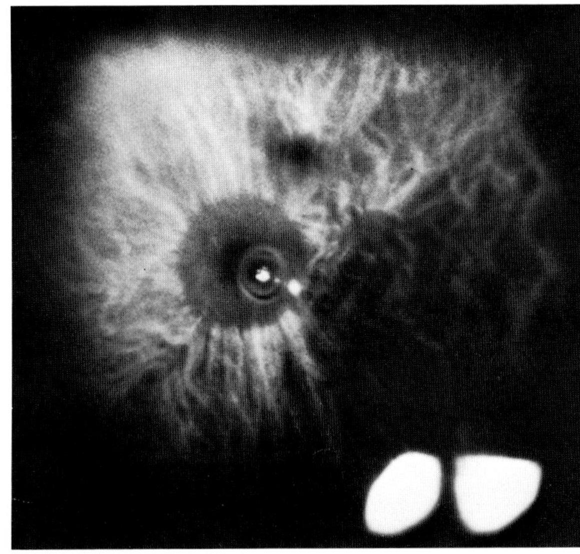

Fig. 24-4. Slit-lamp photograph showing a small vapor bubble created while performing an argon laser iridectomy.

o'clock position, about two thirds out from the pupillary margin. In this way, treatment is fairly peripheral but not far enough to produce problems in an eye with pronounced arcus senilis.

I do not routinely pretreat the iris to create a hump or drumhead, although such a preparatory step may be advantageous on rare occasions. I try to focus the laser energy as sharply as possible on the iris surface (sharp focus is the key to successful argon laser iridectomy), then create a crater in the iris and drill through to the pigment epithelium as quickly as possible. In light-colored irides, a vapor bubble frequently forms (Fig. 24-4). When this occurs, I use the bubble as a condensing lens, aiming subsequent burns through the center of the bubble. In this way, I frequently can penetrate the iris to pigment epithelium with a minimum of burns. In fact, if the iris cannot be penetrated with 20 to 25 burns, I move to a new location or have the patient return another day. In darkly pigmented irides, 50 to 100 burns may be needed to chip through the stroma to the pigment epithelium.

Once the pigment epithelium is reached, I set the duration of the burns at 0.1 second and the power to about 700 to 800 mW, irrespective of the iris color. As the pigment epithelium is penetrated, a plume or shower of pigment often flows out of the hole. I then try to clean the edges of the hole in the pigment epithelium to create an opening in the iris at least 200 μm in diameter. In general, it takes longer to clean and enlarge the iridectomy than to make the initial penetration.

In some eyes it is very difficult to ascertain whether the pigment epithelium has been penetrated. If the laser therapist is not sure of whether the reflex observed represents the lens capsule or simply a small vapor bubble in the depths of the crater that has been created, the iris can be transilluminated; a small bright light is aimed through the

Table 24-1. Treatment Parameters for Argon Laser Iridectomy

	Iris Color		
Treatment Parameters	Blue or Gray	Light Brown	Dark Brown
Spot size (μm)	50	50	50
Power (mW)	750–900	600–750	500
Duration (sec)	0.2	0.1	0.05–0.1
Average number of burns	40–75	25–50	150–300

pupil to make an accurate differentiation. (The laser should be placed on standby during this process to prevent accidental retinal burns.)

Patience is necessary when cleaning pigment clumps from the edge of a laser iridectomy. It is not unusual to have a large clump of pigment float or drop into the opening and occlude a good portion of it. I frequently perform two iridectomies on an eye, one nasally and one temporally, alternating between them to clean up these clumps. During this process (and throughout the entire iridectomy), it is crucial to remember where the laser light is aimed inside the eye. It should always be angled to preclude inadvertent macular burns.[10]

Following treatment, the patient's intraocular pressure (IOP) is monitored hourly for at least 3 hours. If a significant rise in IOP is noted, appropriate therapy (i.e., carbonic anhydrase inhibitors and/or osmotics) is instituted to reduce the pressure. I am more inclined to treat acute pressure elevation in a patient with chronic angle-closure glaucoma who already has field loss and cupping than in the fellow eye of a patient with acute angle closure who has no cupping or field loss. Following the laser session, I prescribe a topical corticosteroid preparation such as 0.1 percent dexamethasone or 1 percent prednisone, four times a day for about 4 or 5 days. Unless there is some overriding reason, I usually do not dilate the pupil until the patient returns for a checkup 1 week after the iridectomy. In approximately one fourth of patients, the laser iridectomy will close, due to proliferation of pigment epithelium or to a clump of pigment epithelium floating into the opening, during the first 4 to 6 weeks after treatment. It is very easy to reopen these holes using 500-mW burns of 0.1- to 0.2-second duration. The same precautions employed during the initial session must be followed for these retreatments. If the iridectomy remains patent after 6 weeks, it is most unusual for it to close over subsequently.

Nd:YAG Laser

A drop of pilocarpine should be instilled about a half-hour before treatment. The eye is anesthetized with topical proparacaine. Either an Abraham iridotomy lens or a special contact lens designed for use with the Nd:YAG laser is placed on the eye. The laser (I use the Lasag laser) is set for about 6 to 7 mJ of energy. I use a Q-switched burst mode, which has two pulses per burst. (Nd:YAG lasers without burst capacity require a higher-energy level, but iridectomies can be created with a single pulse.) Each pulse is approximately 20 nsec in duration and 20 msec apart. One must be careful not to treat too far in the periphery of the angle, or the burst of energy will propagate backward and damage the corneal endothelium. A single laser burst is usually sufficient. In a number of patients, one will see a trickle of blood from the edge of the new iridectomy. To treat this, I press against the eye with the contact lens for about 20 seconds; this generally stops the bleeding. Follow-up care is similar to that for argon laser iridectomies.

The Nd:YAG laser can be used to enlarge an updrawn pupil and thereby create an optical iridectomy in aphakic eyes. Using the same settings as indicated, the laser energy is aimed at the pupillary margin, proceeding peripherally in a linear fashion. Two or more such laser sphincterotomies may be necessary to enlarge the pupil adequately.

COMPLICATIONS

Invasive Technique

Standard invasive surgical iridectomies share the basic potential complications of any procedure involving an incision into the globe, including the possibility of wound leak and resulting flat anterior chamber, infection, inflammation, and hemorrhage. Fortunately, these complications have a rather low incidence with iridectomy, but they can and do occur. Many investigators believe that invasive surgical iridectomy speeds up cataract formation; others deny this claim.

Perhaps one of the more special complications of iridectomy is malignant glaucoma. Following iridectomy, a very small number of patients with angle-closure glaucoma develop very high pressure in the eye a shallow or flat anterior chamber. This problem is thought to be caused by a misdirection of aqueous into the vitreous cavity, which pushes the entire lens–iris diaphragm forward. One of the key differential diagnostic problems in the postoperative iridectomy patient is to determine whether a patient with a flat chamber has a wound leak or malignant glaucoma. The IOP level is usually low in eyes with wound leak and high in those with malignant glaucoma (if it is a good patent iridectomy).

Laser Technique

Many patients develop an acute rise in IOP immediately following laser iridectomy. This is far more serious in an eye that already has glaucomatous damage than in an otherwise healthy eye. Epithelial corneal burns are relatively common but of little import. Endothelial burns, however, cause a permanent scar on the endothelium and represent the loss of irreplaceable endothelial cells. Such burns can arise because (1) the laser energy was aimed too far peripherally, (2) the anterior chamber was too shallow, (3) the power setting was too high, or (4) large vapor bubbles formed at the iris surface and spread to the endothelium. A lot of cellular debris and particulate matter remains in the anterior chamber after a laser iridotomy. There is some disagreement as to whether this represents inflammation or material liberated during the burning or tearing of the iris. Hemorrhages are extremely uncommon with the argon laser technique because the laser burns coagulate the vessels. Hemorrhages are fairly common with the Nd:YAG technique, which tears or disrupts the tissue; it rarely reaches the point of a hyphema, however. Local focal opacities in the lens at the site of a laser treatment are not uncommon with the argon laser, but these seem to be nonprogressive.

In general, an experienced laser therapist can be successful in creating an iridectomy in about 90 percent of cases with a single-treatment session. In some instances, however, a through-and-through hole cannot be created in a single session, and multiple treatments will be required. With Nd:YAG lasers, this is even less common. Under certain circumstances, however, the ability to penetrate the tissue will be somewhat lower, such as with active inflammation in the eye, corneal edema, and similar situations. If a through-and-through hole is essential immediately, this can present a problem. With the argon technique, perhaps 25 percent of the eyes will have reclosure of a patent iridotomy by proliferation of pigment epithelium. If the patient fails to return for adequate follow-up care and the iridectomy closes, serious problems can ensue.

PROGNOSIS

Glaucoma Therapy

The prognosis for glaucoma patients treated with an iridectomy depends on the type of glaucoma being treated and the duration of the problem. In the treatment of acute angle-closure glaucoma that has been present for less than 24 hours, an overwhelming majority of patients will have adequate control after the iridectomy alone. In eyes with an angle-closure episode of longer duration, the percentage of control by the iridectomy alone will drop; still, most cases can be managed adequately by a combination of iridectomy and medical treatment, as necessary. Even in patients with chronic angle-closure glaucoma of long duration associated with advanced cupping and field loss but still some functional angle, iridectomy and medical therapy may be sufficient to bring the glaucoma under control. By contrast, it is unlikely that iridectomy alone or in combination with medical therapy will achieve control of the glaucoma when there is total angle closure of long duration.

Optical Iridectomy Therapy

The prognosis is dependent on the presenting situation. If the patient has progressive lens opacity, it will be a few months to a year or two before cataract surgery becomes necessary. The combination of limited benefit with improved techniques for cataract surgery in infants and in small children has greatly reduced the frequency with which optical iridectomies are performed. In an eye with an updrawn or ectopic pupil, the prognosis is somewhat more favorable, and these cases may show satisfactory improvement with this type of intervention. It is conceivable that the newer techniques for enlarging the pupil by disrupting the iris with Nd:YAG lasers may increase the use of optical iridectomy in the future.

REFERENCES

1. von Graefe A: Uher die iridectomie bei Glaucom und uber den glaucomatosen Prozess. Graefes Arch Clin Exp Ophthalmol 3:456, 1857
2. Barkan O: Glaucoma: Classification, causes and surgical control. Am J Ophthalmol 21:1099, 1938
3. Abraham RK, Miller GL: Outpatient argon laser iridectomy for angle closure glaucoma: A two-year study. Trans Am Acad Ophthalmol Otolaryngol 79:529, 1975
4. Pollack IP, Patz A: Argon laser iridectomy: An experimental and clinical study. Ophthalmic Surg 7:22, 1976
5. Wilensky JT: Current concepts in primary angle closure glaucoma. Ann Ophthalmol 9:963, 1972
6. Wand M, Grant WM, Simmons RJ, Hutchinson BT: Plateau iris syndrome. Trans Am Acad Ophthalmol Otlaryngol 83:122, 1977
7. Wilensky JT: Laser iridectomy: Indications. p. 63. In Wilensky JT (ed): Laser Therapy in Glaucoma. Appleton-Century-Crofts, East Norwalk, CT, 1985
8. Chandler PA: Narrow angle glaucoma. Arch Ophthalmol 47:695, 1952
9. Robin AL, Pollack IP: A comparison of neodymium:YAG and argon laser iridectomies. Ophthalmology 91:1011, 1984
10. Berger BB: Foveal photocoagulation from laser iridotomy. Ophthalmology 91:1029, 1984

Laser Trabeculoplasty

25

Alfred M. Solish
Michael A. Kass

HISTORICAL PERSPECTIVE

During the 1970s several attempts were made to improve outflow facility in open-angle glaucoma using laser energy. Different investigators used conventional ruby lasers, Q-switched ruby lasers, or argon lasers to create a direct communication between the anterior chamber and Schlemm's canal (i.e., a laser trabecular puncture).[1–3] However, it soon became clear that the trabecular punctures healed over a period of weeks and intraocular pressure (IOP) returned to pretreatment levels. Furthermore, adverse effects of laser energy became apparent when Gaasterland and Kupfer[4] were able to produce chronic glaucoma in animal eyes by repeated high-energy argon laser applications to the trabecular meshwork.

In 1979, Wise and Witter[5] reported successful argon laser treatment of open-angle glaucoma. They spaced low energy treatments about the circumference of the trabecular meshwork in an attempt to contract the trabecular ring rather than puncturing into Schlemm's canal. Numerous reports that confirmed the efficacy of this approach followed.

SURGICAL ANATOMY

The trabecular meshwork appears on gonioscopy as a ring of tissue bordered anteriorly by Schwalbe's line and posteriorly by the scleral spur. In cross section, the meshwork is roughly triangular in shape, with its apex at Schwalbe's line and its base along the scleral spur. Schlemm's canal is located deep to the meshwork, approximately midway between these landmarks. The amount of pigment in the trabecular meshwork varies considerably and is related to numerous factors, including patient age, type of glaucoma, and previous surgical procedures.

Microscopically, the meshwork consists of beams of collagenous tissue surrounded by extracellular material containing glycosaminoglycans, proteoglycans, collagen, laminin, and fibronectin. Trabecular endothelial cells line the meshwork.

The trabecular meshwork can be divided into three separate zones: (1) uveal, (2) corneoscleral, and (3) juxtacanalicular. The uveal and corneoscleral zones are fenestrated; that is, there are spaces between the beams. No spaces exist in the juxtacanalicular meshwork.

INDICATIONS

The indications for this procedure are similar to those for filtering surgery, that is, documented or anticipated progressive glaucomatous damage despite maximum tolerated medical therapy. This includes patients whose glaucoma is well controlled on medical therapy but who are intolerant of the medication. Patients who have undergone previous glaucoma surgery (either filtering surgery or iridectomy) but whose IOPs are not well controlled with medication are also candidates for laser trabeculoplasty.

CONTRAINDICATIONS

Laser trabeculoplasty is unlikely to be successful if more than one half the angle is closed by peripheral anterior synechiae or if opacities of the cornea obscure the surgeon's view of the trabecular meshwork. The patient must be able to cooperate sufficiently to hold still at the slit lamp. Retrobulbar anesthesia may be helpful in selected patients who cannot maintain fixation, such as those with nystagmus.

METHODS OF TREATMENT

Medical therapy with miotics, epinephrine, dipivefrin, β-blockers, and carbonic anhydrase inhibitors is often effective in lowering IOP. Some patients, however, do not respond sufficiently to medical treatment. Others are unable to take medication chronically for a variety of reasons, including drug-induced side effects.

When IOP is unacceptably high despite maximum tolerated medical therapy, filtering surgery and cyclocryotherapy can be employed to achieve a lower pressure. These procedures are limited by potential complications and substantial failure rates.

Laser trabeculoplasty increases outflow facility and lowers IOP with minimal risk of systemic side effects, intraocular infection, or substantial intraocular hemorrhage. Laser trabeculoplasty is often acceptable to patients who refuse filtering surgery.

RECOMMENDED TECHNIQUE

The power output of the argon blue-green laser must be calibrated periodically. The power delivered to the eye may be very different from that indicated on the dial. The aiming beam must be parfocal with the treatment beam to ensure accurate focus. This must be checked by each surgeon for each individual laser machine. A piece of orange or red paper is held approximately where the patient's eye will be located. The beam diameter is set at 50 μm. Burns are made on the paper at different focal settings of the microscope oculars. The burns are measured using magnification and the focal setting corresponding to the burn with the smallest diameter is selected for use. A beam of minimum size and power reduces damage to the surrounding trabecular meshwork. A more complete discussion is given by Wise.[6]

A drop of 0.5 percent proparacaine hydrochloride provides adequate anesthesia. A three-mirror Goldmann contact lens with an antireflective coating is applied to the eye with a drop of 2.5 percent methylcellulose. A one-mirror indirect gonioscopy lens may also be used. An elbow support is recommended for the arm holding the contact lens. The gonioscopy mirror of the contact lens usually provides the best view of the angle, but occasionally another mirror is better. Magnification of 25 to 40× is used. Note that different ocular settings may be required at different levels of magnification to maintain the minimum treatment diameter.

It is essential that each surgeon establish a routine pattern of treatment. As the field of view is rather small, it is easy to "get lost" in the angle and forget which areas have already been treated. This is particularly true in eyes with minimal trabecular pigmentation.

The goniolens is placed on the cornea, and the anatomic landmarks of the angle are identified. Accurate identification of these landmarks is of critical importance. Schwalbe's line and the scleral spur are usually the easiest landmarks to identify and can serve as points of reference. They can be traced around the circumference of the angle if the surgeon is uncertain of the location of the meshwork.

If the anterior chamber angle is too narrow, the iris can be retracted (laser gonioplasty) with the use of a few low-power burns. For gonioplasty, the beam size is set at 200 μm, the duration to 0.1 seconds, and the power to 200 to 300 mW. Ten to 30 applications are made to the iris stroma. The burns are more effective in retracting the iris if they are delivered three-fourths of the way between the pupil and the angle rather than immediately adjacent to the angle. The central area of the Goldmann contact lens or the gonioscopy mirror can be used with equal effect in the application of the retracting spots. Laser iridotomy should be performed prior to trabeculoplasty in eyes with critically narrow angles or when iris retraction is unsuccessful.

The correct amount of laser power is then determined using burns made with the mirror at the 12 o'clock position; that is, the burns are made at 6 o'clock in the inferior angle. Treatment is then begun, starting at 3 or 9 o'clock, always rotating the mirror in a single direction, either clockwise or counterclockwise. As a general rule, we treat the inferior meshwork first because this portion of the angle is usually wider and more visible.

The power setting for trabeculoplasty is dependent on the amount of pigment present in the meshwork; more heavily pigmented trabecular meshwork requires less power. In most cases, the surgeon can make the initial test burns with a power setting of 600 mW. The surgeon increases or decreases the power in 100 to 200 mW steps until the desired effect is obtained. The ideal burn is one that produces blanching of the trabecular pigment and perhaps a small vaporization bubble at the point of laser impact. A large explosion is not desirable. Most often, a power setting of 600 to 1,000 mW is adequate to produce the desired effect. Often, the power setting must be adjusted to the variation of pigmentation in different portions of the trabecular meshwork. Lightly pigmented eyes should not be overtreated in an attempt to obtain a vaporization bubble. Specifically, the power setting should not exceed 1200 mW.

Precise focus is absolutely essential, and the focusing beam should appear completely round. This is more easily accomplished if the beam from the laser strikes the central portion of the contact lens mirror. Rotation of the lens during the procedure is necessary to maintain this relationship. Tilting of the lens should be avoided or minimized. The burns should be applied to the anterior portion of the trabecular meshwork. In normally pigmented eyes, the lower edge of the beam should touch the anterior edge of the trabecular pigment stripe (Fig. 25-1).

After the correct power setting and focus are determined, laser burns are applied to the trabecular meshwork approximately 4 degrees apart. We use a 50-μm spot size and 0.1-second laser duration (Fig. 25-1).

We usually treat 180 degrees of the angle at a single session. There is evidence that the incidence and severity of postoperative IOP elevations are reduced when only one-half the circumference is treated at one time.[2-4] In some patients, treatment over 180 degrees produces the desired therapeutic effect. The remaining 180 degrees can be treated at a later time if an additional reduction of IOP is required. If possible, we delay the second treatment for 4 to 6 weeks in order to determine the full impact of the first laser procedure. The following tips will be useful in performing laser trabeculoplasty:

1. Calibrate the laser power.
2. Determine the focal setting for the minimum spot diameter.
3. Carefully identify the angle structures.
4. For a precise focus, keep the aiming beam round, not oval.
5. Center the laser beam in the mirror.
6. Do not tilt the mirror.
7. Determine the proper power setting using test burns.
8. Use either gonioplasty or iridotomy, or both, for narrow angles.

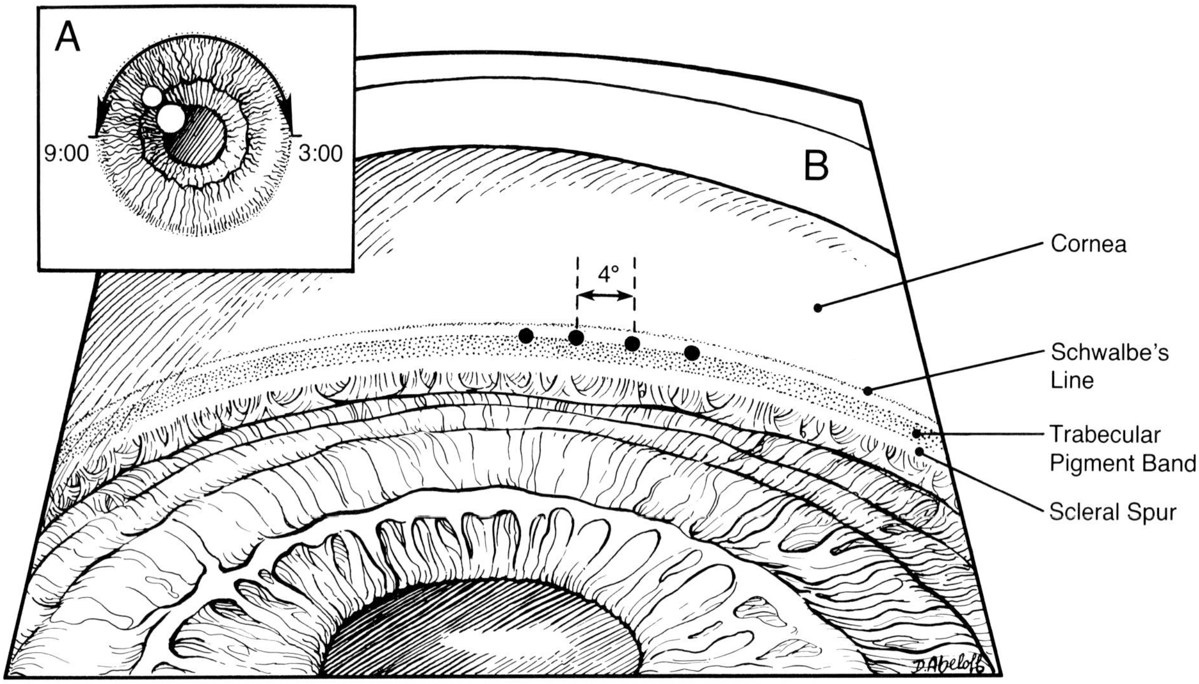

Fig. 25-1. (A,B) Position of argon laser trabeculoplasty treatment in the trabecular meshwork.

9. The laser burn should touch the anterior border of the trabecular pigment stripe.

As yet, we do not know the ideal number of burns, the ideal power setting, nor the ideal amount of the angle to be treated. Most surgeons today use 40 to 50 applications over 180 degrees and 80 to 100 spots when the entire circumference is treated.

Postoperatively, all patients are placed on topical corticosteroids four times daily for 3 to 7 days. All glaucoma medications are continued (including carbonic anhydrase inhibitors) until the results of the procedure are evaluated. The patient's activities are not restricted.

PROGNOSIS AND COMPLICATIONS

The results of laser trabeculoplasty depend primarily on the type of glaucoma being treated. Other factors of importance include patient age, aphakia, previous surgery, and other coexisting ocular conditions (e.g., inflammation).

In general, the best results are achieved in eyes with phakic primary open-angle glaucoma (POAG) and glaucoma associated with senile exfoliation syndrome (pseudoexfoliation, glaucoma capsulare). The average decrease in IOP in these patients is 6 to 10 mmHg, and 75 to 85 percent of these procedures are considered "successful" (defined differently by different authors) (Table 25-1).[7–13]

In aphakic or pseudophakic eyes, eyes with angle recession, eyes that have had angle-closure treated with iridectomy, and eyes that have undergone unsuccessful filtering surgery, laser trabeculoplasty has a somewhat lower "success" rate, in the neighborhood of 45 to 55 percent.[10]

Uveitic glaucoma, congenital glaucoma, juvenile glaucoma, corticosteroid-induced glaucoma, and glaucoma due to the iridocorneal endothelial syndrome (ICE syndrome) rarely respond to laser trabeculoplasty.[8,11] In primary juvenile glaucoma, laser trabeculoplasty is often followed by prolonged inflammation and even higher IOP. Despite the overall lack of success of the laser in these con-

Table 25-1. Prognosis of Laser Trabeculoplasty

Prognosis	Indication
Good	Primary open-angle glaucoma Glaucoma capsulare (senile exfoliation syndrome) Pigmentary glaucoma
Fair	Open-angle glaucoma in aphakic and pseudophakic eyes Angle recession associated with glaucoma Previous failed glaucoma surgery
Poor	Uveitic glaucoma Congenital/juvenile glaucoma Corticosteroid glaucoma Iridocorneal endothelial (ICE) syndrome with glaucoma Retreatment after 360-degree laser trabeculoplasty

ditions, trabeculoplasty may be done if there is no reasonable alternative.

There is controversy surrounding the response of pigmentary glaucoma to laser trabeculoplasty. Various studies have noted 40 percent,[11] 50 percent,[12] 80 percent,[10] and 100 percent[8,13] success rates. Some authorities have noted early success with a high incidence of failure at 10 to 12 months.[14] We believe that most patients with pigmentary glaucoma respond favorably, despite their young age.

Following laser trabeculoplasty, most patients continue to require topical and/or systemic ocular hypotensive agents. Up to 33 percent may require less medication than formerly.[15]

Eyes with higher initial IOPs tend to achieve a greater magnitude of pressure lowering, both in percentage and in absolute value.[8,13] This pressure reduction after trabeculoplasty has been maintained for as long as 10 years. It is important to realize that some patients lose the effect of laser treatment with time.[11,14] After a good initial IOP response, some patients experience a rise in IOP over a period of months. In other patients, a slow upward drift of IOP is noted over a period of years.

Eyes that have undergone 180-degree treatment frequently benefit from treatment of the remaining 180 degrees. Once the entire circumference is treated with 80 to 100 spots, further treatment is rarely of benefit. One report notes a further lowering of IOP in only one-third of patients with retreatment, while 20 percent of these eyes develop a marked postoperative rise in pressure.[10]

Complications of laser trabeculoplasty are relatively infrequent and mild compared with traditional glaucoma surgery (Table 25-2). Corneal complications include abrasion from the contact lens and endothelial burns. These endothelial burns cause transient local opacification but apparently no major loss of endothelial cells. There is a single report of bullous keratopathy following laser trabeculoplasty in a patient with endothelial dystrophy.[16]

Occasionally blood seeps from the meshwork after a burn. This is easily staunched with a cauterizing laser treatment over the same area (100 μm, 200 to 400 mW, 0.1 second) or with tamponade via mechanical pressure to the contact lens.

Peripheral anterior synechiae are seen in up to 30 percent[12] of eyes after the procedure but do not appear to affect the results. They are seen more frequently with posterior treatment and higher-power settings. We therefore recommend treatment to the anterior portion of the trabecular meshwork.

Iritis occurs in nearly all patients but is rarely persistent.[8,10–13,16–18] Postoperative topical corticosteroid treatment four times daily for 3 to 7 days appears to be adequate to treat most of these inflammatory responses.

A mild blurring of vision is reported by many patients following laser trabeculoplasty. This may be due to the methylcellulose, transient corneal edema, a roughening of the corneal epithelium from the contact lens, or iritis. The blurred vision generally clears within 24 hours.

An occasional patient may develop a vasovagal response and syncope during laser trabeculoplasty. Resuscitation equipment should be available for prompt treatment.

The most serious complication of laser trabeculoplasty is a postoperative increase in IOP. Progres-

Table 25-2. Complications of Laser Trabeculoplasty

Degree	Complication
Major	Postoperative rise in intraocular pressure
Minor	Corneal abrasion Corneal endothelial burn Transient blurring of vision Peripheral anterior synechiae Iritis Syncope

sion of visual field loss has occurred, and small residual islands of vision have been "snuffed out" in this manner.[8] Modest pressure rises occur postoperatively in nearly one half of the eyes treated.[8,19] Maximum levels of IOP are reached within 1 to 8 hours after the procedure.[19] It is therefore crucial that IOP be measured 1 to 3 hours after treatment. When a marked elevation of IOP is detected, treatment with either carbonic anhydrase inhibitors or hyperosmotic agents, or both, should be instituted. It is wise to monitor IOP for 24 hours postoperatively in patients with marked glaucomatous damage. Persistent elevations lasting more than 24 hours occur in 3 to 6 percent of treated eyes. An occasional patient may require filtering surgery because of a laser-induced rise in IOP. IOP may be elevated after laser trabeculoplasty:

1. Occurs in 40 percent of eyes
2. Usually reaches maximum in 1 to 8 hours
3. Can produce visual-field loss
4. Can occur days or weeks following procedure (rare)
5. Usually responds to hyperosmotic agents
6. Can rebound after treatment
7. Requires careful follow-up in eyes with advanced damage

Rarely, marked elevation of IOP can occur days to weeks following treatment despite an unremarkable course during the immediate postoperative period. This may occur alone or may be accompanied by pain and marked iritis.

As with other modes of medical and surgical therapy for glaucoma, visual field loss may progress despite reduction of IOP.[17] Continued observation and follow-up of these patients is mandatory. Patients must be warned that laser trabeculoplasty is not a magic cure for their glaucoma.

REFERENCES

1. Hager H: Besondere mikrochirurgische Eingriffe II. Erste Erfahrugen mit dere Argon Laser Gerat 800. Klin Monatsbl Augenheilkd 162:437, 1973
2. Krasnov MM: Laseropuncture of anterior chamber angle in glaucoma. Am J Ophthalmol 75:674, 1973
3. Wickham MG, Worthen DM: Argon laser trabeculotomy: Long-term follow-up. Trans Am Acad Ophthalmol Otolaryngol 86:495, 1979
4. Gaasterland D, Kupfer C: Experimental glaucoma in the rhesus monkey. Invest Ophthalmol 13:455, 1974
5. Wise JB, Witter SL: Argon laser therapy for open angle glaucoma: a pilot study. Arch Ophthalmol 97:319, 1979
6. Wise JB: Errors in laser spot size in laser trabeculoplasty. Ophthalmology 91:186, 1984
7. Weinreb RN, Ruderman J, Juster R, Zweig K: Immediate intraocular pressure response to argon laser trabeculoplasty. Am J Ophthalmol 95:279, 1983
8. Thomas JV, Simmons RJ, Belcher CD III: Argon laser trabeculoplasty in the presurgical glaucoma patient. Ophthalmology 89:187, 1982
9. Schwartz LW, Spaeth GL, Traverso C, Greenidge KC: Variation of techniques on the results of argon laser trabeculoplasty. Ophthalmology 90:781, 1983
10. Kolker AE: Laser therapy for glaucoma. Clinical Modules for Ophthalmologists. Am Acad Ophthalmol Publication, 1984
11. Lieberman MF, Hoskins HD, Hetherington J: Laser trabeculoplasty and the glaucomas. Ophthalmology 90:790, 1983
12. Schwartz AL, Whitten ME, Bleiman B, et al: Argon laser trabecular surgery in uncontrolled phakic open angle glaucoma. Ophthalmology 88:203, 1981
13. Horns DJ, Bellows AR, Hutchinson BT, Allen RC: Argon laser trabeculoplasty for open angle glaucoma. A retrospective study of 300 eyes. Trans Opthalmol Soc UK 103:288, 1983
14. Lunde M: Argon laser trabeculoplasty in the pigment dispersion syndrome with glaucoma. Am J Opthalmol 96:721, 1983
15. Pollack IP, Robin AL, Sax H: The effect of argon laser trabeculoplasty on the medical control of primary open angle glaucoma. Ophthalmology 90:785, 1983
16. Wise JB: Long-term control of adult open angle glaucoma by argon laser treatment. Ophthalmology 88:197, 1981
17. Hoskins HD, Hetherington J Jr, Minckler DS, et al: Complications of laser trabeculoplasty. Ophthalmology 90:796, 1983
18. Schwartz AL, Kopelman J: Four-year experience with argon laser trabecular surgery in uncontrolled open angle glaucoma. Ophthalmology 90:771, 1983
19. Krupin T, Kolker AE, Kass MA, Becker B: Intraocular pressure the day of argon laser trabeculoplasty in primary open-angle glaucoma. Ophthalmology 91:361, 1984

Trabeculotomy, Goniotomy, and Trabeculodialysis

26

H. Dunbar Hoskins, Jr.

Trabeculotomy, goniotomy, and trabeculodialysis are operative techniques whose primary value is in treating young glaucoma patients. Goniotomy is the surgery we prefer in glaucoma associated with isolated trabeculodysgenesis,[1] a condition that usually occurs in primary congenital glaucoma as defined by Shaffer and Weiss.[2] Trabeculotomy is preferred when corneal haze or defects prevent adequate visual control of the goniotomy incision. Trabeculodialysis is a modification of the goniotomy technique; it is used primarily in young patients with inflammatory glaucoma.

In order to highlight the specific aspects of these procedures, each is discussed separately.

TRABECULOTOMY

Indications

Trabeculotomy is indicated in those cases of developmental glaucoma in which corneal haze prevents adequate visualization of the angle recess. It may be more effective in older children and young adults with developmental glaucoma. Some surgeons prefer it over goniotomy because the surgical approach to the eye is more familiar.

Methods of Treatment

The purpose of trabeculotomy is to eliminate the trabecular meshwork as an obstruction to aqueous outflow. The technique was initially described by Burian and Allen[3] and Smith,[4] with further enhancements by Harms and Dannheim.[5]

In the trabeculotomy ab externo procedure, one must locate Schlemm's canal through the external surface of the limbus. A probe is then threaded through the canal; when the probe is in position, it is rotated into the anterior chamber, either tearing the trabecular meshwork or withdrawing it from the scleral sulcus (Fig. 26-1). Most surgeons sweep the probe to the right and to the left of the incision, creating about 120 degrees of trabeculotomy.

Recommended Technique

Although some surgeons prefer a fornix-based conjunctival incision, we have found it simpler to incise the limbal conjunctiva and then raise a

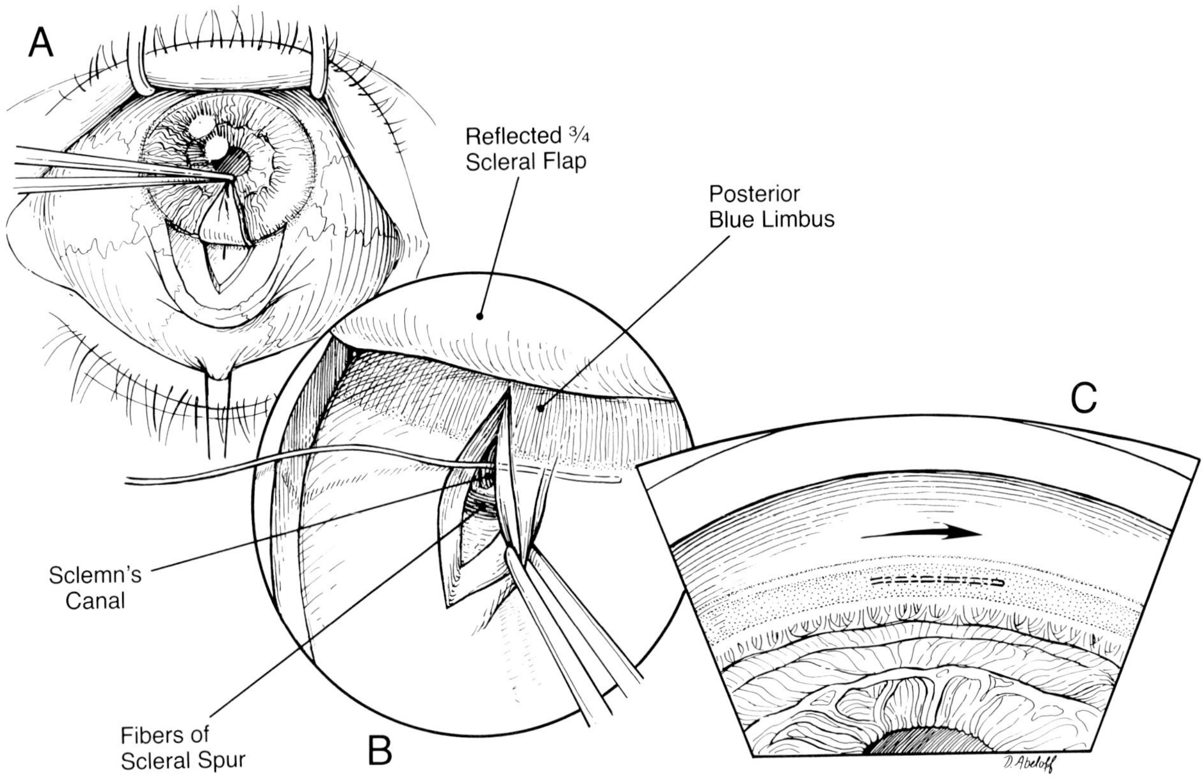

Fig. 26-1. Trabeculotomy. **(A)** A fornix-based conjunctival flap reveals a triangular flap that is $\frac{3}{4}$ of the scleral thickness. A triangular flap is more easily dissected. **(B)** Note the meridional fibers of the scleral spur that lie just posterior to Schlemm's Canal. A 5-0 nylon suture can be inserted into the canal. It should pass with little resistance and can be visualized in the canal (*C*) gonioscopically.

three-quarter-thickness scleral flap. The thick scleral flap facilitates location of the canal because the underlying structures are more easily seen.

A radial incision is then made over the expected site of the canal until the fibers of the scleral spur are recognized. These fibers have the shiny appearance of tendon and are organized circumferentially. The canal appears as a dark space at the anterior edge of these fibers. The canal lies just anterior to this anatomic landmark. The location of the canal can be confirmed by gently incising its roof and introducing a 5-0 nylon suture that can be seen gonioscopically when it is in the canal.

The Harms trabeculotome as modified by McPherson is introduced into the canal and broken through into the anterior chamber. It is important to maintain the probe parallel to the iris throughout the procedure (Fig. 26-2). An anterior deviation can strip Descemet's membrane from the cornea; a posterior misplacement can result in either cyclodialysis, iridodialysis, or both. After sweeping through one direction, the probe is withdrawn, and the opposite curved probe is inserted to complete the sweep in the other direction (Fig. 26-3). The sweeps need not cross the pupillary axis in order to withdraw the trabeculum adequately.

Bleeding and collapse of the anterior chamber generally occur during the second trabeculotomy sweep. The scleral flap must be adequately sutured to maintain the chamber. The chamber can be reformed by injecting balanced salt solution through either the external edges of the scleral flap or a

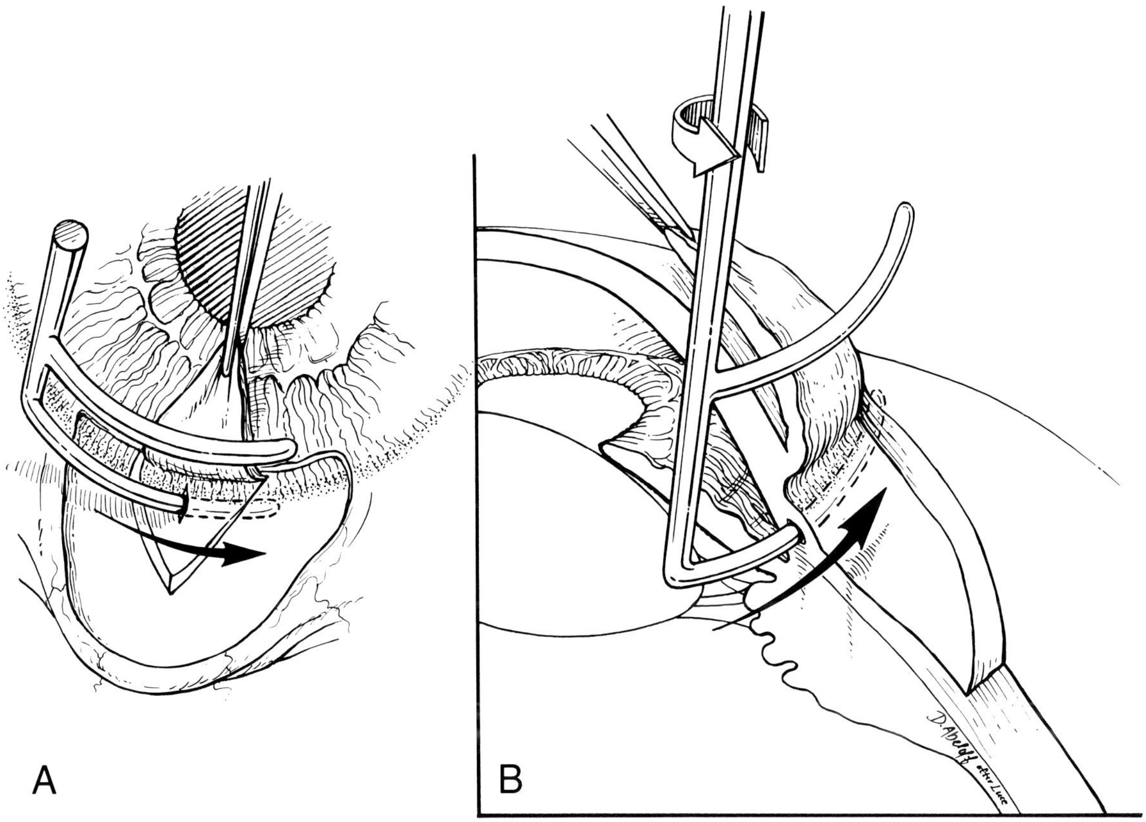

Fig. 26-2. Trabeculotomy. **(A)** The lower arm of the McPherson trabeculotome is inserted into the canal area. It is then passed around the limbus maintaining pressure against the scleral wall. **(B)** Once the probe has been fully inserted, it is rotated into the anterior chamber. Instrument shown larger than actual for clarity.

previously placed paracentesis. Re-formation of the anterior chamber is crucial, since a flat chamber presses the trabecular tissues back against the scleral sulcus and may negate the effects of the surgery.

After closing the scleral flap, the surgeon sutures the conjunctiva. We inject Celestone 1.0 ml subconjunctivally following the procedure and use topical miotics to maintain ciliary muscle contraction in order to keep the trabecular meshwork away from the sclera. This regimen is continued for 2 to 3 weeks. The eye patch is removed as soon as the eye is comfortable. The patient is usually discharged from the hospital on the day of the surgery unless significant bleeding has occurred, in which case overnight observation may be indicated.

After 2 to 3 weeks, the intraocular pressure often rises into the 20 to 30 range. Cessation of steroid drops usually results in a return to normal pressure levels.

Prognosis and Complications

Trabeculotomy works primarily by removing trabecular meshwork as an obstruction to aqueous outflow. In some cases, it also provides filtration to the subconjunctival space. In the hands of experi-

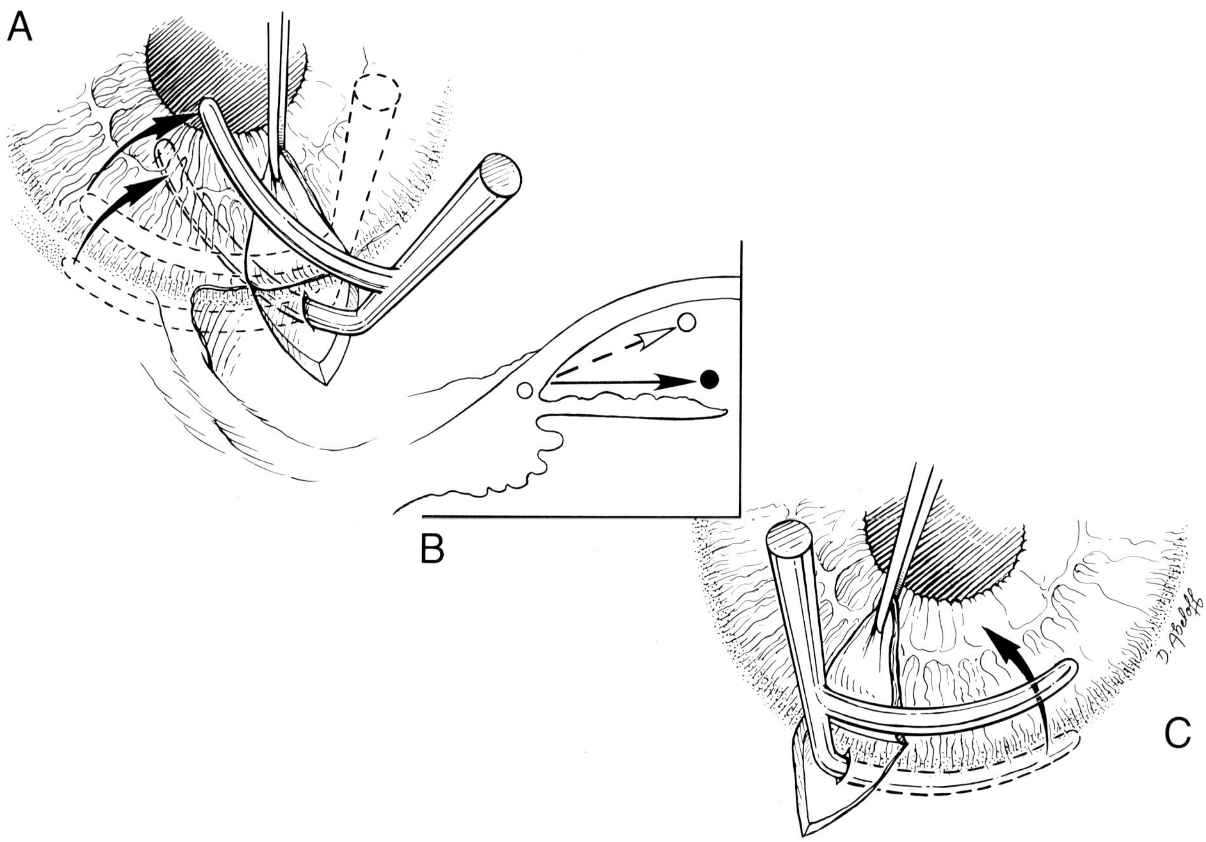

Fig. 26-3. Trabeculotomy. **(A)** The probe should be rotated far enough into the anterior chamber to disrupt the trabecular meshwork. It should not pass across the pupillary area. **(B)** The correct plane of rotation is parallel to the iris toward the black dot. If the probe rides forward toward the open circle, it can disinsert Descemet's membrane. **(C)** The sweep is then made identically in the opposite direction. Instrument shown larger than actual for clarity.

enced physicians, success rates of 80 to 83 percent have been reported in developmental glaucoma.[6,7]

The complications specifically associated with trabeculotomy arise mainly from failure to locate Schlemm's canal accurately. If the probe is not placed within the canal, a nontherapeutic passage into the chamber or the suprachoroidal space results. In the latter case, either cyclodialysis or hemorrhage, or both, may occur.

Other possible complications include stripping Descemet's membrane from the cornea and damage to the ciliary body or iris. Both problems can be avoided by ensuring that the probe is in a plane parallel to the iris at all times during the sweeps.

GONIOTOMY

Indications

This procedure is indicated in all cases of developmental glaucoma with isolated trabeculodysgenesis occurring in children under the age of 3 years. It is also used in cases of Sturge-Weber syndrome, aniridia, Axenfeld's syndrome, and Lowe's syndrome, in which it may lower pressure for weeks, months, or years. The procedure may be repeated as often as three times to achieve therapeutic reduction of intraocular pressure (IOP).

Contraindications

Goniotomy cannot be effectively accomplished if corneal clouding prevents visualization of the goniotomy site. It is less successful in patients over 3 years of age, for whom trabeculotomy is generally preferred. The choice of technique is based on the apparent mechanism of therapeutic result in each of these procedures. Goniotomy is designed to correct the anatomic defect labeled isolated trabeculodysgenesis and is outstandingly successful in treating these cases. These glaucomas generally present for treatment very early in life and fortunately respond well to surgery.

By contrast, we prefer to perform trabeculotomy in older developmental glaucoma patients. In these children, there is usually no obvious defect that the goniotomy knife can correct. In fact, the success rate for goniotomy drops to 30 percent in children over 2 years of age.[8] Rather, in these cases there is a generalized obstruction to outflow, which trabeculotomy can ameliorate.

Methods of Treatment

Goniotomy was introduced by De Vincentiis in the late nineteenth century. In 1938 Otto Barkan[9] described the technique that continues to the present time, with only minor modifications, to take advantage of modern microsurgical instrumentation.

Recommended Technique

An assistant controls eye position by grasping the superior and inferior rectus muscles with locking Elschnig forceps. This maneuver facilitates positioning of the eye to maximize the surgeon's view of the chamber angle.

The modified Barkan lens is held in place on the cornea by means of an angled toothed forceps that grasps the pillar of glass between the two dimples at the top of the lens (Fig. 26-4). After the cornea is irrigated with balanced salt solution, the surgeon positions the lens with one hand while introducing the modified Barkan goniotomy knife into the clear cornea approximately 1.0 mm anterior to the limbus. The assistant must keep the eye immobile during penetration of the cornea. If the surgeon rotates the blade slightly between the fingertips, the entry is usually smoothly accomplished without a sudden breakthrough into the chamber.

With additional gentle pressure and rotation, the surgeon directs the blade across the anterior chamber, parallel to the plane of the iris, to engage the trabecular meshwork opposite the incision. Under direct microscopic visualization at 16× magnification, the superficial layers of the trabecular meshwork are incised at the midpoint of the trabecular band. The iris usually drops posteriorly as this incision is made. The incision is continued circumferentially, first to the right and then to the left. The assistant can facilitate this by rotating the eye first counterclockwise and then clockwise, always maintaining the eye in a position so that the blade is parallel to the iris.

The incision should only be deep enough to part the trabecular fibers, which are very soft and cannot be felt. If the surgeon feels the blade cutting tissue, the blade is too deep and is scratching sclera, causing excessive bleeding.

Once the goniotomy incision is completed, the blade is withdrawn fairly quickly, taking care to avoid touching the iris, lens, or corneal endothelium. There is usually a gush of aqueous from the entry site, and the chamber shallows. This can be avoided by shifting the Barkan lens over the wound as the blade is withdrawn, to allow corneal swelling at the incision, sealing it off. A single 10-0 nylon suture can be used if the wound leaks. The anterior chamber is re-formed by an injection of balanced salt solution through the external lips of the corneal incision.

The entire procedure from initial muscle fixation through completion takes 8 to 10 minutes. The only incision, other than the therapeutic one, is the 1.0-mm corneal paracentesis. The conjunctiva is minimally disturbed by the fixation forceps.

Although there is little intraoperative bleeding, moderate bleeding occurs during the immediate postoperative hypotony. This confirms the estab-

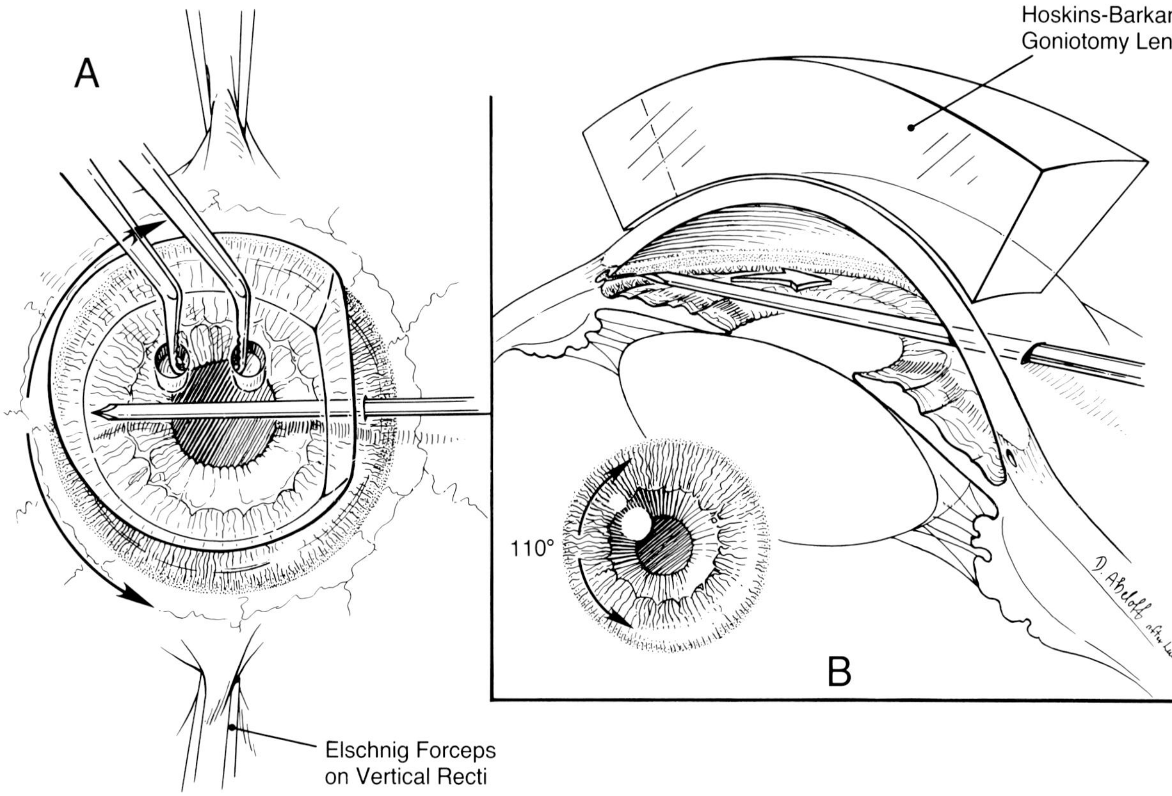

Fig. 26-4. Goniotomy. **(A)** The Barkan operating lens is held in place with angled Bishop–Harmon forceps. The superior and inferior rectus muscles are grasped with Elschnig fixation forceps. The knife passes across the anterior chamber to engage the trabecular meshwork, as seen in **(B)**. An incision is made over approximately 110 degrees. Instrument shown larger than actual for clarity.

lishment of communication to Schlemm's canal. The bleeding generally clears by the following day.

Postoperatively, the eye is patched after instilling an antibiotic steroid preparation. The head is positioned so that any blood drains away from the goniotomy site. The patient may be discharged the same day; the patch may be removed on the following day. Antibiotic steroid drops are usually continued for 3 to 5 days. The corneal suture is removed at reexamination 4 to 6 weeks postoperatively.

Prognosis and Complications

In isolated trabeculodysgenesis with onset of glaucoma between 1 and 24 months of age, the prognosis is excellent. In our office, 94 percent of these patients are successfully treated with one or two goniotomies. Litinsky et al.[10] reviewed 401 goniotomies performed by us and found only six complications (Table 26-1). Clearly, in experienced hands, goniotomy is a safe and effective pro-

Table 26-1. Surgical Complications of Goniotomy Under General Anesthesia[a]

Complication	No. of cases
Iridodialysis	4
Cyclodialysis	2
Postoperative hemorrhage	2

[a] Results are based on a review of 401 goniotomies. In addition, six cases of cardiopulmonary arrest could be attributed to the use of general anesthesia and were not complications specific to the surgical procedure.

(Litinsky SM, Shaffer RN, Hetherington J, et al: Operative complications of goniotomy, Trans Am Acad Ophthalmol 83:78, 1977.)

cedure. The effectiveness of goniotomy in other developmental glaucomas is not as high. The prognosis is somewhat poorer in developmental glaucoma complicated by dysgenesis of the iris or cornea.

TRABECULODIALYSIS

Indications

Trabeculodialysis is a modification of goniotomy used primarily in young patients with inflammatory glaucoma. It has been particularly successful in patients with glaucoma associated with the iritis of juvenile rheumatoid arthritis.

Contraindications

Trabeculodialysis is contraindicated when the chamber angle cannot be adequately visualized.

Recommended Technique

Trabeculodialysis is performed in a manner in every way identical to goniotomy, except for some variations in the actual incision. Once the knife has been passed across the anterior chamber, the trabecular meshwork is engaged at the level of Schwalbe's line, and an incision is made circumferential to Schwalbe's line for approximately 110 degrees. Thus the incision is made at the anterior edge of the trabecular meshwork rather than at the

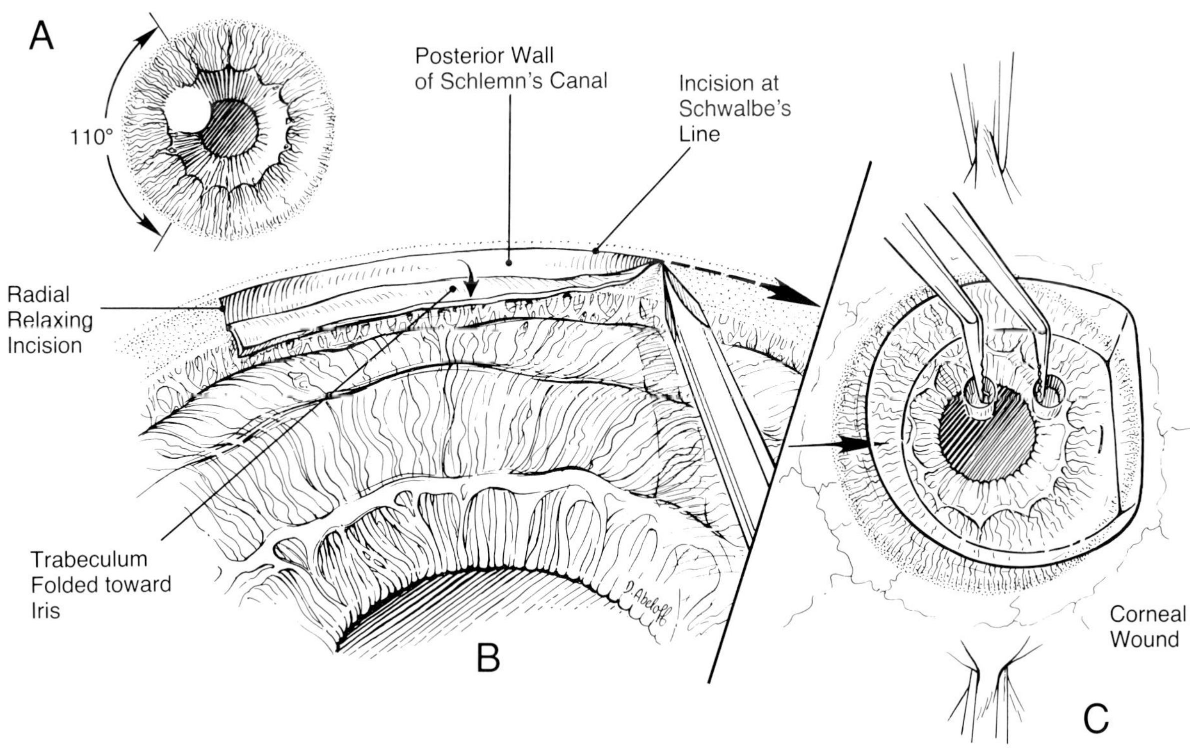

Fig. 26-5. Trabeculodialysis. **(A)** This procedure also incises 110 degrees of the trabecular meshwork by an incision **(B)** at Schwalbe's line that allows the trabeculum to be peeled out of the scleral sulcus with the flat edge of the blade. **(C)** Following removal of the knife in either goniotomy or trabeculodialysis, the lens can be shifted toward the surgeon to cover the corneal entry wound and retain the anterior chamber until swelling of the corneal fibers allows it to remain without further coverage.

midpoint, as is done in a routine goniotomy. The flat side of the blade is then used to push the trabecular meshwork downward toward the surface of the iris. This achieves a complete disinsertion of the meshwork from the scleral sulcus, exposing the outer wall of Schlemm's canal. Vertical relaxing incisions in the trabecular meshwork are then made at either end of the therapeutic incision; thus the trabeculum stays down on the iris and out of the scleral sulcus[11] (Fig. 26-5).

Prognosis and Complications

The theory behind this operation assumes that in a young patient the trabecular meshwork has been clogged by inflammatory debris and that the inner and outer walls of the Schlemm's canal have not been permanently scarred together. Thus, if the trabecular meshwork can be removed as a barrier to the aqueous outflow and the collector channels directly exposed to aqueous, pressure should normalize.

This operation seems to be more successful in children under the age of 20 than in older patients. This again may be related to tissue elasticity that allows retraction of the trabecular meshwork and a more uniform opening of the collector channels.[12]

Complications of this procedure are minimal. If the incision is made too deeply, the surgeon feels the scleral contact, and bleeding occurs during the postoperative period. The usual precautions exercised during goniotomy are necessary to prevent damage to the lens.

The operation seems to be ideal for those young patients who have glaucoma secondary to inflammation, since it is effective and causes minimal trauma to the eye.[13]

REFERENCES

1. Hoskins HD Jr, Shaffer RN, Hetherington J: An anatomic classification of the developmental glaucomas. Arch Ophthalmol 102:1331–1336, 1984
2. Shaffer RN, Weiss DI: Congenital and Pediatric Glaucomas. CV Mosby, St. Louis, 1970
3. Burian HM, Allen L: Trabeculotomy ab externo, a new glaucoma operation. Am J Ophthalmol 53:19, 1962
4. Smith R: A new technique for opening the canal of Schlemm. Preliminary report. Br J Ophthalmol 44:370, 1960
5. Harms H, Dannheim R: Epicritical consideration of 300 cases of trabeculotomy ab externo. Trans Ophthalmol Soc UK 89:491, 1970
6. McPherson SD Jr, Berry DP: Goniotomy vs. external trabeculotomy for developmental glaucoma. Am J Ophthalmol 95:427, 1983
7. Quigley HA: Childhood glaucoma: Results with trabeculotomy and study of reversible cupping. Ophthalmology 89:219, 1982
8. Shaffer RN: Prognosis of goniotomy in primary infantile glaucoma (trabeculodysgenesis). Trans Am Ophthalmol Soc 80:321, 1982
9. Barkan O: Technique of goniotomy. Arch Ophthalmol 19:217, 1938
10. Litinsky SM, Shaffer RN, Hetherington J, et al: Operative complications of goniotomy. Trans Am Acad Ophthalmol 83:78, 1977
11. Hoskins HD Jr, Hetherington J, Shaffer RN: Surgical management of the inflammatory glaucomas. Perspect Ophthalmol 1:173, 1977
12. Herschler J, Davis EB: Modified gonitomy for inflammatory glaucoma. Histologic evidence for the mechanism of pressure reduction. Arch Ophthalmol 98:684, 1980
13. Kanski JJ, McAllister JA: Trabeculodialysis for inflammatory glaucoma in children and young adults. Ophthalmology 92:927, 1985

Filtering Surgery

27

Jonathan Herschler

Almost since glaucomatous damage to the optic nerve was discovered to be caused by increased intraocular pressure (IOP), fistulizing procedures have been performed. By establishing a communication between the anterior chamber and the subconjunctival space, "decompression" of the globe was accomplished.[1] Holes of all sizes and shapes have been created: circular (trephine), semicircular (posterior or anterior lip sclerectomy), linear (thermal sclerostomy), and with a wick (iridencleisis).[2-6] All through-and-through or unprotected filtering operations suffered from the problems associated with early hypotony due to overfiltration during the early postoperative period.

Two kinds of filtering cicatrices have been noted. A localized thin cystic bleb is often associated with low IOP. Kronfeld[7] showed that the major avenue of egress of aqueous is via transconjunctival drainage. He measured ascorbate concentrations in the tear fluid of postfiltering surgery patients with thin cystic blebs. Ascorbate was found to be much higher in the tear fluid of the postoperative patients than in that of controls.[7]

Another type of filtering scar is the diffuse bleb; it is assumed that filtration in these cases occurs primarily by subconjunctival absorption of aqueous, perhaps by the formation of new aqueous veins, as demonstrated by Benedikt.[8]

The diffuse scar has been favored for decades because of a lower incidence of late complications, such as endophthalmitis, late hypotony from pinhole leaks or bleb rupture, or discomfort from localized elevation and dellen formation.

Iridencleisis was favored over other through-and-through filtering procedures because it tended to produce the more diffuse type of bleb and lessened the risk of early postoperative hypotony and flat chamber. Slitlike openings, such as with thermal sclerostomy, were associated with fewer early difficulties than were large symmetric sclerectomies, such as the Elliot trephine.

All filtering operations, when compared in large series limited to chronic open-angle glaucoma, report success rates that vary between 80 and 90 percent. Through-and-through procedures, on the average, will produce lower postoperative IOP without medication, but this advantage may be neutralized by increased surgical complications. Only in cases in which extremely low IOP is desired (8 to 12 mmHg) should these types of procedures be considered.

In 1968, Cairns[9] presented his trabeculectomy technique. This operation was designed to remove a block of trabecular meshwork to facilitate circumferential flow in Schlemm's canal and thereby lower IOP. The operation removed a block of trabecular tissue beneath a sutured half-thickness scleral flap in addition to a conjunctival flap.

Success rates similar to those associated with through-and-through procedures were thus obtained. It gradually became clear that the mechanism of success for trabeculectomy was subconjunctival filtration and not flow through the cut ends of Schlemm's canal. Grant had previously shown that circumferential flow in Schlemm's canal did not occur in glaucomatous eyes.

The success or failure of filtering operations has been correlated with the biologic properties in a given patient's aqueous humor.[10] The interaction of patients' subconjunctival fibroblasts with their own aqueous was studied. Patients who tended to have successful outcomes from filtering surgery had aqueous that inhibited the growth of their subconjunctival fibroblasts in tissue culture. On the basis of this research and my own clinical experience, I believe that the patient's own biologic properties, as well as the glaucoma type, are the major determining factors in the success or failure of glaucoma filtering operations. Clearly the safest and simplest procedure that avoids immediate intra- and postoperative problems is the most desirable. I have not been impressed that modifying the simplest technique improves success rates, except where the modification is designed to address a specific cause for failure in certain glaucoma types. For primary phakic open-angle glaucoma, the following trabeculectomy technique is my preferred method.

RECOMMENDED TECHNIQUE

The procedure can safely be performed on an outpatient basis. Local anesthesia with retrobulbar block and lid akinesia is preferred. The operation should be performed in as little time as possible to avoid intraoperative hypotony—normally the procedure can be completed within 30 to 40 minutes. The pupil should be miotic preoperatively. Long-acting anticholinesterases should be stopped at least 2 weeks prior to operation.

The technique of conjunctival dissection that I prefer to use is a limbus-based flap. Following insertion of a superior rectus traction suture, 10 to 12 mm behind the limbus, the globe is rotated slightly temporally, exposing the superior nasal quadrant. A small cut through the conjunctiva and Tenon's capsule is made with a blunt Westcott scissors. The initial cut is made directly in front of the traction suture, overlying the superior rectus muscle. The incision is made here so that the surgeon takes particular care not to incise the superior rectus or its sheath.

The incision through the conjunctiva and Tenon's capsule is enlarged temporally just beyond the margin of the superior rectus (about 2 mm). The incision is then extended nasally 6 to 7 mm, care being taken to maintain an orientation parallel to the limbus.

A sharp dissection with blunt-tipped Westcott scissors is performed. The scissors should be visualized through the overlying conjunctiva rather than directly through a reflected conjunctiva, so as to lessen the chance of inadvertent buttonholing (Fig. 27-1). The conjunctival and Tenon's flap should be freed of any underlying adhesions so that the closed Westcott scissors can now be freely passed beneath the full extent of the flap. The flap is then retracted with a Weck-cel sponge and the limbus inspected. A No. 67 Beaver blade is then used to gently push forward the underlying Tenon's capsule and conjunctiva. Care is taken not to disinsert Tenon's capsule.

A straight McPherson forceps attached to a bipolar cautery is then used to outline the scleral flap to be dissected (Fig. 27-2). Cautery setting is light (15 to 20 on Codman Mentor), in order to lessen bleeding during the dissection without shrinking tissue. Excessive cautery also causes charring, which can result in inflammation and ultimately a higher incidence of failure. A 5-mm equilateral triangular scleral flap is outlined, hinged at the limbus. The sclera adjacent to the outlined flap is grasped with a 0.12-mm Colibri forceps and the globe rotated slightly superiorly. The assistant retracts the con-

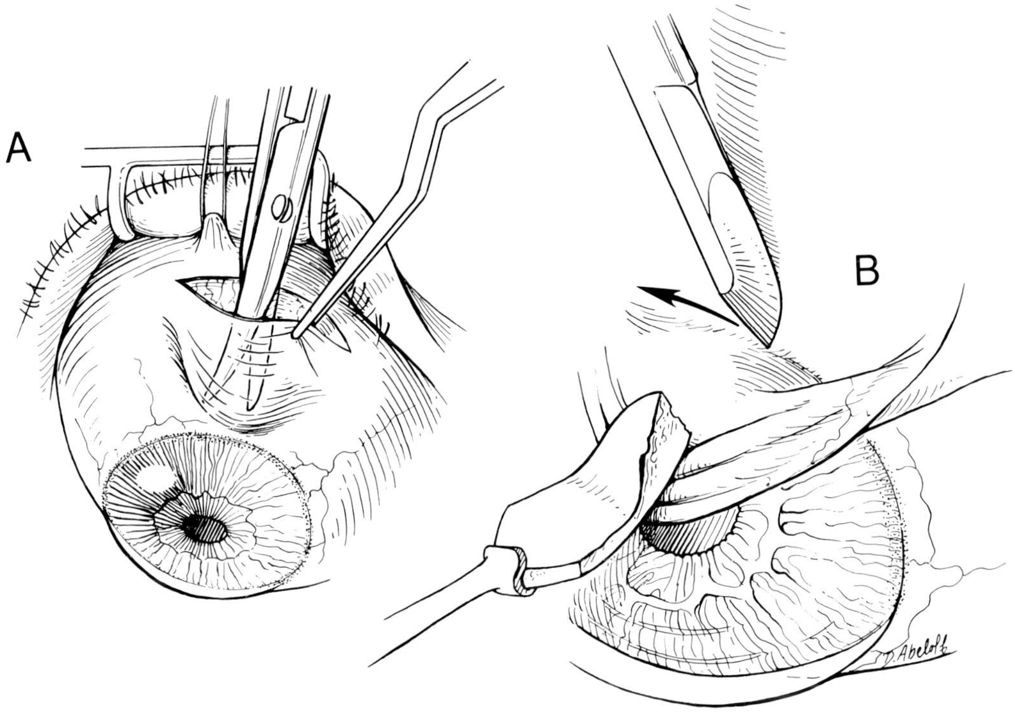

Fig. 27-1. Conjunctival dissection. **(A)** Visualizing the scissor tips at all times through the overlying conjunctiva helps avoid inadvertant buttonholes. This technique is especially useful when dissecting through previous scar tissue. **(B)** Gentle and minimal reflection of the insertion of the Tenon's capsule should be employed so as not to disinsert Tenon's capsule, which would produce a thin and cystic bleb.

junctiva gently with a Weck-cel sponge. A one-half to three-quarter depth incision is made with a No. 67 blade. It should start as anteriorly as possible behind the reflected Tenon's capsule and conjunctiva. The incision should be made in one continuous movement from the limbus to the apex of the triangle. A similar cut is then made on the other leg of the triangle (Fig. 27-2).

The No. 67 blade is then used to dissect the scleral flap. The tip of the triangle is elevated with the blade. Once a half-depth plane is found, tension with the Colibri forceps on the tip of the flap is directed up and forward toward the pupil. The No. 67 blade is held flat against the sclera, and the rounded portion of the blade is used to separate the adhering strands of sclera with a wiping motion (Fig. 27-3). Most of the dissection is performed by the tension on the flap by the Colibri forceps. As the corneoscleral limbus is approached, it will be necessary to tip the heal of the blade slightly inferiorly so that it is now parallel to the new curve of the cornea. Failure to do this will cause a loss of the plane of dissection—a deepening of the incision—and, on occasion, inadvertent entering of the anterior chamber.

The dissection is carried forward about 1.5 to 2 mm anterior to the scleral spur. A block of tissue 1 mm in AP measurement and 3 mm in horizontal measurement is outlined with the point of the No. 67 blade. At this point, a fixation forceps (0.3 mm Castroviejo) is used to grasp an edge of the scleral bed and a 25-gauge $\frac{5}{8}$-inch needle on a tuberculin syringe is used to make a paracentesis in clear cornea, temporally. The needle is beveled toward the

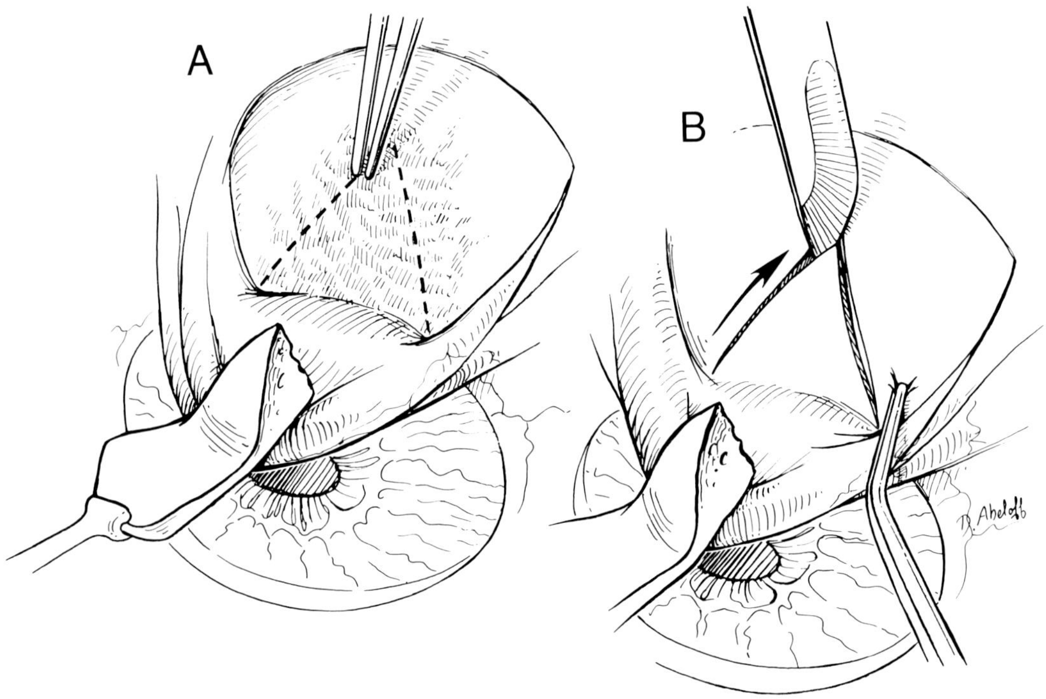

Fig. 27-2. Scleral incision. **(A)** Prior to the scleral incision, gentle use of bipolar cautery to outline the scleral flap to be dissected will decrease bleeding and prevent shrinking during dissection. A 5-mm equilateral triangular flap is outlined, hinged at the limbus. Adjacent sclera is grasped with a 0.12-mm Colibri forceps and the globe is rotated slightly superiorly. Assistant retracts the conjunctiva with a Weck-cel sponge. **(B)** A one-half to three-quarter depth incision with a No. 67 blade is started anteriorly just behind the reflected Tenon's capsule and conjunctiva. The incision should be one continuous cut from the limbus to the apex of the triangle. Repeat incision for other side of triangle. The flap should be half-thickness for ease in handling.

inferior temporal angle. The needle is rotated gently so as to ease the penetration through Descemet's membrane, thereby lessening the risk of sudden forceful perforation and resultant lens injury. If IOP is high, a small amount of aqueous is withdrawn.

The assistant then grasps the apex of the triangular scleral flap and gently retracts it toward the pupil. Using the No. 67 blade, with the blade facing upward, the surgeon incises the anterior edge of the previously marked 1 × 3 rectangle. Care is taken to cut along the full extent of the 3 mm with an upward motion away from the underlying tissues.

A right-angled Vannas scissors is then carefully inserted into the anterior chamber and directed posteriorly toward the scleral spur. The lower blade is parallel to the iris and gently elevated. One side of the 1 × 3 rectangle is cut. The Colibri forceps is used to grasp the free corner of the rectangle, which is rotated posteriorly. The lower blade of the Vannas scissors is then placed beneath the 1 × 3 rectangle and moved to the posterior incision. A single vertical cut is used for the full 3-mm length. The 1 × 3 rectangle is then lifted, and the hinged end is cut with the scissors (Fig. 27-4).

Should the iris prolapse during any phase of this procedure, a tiny iridotomy is made and the iris gently reposited. The iris is now grasped with the Colibri forceps in the middle of the exposed window. It is gently lifted and rotated posteriorly. It is important to avoid pulling anteriorly, as this may cause iridodialysis and bleeding. The blunt-edged iris scissors (Barraquer or DeWecker) is used to

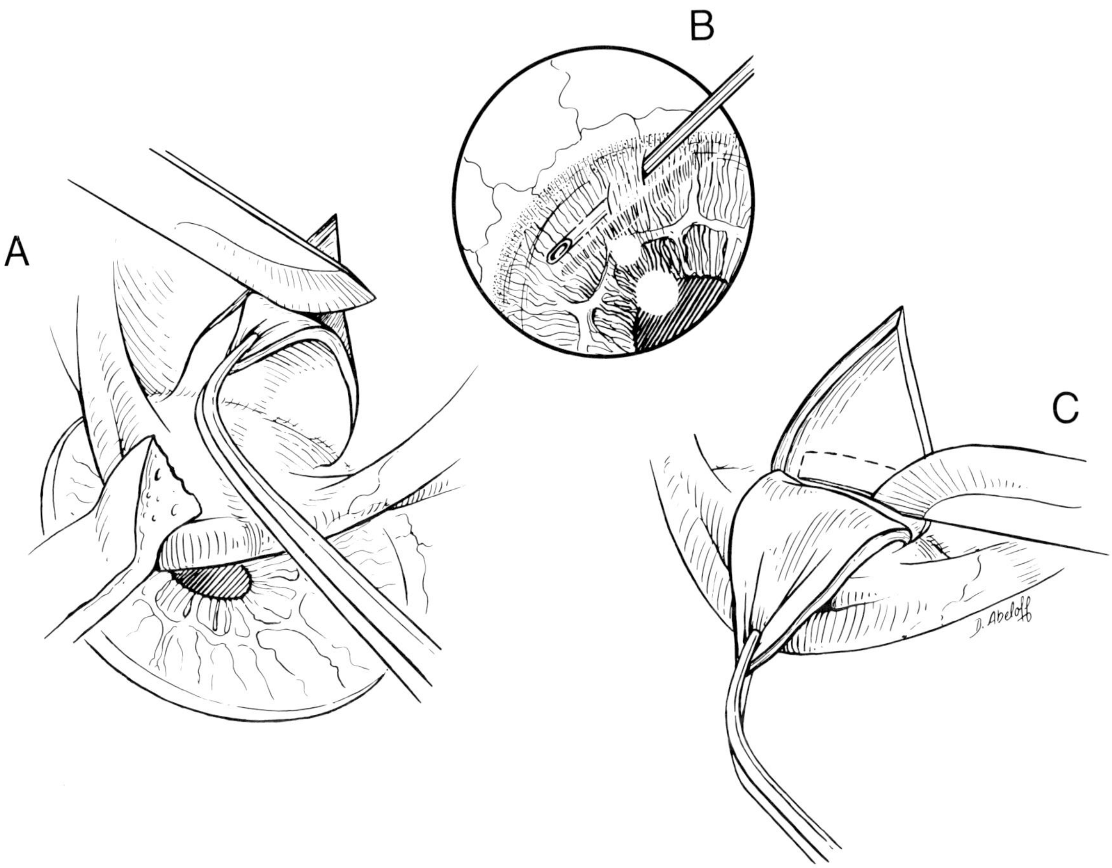

Fig. 27-3. Scleral dissection. **(A)** Tension on the forceps retracting the tip of the flap greatly facilitates the dissection. The No. 67 blade is placed flat on the scleral bed. Once a half-depth thickness is found, the belly of the blade gently cuts the scleral fibers stretched by the retracting forceps. **(B)** Prior to entering the anterior chamber at the trabeculectomy site, a paracentesis tract is placed in the temporal cornea. **(C)** A No. 67 blade is used vertically to cut the anterior edge of the 1-mm × 3-mm trabeculectomy window.

make a 45-degree cut in the iris. The scissors is then turned, and a 45-degree cut in the opposite direction is made. This makes for a large yet very basal iridectomy that is larger in its dimensions than the window of excised limbal tissue. This is done so that the iris will not block the internal fistula opening if shallowing of the anterior chamber occurs postoperatively. A single 10-0 nylon suture is then placed in the apex of the scleral triangle and the flap is secured in place. Additional sutures are placed 1 mm posterior to the anterior limits of the scleral dissection on either side of the scleral triangle. The sutures are oriented perpendicular to the scleral incisions (Fig. 27-5). At this point, if the anterior chamber is not fully formed, balanced salt solution is injected with a blunt 27 cannula through the previously placed paracentesis tract in the cornea. The object of scleral closure is to ensure that the anterior chamber will remain formed at this point. One need not be concerned with the rate of fluid flow beneath the scleral flap as long as the anterior chamber stays nicely formed. Attempts at loosening or cutting sutures because of poor fluid flow are unwarranted, since the aqueous is of very high protein content and is quite viscous and sticky at this point. Removal of sutures frequently leads to postoperative complications related to hypotony and postoperative shallowing of the anterior chamber.

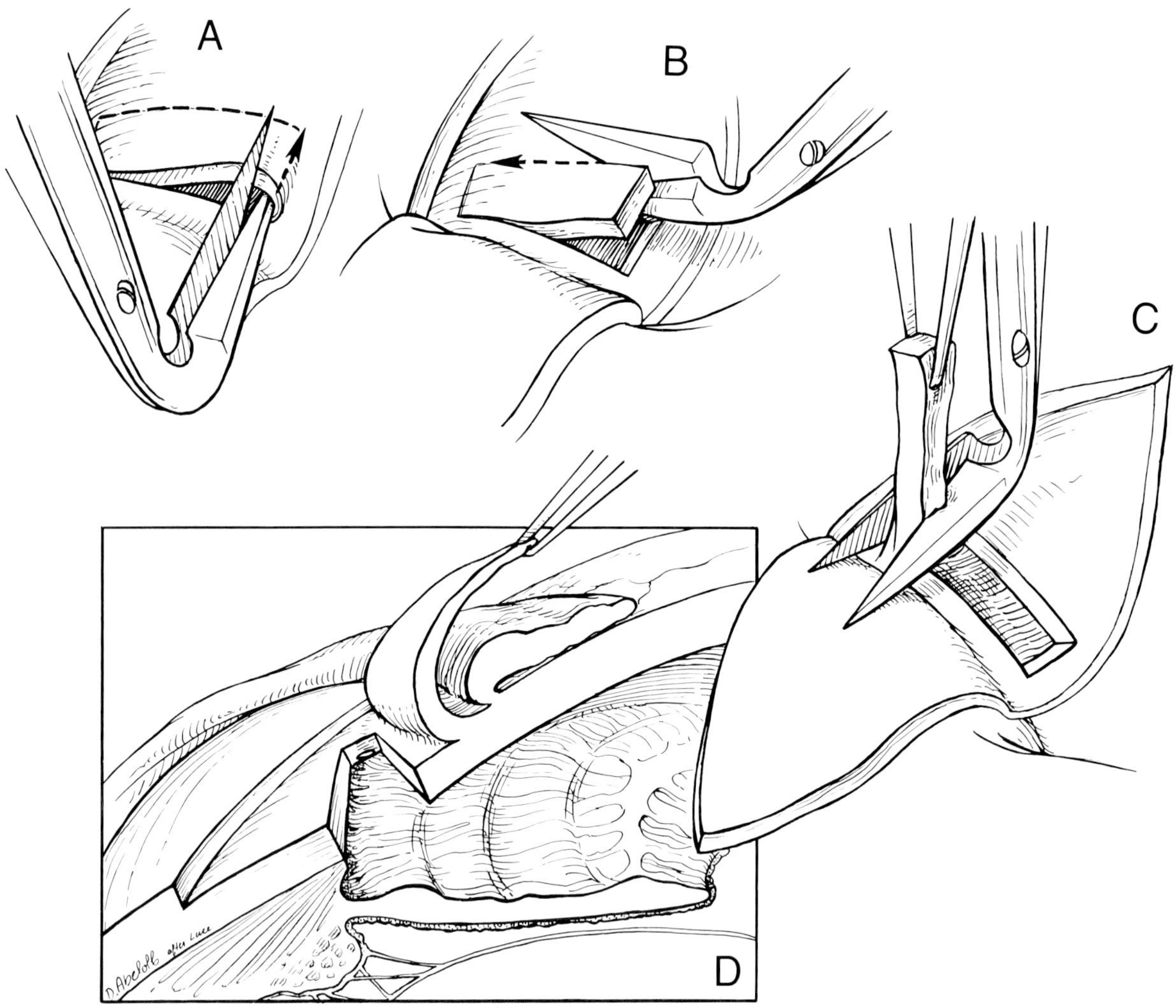

Fig. 27-4. (A) Right-angled Vannas scissors are held vertically and inserted carefully to cut the 1-mm first side of the trabeculectomy window. **(B)** A single vertical cut is used for the full 3-mm posterior side of the window, and **(C)** the Colibri forceps is used to grasp and lift the free corner of the rectangle. The lower blade of the scissors is then placed beneath the rectangle, and the hinged end is cut. **(D)** Cross-section view of trabeculectomy window and scleral flap.

If the anterior chamber remains formed, the conjunctival and Tenon's flap is closed carefully with 5-0 plain catgut suture used in a running, unlocked, fashion. Care is taken to suture only the edges of the cut conjunctiva and Tenon's capsule, but to be sure, both layers are included in all bites.

The proper appearance at this point is a deep anterior chamber and diffuse bleb. If the anterior chamber is not fully formed, BSS is again injected through the paracentesis tract. The anterior chamber should remain nicely formed. In the rare circumstance in which it does not, air is injected into the anterior chamber, leaving a 6-mm air bubble. An injection of 1 ml containing 20 mg triamcinolone diacetate (Aristocort) and 2 mg dexamethasone phosphate (Decadron) is made inferotemporally in the sub-Tenon's space; 10 percent Neo-Synephrine and 1 percent Cyclogyl drops and a steroid or antibiotic-steroid ointment are instilled. A loose patch and Fox shield are applied.

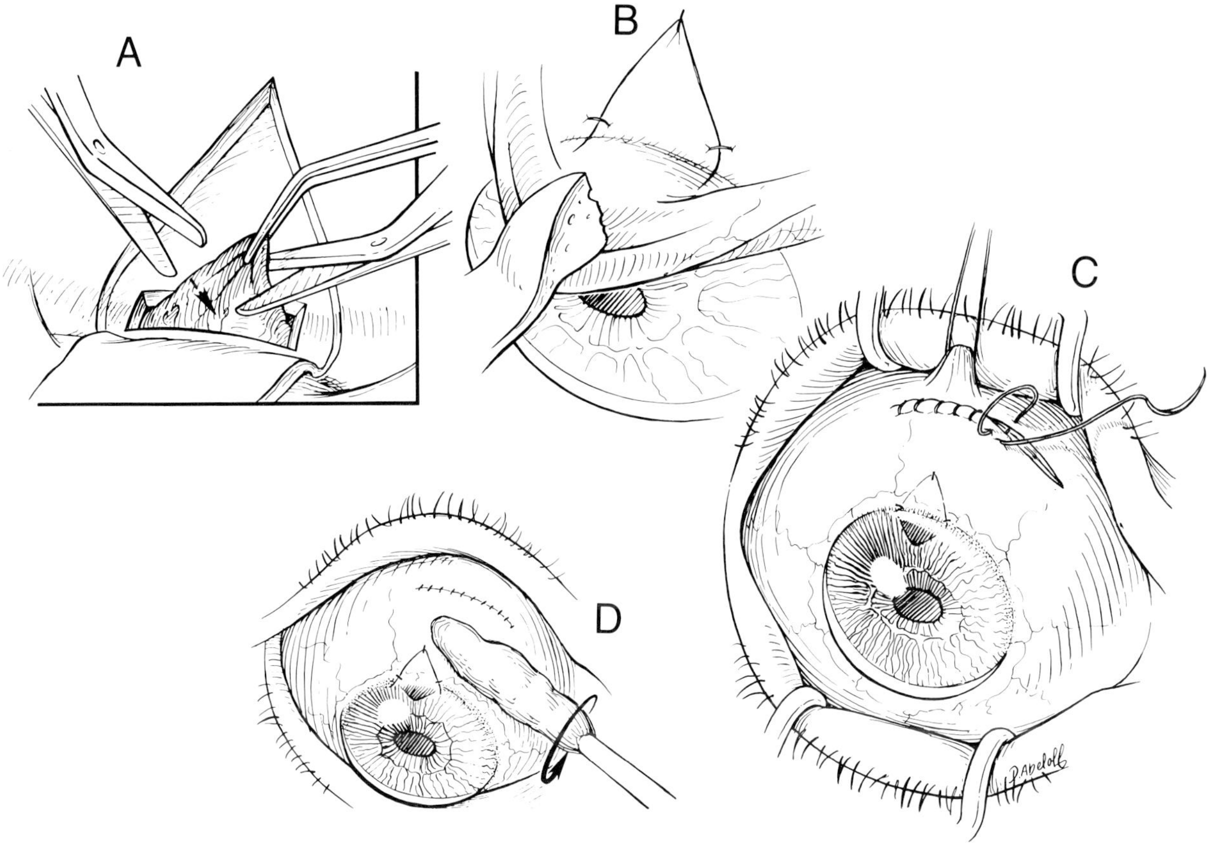

Fig. 27-5. Iridectomy. **(A)** The hole in the iris should be larger than the overlying trabeculectomy window. To prevent the iridectomy from extending too far toward the pupil, the incision in the iris is made in two steps, 45 degrees toward the pupil. This accomplishes a broad-based but short iridectomy. **(B)** The scleral flap is closed with three interrupted 10-0 nylon sutures. The sutures near the limbus are the keys to avoiding hypotony during the immediate postoperative period. **(C)** Careful closure of the conjunctiva is accomplished with 5-0 plain gut suture placed in a running, nonlocking, fashion. **(D)** If IOP is high without a bleb during the immediate postoperative period (1 to 3 days), a moist cotton-tipped applicator is used to apply gentle pressure on the host sides of the triangle. An immediate large bleb should form.

POSTOPERATIVE MANAGEMENT

On the first postoperative day, a large bleb and normal-depth anterior chamber should be present. A typical anterior chamber reaction is one to two plus cell with minimal or no flare. If a small hyphema occurred at surgery, a greater cellular count will be observed. The pupil should be 4 to 5 mm or greater and round.

Intraocular pressure is typically 5 to 20 mmHg. If it is lower, but the anterior chamber is full depth, no particular concern is warranted. If the anterior chamber is less than full depth with very low IOP, topical steroids should be withheld, as they would aggravate the overfiltration or wound leak problem. The eye is again dilated with Neo-Synephrine and cycloplegic (atropine, scopolamine, or Cyclogyl) and the shield reapplied, this time without a patch. If the next day the anterior chamber is continuing to shallow, air can be injected through the operatively placed paracentesis tract to create a deeply formed anterior chamber. This maneuver is most effective before large choroidal separations have occurred and should therefore be employed prior to total anterior chamber flattening.

If the anterior chamber shows full depth, topical steroids in maximal strength (i.e., 1 percent Pred-forte) should be prescribed every 2 hours while awake and steroid ointment at night. A shield is worn at all times in the first week and nightly for 1 month. No patch is employed. Mydriasis is continued two times daily for 4 weeks. Steroids are tapered beginning at 3 weeks if the anterior chamber has no reaction and should be discontinued before 6 weeks.

Massage is an extremely useful and effective technique and is employed in two ways. If IOP is high without a bleb during the immediate postoperative period (1 to 3 days), a moist cotton-tipped applicator is used to apply gentle pressure on the host side of the scleral triangle (Fig. 27-5D). Both sides are manipulated. The cotton-tipped applicator may be rolled across the edges of the flap. An immediate large bleb should form. Often the anterior chamber will shallow markedly. While the patient is awake, topical steroids are employed every hour with steroid ointment at night. The patient should be seen daily and the massage maneuver employed if a bleb is not present on examination.

If a diffuse bleb is present, a different massage technique can be employed if IOP is too high (≥30 mmHg) after the first postoperative week. The patient closes the eyelid and looks straight ahead. Direct pumping on the cornea through the lid is performed 15 to 20 times. The bleb should increase, and the IOP should drop. If the anterior chamber remains deeply formed, the patient can be instructed in this technique to be used two to three times daily at home. If the anterior chamber shallows, it is too dangerous to allow the patient to employ this technique at home.

No antiglaucoma drops should be employed for 6 weeks postoperatively. Aqueous suppressors should not be employed unless the surgeon has totally given up on any hope of successful filtration.

If bleb localization and vascularization begin 4 to 6 weeks postoperatively, steroids should be rapidly tapered and active massage started. Fifty percent of blebs can be saved by this technique.

Bleb Revision

The question of when to reintervene surgically in a failing or failed filtering operation is somewhat controversial. In my experience, early revision—within the first 6 weeks—is almost never appropriate, unless a mechanical blockage of the internal filtration ostia is detected by gonioscopy. It is preferable to allow postoperative inflammation to resolve entirely before reintervention is undertaken.

One indication for revision is the development of an encysted bleb (i.e., an externalized anterior chamber). This development is caused by a rapid proliferation of fibroblasts forming a syncytium of relatively impermeable cells. This is not hypertrophied Tenon's tissue. Once a continuous cell-to-cell lining has been formed, fibroblastic activity stops. However due to stagnation of aqueous flow through the impermeable lining, a gradual decrease in size of the encysted bleb occurs. Once the eye appears totally quiet with all antiinflammatory agents discontinued, surgical revision can be attempted, and at least a 50 percent success rate should be expected.

REVISION TECHNIQUE

A paracentesis tract is made, and fluorescein-stained BSS is injected into the anterior chamber. An incision is made in the conjunctiva only, posterior to the original conjunctival incision. Using a blunt Westcott scissors, a gentle sharp and blunt dissection technique is used to separate the conjunctiva from the underlying Tenon's capsule and fibroblastic scar tissue. This dissection is carried anteriorly just beyond the insertion of the Tenon's capsule. At this stage, a dome of thick impermeable tissues is observed. This dome is then completely excised using a No. 67 blade. At this point, the limbs of the underlying scleral flap are observed.

Commonly free aqueous can be seen flowing between the nonhealed scleral incisions. If this is the case, no further dissection is indicated, and the conjunctiva is closed as described in the earlier description of the primary trabeculectomy.

If no flow of fluorescein-stained aqueous is noted, the scleral flap is gently elevated from posterior to anterior. This is done by removing the apical suture, incising with a No. 67 blade along the original scleral incisions and lifting the scleral flap firmly with a Colibri-type forceps. The end point of the scleral dissection is to uncover a fistulous tract wherein free flow of aqueous is obtained. Once free flow is achieved, a single 10-0 nylon suture is placed at the apex of the scleral flap, loosely closing the flap. BSS injected through the paracentesis should cause free flow under the scleral flap. The conjunctiva is then closed. Postoperative measures are as for the primary operation.

MODIFICATIONS OF THE TRABECULECTOMY PROCEDURE

Fornix-Based Flap

During the 1980s, proponents of this method of conjunctival dissection have suggested the fornix-based approach of conjunctival incision and closure as safe and easier to perform than the classic limbus-based approach. In the hands of experienced glaucoma specialists, this appears to be true. Nevertheless, because of the obvious increased risk of direct fistula to the outside and increased chance of hypotony and flat anterior chamber, I am reluctant to recommend this as the preferred technique for a nonglaucoma specialist. Since I have had no difficulties with the limbus-based approach, I rarely employ the fornix-based technique.

Excision of Tenon's Capsule

Some authorities suggest that the excision of Tenon's capsule might increase the chance of success in young or black patients. I do not recommend this modification, as I believe it is based on the erroneous hypothesis that Tenon's tissue is a cause for bleb failure. Rather, I believe that the additional trauma of Tenon's excision with the raw edges left behind will increase chances of fibroblastic proliferation and bleb failure. In fact, excision of Tenon's capsule will lead to thinner blebs, with the increased risk of late complications such as endophthalmitis and bleb perforation or rupture.

Size and Shape of Scleral Flap or Inner Window

The size or shape of the scleral flap probably has little or no effect on the ultimate success or failure of an operation.[11] The size of the inner window is also probably not crucial unless an edge of the inner window gets close (<0.5 mm) to the external scleral incision. This leads to a direct "uncovered" communication and, if that is what was initially desired, I believe that a more standard through-and-through procedure should be chosen.

Medications

The greatest chance of increasing the success with filtration operations lies with the hope for modifying the scarring response of the patient. Corticosteroids have been our only useful drug adjunct in the past. Recent work with antimetabolites offers promise for the future, but their use remains investigational. Better delivery systems and more firm data on the best agents to be employed are needed before they can be recommended for routine use in high-risk patients.

One such experimental method of antimetabolite delivery that seems to have potential for clinical value employs the use of an absorbable collagen sponge. Studying the release rates of radiolabeled agents using varying strategies for drug delivery, Kay et al.[12] found that a collagen sponge or silicone wafer was best able to prolong contact time with the desired target site. Pilot experiments in rabbits[13] and a preliminary clinical trial in high-risk glaucoma patients confirm the efficacy of this approach.[14] The technique of collagen sponge implantation at the time of trabeculectomy is shown

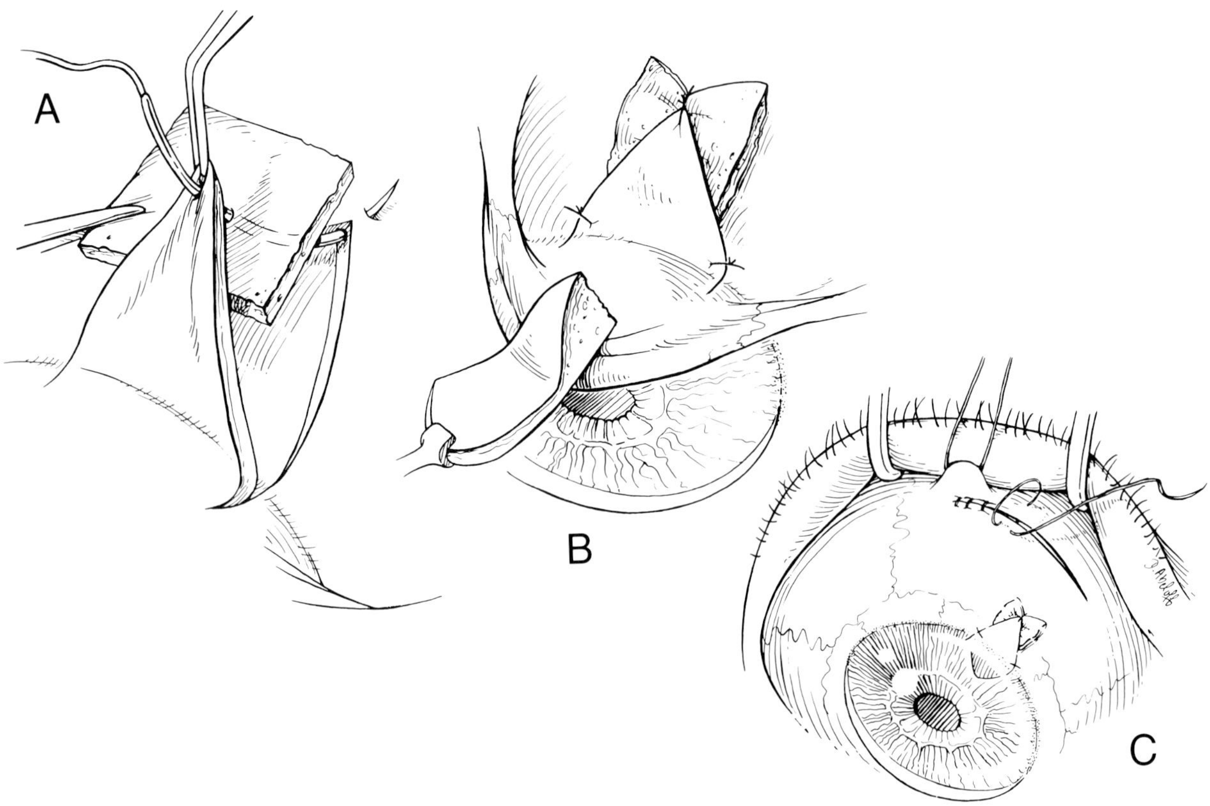

Fig. 27-6. (A–C) Technique of implantation of the collagen sponge. The apical scleral suture includes the sponge. Use of an antimetabolite will delay healing of the conjunctival incision. Thus, closure of the conjunctiva is accomplished with a running, nonabsorbable suture, such as 10-0 nylon. Watertight closure is especially important when antimetabolites are employed.

in Figure 27-6. Since the sponge is sewn into place under the scleral and conjunctival flaps, the complications associated with release of the antimetabolite into the tear film are not encountered. In addition, the dosage of antimetabolite required to obtain the desired inhibition of wound healing is greatly reduced.

Bipolar Cautery to Iris and Ciliary Body for Neovascular Glaucoma

This technique is identical to standard trabeculectomy except that prior to performing iridectomy, light bipolar cautery is applied to the iris surface exposed in the limbal window. Following the bloodless iridectomy, light bipolar cautery is applied to the two or three ciliary processes exposed by iridectomy. First, cautery is applied to the base of the process, retracting the tip from the lens equator. The tip can then be safely cauterized without causing injury to the lens.[15]

Vitrectomy for Aphakia

The success of trabeculectomy can be improved in aphakic patients who have had previous intracapsular extraction, by combining the trabeculectomy with total vitrectomy performed through the trabeculectomy incision. This complex and potentially dangerous modification of a trabeculectomy procedure should be undertaken only by an experienced vitrectomist. Details of the procedure are described by Herschler.[16]

THROUGH-AND-THROUGH FILTERING OPERATIONS

The primary indication for the through-and-through filtering operation is lower tension glaucoma with moderate to severe field loss, wherein extremely low IOP of 10 to 12 mmHg is considered necessary to halt further visual-field loss. The secondary indication is failure of a previous well-performed trabeculectomy.

Technique

Thermal Sclerostomy (Scheie)

The preparation of the conjunctival flap is identical to that for primary trabeculectomy, except that the Tenon's insertion will need to be pushed slightly more anteriorly. A paracentesis is made in the temporal cornea. A 2- to 3-mm scratch incision perpendicular to the sclera is made parallel to the limbus just anterior to the pure white-to-gray transition zone — the surgical limbus. A No. 67 blade is used; between cuts, bipolar cautery is applied by a McPherson forceps to the full extent of the incision, including the very deepest aspect. Alternative cut and cautery is used until the anterior chamber is reached. A last application of cautery is applied to the inner posterior lip of the wound. Pressure on the posterior wound margin with a closed DeWecker scissors enables the iris to prolapse; it is grasped with a Colibri forceps and elevated, and an iridectomy is performed, as in trabeculectomy. Gentle irrigation of the wound with stroking of the cornea in a downward fashion will reposit the iris. The conjunctiva is closed as in trabeculectomy. The anterior chamber is reformed with BSS and air through the paracentesis tract. During this procedure, the sutured conjunctival incision is checked for watertightness. If any leakage is noted, additional interrupted 6-0 plain gut sutures are placed. Postoperatively, steroids are gingerly employed, as long as the anterior chamber remains fully formed.

Corneoscleral Trephination

Corneoscleral trephination is identical to thermal sclerostomy, except that a sharp 1.5-mm Elliot trephine is used to make the through-and-through scleral entry. The trephine is positioned perpendicular to the sclera with its anterior edge as close to the limit of the retracted conjunctiva and Tenon's capsule as possible. A gentle to-and-fro twisting motion is made until the aqueous presents. It is best to tilt the trephine slightly anteriorly so that the entry into the anterior chamber is in the deepest portion. The trephine is removed, and an angled Vannas scissors is used to cut free the plug of limbal tissue. Iridectomy is performed as previously described. The conjunctival and Tenon's flap is closed and the anterior chamber is deeply formed with air. Medical treatment is the same as for thermal sclerostomy.

Postoperative Complications

A flat anterior chamber with hypotony and large choroidals are complications of filtering surgery, more commonly seen after the through-and-through technique. If the air injection at the slit lamp has not been successful or failed to be performed, and the anterior chamber is absent (i.e., lens–corneal touch), immediate intervention is necessary.

The operation should be done under general anesthesia. The superior rectus suture is carefully placed high in the fornix. The sclera is grasped, at the temporal limbus, with a 0.3-mm Castroviejo fixation forceps. A short sharp 27- or 30-gauge needle attached to a 3-cc glass syringe filled with sterile air is used to make a paracentesis entry adjacent to the point of fixation. The needle is pointed toward the lower temporal angle, and a beveled entry is slowly accomplished with a gentle twisting motion. As soon as entry into the anterior chamber is suspected, gentle positive pressure on the syringe plunger allows air to form the anterior chamber. If intracorneal lamellar air is noted, pressure on the plunger must be released. The anterior chamber is deeply formed, and the eye is made firm. Next, attention is directed to the inferotemporal quadrant. A 2- to 3-mm radial incision is made in the conjunctiva to the sclera. A scratch incision, through the sclera, is accomplished with a No. 67 blade. The incision is 2 to 3 mm in length and vertical. As soon as entry into the suprachoroidal space is achieved, yellow fluid should be observed. The incision is extended at its base, to the full limit, so as to permit free flow of suprachoroidal fluid. No attempt is made to drain the fluid fully at this point. BSS is injected into the anterior chamber through the corneal tract until the eye is again firm. Suprachoroidal fluid is again allowed to drain. An alternate filling of the anterior chamber and draining of fluid is accomplished until no more fluid remains in the suprachoroidal space. Patience is required, and the draining and filling can take up to 15 to 20 minutes, since all four quadrants must be allowed to drain. The anterior chamber is left deeply formed with air.

The conjunctival incision is closed with a running 6-0 gut suture. The sclera is left unclosed. Postoperative management is identical to the original description for through-and-through procedures. *Do not reopen the original conjunctival incision in an attempt to close the sclerostomy — this will not solve the problem and will likely lead to failure of the original operation.*

SUMMARY

The ultimate success or failure of a filtering operation is, in the end, determined by the patients own healing properties. The role of the glaucoma surgeon is to maximize the opportunities for that individual patient's success by performing a quick, simple, technically correct and appropriate filtering operation.

Careful and appropriate postoperative management, including medications and massage, as well as surgical reintervention when required, will contribute to the attainment of this goal. No operation will be 100 percent effective, however, and visually threatening complications can occur. Both the surgeon and patient must be fully aware of these facts before a filtering procedure is performed.

REFERENCES

1. DeWecker L: Traité Théoretique et pratique des maladies des yeux. Vol. 2. Delahaye, Paris, 1867
2. Herbert H: Subconjunctival fistula formation in the treatment of primary chronic glaucoma. Trans Ophthalmol Soc UK 23:324, 1903
3. La Grange F: Production of a cicatrix in chronic glaucoma. Ophthalmoscope 5:467, 1907
4. Holth S: Iridencleisis cum iridotomia meridionali. Arch Ophthalmol 4:803, 1930
5. Elliot RH: A preliminary note on a new operative procedure for the establishment of a filtering cicatrix in the treatment of glaucoma. Ophthalmoscope 7:804, 1909
6. Scheie HG: Peripheral iridectomy with scleral cautery for glaucoma. Arch Ophthalmol 61:291, 1959
7. Kronfeld PC: Chemical demonstration of transconjunctival passage after antiglaucomatous operations. Am J Ophthalmol 35:38, 1952
8. Benedikt O: Die Darstellung des Kammerwasserabflusses Normaler und Glaucomkranker Menschlicher Augen Durch Fullung der Vorderkammer mit Fluorescein. Von Graefes Arch Klin Ophthalmol 199:45, 1976
9. Cairns JE: Trabeculectomy. Preliminary report of a new method. Am J Ophthalmol 66:673, 1968
10. Herschler J, Claflin AJ, Fiorentino G: The effect of aqueous humor on the growth of subconjunctival fibroblasts in tissue culture and its implications for glaucoma surgery. Am J Ophthalmol 89:245, 1980
11. Starita RJ, Fellman RL, Spaeth GL, Poryzees E: Effect of varying size of scleral flap and corneal block on trabeculectomy. Ophthalmic Surg 15:484, 1984
12. Kay JS, Litin BS, Woolfenden JM, et al: Delivery of antifibroblast agents as adjuncts to filtration surgery. Part I. Periocular clearance of Cobalt-57 Bleomycin in experimental drug delivery: Pilot study in rabbits. Ophthalmic Surg 17:626, 1986
13. Kay JS, Litin BS, Jones MA, et al: Delivery of antifibroblast agents as adjuncts to filtration surgery. Part II. Delivery of 5-fluorouracil and bleomycin in a collagen implant. Pilot study in the rabbit. Ophthalmic Surg 17:796, 1986

14. Herschler J, Kay JS, Litin BS, Chvapil M: Drug delivery of antimetabolites as adjuncts to glaucoma filtration surgery: Preliminary clinical experience. p. 215. In Glaucoma Update. III. Springer Verlag, New York, 1986
15. Herschler J, Agness D: A modified filtering operation for neovascular glaucoma. Arch Ophthalmol 97:2339, 1979
16. Herschler J: The effect of total vitrectomy on filtration surgery in the aphakic eye. Ophthalmology 88:229, 1981

Combined Procedures for Glaucoma and Cataracts

28

George L. Spaeth

When considering the surgical management of the patient who has both glaucoma and cataract, the major governing principles are to be clear regarding the specific goals of the surgery and to realize that the likelihood of accomplishing the goals is a function of how completely the patient's condition is understood preoperatively and how thoroughly the surgeon knows the full range of effects induced by the surgery. There is no single "right" management. However, there are methods of management that are more reasonable, and those that are less reasonable. The more reasonable the management, the more likely the result will be pleasing to the patient and to the surgeon. The following principles, upon which reasonable surgery is based, are derived both from the literature and from the author's personal experience.

PRINCIPLES GOVERNING REASONABLE SURGERY

1. The usual, immediate, postoperative response of intraocular pressure (IOP) to an uncomplicated cataract extraction is a transient elevation.[1,2] This rise of IOP occurs regardless of the technique employed. Previous comments that IOP following uncomplicated cataract extraction tended to fall may have been valid for previously utilized techniques.[3,4] They referred, however, more to the long-term effect on IOP of cataract extraction, rather than the pressure changes that occur in the immediate postoperative period. Furthermore, they are not valid in considering the first weeks following uncomplicated surgery, in which the incision is tightly closed with multiple fine sutures.
2. The "sick disc," that is, the badly damaged optic nerve head, is extremely vulnerable. Elevation of intraocular pressure (IOP), even when transient or of small magnitude, causes rapid further damage. This may result in serious deterioration of vision, particularly when preoperative visual field loss is severe and cuts close to fixation. Such sick discs are also vulnerable to changes in nourishment, as occur with a fall in systemic blood pressure, etc. Probably the most common cause of "unexplained" poor vision in patients with glaucoma having cataract extraction is the further deterioration of the optic nerve, this deterioration occurring around the time of surgery, usually due to an elevation of IOP.

Some of the factors that appear to make the optic nerve more sensitive to rapid deterioration include the following: thinness of the rim and extent of cupping, low vascular perfusional pressure, S-hemoglobinopathy, large scleral ring, large laminar tunnels, history of "low-tension glaucoma."[5–8]

3. The healthy optic nerve without cupping can withstand pressure elevations lasting up to a week (or longer), and up to a level of 40 to 60 mmHg (or higher) without apparent difficulty.
4a. The degree of elevation of intraocular pressure (IOP) following uncomplicated cataract extraction is related to the preoperative functional ability of the outflow mechanisms of the eye. Preoperative IOP on medications is only a fair estimate of this outflow ability. By and large the older the patient, the longer the history of elevated and unstable intraocular pressure, the greater the extent of the exfoliation syndrome, and the greater the proportion of anterior chamber closure due to peripheral anterior synechiae, the more damage has been done to the outflow channels, and the greater will be the likelihood of pressure rise at the time of cataract extraction. Additionally, eyes with poorly functioning outflow channels will have their IOP decompensated by factors that do not ordinarily affect eyes with normal outflow mechanisms. Thus, small amounts of red blood cells in the aqueous, among other factors, can cause marked elevation of pressure in vulnerable eyes.
4b. Sodium hyaluronate in the anterior chamber tends to cause the IOP to be elevated, especially in patients with increased resistance to outflow.[9]
5a. Meticulously correct apposition of the corneoscleral incision predisposes to the best optical result following cataract extraction, whereas an incompletely closed corneoscleral incision predisposes to increased amounts of astigmatism and a poorer final optical result.
5b. Postoperative astigmatism tends to be less with scleral incisions than with corneal incisions.
6. The iris of the patient who has had marked elevation of IOP and in whom there is a dilated, fixed pupil is atrophic, flaccid, and atonic. The pupil of the patient who has been on miotics for many years is rigid and extremely difficult to dilate; it may be fibrotic. The iris of the patient with a long history of glaucoma is flaccid. Cut or traumatized surfaces of the iris of patients with long-standing glaucoma or glaucomatous iris atrophy or sphincter rigidity will become adherent to whatever they touch; this is true regardless of how and with what instrument the iris is touched.
7. The lens zonules of patients with long-standing glaucoma on therapy can be fragile; "loose lenses" are not uncommon in such patients.
8. Pigment release in patients with the exfoliation syndrome tends to be marked at the time of cataract extraction and may continue to occur in a postoperative period, especially if an intraocular lens traumatizes the posterior pigment epithelium; this pigment release may be confused with a chronic anterior uveitis, and characteristically causes elevation of intraocular pressure.[10]
9. In a patient with peripheral anterior synechiae due to secondary angle closure, the angle tends to continue to close if there is a continuing stimulus to the development of adhesions.[11]
10. In some individuals there is a real urgency to accomplish visual rehabilitation promptly. This is especially so in the elderly person who is failing physically and spiritually. In such situations, the interval between the decision to perform a cataract extraction and the time when visual improvement usually occurs should be as brief as feasible.
11. The elderly individual with glaucomatous field loss is not easily visually rehabilitated with aphakic spectacles.
12a. Contact lenses are often not well tolerated by patients with long-standing glaucoma.
12b. Contact lenses are less well tolerated in patients with filtering blebs than with those without.
13. Soft contact lenses are stained by epinephrine products or echothiophate iodide. Topical timolol not infrequently causes superficial punctate keratitis, deficient tearing, and corneal anesthesia.[12]

14. The corneal endothelium of patients who have had significant elevations of intraocular pressure is diseased; corneal decompensation following uncomplicated cataract extraction in patients with such a history, especially those with previous severe acute primary angle closure glaucoma, is common.[13]
15. Expulsive suprachoroidal hemorrhages are around 10 times as common in patients with glaucoma as in those without.[14] The prognosis after expulsive choroidal hemorrhage is strongly affected by ability to contain the bleeding within the eye promptly, and to retain all internal contents within the eye globe (except the vitreous). The outlook for preservation of vision is excellent when these objectives are accomplished; prognosis for maintenance of visual function is extremely poor when expulsive choroidal hemorrhage occurs in an open eye that cannot be immediately closed. The presence of preplaced, mattress-type, incisional sutures, size 7-0 or larger, allows almost immediate closure of an incision, even in the face of an expulsive choroidal hemorrhage.
16. No matter what technique is employed, filtering blebs generally work less well after cataract extraction; a significant number of patients, perhaps 50 percent, will have clinically important deterioration of IOP control as a result.
17. Cystoid macular edema is at least partially related to intraocular inflammation.

HISTORICAL REVIEW

How best to remove a cataract in a patient with glaucoma has intrigued ophthalmologists for generations.[15–20] The major choices were: cataract extraction first and management of glaucoma later, surgical if needed[3,4]; surgical control of glaucoma first, with cataract extraction later[2,21–23]; or combined "simultaneous" cataract extraction with glaucoma surgery.[24–35] When glaucoma was defined as IOP above an absolute level, say 24 mmHg, before years of treatment with medical therapy had become the usual condition of the glaucoma patient, and before surgical techniques were likely to result in truly watertight incisional closures, it was logical to choose the first option, performing a cataract extraction before a glaucoma procedure. Nevertheless, performing glaucoma surgery first was usually recommended by those whose practices were weighted with glaucoma patients who were seen to do poorly with cataract extraction alone, usually because of progressive optic nerve damage, joined with the high failure rate of most surgical procedures for glaucoma in aphakic patients. While there is a long history of suggestions for combined surgery (the third option), most surgeons eschewed the choice because of the higher complication rate, the lower success rate, and the poorer visual result.

The return to planned extracapsular cataract extraction, associated improvements in surgical technique made possible by the operating microscope, finer sutures and needles, and better instruments, new understanding of the course of IOP around the time of cataract extraction, and a new concept that glaucoma damage can progress despite IOP formerly considered "normal," along with the continued absence of a satisfactory surgical procedure for control of glaucoma in the aphakic patient, have united to lead to a new popularity for the "combined procedure." Additionally, the remarkable rarity of glaucoma problems caused by the posterior chamber intraocular lens implant, joined with the dramatic improvement in visual rehabilitation such a lens provides, especially for glaucoma patients, has resulted in posterior chamber lens implantation becoming the preferred procedure in most glaucoma patients. A continuing and still unsettled difficulty, however, rests with how best to perform such lens implantations in glaucoma patients, who have all the very real surgical problems enumerated in the first section of this chapter. For example, postoperatively does one dilate and get pupillary capture, or constrict and get poor vision due to iris stuck to the central portion of the intraocular lens?

While it is obvious that the technique of the removal of a cataract (still the most common correctable cause of visual loss around the world) in patients with glaucoma (still one of the commonest preventable causes of blindness around the world) will continue to evolve, one principle seems certain to this author: specifically, *there is no single "best" way to remove a cataract in a patient with glaucoma; to give patients the best care demands: familiarity and competency with those diagnostic techniques needed to characterize the patient correctly; familiarity and competency with a wide variety of surgical approaches to the management of patients with both glaucoma and cataract; and knowledge, judgement and skill to select and perform the particular procedure "best" for the particular patient under consideration.*[36]

PRACTICE

Using these principles as guidelines, one can devise a reasonable strategy for the management of patients with combined cataract and glaucoma. The principles are clearly quite different than those for cataract extraction alone or for glaucoma alone. In the detailed discussion of a surgical technique that follows, several of these principles will be seen as the basis for the suggested procedure. However, individualization of care is absolutely essential in the patient with glaucoma and cataract. Thus, no single technique is appropriate for even the majority much less all of such cases. It is the principles that must guide the practice. The reader eager to get on with the work of surgery, and thus, tending to skip over the "theoretical" introductory comments to a chapter, is urged to stop at this point, and go back and reread the section on principles.

The reason for removing a cataract in a patient with glaucoma is, with the uncommon exceptions mentioned below, the same as in a person without glaucoma, specifically, improvement in vision.

The patient must have sufficiently reduced visual function that quality of life is significantly impaired from the patient's point of view, and there must be a sufficiently great likelihood that removal of the cataract will improve the patient's quality of life to justify the inconvenience, risk, and expense of surgery.

There are two occasions where improvement in vision is not the primary indication for cataract extraction in the patient with glaucoma. Phacolytic glaucoma is, in the United States, a rare condition in which leakage of lens protein through a ruptured capsule results in a severe uveitis.[37,38] The proteinaceous material is ingested by macrophages. There is usually little difficulty in making the diagnosis. The combination of a high pressure in association with a milky anterior chamber and a hypermature lens is highly characteristic. Where there is a question about the correct diagnosis, it is helpful to examine the aqueous humor microscopically. The presence of protein-filled macrophages is diagnostic. Visual acuity in patients with phacolytic glaucoma is often very poor; it may be limited to light perception with inaccurate projection. Patients are even occasionally referred for enucleation of "blind, painful eyes." However, the prognosis for recovery of vision in patients with phacolytic glaucoma is excellent. As the condition is usually painful and therefore brings the patient to the physician promptly, the glaucoma is rarely of long duration, and it is unusual for the optic nerve to become damaged. A standard extracapsular extraction is probably the procedure of choice. This is best done with copious irrigation of the anterior chamber to enhance visibility. During the capsulotomy, the surgeon may be concerned about poor visibility; however, if irrigation is continued for a few minutes, soon the milky cortical material will all be removed, leaving an entirely satisfactory view, and permitting an excellent surgical result. As phacolytic glaucoma is not associated with the development of peripheral anterior synechias or permanent interference with the function of the trabecular meshwork, no glaucoma procedure needs to be done in conjunction with the cataract extraction. As soon as the fluid cortical material has been removed, the pressure will fall spontaneously.

The other condition where the lens itself is the reason for cataract extraction in a patient with glaucoma is angle closure glaucoma caused by a dislocated, swollen, or dislocated and swollen lens. In the overwhelming majority of patients whose glaucoma is caused by a dislocated lens, the problem is pupillary block, and the treatment for the glaucoma is iridectomy.[39] In occasional cases, however, in addition to the glaucoma, vision is reduced by the dislocated lens having become cataractous. In such cases cataract extraction, usually by the intracapsular route, is appropriate. Lens-induced angle closure glaucoma, in the author's experience, is usually caused by a partially dislocated lens. The diagnostic clue is a difference in anterior chamber depth. In addition, "primary" angle closure glaucoma can be triggered by the development of a swollen lens in a patient with a narrow angle; in such cases, the lens plays a significant role in the pathogenesis of the glaucoma. In these instances, especially when associated with marked elevation of IOP, treatment is best directed at the acute elevation of IOP itself, in hopes of deferring cataract extraction until the eye has quieted, the cornea cleared, the anterior chamber angle properly evaluated, and a more rational decision made regarding the possible need for cataract extraction or for combined cataract extraction-glaucoma surgery. Thus, iridectomy, either incisional or laser, is the initial surgery in the vast majority of cases, the cataract operation being performed at a later date if necessary and as appropriate.

Cataract extraction can in some patients with glaucoma be deferred by modification of therapy. Specifically, patients having axial cataracts often have satisfactory visual function if their pupils are not miotic. This can be accomplished, obviously, by avoiding the use of miotics in such cases. Where miotics are needed to control pressure, it may be possible to eliminate the need for the miotic by performing an argon laser trabeculoplasty. In other cases pressure can be controlled satisfactorily by using the three other classes of glaucoma agents, specifically epinephrine, beta-blockers, and carbonic anhydrase inhibitors. The combination of topical epinephrine with a topical beta-blocker is especially effective from one point of view in such patients, as it may produce significant pupillary dilatation.

If, despite appropriate medical treatment, the patient with glaucoma has a sufficient reduction of vision due to cataract that she or he needs to see

Table 28-1. Preferred Procedure in Patient with Conjoint Cataract and Glaucoma in Whom a Cataract Extraction is Indicated

Stage of disease	State of Control	Diagnostic Entity	Prefered Procedure
Far-advanced	Any	Low-tension glaucoma	Filtering procedure 1st, with ECCE[a] later, preferably with PC IOL[b]
Far-advanced	Poor	POAGL[c]	Filtering procedure 1st, with ECCE later, preferably with PC IOL
Far-advanced	Good	POAGL	Combined ECCE with trabeculectomy with limbus-based flap and PC IOL
Moderate or advanced	Any	Any noninflammatory glaucoma	ECCE, with trabeculectomy fornix-based flap, & preferably with PC IOL
Early	Poor	Any noninflammatory glaucoma	ECCE, with trabeculectomy, fornix-based flap, & preferably PC IOL
Early	Good	Any noninflammatory glaucoma	ECCE, with PC IOL
Early	Good	1 ° or 2° glaucoma with dislocated lens	ICCE[d] or pars plana lensectomy
Advanced	Any	1° or 2° glaucoma with dislocated lens	ICCE with trabeculectomy or cyclodialysis
Early	Good	Inflammatory glaucoma	ICCE or ECCE with no implant
Advanced	Any	Inflammatory glaucoma	ICCE with trabeculectomy & no implant; often cyclocyrotherapy or similar treatment in postoperative period

[a] ECCE: Extracapsular cataract extraction.
[b] PC IOL: Posterior chamber intraocular lens.
[c] POAGL: Primary open-angle glaucoma.
[d] ICCE: Intracapsular cataract extraction.

better and understands the potential risks of surgery, then a cataract extraction is usually indicated. Obviously the surgeon's and the patient's goal is to achieve the best possible visual rehabilitation in the safest and most convenient manner. This is accomplished by accurate diagnosis, full discussion with the patient so that the patient's needs and expectations can be most fully satisfied, and knowledgeable attention to the principles given earlier in this chapter. Table 23-1 provides a framework for helping decide upon which procedure is preferable in the patient under consideration.

Probably the single most critical criterion determining the type of procedure to be done is the stage of the glaucoma. Where the optic nerve is badly damaged, especially in the individual where that damage has occurred with low intraocular pressure, the damaging effects of the rise of intraocular pressure that characteristically follows cataract extraction must be avoided if the health of the eye is to be preserved. On the other hand, in the patient who has an optic nerve with only mild glaucomatous cupping, the likelihood that a transient pressure rise will damage the eye is so small that the surgeon does not have to guard against it to the same degree as in the patient with advanced glaucomatous damage. All surgical efforts, whether cyclodialysis, trabeculectomy, full thickness filtering procedure, or ciliary body destructive procedure, increase complications (astigmatism, cystoid macular edema, hemorrhage, etc.); consequently, they should only be employed if their potential benefit justifies the increased risk. They should not be done with the misguided idea that "adding a glaucoma procedure" will necessarily make the cataract extraction safer in a patient with glaucoma.

SURGICAL TECHNIQUE: COMBINED CATARACT EXTRACTION AND TRABECULECTOMY

Because the procedure of a combined cataract extraction and trabeculectomy tends to be a long one, the surgeon must be especially careful of the problem of light toxicity. The author performs all those portions of the operation not related to the cataract extraction itself using illumination supplied by two overhead operating lamps. The light of the microscope is not turned on until that portion of the surgery requiring axial illumination.

Similarly, anesthesia must be of adequate duration. General anesthesia is occasionally employed. However, local anesthesia with long-acting agents such as bupivacaine 0.75 percent offers advantages to the surgeon who does not know whether he or she will be able to complete the surgery within a period of an hour. If the surgeon is not fully familiar with the technique of surgery, or if he or she tends to operate slowly, probably bupivacaine should be employed. The author prefers the shorter acting agent mepivacaine 2 percent for reasons detailed later. A modified O'Brien block, using 10 cc of mepivacaine, is employed to obtain complete akinesia of the muscles controlled by the facial nerve.[40] Two cc of mepivacaine 2 percent without hyaluronidase are injected in the retrobulbar space, entering at the inferotemporal edge of the orbit; 2 cc are also injected in the area of the supraorbital notch, to permit adequate anesthesia of the superior conjunctiva. Pressure is applied with the palm of the hand over the closed lids, to produce an adequately softened globe. This is done by applying pressure for 20 seconds, and then releasing for 10 seconds, for as long as is required to soften the globe adequately. The technique of pressure employed must be sure not to cause ischemia of the optic nerve.

Betamethasone, 3 mg (0.5 ml) and gentamycin, 40 mg (0.5 ml) are injected deep into the inferior sub-Tenon's space.

Limbus-Based Flap

The initial portion of the surgery is performed with illumination provided by oblique light to the microscope or overhead lamps.

A 4-0 black silk bridle suture is placed under the superior rectus muscle. A similar suture is placed in the inferior rectus; the needle should be of the tapered type used in vascular surgery; it should not be a cutting or spatula needle.

A conjunctival–Tenon's flap is developed in the standard fashion (Fig. 28-1). The initial incision is

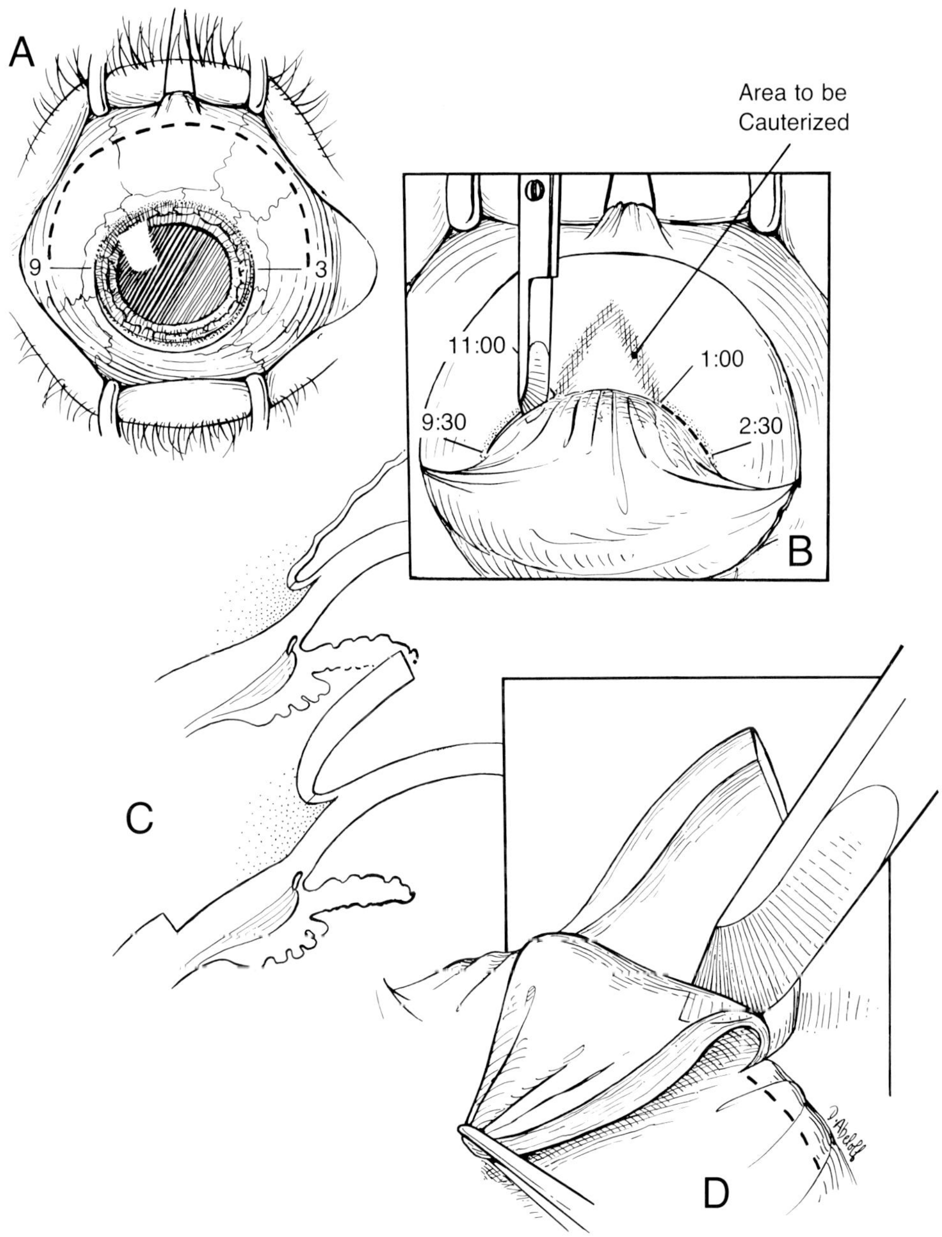

Fig. 28-1. (A) A limbus-based conjunctival flap is prepared. The conjunctiva is incised as high in the cul-de-sac as possible, and the incision is extended 180 degrees. **(B)** The conjunctival-Tenon's flap is extended all the way to the corneoscleral sulcus. It is essential that the sulcus be cleaned meticulously so that there will be an adequate lip remaining on the corneal side of the incision to permit satisfactory placement of buried sutures. **(C)** The cornea is partially split as shown in the upper drawing. A trabeculectomy flap is developed. **(D)** The shape of the corneoscleral flap is unimportant; a triangular flap may be more easily prepared and closed than a traditional rectangular flap. After the scleral flap has been fashioned, a paracentesis is always placed in every case, using a sharp, short 25-gauge needle.

made just anterior to the bridle suture, as high in the cul-de-sac as possible (Fig. 28-1A). This is extended almost 90 degrees in both directions, so that the final incision extends from just superior to the medial rectus (at 3 o'clock in the left eye) to just superior to the lateral rectus (at 9 o'clock in the left eye). This incision reaches all the way to the sclera and should include the full thickness of Tenon's capsule as well as conjunctiva. As the incision is extended toward the edges of the rectus muscles, the surgeon must be careful not to cut into one of the rectus muscles inadvertently. The limbus-based flap is bluntly extended as far towards the corneoscleral as possible, reflecting the tissue over the cornea. A #67 Beaver blade is then employed to continue the dissection until the corneoscleral sulcus is reached. As Tenon's capsule is most adherent at the 10 and 2 o'clock positions, the surgeon must be most careful in these areas. Every reasonable effort should be made to avoid buttonholing the conjunctiva as this flap is developed. The tissue may be extremely thin, especially toward the edges of the flap, and extreme care must be employed. A nontoothed forceps, such as a Wills Eye Hospital utility forceps, should always be used to hold the conjunctiva. Dissection of the flap toward the corneoscleral sulcus can not be reliably performed with the scissors. The use of knife is essential.

Once the corneoscleral sulcus has been reached, the cornea is split from the 9:30 to 11 o'clock positions, and from the 1 to 2:30 o'clock positions (Fig. 28-1B). Splitting of the cornea is best done so that the external layer is extremely thin (Fig. 28-1C, top), preferably only slightly thicker than the conjunctival flap, which is reflected back over the cornea in these areas.

After the conjunctiva has been dissected to the corneoscleral sulcus, and the superficial cornea split as described, the cornea and sclera are cauterized where the radial incisions for the trabeculectomy scleral flap are to be placed. *All* bleeders are coagulated. Bipolar cautery is useful for this. The power must be sufficiently high to coagulate, but the tissue should not be charred or caused to shrink. Every bleeding vessel is coagulated; the sclera in the area where fixation is to occur, where the sutures are to be placed, and where the scleral incision is to be made is also cauterized so that there will be no bleeding, and no need to cauterize the tissue after an incision has been made (Fig. 28-1B). Cautery is definitely preferable prior to the incision, because when used later near the edge of an incision, it will cause tissue shrinkage, making closure difficult. The incisions for the scleral flap are made in the shape of a triangle, roughly equilateral, the base being the area at the 12 o'clock position where the cornea was not split, and the two arms of the apex proceeding posteriorly from the 11 o'clock and 1 o'clock edges.

The incisions are made deeply into the sclera, to a depth of approximately three-quarters of the thickness of the sclera. The posterior tip of the triangular flap is held with a Pierse–Hoskins forceps or other similar serrated, nontoothed forceps, and the triangular flap developed. In order to assist visualization, the microscope power is usually increased at this point. The surgeon should be careful to keep the flap thick, approximately one-half to three-quarters the thickness of the sclera. Dissection is carried well past the junction between light sclera and clear cornea, so that the scleral flap extends well past Schlemm's canal, allowing further excision of a block containing only clear cornea. As the scleral flap is developed, it should become contiguous with the more lateral areas of previously split cornea (Fig. 28-1C, bottom, 28-1D).

A paracentesis track is placed using a short, sharp, 25-gauge disposable needle. This should always be put in exactly the same place, so it can be easily found at a later date, if necessary. It should also be placed sufficiently anterior to the limbus so that it will not be involved in the suture line or the sutures, and will not be hidden by a large overhanging bleb at a later date. I place the paracentesis in a perfectly horizontal direction, starting 3 mm anterior to the limbus, in the far temporal portion of the cornea. If the plane of the needle is always held exactly parallel to the plane of the iris, the complication rate from such paracentesis is very close to zero. Penetration through the cornea is achieved by pushing the entire syringe and needle downwards toward the operating table, at the same time making sure that the needle is held parallel to the iris. The bevel of the needle should be up toward the microscope.

A 25-gauge sharp disposable needle is bent in preparation for performing the anterior capsulotomy.

The anterior chamber is entered with a sharp blade, such as a #75 Beaver, or an Alcon "Sharp." The incision into the anterior chamber is made in the region of Schlemm's canal, at the junction between clear cornea and opaque sclera. This is done in the bed of the trabeculectomy, as far anteriorly as possible and usually at the temporal edge of the bed. This incision is made parallel to the edge of the trabeculectomy flap, leaving about a 0.25-mm ledge at the base. The incision is made just large enough to allow entrance of the capsulotomy instrument.

At this point in the procedure, the overhead lights are turned off and the axial illumination of the microscope turned on.

A "standard can-opener" capsulotomy is done (Fig. 28-2A,B), making sure that the incisions into the anterior capsule are placed very close together and performed gently so as not to dislocate the lens. I do this by rotating the handle so that cuts into the capsule are made by the rotating edge of the bent needle. If a second bend is placed in the needle at its base, as recommended by some, this maneuver

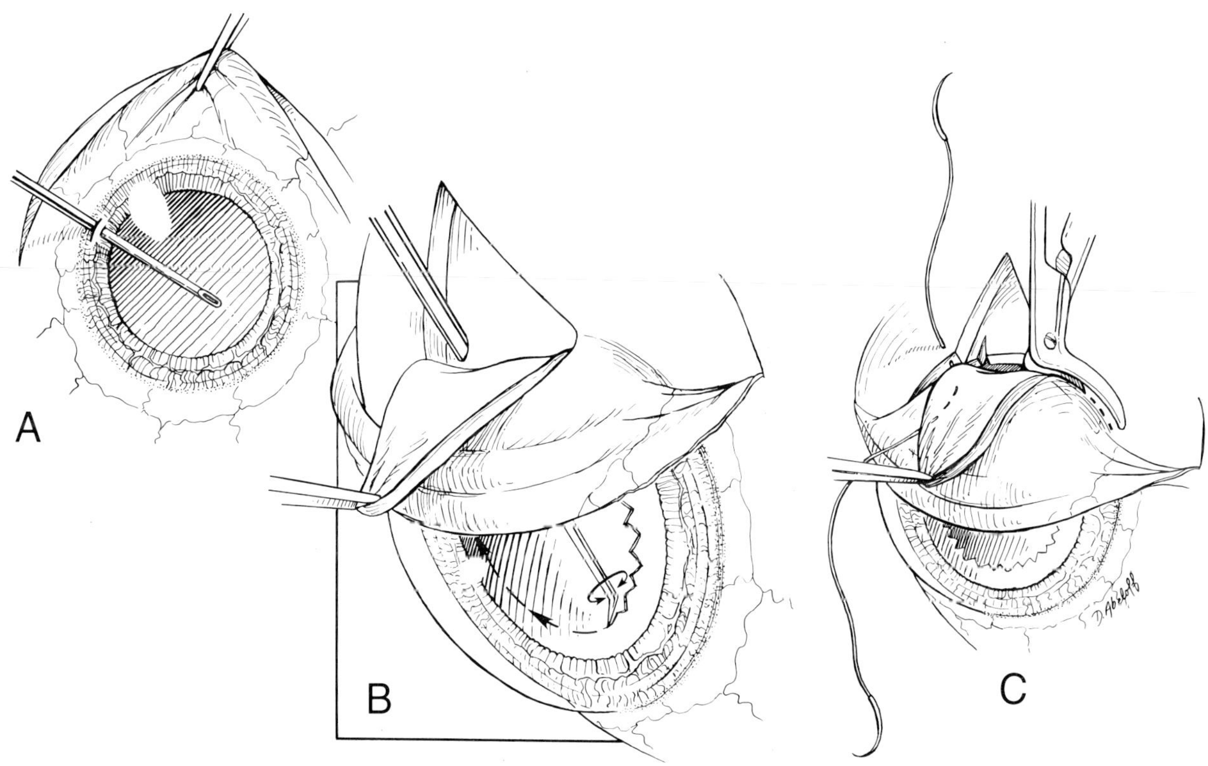

Fig. 28-2. (A) Anterior capsulotomy. An anterior capsulotomy is performed tenderly. The zonules are frequently weak in patients with glaucoma. Some authors perform a capsulotomy through a separate stab incision in the cornea. **(B)** I prefer performing the capsulotomy through the radial incision that will be used later to excise the corneoscleral block. The capsulotomy is best performed by rotating an extremely sharp instrument such as a bent 25-gauge sharp needle. Traction should not be placed on the zonules. **(C)** After the corneoscleral incision is made in one direction, a suture is placed to allow rapid closure of the eye should an expulsive hemorrhage occur. The corneoscleral incision is completed by cutting in the other direction, leaving sufficient space between the conjunctival reflection to permit placement of sutures.

of rotating the handle in order to cut with the edge of the needle is made almost impossible. If the pupil can not be dilated (because of a rigid sphincter secondary to long use of miotics, or to posterior synechias caused by previous surgery, or for any other reason), the incision into the anterior chamber is enlarged to permit performance of a sector iridectomy at this point. If the sphincter is fibrotic and the pupil likely to be updrawn, one sphincterotomy at the 6 o'clock position is performed with a Vannas scissors. If it is necessary to perform a sphincterotomy or sector iridectomy, it will probably be difficult to keep the anterior chamber formed with irrigating solution, and the capsulotomy is usually best performed with the anterior chamber filled with a viscous substance such as sodium hyaluronate.

After the anterior capsulotomy is completed, the nucleus is loosened by pulling it with the capsulotomy instrument, rocking it, and rotating it until it is clearly separated from the posterior capsule. A corneoscleral incision is made with corneoscleral scissors, cutting from the point of entry into the anterior chamber, cutting in the temporal direction. The incisions should be shelved, and should be sufficiently posterior to the corneoscleral sulcus to permit the development of a 1- to 2-mm ledge on the corneal side of the incision. The incision, therefore, is usually made close to Schlemm's canal. The corneoscleral incision is made for a distance of about 70 degrees, or around 4 mm. A husky suture, such as 7-0 polyglactin, is placed across the corneoscleral incision, just temporal to the trabeculectomy bed; this is left double-armed so that when the second bite is placed later in a mattress fashion, it becomes possible to close the corneoscleral incision promptly and completely in case of an expulsive hemorrhage (Fig. 28-2C).

The other corneoscleral scissors is then used to complete the corneoscleral incision in the nasal direction. The incision should be well posterior to the corneoscleral sulcus, again creating a ledge. This incision is made so that the total length of the incision, so that the chord is around 12 mm, or about 160 degrees. The other half of the 7-0 polyglactin suture is placed in the corneoscleral sulcus just nasal to the trabeculectomy bed, in a horizontal mattress suture fashion.

The corneoscleral mattress sutures are loosened (Fig. 28-3A). The nucleus is removed as atraumatically as possible. It is important that the incision be sufficiently large; excessive pressure must not be used to "express" the lens nucleus. Methods that rely on transmission of external pressure to the vitreous are probably best *not* used, as these will often result in expression of vitreous at the 12 o'clock position.

My preferred technique is to have the assistant lift the cornea at the 12 o'clock position, while holding a lens hook with the other hand close to the incision. The surgeon then depresses the iris at the 12 o'clock position with a lens loop, indenting the sclera very slightly, if necessary, in order to get the loop under the edge of the nucleus at the 12 o'clock position. The surgeon's other hand applies very gentle pressure, with the smooth portion of a curved Pierse–Hoskins forceps (or a similar instrument) on the sclera at 6 o'clock, lifting the nucleus onto the loop. Once the nucleus is sufficiently in view, it is caught with the lens hook, being careful to keep the lens hook parallel to the surface of the iris so as to avoid the posterior capsule. The nucleus is then pulled out by the hook. The hook may not be able to complete this, but once the removal has been started, the Pierse–Hoskins forceps can be used to complete the removal.

The suture on each side of the trabeculectomy bleb is then tied. Additional sutures are placed in order to assure a tight incision at the time of irrigation–aspiration (Fig. 28-3B). This usually requires a suture at the 12 o'clock position at the end of the scleral flap of the trabeculectomy, and two or three additional sutures, one at about the 10 o'clock position and the other about the 2 o'clock position. The 12 o'clock suture may be 7-0 polyglactin (or whatever other husky suture was used prior to delivery of the nucleus). The nasal and temporally placed sutures need not be removed later, and thus, 10-0 nylon is appropriate. If 10-0 nylon is employed, it may have to be replaced later if it becomes loosened during the aspiration manipulation. The suture temporally is placed far enough from the temporal end of the corneoscleral incision to allow the irrigation–aspiration tip to enter as far temporally as possible (Fig. 28-3C).

After removal of the lens nucleus, the cortex is removed by a standard irrigation–aspiration technique. The posterior capsule should be well, but

start appropriate postoperative medication at that time. It is because of this desire to be able to remove the patch promptly following surgery in patients in whom this seems appropriate that the author routinely uses a relatively short-lasting anesthetic agent in patients in whom the procedure is performed under local anesthesia (which is the overwhelming majority of patients). Specially, mepivacaine hydrochloride (Carbocaine) 2 percent is used to perform the facial nerve block.

A topical antibiotic and an anti-inflammatory corticosteroid are employed. Type, dosage, and frequency will vary with the surgeon's experience. In most cases the minimum dose would be prednisolone acetate 1 percent four times daily. This is increased to a higher dosage if inflammation is marked. In most cases neither a cycloplegic nor a mydriatic is routinely employed during the first postoperative week. The goal should be to keep the pupil small enough to make sure that the iris stays anterior to the intraocular lens, but does not adhere to the intraocular lens or the pupil in a miotic position. If the latter appears to be occurring, then pupillary dilatation is mandatory.

The postoperative management of the trabeculectomy is essentially the same as if a cataract extraction had not been performed. Specifically, techniques are employed to assure continued filtration with the development of a subconjunctival filtering bleb, without the complication of collapse of the anterior chamber. If the bleb is flat and the pressure is high, clearly filtration needs to be encouraged. On the other hand, if the bleb is high and the pressure below 5 mmHg and the chamber flat, one can justifiably assume that the problem is excessive filtration.

REFERENCES

1. Rich WJ, Radtke ND, Cohan BE: Early ocular hypertension after cataract extraction. Br J Ophthalmol 58:725, 1974
2. Spaeth GL: The management of patients with cataract and glaucoma. Ophthal Surg 11:780, 1980
3. Linn JG: Cataract extraction in management of glaucoma. Trans Am Acad Ophthalmol Otolaryngol 75:273, 1971
4. Bigger JF, Becker B: Cataracts and primary open-angle glaucoma: the effect of uncomplicated cataract extraction on glaucoma control. Trans Am Acad Ophthalmol Otolaryngol 75:260, 1971
5. Spaeth GL: Low tension glaucoma: its diagnosis and management, p. 263. In Greve EL (ed): Documenta Ophthalmologica Proceedings, Series 22, Glaucoma Symposium, Diagnosis and Therapy, Amsterdam, 1979. Dr W Junk Publishers, The Hague, 1980
6. Levene RZ: Low tension glaucoma: a critical review and new material. Survey Ophthalmol 24:621, 1980
7. Moller HV: Excessive myopia and glaucoma. Arch Ophthalmol 26:185, 1948
8. Wax MB, Ridley ME, Magargal LE: Reversal of retinal and optic disc ischemia in a patient with sickle cell trait and glaucoma secondary to traumatic hyphema. Ophthalmol 89:845, 1982
9. Cherfan GM, Rich WJ, Wright G: Raised intraocular pressure and other problems with sodium hyaluronate and cataract surgery. Trans Ophthal Soc UK 103:277, 1983
10. Spaeth GL, Kline OR: Secondary glaucoma caused by posterior chamber lens implantation in patients with the exfoliation syndrome: a new syndrome. Ophthal Surg (in press)
11. Rowsey JJ, Gaylor JR: Intraocular lens disasters: peripheral anterior synechiae. Ophthalmology 87:646, 1980
12. Van Buskirk EM: Adverse reactions from timolol administration. Ophthalmology 87:447, 1980
13. Bigar F, Witmer R: Corneal endothelial changes in primary acute angle-closure glaucoma. Ophthalmology 89:596, 1982
14. Cantor L, Katz LJ, Spaeth GL: Complications in glaucoma surgery I: suprachoroidal expulsive hemorrhage in glaucoma patients undergoing intraocular surgery. Ophthalmology (in press)
15. Kolker AE: Cataract surgery in glaucoma, p. 148. In Becker B, Drews RC (eds): Current Concepts in Ophthalmology. CV Mosby, St. Louis, 1967
16. Laatikainen L: Late results of surgery on eyes with primary glaucoma and cataract. Acta Ophthalmol 49:281, 1971
17. Harrington DO: Cataract and glaucoma. Management of the coexistent conditions and a description of a new operation combining lens extraction with reverse cyclodialysis. Am J Ophthalmol 61:1134, 1966
18. Bessiere E, Verin P, LeRebeller MJ: Combined cataract and glaucoma surgery: techniques and results. Arch Ophthalmol 29:7, 1969

19. Shields MB, Simmons RJ: Combined cataract extraction and glaucoma surgery. Ophthalmol 89:231, 1982
20. Kass, MA: Cataract extraction in an eye with a filtering bleb. Ophthalmol 89:871, 1982
21. Frankelson EN, Shaffer RN: The management of coexisting cataract and glaucoma. Can J Ophthalmol 9:298, 1974
22. Kondo T: Cataract extraction after filtering operation. Glaucoma 1979; 1:165
23. Weekers R: Indikation und Kontraindikation der kombinierten Operation (fistulierende Operation und Kataraktextraktion) beim Weitwinkelglaukom und beim Engwinkelglaudom. Klin Mbl Augenheilk 179:831, 1977
24. Francois J: A combined operation for glaucoma and cataract. Ophthal Surg 1:9, 1970
25. Eustace P, Harun AQSM: Trabeculectomy combined with cataract extraction. Trans Ophthal Soc UK 94:1058, 1974
26. Edwards RS: Trabeculectomy combined with cataract extraction: a follow-up study. Br J Ophthalmol 64:720, 1980
27. Johns GE, Layden WE: Combined trabeculectomy and cataract extraction. Am J Ophthalmol 88:973, 1979
28. Mackensen G, Orsoni GJ: Mit trabekulotomie kombinierte Kataraktextraktion. Klin Mbl Augenheilk 173:756, 1978
29. Galin MA, Baras I, Sambursky J: Glaucoma and cataract. A study of cyclodialysis lens extraction. Am J Ophthal 67:522, 1969
30. Shields MB, Simmons RJ: Combined cyclodialysis and cataract extraction. Trans Am Acad Ophth Otol 81:286, 1976
31. Spaeth GL, Sivalingam E: The partial-punch: A new combined cataract-glaucoma operation. Ophthal Surg 7:53, 1976
32. Stewart RH, Loftis MD: Combined cataract extraction and thermal sclerostomy versus combined cataract extraction and trabeculectomy. Ophthal Surg 7:93, 1976
33. Sautter H, Demeler U, Naumann G: Simultaneous trabeculotomy and intracapsular cataract extraction. Klin Mbl Augenheilk 164:65, 1974
34. McPherson Jr, SD: Combined trabeculotomy and cataract extraction as a single operation. Trans Am Ophthal Soc 74:251, 1976
35. Papst W: Zur kombinierten Trepanation mit Skleradeckel (Elliot-Fronimopoulos) und intrakapsulären Kataraktextraktion. Klin Mbl Augenheilk 171:343, 1977
36. Spaeth GL: Glaucoma surgery, p. 215. In Spaeth GL (ed): Ophthalmic Surgery—Principles and Practice. WB Saunders, Philadelphia, 1982
37. Goldberg MF: Cytological diagnosis of phacolytic glaucoma utilizing Millipore filtration of the aqueous. Br J Ophthalmol 51:847, 1967
38. Epstein DL, Jedziniak JA, Grant WM: Identification of heavy-molecular-weight soluble protein in aqueous humor in human phacolytic glaucoma. Invest Ophthalmol Vis Sci 17:398, 1978
39. Chandler PA: Choice of treatment in dislocation of the lens. Arch Ophthalmol 71:765, 1964
40. Wilson RP: Anesthesia. p. 81. In Spaeth GL (ed): Ophthalmic Surgery—Principles and Practice. WB Saunders, Philadelphia, 1982
41. Weinstein GW: Implantation of the C-Loop Simcoe posterior chamber lens. Ophthal Surg 15:25, 1984

Setons in Glaucoma Surgery

29

Theodore Krupin

Various foreign materials have been used as an aid to promote drainage in glaucoma surgery. Alloplastic devices that have been used to maintain patency of the sclerostomy include horse hair, stainless steel wires, nylon and silk threads, gold foil, platinum and tantalum wire, and acrylic plates. In addition, these materials have been placed between the anterior chamber and a cyclodialysis cleft. In spite of good drainage with the formation of a large filtration bleb during the early postoperative period, later foreign-body reaction has led to bleb scarring and failure of the procedure in spite of an often patent fistula.

Three plastic implants have given encouraging results and are being used in patients with previous failed filtration surgery. In addition, these implants have been used as a primary procedure in eyes with neovascular glaucoma, a condition with a relatively low success rate following standard filtration surgery. These implants are those described by Krupin et al., Molteno et al., and Schocket et al. The wide variations in surgical results with these devices may be secondary to differences in patient selection, length of postoperative follow-up, and the criteria used for success (Table 29-1).[1] Use of these devices requires specialized technical skills. The complication rate in these patients with complicated disease is higher than that associated with routine filtration surgery. However, these devices offer a means to obtain an increased incidence of surgical glaucoma control in patients unresponsive to our more conservative surgical techniques.

GLAUCOMA VALVE IMPLANT

Description of Device

This implant[2,3] (Fig. 29-1) consists of an open Supramid tube with an outer diameter (OD) of 0.58 mm and an inner diameter (ID) of 0.38 mm, placed in the anterior chamber. This tube is cemented to a Silastic tube. The end of this tube is sealed; it contains horizontal and vertical slits that function as a unidirectional and pressure-sensitive valve. The opening pressure of the valve is approximately 11 mmHg, with a closing pressure that is 1 to 2 mmHg lower. The Silastic valve portion remains outside the eye. Supramid side arms are attached in order to provide stability of the device as well as a means of fixating the implant.

The original valve implant has a short Silastic portion designed to be placed under a limbus-ori-

Table 29-1. Results of Drainage Implants for Neovascular Glaucoma

Type of Implant	Investigators	No. of Eyes	Success Rate (≤24 mmHg)
Valve implant	Krupin et al.[2]	79	67%
Standard			(51% without med) (49% with med)
Long with encircling band	Krupin et al.[3]	22	85% (68% without med) (32% with med)
Molteno implant	Molteno et al.[5]	21	94%
	Cairns	16	75%
ACTSEB	Schocket et al.[7]	19	95% (83% without med) (17% with med)

ACTSEB = anterior chamber tube shunt to an encircling band; med = medication.

ented scleral flap. A recent modification (Fig. 29-1B) has a 20-mm Silastic tube with the valve portion at the end of the tube. This is designed to extend posterior to the limbus and open into a 180-degree inverted No. 220 Silastic band.

Surgical Implantation

The original valve implant (Fig. 29-1) is placed within the bed of a 5 × 5 mm lamellar scleral flap. This portion of the procedure, as well as the conjunctival flap, is performed as described for a trabeculectomy procedure. I routinely use a fornix-based conjunctival flap.[4] The lamellar scleral flap is dissected into clear cornea. A paracentesis is performed away from the surgical site. Fluorescein is placed on the paracentesis knifeblade to mark the tract for later reformation of the anterior chamber. Entry is then made into the anterior chamber at the site of the scleral flap. This entry is critical. It must be parallel to the iris plane to avoid directing the Supramid tube into the iris or cornea. Too large an opening can permit leakage of aqueous around the

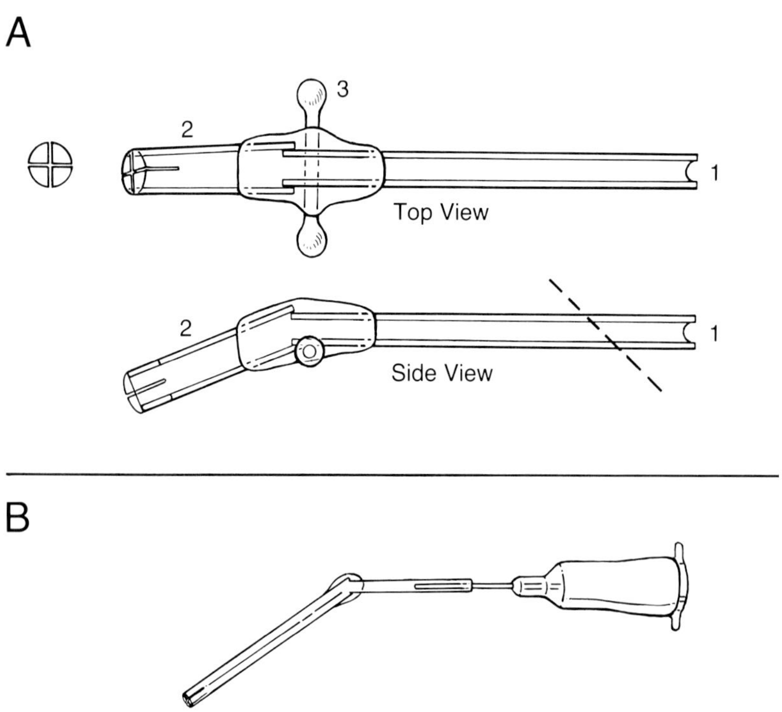

Fig. 29-1. (A) The standard glaucoma valve implant consists of (1) an open Supramid tube which is cut to length at surgery, (2) a Silastic tube with sealed end containing horizontal and vertical slit valves, and (3) Supramid side arms for fixation of the device. Top and side views are shown. **(B)** A modification of the standard glaucoma valve implant, consisting of an open Supramid tube on a 27-gauge needle, and a longer Silastic tube with horizontal and vertical slit valves at the end. (Drawings by Diane Abeloff, after Craig Luce.)

tube and can result in a flat anterior chamber. This bypasses the advantage of implant in which the resistance to aqueous flow is controlled by the valve portion, and not the scleral flap. This opening should be approximately 1.5 mm wide and is best made using a sharp disposable knife or a goniotomy needle knife. The Supramid tube is cut to a proper length so the open end rests within the chamber without iris or cornea contact. The tube is cut with a bevel facing the corneal surface (Fig. 29-1, side view). The tube length is dependent on the location and intracorneal extent of the entry incision. The device is sutured at the wound with a 10-0 nonadsorbable material using the side arms as anchor points (Fig. 29-2). This prevents anterior–posterior (AP) movement of the implant. The anterior chamber is reformed through the paracentesis site with balanced salt solution. This confirms proper position of the tube in the anterior chamber as well as flow of fluid through the valve end. If fluid flows around the tube at the entry site, a mattress 10-0 nonadsorbable suture is placed to close the wound completely. The scleral flap is closed with a 10-0 suture at either corner of the scleral flap. This closure advances the flap edge inward to avoid tension of the scleral flap on the implant. The conjunctiva is closed and balanced salt solution is again injected into the anterior chamber to create a bleb and ensure the adequacy of a fluid tight conjunctival closure.[4]

The long glaucoma valve implant requires preparation of the conjunctiva and scleral flap similar to that for the standard glaucoma valve implant. However, the valve end of this implant is first sutured within the groove of a No. 220 Silastic band (Fig. 29-3). A 1- to 2-mm-wide notch is excised in one

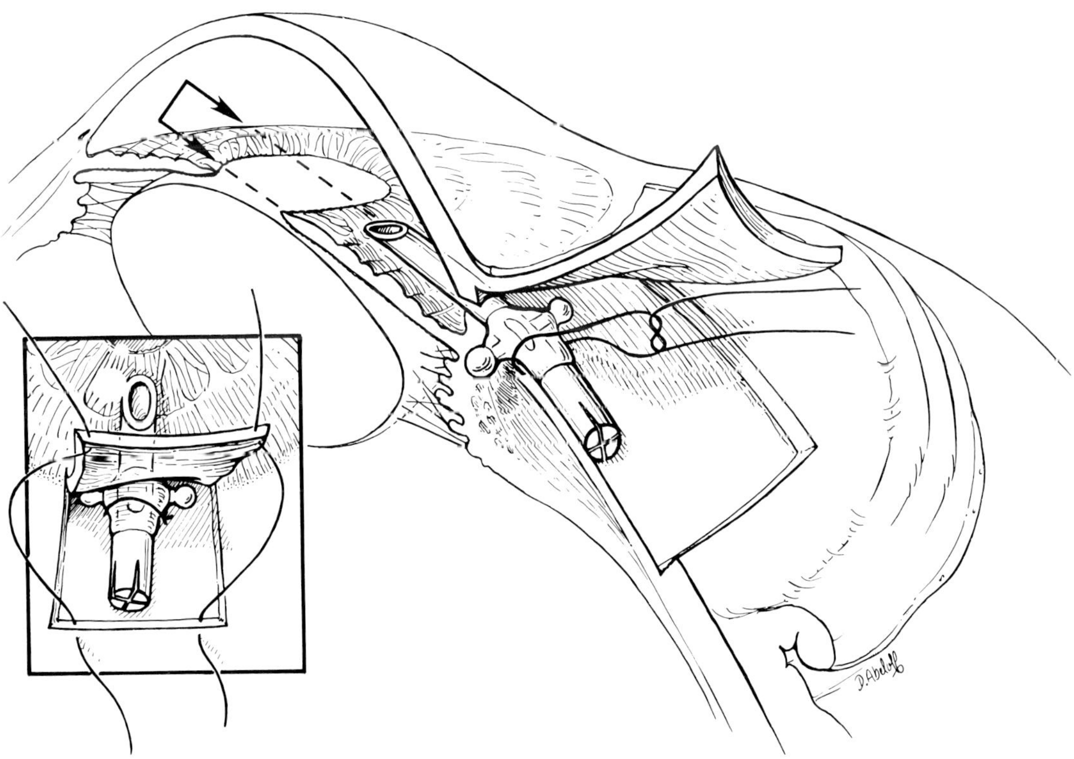

Fig. 29-2. A glaucoma valve implant in place with the two sides of the fixation suture behind the side arms. The fixation suture is tied posterior to the side arms and over the top of the implant. **Inset:** The interrupted sutures for closure of the scleral flap are recessed approximately 0.5 mm inward from the corners of the scleral bed flap closure. (Drawing by Diane Abeloff, after Craig Luce.)

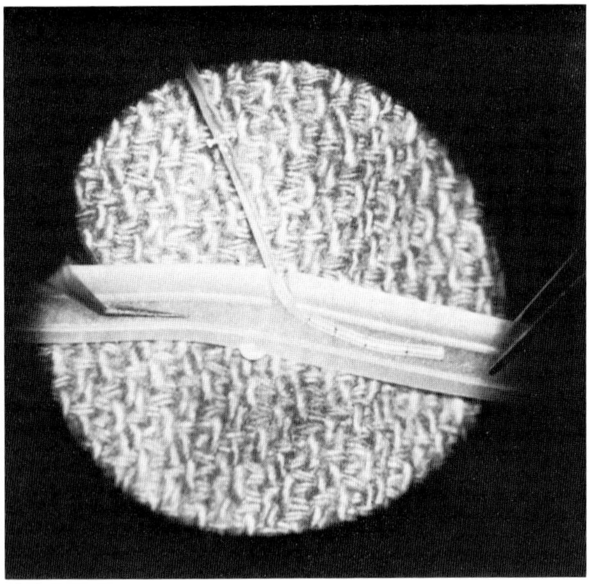

Fig. 29-3. Long glaucoma valve implant sutured within the groove of a No. 220 Silastic band (modification of the standard glaucoma valve implant). (Krupin T, Kaufman P, Mandell A et al: Filtering valve implant surgery for eyes with neovascular glaucoma. Am J Ophthalmol 89:340, 1980, Published with permission from the American Journal of Ophthalmology. Copyright by the Ophthalmic Publishing Company.)

side wall of the band (Fig. 29-4A), and the valve end sutured within the groove with two 10-0 nylon sutures and tied on the groove side. The band is placed beneath the superior or inferior rectus muscles and is cut to a length to extend to or just beneath both horizontal rectus muscles (Fig. 29-4B). Mattress sutures fixate the band to the sclera with the valve implant exiting on the appropriate side of the vertical muscle to be directed toward the scleral flap. The side arms should reach the entry site. Entry into the anterior chamber, preparation of the Supramid tube, and closure of the scleral flap, are similar to the technique described for the standard valve implant (Fig. 29-2). A mattress 10-0 nonadsorbable suture is placed episclerally around the tube between the scleral flap and the band to prevent tube movement. The conjunctival incision is closed and the anterior chamber reformed with balanced salt solution.

Subconjunctival steroid and antibiotic injections are performed at the conclusion of the surgery. Topical atropine and corticosteroids are administered postoperatively. Ocular massage is initiated when intraocular pressure (IOP) reaches a level of 15 mmHg.

Prognosis Results

The standard glaucoma valve implant is successful in controlling IOP (≤24 mmHg) in 65 to 70 percent of eyes with neovascular glaucoma (360 degrees of angle closure) and in eyes with previously failed filtration surgery. Approximately one half of successful cases are controlled without glaucoma medication.

Preliminary short-term follow-up results with the long implant placed under an inverted Silastic retinal band have resulted in higher success rates. Approximately 80 percent of eyes with neovascular glaucoma and 85 to 90 percent of eyes with previous filtration failures are controlled with this implant. Only a small proportion of these eyes require additional medical therapy.

Complications

External Bleb Scarring

The valve implant places the effective sclerostomy opening (the open end of the Supramid tube) into the anterior chamber, away from the iridocorneal angle, thereby reduces internal sclerostomy closure. However, the standard implant does not eliminate external scarring of the conjunctival bleb.

External bleb scarring with increased IOP requires bleb revision. The conjunctiva is incised 6 to 8 mm posterior to the limbus in the area of the original scleral flap. A paracentesis incision is made in a clear cornea. Subconjunctival scar tissue is excised and the scleral flap identified and redissected until the end of the Silastic valve is located. Excision of scar tissue from this end is accompanied by free flow of aqueous humor. The scleral flap is not resutured. The conjunctiva is closed and the anterior chamber re-formed through the paracentesis site. Postoperative management is similar to that used after the original surgery. Revision is successful in approximately 60 percent of cases.

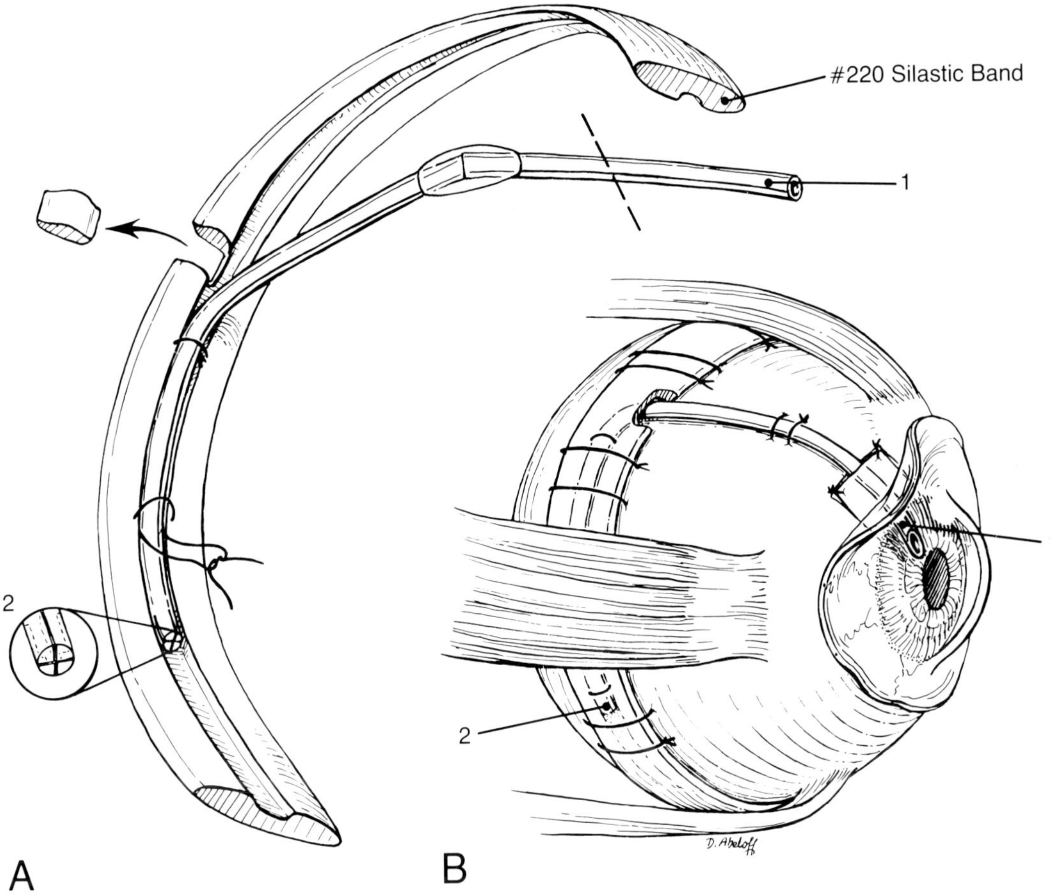

Fig. 29-4. (A) Long glaucoma valve implant sutured within the groove of a No. 220 Silastic band. The valve portion (2) is sutured within the groove and against the sclera. A 1- to 2-mm-wide notch is excised in one side wall of the band to permit exit of the open end of the tube for insertion into the anterior chamber. **(B)** The Supramid open end (1) is placed into the anterior chamber and the band (2) is placed beneath the superior and inferior rectus muscles. The band is cut to a length to extend to, or just beneath, both horizontal rectus muscles. See text for procedure. (Drawings by Diane Abeloff, after Craig Luce.)

Limbal Conjunctival Scarring

Limbal conjunctival scarring is not a problem with the long valve implant, since filtration does not occur at this location. Scarring is a normal process over the Silastic retinal band. Aqueous humor appears to pass through, or be adsorbed by, the vascular component of this capsule.

Flat Anterior Chamber

A flat anterior chamber with hypotony indicates too large an opening with leakage of aqueous humor around the tube. This complication is avoided with proper operative technique, including placing a suture across the wound if fluid is noted to leak around the tube during re-formation of the chamber. A prolonged flat anterior chamber is usually associated with choroidal detachment. Consequently, if surgical reformation is necessary, choroidal fluid should also be drained.

Internal Tube Complications

Improper placement of the anterior chamber tube can result in damage to the cornea, lens, or iris as well as blockage of flow through the tube. Iris tissue or pigmented debris can be removed from the tube opening using an argon laser (50-μm spot, 0.1-second duration, 300- to 800-mW power). I have also used the Nd:YAG laser to vaporize nonpigmented tissue occluding the internal opening.

Conjunctival Erosion

External erosion of the Silastic valve end has occurred in the original design. This complication is reduced if the external portion is flat against the sclera and within the scleral dissection bed. The scleral flap should cover the device and be sutured in place without placing tension on the end of the Silastic tube.

MOLTENO IMPLANT

Description of Device

The Molteno drainage implant[5,6] (Fig. 29-5) consists of an open silicone rubber tube (OD 0.63 mm, ID 0.3 mm) extending 2 to 4 mm into the anterior chamber. The tube is attached to, and opens onto, the upper surface of a thin acrylic episcleral plate 13 mm in diameter. The edge of the plate has a thickened rim 0.7 mm in height that is perforated to permit attachment of the tube by suturing the plate to the sclera.

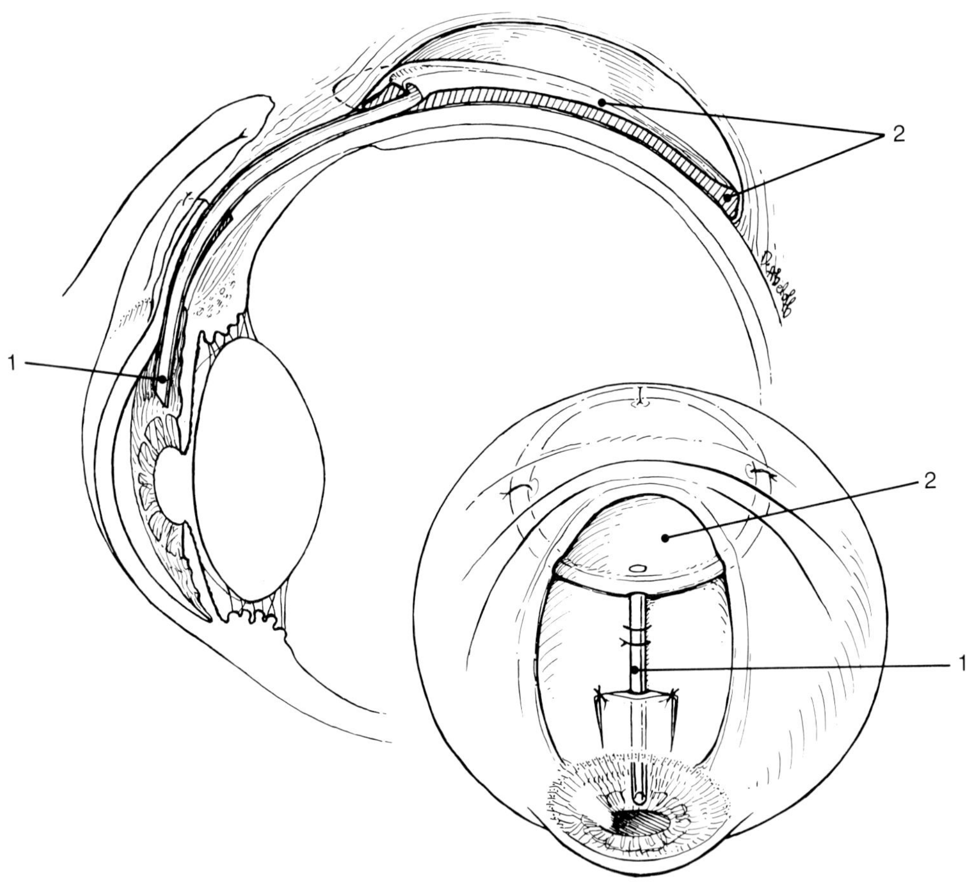

Fig. 29-5. The Molteno drainage implant consists of an open silicone rubber tube extending 2 to 4 mm into the anterior chamber (1). The tube is attached to, and opens onto, the upper surface of a thin acrylic episcleral plate 13 mm in diameter (2). See text for procedure. (Drawing by Diane Abeloff, after Craig Luce.)

The scleral plate functions as a limiting boundary over which vascular connective tissue can grow. Intraocular fluid pressure within this cavity results in distention and stretching of the bleb cavity. Long-term pressure control depends directly on the area of bleb available for drainage and inversely on the thickness of the fibrous inner bleb lining.

Surgical Implantation

A fornix-based conjunctival flap is prepared with Tenon's space exposed to the equator of the globe. A rectangular half-thickness limbal-based 8-mm scleral flap is prepared. The implant is placed into Tenon's space and sutured to the sclera at the posterior edge of the scleral flap. The silicone tube is laid radially across the scleral flap, and excess tube is cut off such that the tube overlaps the limbus by 2 mm. The anterior chamber is entered parallel to the iris plane with a 2-mm keratome. The tube is inserted into the anterior chamber and the scleral flap sutured. Tenon's tissue and conjunctiva are drawn forward and sutured to the limbus.

Molteno recommends a two-stage operation for eyes with neovascular glaucoma. In the first stage, the episcleral plate is inserted beneath Tenon's capsule and the tube buried beneath the scleral flap with the anterior portion tucked underneath the medial rectus muscle. The conjunctiva is closed. At a later time, the conjunctiva is reopened, the tube is identified, and the second stage of insertion of the silicone tube into the anterior chamber is carried out. Other surgeons still perform a one-stage implantation in eyes with neovascular glaucoma.

Subconjunctival methylprednisolone, 40 mg, is injected at the end of the procedure. Postoperative therapy is directed to prevent excessive drainage bleb fibrosis. Molteno recommends a combination of systemic prednisone (10 mg TID), fluphenamic acid (200 mg TID), and colchicine (0.5 mg TID) as well as four times a day topical epinephrine 2 percent, atropine 1 percent, and dexamethasone 0.1 percent for 6 weeks.

Results

The success rate in neovascular glaucoma ranges from 60 to 94 percent. Approximately 67 percent of these eyes are controlled <20 mmHg without medication.

Complications

Hyphema

This frequent complication is associated with tube implantation. Blood and fibrin can occlude the anterior chamber tube.

Hypotony

This frequent early complication can persist for up to 3 weeks. An open chamber tube without resistance can lead to a flat anterior chamber with subsequent choroidal detachment.

Implant Erosion

Conjunctival erosion with exposure of the implant can occur. This complication requires removal of the device.

ANTERIOR CHAMBER TUBE SHUNT TO AN ENCIRCLING BAND

Description of Device

Schocket and co-workers[7] described a device whereby aqueous could be shunted to the reservoir of an encircling No. 20 silicone band, that is, the anterior chamber tube shunt to an encircling band (ACTSEB) (Fig. 29-6). A 30-mm-long Silastic tube (OD 0.64 mm, ID 0.30 mm) is sutured into the grooved portion of a No. 20 silicone band such that 15 mm extends from the wall of the band.

Surgical Implantation

A 360-degree peritomy is made 4 to 5 mm posterior to the limbus, except for the superior nasal quadrant, where the conjunctival incision is extended posteriorly 8 to 10 mm. A vitreous tap is performed 4 to 5 mm from the limbus, using a 25-gauge needle to prevent excessive IOP increase

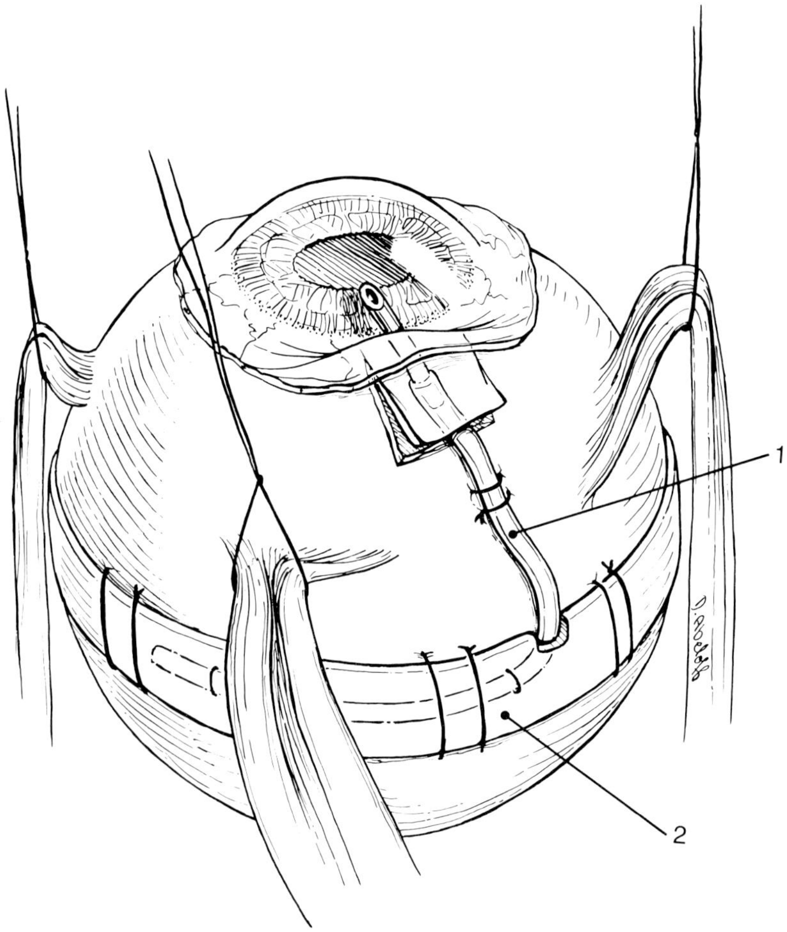

Fig. 29-6. The anterior chamber tube shunt to an encircling band (ACTSEB) is used to shunt aqueous to a reservoir of an encircling band of No. 20 silicone (2). The 30-mm-long Silastic tube (1) is sutured into the grooved portion of the band so that 15 mm extends from the wall of the band. See text for procedure. (Drawing by Diane Abeloff.)

after securing the band. The 360-degree band is placed grooved side toward the sclera beneath the rectus muscles. Scleral 5-0 Supramid mattress sutures are placed in each quadrant so that the anterior band edge is 10 to 12 mm from the limbus. The tube emerges nasal to the superior rectus muscle. The ends of the band are united with a mattress sutures. A 4 × 4-mm scleral flap is prepared. The tube is cut obliquely to a length to extend 3 mm into the anterior chamber. Entry is made into the chamber, and the tube is placed so that it lies over the iris surface. Schocket et al.[7] suggest that the chamber be filled with hyaluronic acid. The scleral flap is closed with 10-0 nylon sutures. The conjunctiva incision is closed with a running suture. Subconjunctival gentamicin sulfate 40 mg and dexamethasone sulfate 4 mg are injected.

Results

Surgical success with the ACTSEB procedure is very high as reported by Schocket and co-workers. Success in the range of 95 percent is stated to occur in eyes with neovascular glaucoma or with previously failed glaucoma surgery. Most of these cases are controlled without glaucoma medications.

Complications

Flat Anterior Chamber

Prolonged (i.e., 5 to 16 days) flat anterior chamber occurs in 74 percent of cases. This complication is expected in face of an open anterior chamber tube. Refilling the anterior chamber with hyaluronic acid at the end of the procedure may result in less shallowing of shorter duration. The prolonged flat chamber may increase the occurrence of cataract formation. A flat chamber increases the risk of tube contact with the cornea, lens, or iris.

Hyphema

This complication occurs in 21 percent of operated cases. While most hyphemas are small, large hyphemas requiring additional surgery can occur. In addition, blood and fibrin can occlude the anterior chamber tube.

Internal Tube Complications

Blockage of the tube with blood or protein debris can occur. Laser or surgical intervention is indicated to bring about return of function of the implant. Improper position of the tube can result in corneal contact and decompensation. This problem necessitates surgical modification or removal of the tube.

REFERENCES

1. Luntz MH: A review of alloplastic devices (setons) in glaucoma surgery. Presented at the Annual Meeting of the American Academy of Ophthalmology, 1983
2. Krupin T, Podos SM, Becker B, Newkirk JB: Valve implants in filtering surgery. Am J Ophthalmol 81:232, 1976
3. Krupin T, Kaufman P, Mandell AI, et al: Long-term results of valve implants in filtering surgery for eyes with neovascular glaucoma. Am J Ophthalmol 95:775, 1983
4. Shuster JN, Krupin T, Kolker AE, Becker B: Limbus-versus fornix-based conjunctival flap in trabeculectomy: A long-term randomized study. Arch Ophthalmol 102:361, 1984
5. Molteno ACB, VanRooyen MMB, Bartholomew RS: Implants for draining neovascular glaucoma. Br J Ophthalmol 61:120, 1977
6. Ancker E, Molteno ACB: Molteno drainage implant for neovascular glaucoma. Trans Ophthalmol Soc UK 102:122, 1982
7. Schocket SS, Lakhanpal V, Richards RD: Anterior chamber tube shunt to an encircling band in the treatment of neovascular glaucoma. Ophthalmology 89:1188, 1982

Cyclocryotherapy, Therapeutic Ultrasound, and Laser Treatment to the Ciliary Body

30

Hugh Beckman

CILIODESTRUCTIVE PROCEDURES

Having failed to control elevated intraocular pressure (IOP) with the use of either topical or systemic medications, or both, the ophthalmologist generally escalates therapy using surgical procedures aimed at increasing aqueous outflow. In recent years, argon laser trabeculoplasty has been used in many cases to forestall surgical ocular procedures. Eventually, however, many of the eyes undergo full-thickness filtration procedures or guarded filtration procedures such as trabeculectomy in an attempt to control IOP at a level compatible with retaining visual function. In selected situations, procedures such as goniotomy for congenital glaucoma, cyclodialysis for glaucoma with aphakia, and setons for neovascular glaucoma have come into vogue. There are, however, many eyes in which all efforts to increase outflow fail. Historically, in this group of conventionally intractable glaucomas we find the vast majority of those eyes in which the various ciliary-destructive procedures have been used to decrease aqueous production as a means of pressure control.

The first ciliodestructive procedure, introduced by Vogt,[1] entails the use of electrodiathermy. Electrodiathermy was administered either through intact conjunctiva, subconjunctivally, or beneath scleral flaps to destroy portions or all of the ciliary body. This approach led to atrophy and subsequently decreased aqueous secretion. As detailed by Berens and Sheppard,[2] the success rate was low and, perhaps as important, the incidence of phthisis was close to 10 percent. This high incidence of failures and phthisis is reported throughout the literature on the ciliodestructive procedures and is certainly due in part to the generally intractable nature of the glaucomas (e.g., neovascular glaucoma), in which these modalities have been used. The high incidence of phthisis and chronic hypotony that occurs in these procedures is probably the single factor that has kept aqueous flow-decreasing procedures in a secondary position to outflow-increasing procedures over the years. Certainly the outflow in these eyes is often so impaired that even slight incremental changes in inflow may result in a considerable drop in IOP, leaving less margin for error with resultant hypotony. It may or may not be that this is an overemphasized complication, but certainly most series have been biased by the high number of neovascular glaucoma eyes on which these procedures have been tested.

CYCLOCRYOTHERAPY

Transscleral cyclocryotherapy was first performed by Bietti[3] in 1950 and popularized by de Roetth[4] in 1968. It has since become the standard modality for ablation of the ciliary body. Cyclocryotherapy is the use of some type of freezing probe applied transconjunctivally in an attempt to lower the temperature in the ciliary body. This lowering of temperature causes destruction of the pigmented cells within the ciliary body—notably the pigment epithelium—with resultant stromal necrosis due to embarrassment of the vascular supply. Many protocols for treatment have been used. The various instruments used, temperatures, and varying numbers of lesions, together with changes in duration of freezing and location of application, have resulted in many varying reports regarding its efficacy and safety (Fig. 30-1).

Beitti used a solid CO_2 cylinder for $\frac{1}{2}$ to 1 minute in the rabbit, demonstrating the resultant hypotony. He used a similar method in human subjects; in 21 eyes, he found that 16 had decreases in IOP. In two of these eyes, chronic hypotony had occurred. McClean and Lincoff[5] applied a liquid nitrogen probe for up to 1 minute in seven eyes, producing a transient lowering of IOP in five and a significant lowering of IOP in two. de Roetth, who popularized cyclocryotherapy, treated 165 eyes with six 1-minute applications at a temperature of $-80°C$. In his overall series, de Roetth produced a normalization of IOP in 40 percent of eyes, and in a separate group of primary open-angle glaucoma patients he reported reduction of IOP to normal in 75 percent. He reported mostly minor complications, such as mild iritis, with the exception of choroidal hemorrhages in two cases. No major complications were reported.

Chenoweth[6] was the first to describe sequential cyclocryotherapy, on 35 glaucomatous human

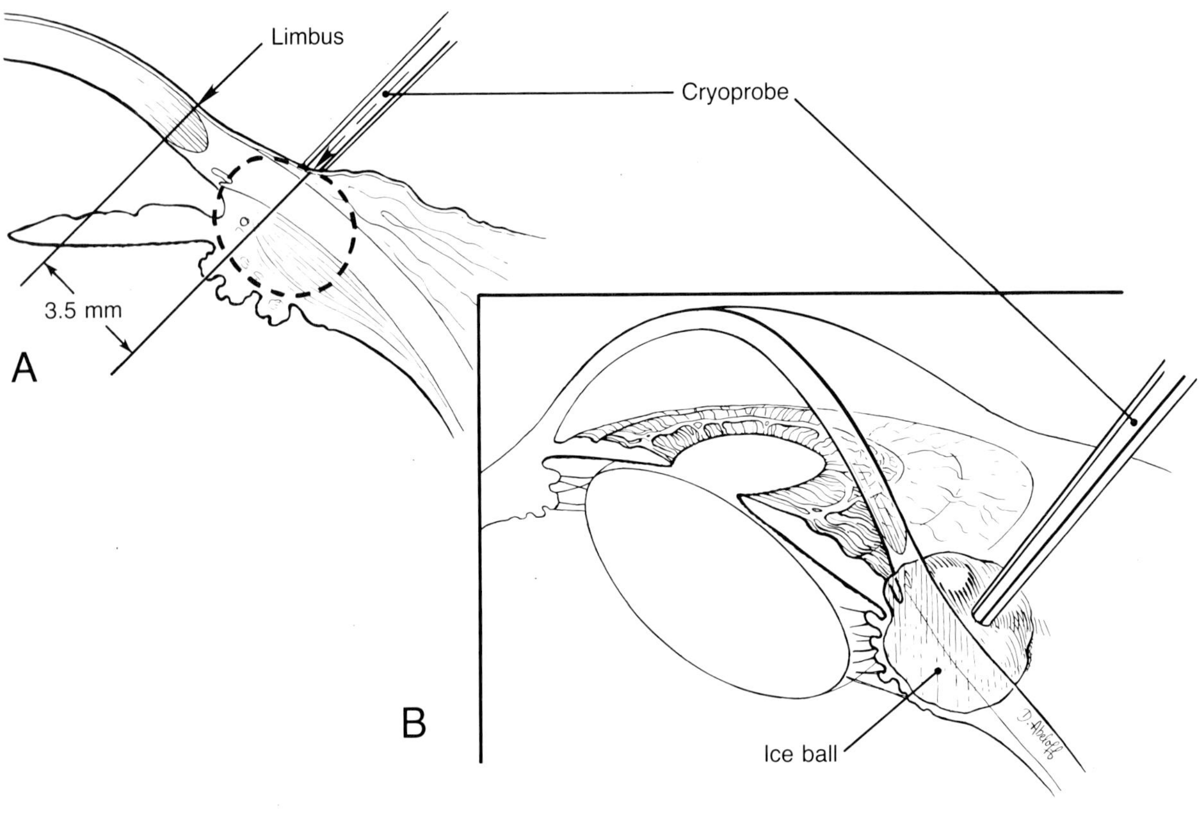

Fig. 30-1. (A,B) The proliferation of ice ball with cryoprobe centered 3.5 mm from limbus.

eyes. He initially treated 180 degrees of the ciliary body at −60°C initially. After waiting at least 1 month, he treated the same area at −80°C, and again 1 month later a third treatment at −80°C. Chenowith believed that sequential treatment permitted use of the −80°C temperature necessary for ciliary body destruction without causing hemorrhagic uveitis. His series had only one case of choroidal separation, his only reported complication.

Feibel and Bigger[7] reported a retrospective study of 38 eyes treated for neovascular glaucoma. These investigators found no difference between −60° and −80°C lesions. Sixty-three percent of the eyes were controlled with an IOP of less than 20 mmHg, but the visual acuity results were extremely poor, with dense cataracts developing in 25 percent of cases and hypotony developing in more than one-third of cases.

Boniuk[8] found a 10 percent incidence of phthisis in 19 eyes with neovascular glaucoma treated with eight circumferential applications of cyclocryotherapy of −85° to −100°C, 3.5 mm posterior to the limbus. Of nine eyes with diabetic neovascular glaucoma, there was control of pain in all cases. Six of the eyes became completely blind and four developed hypotony. Two became phthisical. Of 10 eyes with nondiabetic neovascular glaucoma, pain control was achieved in 7, and 3 developed hypotony. No phthisis was found in this group. Boniuk advocated the use of transillumination in determining whether previous therapy had been adequate or properly placed. He recommended cyclocryotherapy as the surgical treatment of choice for neovascular glaucoma.

In a prospective study, Bellows and Grant[9] created six lesions using a CO_2 gas instrument over the inferior 180 degrees of the ciliary body, at a temperature of −60°C for 60 seconds. Success by a criterion of an IOP of less than 20 mmHg without medical treatment, was 76.6 percent in open-angle glaucoma in aphakia, 57 percent in secondary glaucoma, 30 percent in neovascular glaucoma, and 38 percent in the glaucoma of childhood. Sixteen percent of cases had complications, including hyphema, choroidal detachment, and retinal detachment. Other complications included unexplained loss of vision, absolute glaucoma secondary to chronic uveitis, and dellen.

In a later analysis of this group of patients, a long-term complication of uveitis with macular edema was found that resulted in frequent decreases in vision. In the glaucoma in aphakia group, which had the best success rate in the series, there were 26 eyes of which 92 percent were deemed successful. Twenty-two of these patients were on medication, and nine had been treated twice.

Probably the worst reported results were those of Krupin et al.[10] These workers used the heaviest reported amount of cyclocryotherapy, that is, 12 circumferential applications 3 mm from the limbus, with temperatures of −60° to −80°C for 60 seconds. Thus, in one-third of the eyes IOP was controlled to less than 26 mmHg, one-third had pressures greater than 26 mmHg, and, significantly, one-third developed phthisis. Close to 60 percent of these patients lost light perception.

The most encouraging results were obtained by Wesley and Kielar,[11] who treated 31 eyes, achieving control of IOP to below 20 mmHg in 74 percent of cases. Eight circumferential applications were used approximately 3 mm from the limbus, at −80°C for 1 minute. The success rate was 84 percent when transillumination was used as compared with 58 percent without transillumination. Better results were achieved when the probe was applied at 3.5 mm from the limbus (85 percent success as opposed to greater than 4 mm from the limbus, in which there was a 20 percent success rate). The success rate was 85 percent using −80°C as opposed to 46 percent when −60°C lesions were produced. An IOP of less than 5 mmHg was obtained in 10 percent of cases.

Aminlari[12] compared goniotomy and goniopuncture with cyclocryotherapy. He used at least six applications at 180 degrees; −60°C cold was applied for about 60 seconds. His success rate was 60 percent in the operated group and only 18 percent in the cyclocryotherapy group. Aminlari concluded that cyclocryotherapy is not effective in treating congenital glaucoma.

Yeo and Quigley[13] presented a paper at the Association for Research in Vision and Opthalmology meeting in 1984, in which they gave a retrospective review of 25 eyes of 21 patients treated with eight applications over a 180-degree area, using −70°C for 1 minute. A final IOP value of less than 25 mmHg was achieved in 56 percent of patients.

Visual acuity of better than 20/400 was preserved in 9 of 11 patients who had good preoperative vision. Repeat therapy was found necessary in 48 percent of the eyes. Four eyes lost light perception, two eyes became phthisical, and two eyes were enucleated. Antiglaucoma medication was required in 18 of the eyes.

In 1974, Paton and Butner[14] outlined no less than seven different techniques of cryotherapy, using eight combinations of probe tips and freezing temperatures. A perusal of the literature would seem to indicate that the method of therapy as described by Wesley and Kielar probably approximates the most widespread and safest protocol: after retrobulbar anesthesia, a lid speculum is inserted. A fiberoptic transilluminating device is placed directed on the cornea in a darkened room. After locating the pars plicata, a N_2O cryoprobe with a 4-mm probe tip is applied. Eight applications of −80°C cold are used either 360 degrees circumferentially or for 180 degrees. The center of the probe is placed 3 to 4 mm from the limbus, with the edge of the probe 1 to 2 mm from the limbus (Fig. 30-1). This distance may vary according to the findings of the transillumination. The iceball usually extends onto the cornea. At the end of 1 minute, the tip is irrigated to remove the probe. Postoperative therapy consists of topical atropine and steroids for a variable period of time. Oral analgesics are prescribed. Occasionally narcotics are necessary.

THERAPEUTIC ULTRASOUND

Therapeutic ultrasound was first used by Donn[15] to disrupt the vitreous. In 1964, Purnell et al.[16] developed an ultrasonic device and proposed destroying ciliary epithelium as a means of treating high IOP. During the late 1970s, Lizzi and Coleman and colleagues[17–20] described the use of ultrasound to coagulate the lens, produce lesions of the choroid and retina, and disrupt vitreal membranes. These investigators continued the development of therapeutic ultrasound, and in 1985 reported it as a transconjunctival transscleral means of therapy for otherwise intractable glaucoma.[21,22] The therapeutic transducer is wedded to a central fiberoptic light source that serves as a guidebeam, illuminating the area selected for treatment. A diagnostic ultrasound transducer is incorporated into the system so that the distance from the sclera can be measured accurately for purposes of positioning the probe. The transducer is designed to provide a focal spot 0.4 mm in diameter and 3 mm in length at a distance 25 mm from the cone tip (90 mm from the transducer), using 4.5-MHz ultrasonic pulses of 5 seconds duration. These are focused onto the sclera 1.5 mm from the limbus. Powers in excess of 2,000 watts (W)/cm are used (Figs. 30-2, 30-3).

Initially, this procedure was performed under topical anesthesia. However, patient discomfort as well as ocular movement have dictated the use of a retrobulbar anesthetic when performing the procedure. Initially the treatment regimen consisted of an average of 10 lesions. However, further experience led to the utilization of six or seven lesions per treatment. A recent paper by Burgess et al.,[23] reported the use of two levels of ultrasound. For the earlier cases (78 eyes), used levels exceeding 10 kWlcm^2 were used. In later cases (50 eyes), the intensity was reduced 50 to 80 percent from the original eye, while in the last 43 eyes, the higher-intensity level was again used after it was observed that the diminished intensity was less effective.

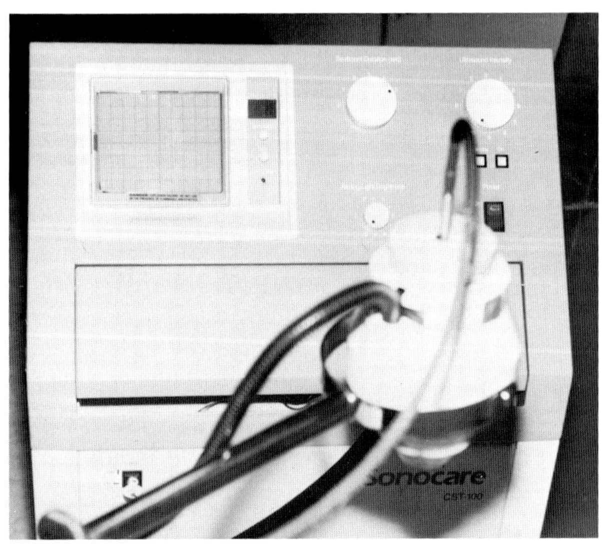

Fig. 30-2. Therapeutic ultrasound.

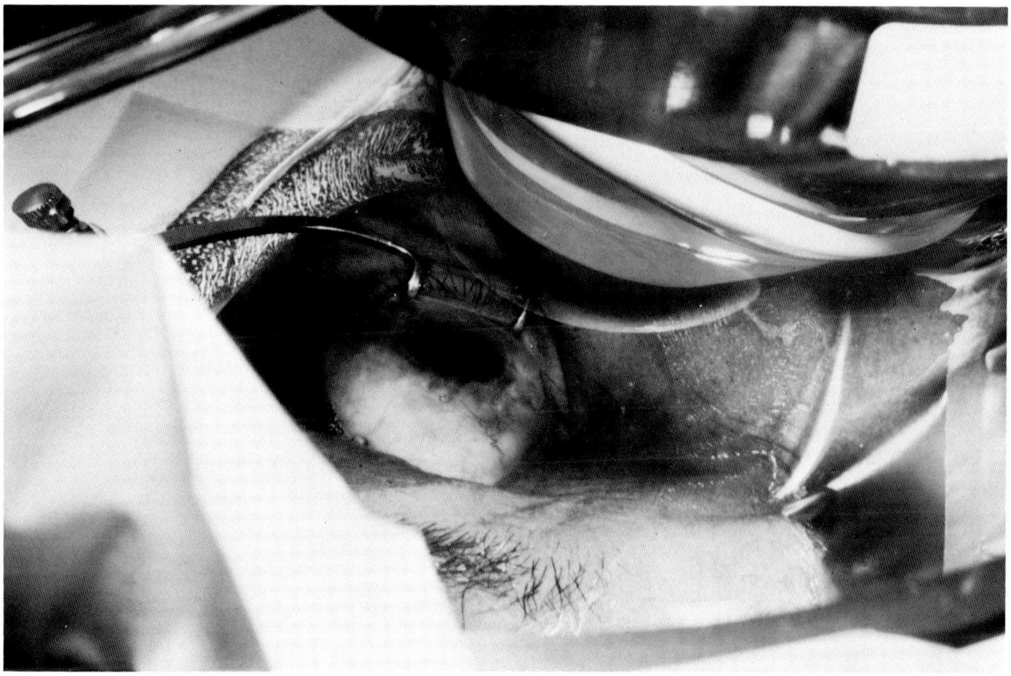

Fig. 30-3. Water bath drape for ultrasound glaucoma therapy with transducer in position.

Post-therapy care is aimed at control of iridocyclitis with topical steroids and cycloplegics.

Burgess treated 121 eyes at optimal levels. The mean IOP was 39 mm prior to treatment. Thirty days after treatment, an average drop of 19 mmHg was observed. Using a criterion of 25 mmHg or less, a success rate of 71 percent was achieved at 1 year. When using a success criterion of 22 mmHg or less, a 64 percent success rate was achieved at 1 year. These figures did not exclude eyes with IOP of less than 5 mmHg, which constituted 13 of the 121 cases. This would decrease the success rate for 25 mmHg or less to approximately 62 percent, and for 22 mmHg or less to approximately 55 percent, assuming that chronically hypotonic eyes were eliminated from consideration as successes, as has been commonly done in other ciliodestructive therapy series.

It should be noted that the cases of hypotony were less in the series in which lower power levels were used, but the decrease in the incidence of hypotony was counterbalanced by a decrease in the incidence of successful control of IOP. Four of the eyes with hypotony had end-stage neovascular glaucoma, and two were cases of uveitic secondary angle-closure glaucoma. Twenty-seven of the eyes treated with therapeutic ultrasound required retreatment. Of these cases, 20 were successful, while five failed to respond.

Burgess and co-workers noted that 46 of the 171 eyes in the series demonstrated some changes severe enough to be considered complications. Generally, they were divided into two categories: (1) complications associated with uveal reaction and hypotony, and (2) complications related to corneal and scleral damage. Hypotony was observed in 15 of the 171 cases, with only two of the cases occurring among those treated at reduced power levels.

Some eyes developed scleral thinning. This most commonly occurred in children and was seen in 4 of 19 cases (21 percent). Staphyloma formation occurred in two cases, but no perforation was observed. Seven patients had corneal problems after therapy, two of which were limbal corneal burns. One had marked astigmatism and two developed corneal abrasions. Cystoid edema was present in one case and choroidal effusions developed in three cases. Other complications included two lid burns and one ciliary body hemorrhage. Visual acuity data were available for 83 cases, showing improvement in visual acuity in 13 percent, no change in 42 percent, and decreased acuity in 45 percent.

It was clinically observed, although not statistically defined, that there was a synergistic effect between therapeutic ultrasound and the use of post-therapy topical phospholine iodide. This empirical observation gave rise to speculation that not only does the procedure decrease aqueous production but that it might increase uveal scleral outflow as well.

Therapeutic ultrasound, a procedure recommended for severe intractable neovascular and complicated glaucomas, is undergoing clinical trials. A full statement as to its efficacy should be forthcoming.

TRANSSCLERAL LASER CYCLOCOAGULATION

Ruby and Neodymium

In 1968 Beckman et al.[24] designed a solid-state ruby laser delivery system (Fig. 30-4), and with it initially performed laser iridectomies. After reading reports of the successful use of cyclocryotherapy for ciliary destruction, these workers used this laser to perform transconjunctival transscleral cyclocoagulation.[25] The laser beam is focused through the relatively transparent conjunctiva and sclera into the ciliary body, where the energy is absorbed by melanin-containing tissue (Fig. 30-5).

Histopathologic studies of rabbit eyes showed an initial hyperemia ensuing within 24 hours, followed by a rather massive inflammatory response in the ciliary body. One month after treatment, atrophy of the ciliary processes was demonstrated at the site of the lesions.

In 1984, Beckman and Waelterman[26] reported the results of a series of 241 eyes treated by transscleral ruby laser cyclocoagulation over a 10-year period. All these eyes had a minimum follow-up of 6 months, with an average follow-up of 2 years. The treatment method was as follows: After a retrobulbar anesthetic is given, the eye is marked into eight sectors by marks 3.5 mm from the limbus. Following this, either 6 or 7.5 joules (J) of ruby laser energy are impacted through the intact conjunctiva onto the ciliary body, creating a total of 32 lesions in each eye. A silver contact lens was placed over the cornea in each case to protect the retina from inadvertent impact with the high-energy ruby beam (Figs. 30-6, 30-7).

A total of 122 eyes received 7.5 J per lesion, and 119 eyes received 6 J per lesion. Following all treatments, the patients were given a sulfa–steroid combination drop, three times daily, and atropine once a day for 2 weeks. After this period, the atropine was discontinued, and the sulfa–steroid combination was replaced by fluoromethalone solution until the intraocular inflammation had subsided. All antiglaucoma medications, with the exception of carbonic anhydrase inhibitors, were discontinued at the time of therapy. The carbonic anhydrase inhibitors (CAI) were discontinued 2 days to 1 week after the therapy.

Immediately following treatment, conjunctival burns can be seen at the site of each laser impact. These generally disappear within 72 hours. Interestingly enough, they do not result in scarring down of the conjunctiva, as in the few cases in which filtering procedures were performed on previously laser-treated eyes, dissection of the conjunctival flaps could be performed without difficulty. The anterior chamber reaction is generally moderate (1+ cell, 3–4+ flare) and usually persists for several weeks.

Postoperative pain varies from mild to moderately severe but generally does not last longer than 24 hours. In general, the pain following ruby laser cyclocoagulation is much less than that which occurs following cyclocryotherapy. The IOP falls within 48 hours of treatment and continues to fall for 2 weeks. At that time, it tends to rise as the eye whitens, and the inflammatory process subsides.

We have used a 6-month post-treatment IOP of 5 to 22 mmHg as a criterion for successful control of IOP. The results for 122 eyes using 7.5 J per spot are shown in Table 30-1; these results can be compared with those using 6 J per spot, shown in Table 30-2. The overall success rate of both series was 62 percent. This varied from a high of 86 percent in open-angle glaucoma in aphakia to a low of 53 percent in cases of neovascular glaucoma. Many of the

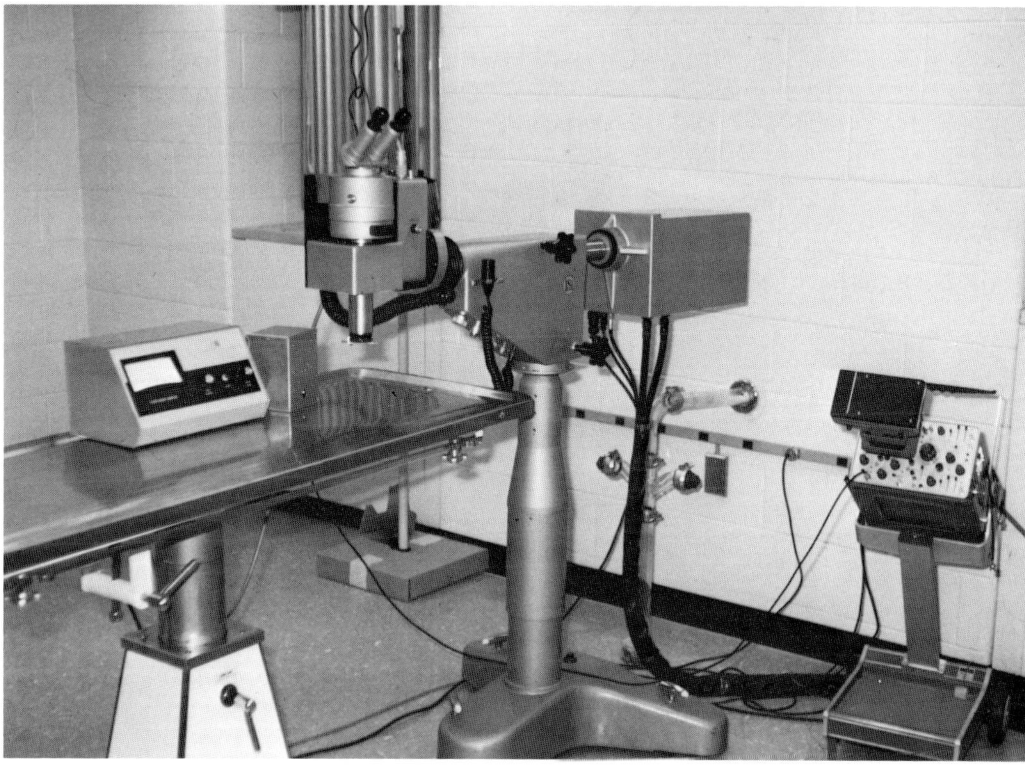

Fig. 30-4. Ruby laser used for transscleral cyclocoagulation.

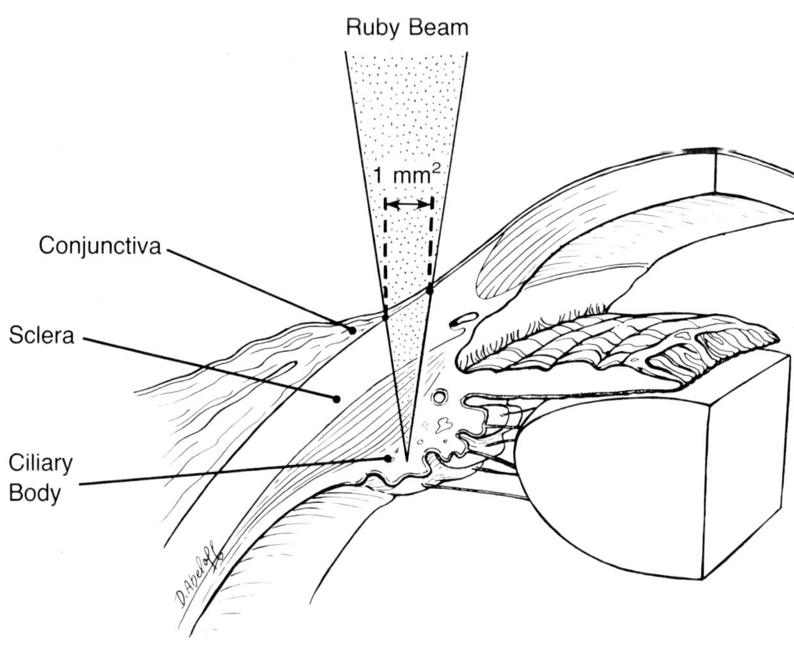

Fig. 30-5. Ruby laser beam focused onto the sclera and well-transmitted by the sclera into the ciliary body.

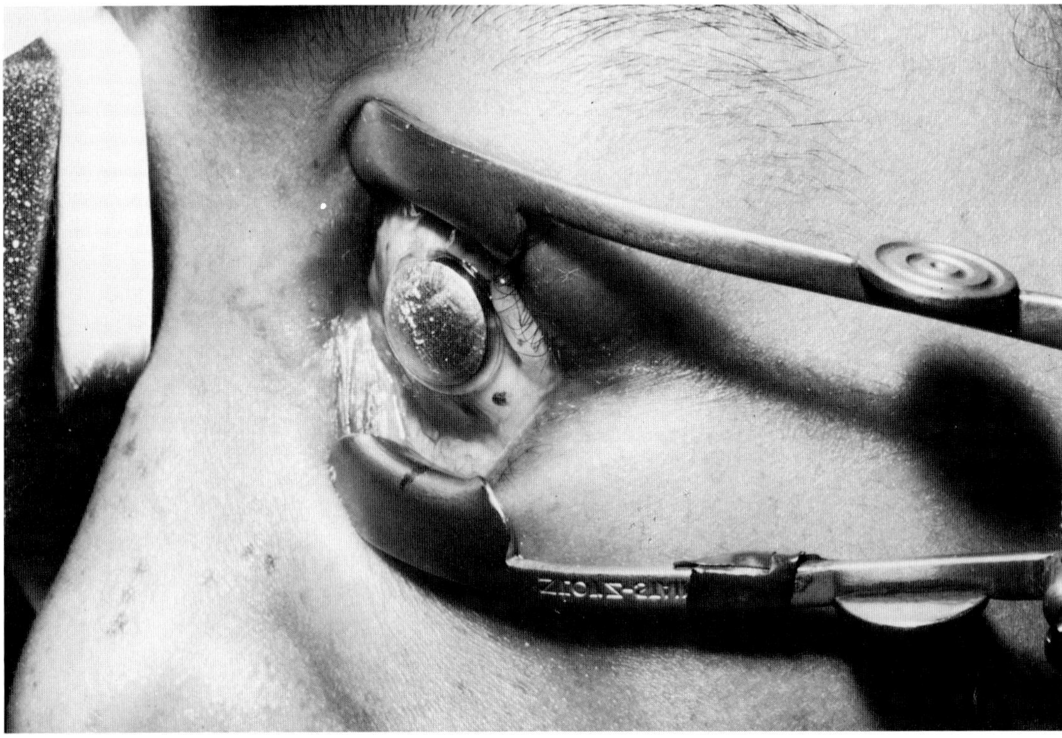

Fig. 30-6. Eye with marks on sclera and silvered contact lens in place prior to Nd:YAG laser cyclocoagulation.

eyes treated had had multiple previous procedures including filtering surgery, cyclocryotherapy, and conventional antiglaucoma medical therapy. For most of the eyes treated, this was either their last or nearly last resort.

In 54 of 135 eyes with neovascular glaucoma, visual acuity consisted of counting fingers or less. Of these, 24 percent progressed to no light perception during the follow-up period. Visual loss in these cases was due to varying causes: phthisis (6), vitreous hemorrhage (3), and hyphema (4). Eight eyes in this group had a useful pretreatment visual acuity of better than 20/200. Four of these eyes deteriorated to no more than the ability to count fingers. Three eyes had vitreous hemorrhage unrelated to treatment. The remaining four eyes retained prelaser acuity. Five eyes that had visual acuity of less than 20/400 recovered useful vision

Table 30-1. 7.5-Joule Ruby Laser Series: Success Rates for 122 Eyes[a]

Type of Glaucoma	Success	Failure	Success Rate (%)
Neovascular	38	39	49
Open-angle glaucoma in aphakia	11	2	85
Secondary	8	3	73
Traumatic	4	5	44
Chronic open-angle glaucoma	5	3	62
Congenital	2	2	50
Totals	68	54	56

[a] Intraocular pressure: 5 to 22 mmHg.

Table 30-2. 6.0-Joule Ruby Laser Series: Success Rates for 119 Eyes[a]

Type of Glaucoma	Success	Failure	Success Rate (%)
Neovascular	34	24	59
Open-angle glaucoma in aphakia	21	3	88
Secondary	13	6	68
Traumatic	10	2	83
Chronic open-angle glaucoma	3	2	60
Congenital	1	0	100
Totals	82	37	69

[a] Intraocular pressure: 5 to 22 mmHg.

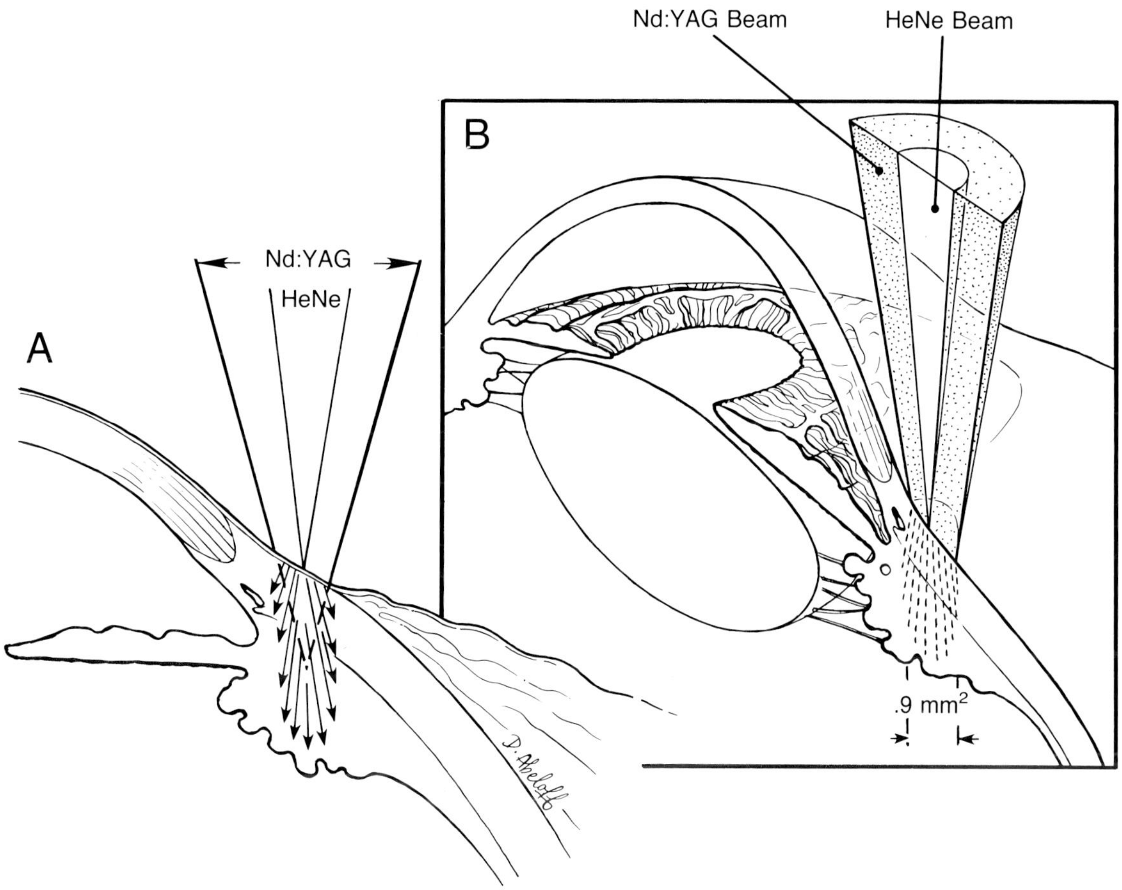

Fig. 30-7. (A,B) Increasing the spot size on the sclera by defocusing the Nd:YAG beam in relation to the HeNe aiming beam is shown. The Nd:YAG beam then scatters through the sclera into the ciliary body.

due to resolution of preexisting conditions such as corneal edema. Three eyes were better than 20/100, and one attained 20/50 vision.

In the other large group of patients, that is, those aphakic eyes with chronic open-angle glaucoma, 16 had pretreatment acuity of 20/200 or better. Three of those eyes had decrease in vision. The remaining 13 eyes either maintained prelaser acuity or improved. Two of 21 eyes with acuity of less than 20/200 fell to light perception. No eye with pretreatment vision better than 20/200 decreased to light perception.

Lumping all the other glaucomatous eyes together, 23 eyes out of 69 had 20/200 vision or better. Seventy-eight percent of these eyes maintained visual acuity after laser treatment. Five eyes dropped in acuity but maintained 20/400 vision or better. Of 46 eyes with less than 20/200 vision, only three went on to nil vision. All these eyes had had light perception and developed phthisis. In all, 70 percent of those eyes with useful vision better than 20/200 maintained useful vision following treatment. This is much better than any series reported with cyclocryotherapy.

As with cyclocryotherapy and cyclodiathermy, the most common complication was chronic hypotony. Phthisis also occurred, common only in the neovascular glaucoma group.

The postoperative morbidity and pain are less than with cyclocryotherapy. The visual results and requirement for retreatment are statistically more favorable than cyclocryotherapy. The incidence of complications, both early and late, is less with the laser procedure.

Table 30-3. Results of Nd:YAG Cyclocoagulation

	Total		Aphakia		Neovascular		Other	
Success[a]	*N*	%	*N*	%	*N*	%	*N*	%
5–22 mmHg	19	44	5	50	11	52	3	25
5–25 mmHg	24	56	8	80	11	52	5	42

[a] Reduced IOP.

Neodymium:YAG

The beneficial effects of transscleral ruby laser cyclocoagulation suggested the investigation of glass:neodymium (1.06 μm) wavelength to perform the same task. In 1973, Beckman and Sugar[27] reported an encouraging series of intractable glaucoma cases treated in this manner. Neither procedure gained in popularity primarily due to the unavailability of commercial lasers capable of performing them.

With the influx of high-powered ND:YAG lasers in ophthalmology, we began performing cyclocoagulation on a group of intractable glaucoma cases, with generally encouraging results. The Lasag II Microrupter Laser was chosen as the delivery system, as the only Q-switched laser that has provision for external defeat of the Q-switching system, enabling the laser to run in what is called the thermal or free-running mode.

Our laser was specifically designed to run at a 10-msec pulsewidth, thus approximating the 6-msec pulsewidth used in our prior work. All cases were done with 32 bursts of energy arranged circumlimbally 3.5 mm from the limbus. The laser was defocused to the #9 position, moving the focal point 3.6 mm posterior into the eye and creating approximately a 0.9-mm spot on the conjunctiva (Fig. 30-7). Our laser, which started out delivering a maximum 9 J per pulse, degraded over the course of the study until at the end of this particular series it was yielding only 6 J per pulse. Animal studies performed by Wilensky et al.,[28] van der Zyphen et al.,[29] and Fankhauser (Fankhauser F: personal communication) confirm the ability of the Nd:YAG laser to cause transscleral thermal destruction in the ciliary body.

A group of 39 eyes were treated once in this manner. With a minimal follow-up of 6 months, the mean preoperative IOP in the eyes fell from 45 mmHg to a mean postoperative IOP of 17.7. The results, as shown in Table 30-3, using a criterion for a successful IOP of greater than 5 mmHg and less than 25 mmHg, are 57 percent for the entire series. Using 22 mmHg as a criterion for success, it falls to 47 percent. The rate of hypotony was 11 percent and, with the exception of one patient, all these eyes are doing well.

As can be seen in Table 30-4, the results in open-angle glaucoma in aphakia and neovascular glaucoma approximate those of the other laser series. The Nd:YAG laser does seem slightly less effective. This is probably due to the decreased-from-optimal power levels available through much of the series.

In terms of visual acuity, four of the neovascular glaucoma patients had decreased acuity as a result of intercurrent disease processes and vitreal hemorrhages, and one LP eye became phthisical. One nonneovascular eye developed cystoid macular edema (CME). Five had improvement in vision and 28 showed no significant change.

Table 30-4.

Success[a]		Total		Aphakia		Neovasc	
Laser	J	*N*	%	*N*	%	*N*	%
Ruby	7.5	(68/122)	56	(11/13)	85	38/77	49
Ruby	6.0	(82/119)	69	(21/24)	88	34/58	59
Nd:Glass	7.0	(8/19)	42	(1/2)	50	5/14	36
Nd:Glass	14.0	(17/28)	61	(1/1)	100	11/20	55
Nd:YAG	8.0	(19/43)	44	(5/40)	50	11/21	52
TN	5–25	(24/43)	56	(8/10)	80	11/21	52

[a] Reduced IOP to 5 to 22 mmHg.

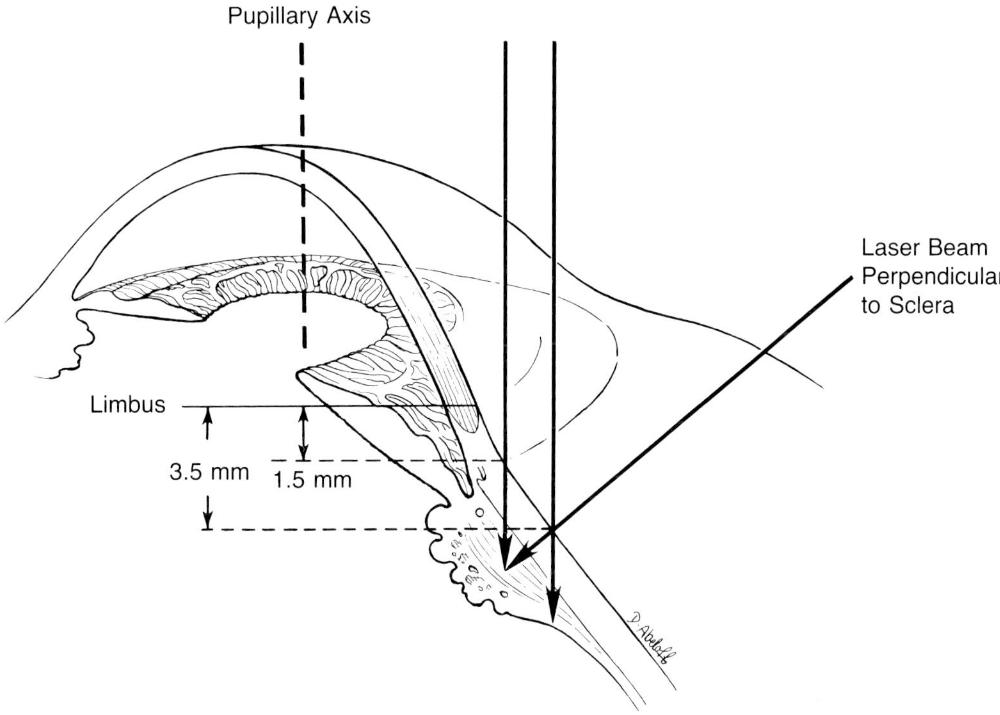

Fig. 30-8. The difference in target site as a factor of the distance from the limbus and the angle of beam incidence.

Other investigators (Fankhauser F: personal communication; Hamburger H: personal communication) have performed experiments, mapping the course of the laser energy when it is applied tangentially to the sclera. These workers estimate that for placement into the ciliary body, one must transmit the energy from a point 1.5 mm from the limbus if aimed at the sclera tangentially on an axis parallel to the pupillary axis. Future work will be performed to corroborate or deny this in an effort to optimize the therapeutic effect. All our work has been done aiming at 3.5 mm from the limbus parallel to the pupillary axis, which may mean that our lesions were posterior to the center of the pars ciliaris (Fig. 30-8).

It would seem that our laser had an optimal therapeutic effect at energy settings of 7.5 to 8 J. Communication with other investigators in the field reveals beneficial effects with as little as 2 J per spot. It is possible that the energy outputs of individual lasers are not comparable as determined by the energy-meters provided.

SUMMARY

It is somewhat difficult to compare these modalities, as (1) the cyclocryotherapy series are quite varied, both in technique and in results; and (2) the ruby and Nd:YAG laser cyclocoagulation series, as well as the ultrasound series, represent work based on the results of a few investigators using specialized equipment. Nevertheless, if one compares what is probably the most favorable series of cyclocryotherapy, that of Wesley and Kielar, with the series of ultrasound (Burgess et al.[23]), with our ruby

Table 30-5. Comparison of Ciliodestructive Modalities

Modality	Cost ($)	Versatility	Pain	Vision
Cyclotherapy	3,000 (1)	Yes (1)	++++(3)	Poor (2)
Ultrasound	60,000 (2)	? (2)	+(1)	Good (1)
Ruby laser	60,000 (3)	No (3)	++(2)	Good (1)
Nd:YAG laser	100,000 (4)	Yes (1)	+(1)	Good (1)

Table 30-6. Comparison of Ciliodestructive Modalities

Modality	Ease	Results	Availability	Total
Cyclotherapy	+++(2)	3	1	13
Ultrasound	+(4)	2	3	15
Ruby laser	++++(1)	1	4	15
Nd:YAG laser	++++(1)	2	2	12

laser and Nd:YAG laser series (Tables 30-5, 30-6) and combines that with some practical and clinical observations, the following statements might be made:

1. Cyclocryotherapy is the most available modality, using the least expensive equipment.
2. Cyclocryotherapy is the least controllable and most painful of the three modalities, having the greatest incidence of visual loss, and probably in most hands, the lowest incidence of successful control of IOP.
3. Both the therapeutic ultrasound equipment and the Nd:YAG laser equipment are just becoming reasonably available at major centers, and both appear promising for ciliodestructive therapy.
4. The laser, with its ability to be focused through air, is more easily delivered than the therapeutic ultrasound, which requires a waterbath interface.
5. The ruby laser, which is the least available, may be the best modality, as its wavelength is more suitable for maximal scleral transmission and ciliary body melanin absorption.
6. Ciliodestructive procedures, in general, are more efficacious than commonly believed. A great deal of the negative comments attributed to them is based on their use in neovascular glaucoma or in other severe intractable glaucomas in which the outflow is so impeded that the incremental changes in inflow required to normalize IOP are very close to those that create chronic hypotony and phthisis.
7. All the modalities may have success rates in the treatment of aphakic open-angle glaucoma that are better than conventional filtering procedures.
8. Any of these modalities may exceed the success rate of filtering surgery. The complication rate in complicated glaucomas is actually reasonably low; in time, these procedures may become useful in the treatment of open-angle glaucoma, especially of low-tension glaucoma.

REFERENCES

1. Vogt A: Versuche zue intraokularen Druckherabsetzung mittelst Diathermieschadigung des Corpus ciliare (Zyklodiathermiestichelung). Klin Monatsbl Augenheilkd 97:672, 1936
2. Berens C, Sheppard LB: Clinical and experimental consideration of cycloelectrolysis and cyclodiathermy. Am J Ophthalmol 50:599, 1960
3. Bietti G: Surgical intervention on the ciliary body. JAMA 142:889, 1950
4. de Roetth A Jr: Cryosurgery for the treatment of advanced chronic simple glaucoma. Am J Ophthalmol 66:1034, 1968
5. McLean JM, Lincoff HA: Cryosurgery of the ciliary body. Trans Am Ophthalmol Soc 62:385, 1964
6. Chenoweth RG: Proper techniques of cyclocryosurgery for glaucoma. p. 555. In Welsh RC, Welsh J (eds): The Second Report on Cataract Surgery. Miami Educational Press, Miami, FL, 1971
7. Fiebel RM, Bigger JF: Rubeosis iridis and neovascular glaucoma. Am J Ophthalmol 74:862, 1972
8. Boniuk M: Cryotherapy in neovascular glaucoma. Trans Am Acad Ophthalmol Otolaryngol 78:337, 1974
9. Bellows AR, Grant WM: Cycryotherapy in advanced inadequately controlled glaucoma. Am J Ophthalmol 75:697, 1973
10. Krupin T, Mitchell B, Becker B: Cyclocryotherapy in neovascular glaucoma. Am J Ophthalmol 86(1):24, 1978
11. Wesley RE, Kielar RA: Cyclocryotherapy in the treatment of glaucoma. 3:533, 1980
12. Aminlari A: Cyclocryotherapy in congenital glaucoma. Glaucoma Nov–Dec:331, 1981
13. Yeo JH, Quigley HA: Cyclocryotherapy: Recent experience using a standardized technique. Presented at The Association for Research in Vision and Ophthalmology, Annual Meeting, 1984
14. Paton D, Butner R: Cyclocryotherapy. Ophthalmic Surg 5:24, 1974
15. Donn A: Ultrasonic wave liquefaction of vitreous humor in living rabbits. Arch Ophthalmol 53:215, 1955
16. Purnell EW, Sokollu A, Torchia R, Taner N: Focal

chorioretinitis produced by ultrasound. Invest Ophthalmol 3:657, 1964
17. Lizzi FL, Packer AJ, Coleman DJ: Experimental cataract production by high frequency ultrasound. Ann Ophthalmol 10:934, 1978
18. Lizzi FL, Coleman DJ, Driller J, et al: Experimental, ultrasonically induced lesions in the retina, choroid and sclera. Invest Ophthalmol Vis Sci 17:350, 1978
19. Coleman DJ, Lizzi FL, El-Mofty AAM, et al: Ultrasonically accelerated resorption of vitreous membranes. Am J Ophthalmol 89:490, 1980
20. Coleman DJ, Lizzi FL, Jakobiec FA: Therapeutic ultrasound in the production of ocular lesions. Am J Ophthalmol 86:185, 1978
21. Coleman DJ, Lizzi FL, Driller J, et al: Therapeutic ultrasound in the treatment of glaucoma I (experimental model). Ophthalmology 92:339, 1985
22. Coleman DJ, Lizzi FL, Driller J, et al: Therapeutic ultrasound in the treatment of glaucoma I (clinical applications). Ophthalmology 92:347, 1985
23. Burgess SEP, Silverman RH, Coleman DJ, et al: Treatment of glaucoma with high intensity focused ultrasound. Parts I and II. Ophthalmology 92:339, 1985
24. Beckman H, Barraco R, Sugar HS, et al: Laser iridectomies. Am J Ophthalmol 72:393, 1971
25. Beckman H, Kinoshita A, Rota A, Sugar HS: Transscleral ruby laser irradiation of the ciliary body in the treatment of intractable glaucoma. p. 423. In Transactions of the American Academy of Ophthalmology and Otolaryngology, March–April, 1972
26. Beckman H, Waeltermann J: Transscleral ruby laser cyclocoagulation. Am J Ophthalmol 98:788, 1984
27. Beckman H, Sugar HS: Neodymium laser cyclocoagulation. Arch Ophthalmol 90:27, 1973
28. Wilensky JT, Welch D, Mirolovich M: Transscleral cyclocoagulation using a neodymium:YAG laser. Ophthalmol Surg 16:95, 1985
29. Van der Zyphen E, England C, Fankhauser F, Kwasniewska S: Ultrastructural effects of transscleral cyclophotocoagulation.

Cyclodialysis

31

Omah S. Singh
Richard J. Simmons

Late-stage operations such as cyclodialysis have proved beneficial in the aphakic eye that has not responded previously to multiple operations, including new techniques such as trabeculectomy, in an attempt to control intraocular pressure (IOP) and prevent progressive disc and field damage.[1-5] The art of glaucoma surgery has been modified over the years with the advent of new instrumentation[6] as well as techniques designed to improve the success rate and minimize complications, especially those of hypotony and phthisis.[7] Included are various types of implants to maintain an open cleft[8-23] cyclodialysis in combination with other operations,[24-33] modifications of the actual operation,[15,34-43] or postoperative care.[3,39]

Cyclodialysis, performed since 1905,[39-44] is a procedure to be considered in the end-stage glaucomatous eye. It has been limited to desperate eyes in which numerous previously unsuccessful glaucoma operations have been performed. Nevertheless, there remains an aura of distrust for this procedure, possibly stemming from a reputation for unpredictability (an all-or-none mechanism), a variable success rate,[1-3,5,41-47] and a reputation for a high incidence of complications including hypotony and its sequelae, such as cataract,[46] and phthisis. The prognosis for functional improvement following this operation has appeared to be poor. However, the eyes usually subjected to this procedure are complicated end-stage eyes in which the surgical options are limited, and the potential for phthisis is high with any form of surgical therapy.

For all practical purposes, cyclodialysis has been abandoned by many glaucoma experts. However, the relative simplicity of the procedure, with minimal complications when it is employed with proper technique, and the ability to repeat the operation make us reluctant to abandon it in eyes in which the chance of success with other procedures is extremely low.[47] Cyclodialysis has a significant chance of success in these eyes when the appropriate indications are observed.[3,5,27,41] Debate about the precise mechanism of action continues and the physiology is yet to be determined with certainty.[12,14,47-63]

In our experience, the alternative procedure of cyclocryotherapy is often accompanied by extensive exudates of fibrin and blood, cells and flare, vitreous debris, and in a substantial number of cases, there is a decrease in visual acuity. We have found this problem less common with cyclodialysis, our clinical experience (with surgery performed by members of our group from 1956 to 1984) supports the belief that the retention of cyclodialysis as an option for these difficult cases is justified. This appears to be supported by our results in the retrospective analysis of 96 cyclodialysis operations in 86 eyes of 78 patients. In the interests of reliability, we excluded those eyes in which follow-up management was inadequate for at least 6 months or in which penetrating cyclodiathermy was combined, as was frequently done several years ago.

SURGICAL TECHNIQUE

As with any other surgical procedure, there have been many modifications with varying degrees of success reported.[1,22,24,26,38] The basic aim of the operation is to disinsert an area of ciliary body from the overlying sclera in order to create a cleft communicating between the anterior chamber and the suprachoroidal space.

Our standard procedure is as follows. A beveled paracentesis wound is made with a Wheeler knife in the paralimbal area of the cornea at a site away from the location of the proposed operation. This provides access to the anterior chamber for later injection of air or balanced salt solution (BSS) (Fig. 31-1). The proposed quadrant is exposed, and a radial conjunctival incision is made in the center of this quadrant, approximately 5 to 6 mm long. Careful attention is paid to hemostasis, for which we use the monopolar underwater diathermy. A #15 Bard-Parker blade is then used to create a 3-mm incision through bare sclera 3.5 mm from the cor-

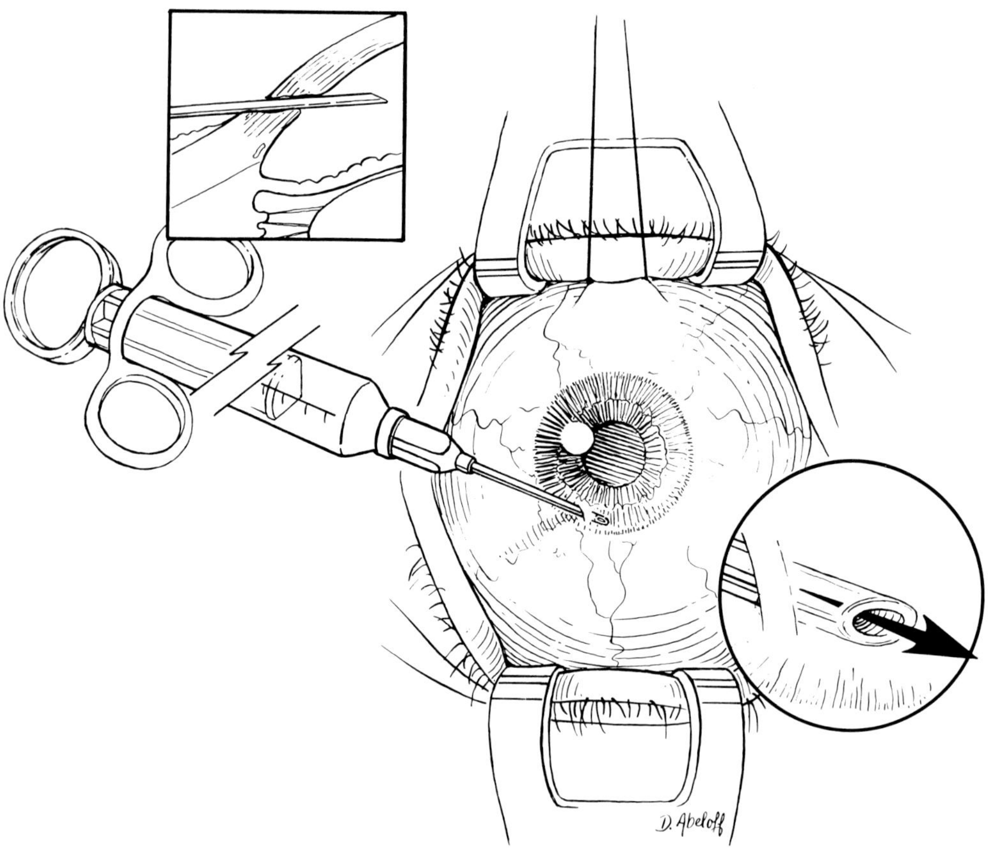

Fig. 31-1. A beveled paracentesis incision is made through the cornea into the anterior chamber using a thin blade. This permits injection of balanced salt solution (BSS) or air through a beveled, full, smooth needle (bottom inset) into the anterior chamber. The corneal wound is sloping and self-sealing (upper inset). A #23 blunt needle is used for injection into the anterior chamber.

neal limbus to the anterior edge of the wound. The #15 Bard-Parker blade is ideal because sharper blades such as the Beaver, Diamond, or Super blades are more likely to cut the uvea; we have found the blunt blade satisfactory in opening the sclera without damaging the underlying uvea, which should not bleed at all during the procedure (Fig. 31-2).

The sclera is slowly dissected until the choroidal tissue is visualized through the base of the incision, taking care to avoid cutting into the choroidal tissue (Fig. 31-2). A cyclodialysis spatula is then inserted into the supraciliary space with the tip of the spatula tightly pressed against the sclera to prevent perforation of the choroid (Fig. 31-3). The aim is to separate the tissue planes bluntly at the scleral spur. We find the Simmons-Kimbrough spatula[6] ideal, since it is blunt, strong, and short; thus, when swept into the anterior chamber, it will not rub the endothelium or Descemet's membrane, except in the far periphery. A sharp instrument is not appropriate, as it can cut the uvea. A long spatula is also undesirable, since the heel can abut the fornix and decrease control of the spatula and its motion, or it can sweep far into the anterior chamber and disrupt the endothelium and Descemet's membrane of the cornea. If this occurs within the peripheral 1 mm of the cornea, there is no significant functional effect; if the central cornea is injured, however, visual difficulty can result. The spatula is

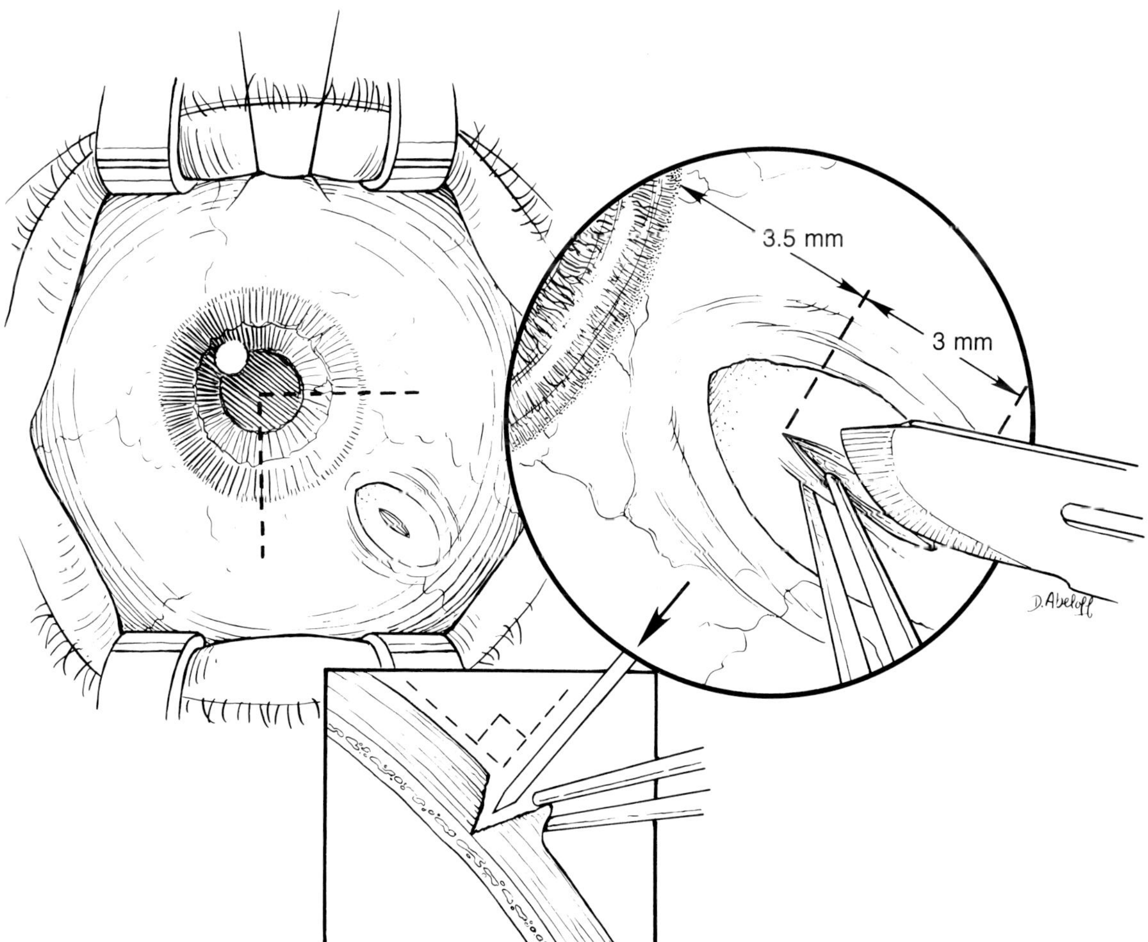

Fig. 31-2. Full-thickness scleral dissection with a #15 Bard-Parker blade to the uvea. The incision is 3 mm long and 3.5 mm from the corneal limbus to the anterior edge of the wound. The sclera is cut perpendicularly to the choroid.

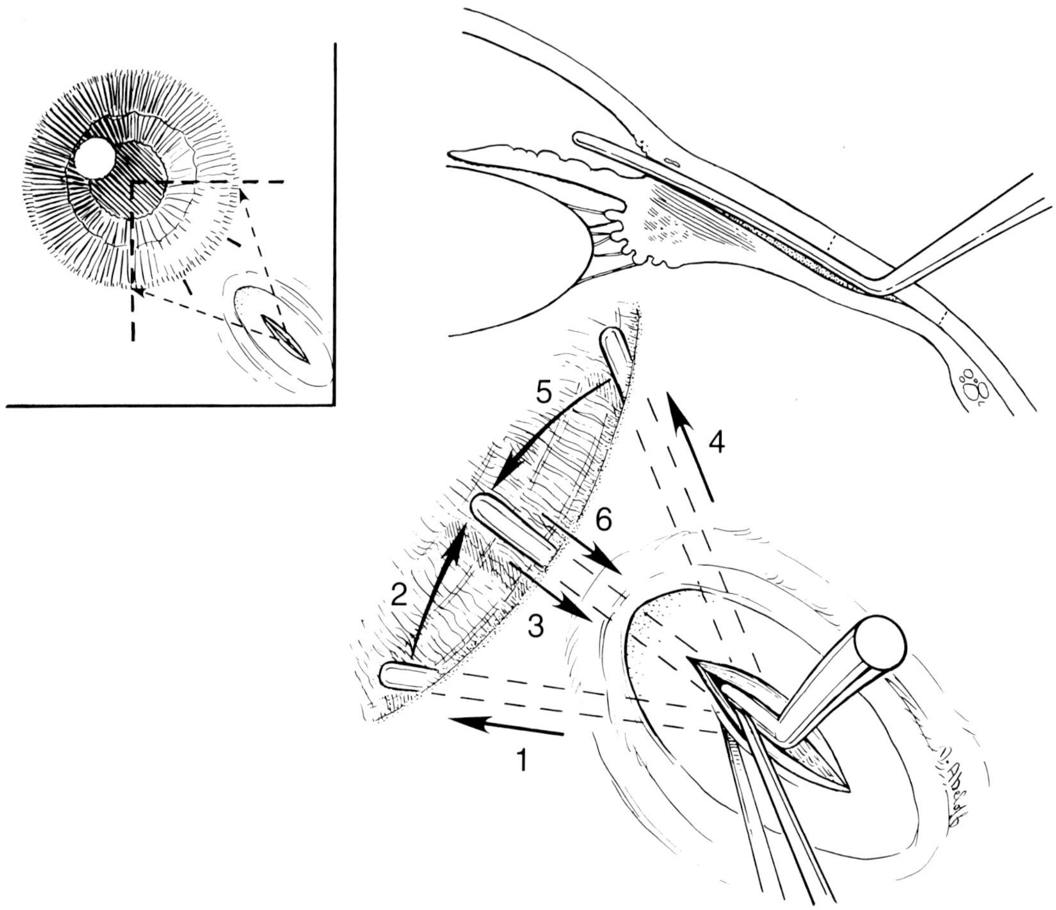

Fig. 31-3. Cyclodialysis performed to include one quadrant (upper inset). The spatula tip is pressed against sclera into anterior chamber at scleral spur. Insert spatula at 1, sweep to 2, and withdraw at 3. Reinsert at 4, sweep in opposite direction, and withdraw at 6. Repeat this procedure to ensure that all attachments of uvea to scleral spur are separated.

then guided forward with pressure against the sclera until it causes visible bulging, to a position approximately at the 2 o'clock position away from the incision, and is gradually advanced until the tip appears at the limbus in the anterior chamber (Fig. 31-3). This helps ensure that the tip remains in the proper plane when it enters the anterior chamber. The spatula is then slowly and carefully swept from one side to the center of the wound in a position radial to the limbus, dialyzing the ciliary body with slight downward pressure of the tip of the spatula, taking care not to injure Descemet's membrane. It is crucial to achieve a plane not in or behind the iris. If the tip enters in or behind the iris, it should be withdrawn and another attempt made to achieve the proper plane. The spatula is withdrawn, re-inserted into the suprachoroidal space to enter the anterior chamber in the opposite direction 2 clock hours away from the incision, sweeping in from the other side across the anterior chamber, to join the previous portion of the cleft. The spatula is then carefully withdrawn, keeping the tip close to the sclera and avoiding injury to the choroid. On completion, there is a separation in the form of a cleft; at this point, the spatula is passed back and forth from side to side, in order to allow clean separation of the ciliary body from the scleral spur and separate any strands or attachments that may remain in this area. Finally, the spatula is withdrawn.

At this time, there is usually a small amount of

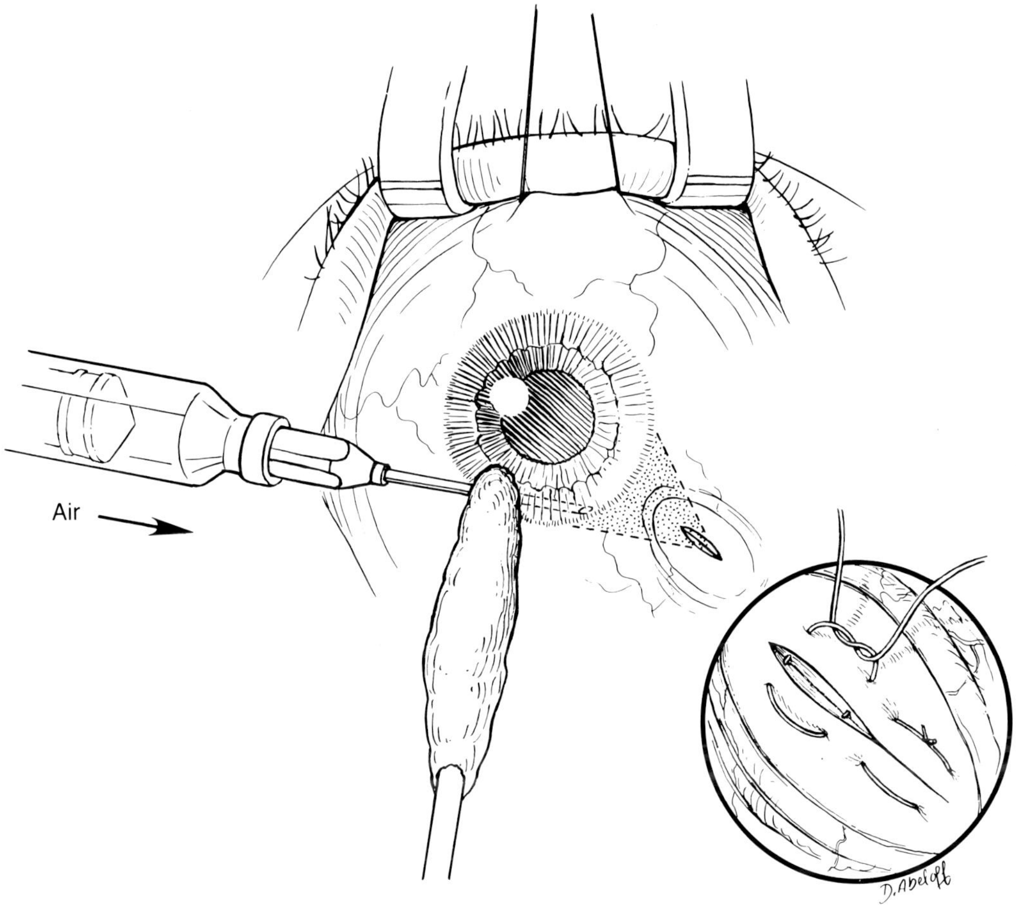

Fig. 31-4. Air injected into the anterior chamber (AC) through paracentesis wound until firm. Tamponade is applied when needle withdrawn to keep air in the AC.

oozing into the anterior chamber, but bleeding may be brisk. Air is quickly injected into the anterior chamber through the paracentesis wound (Fig. 31-4) until the eye is firm (on testing with gentle compression with a muscle hook), and the bleeding stops. The scleral incision is then closed using one or two 10-0 nylon mattress sutures (Fig. 31-4). The conjunctival edges are reapposed with two interrupted 10-0 nylon mattress sutures. After 3 to 4 minutes, the air is partially replaced with BSS, leaving an air bubble that fills approximately a third of the anterior chamber (Fig. 31-5).

At the end of the procedure, a drop of phospholine iodide, 0.25 percent, is instilled into the conjunctival sac, antibiotic ointment is applied, and an eyepad and shield are applied.

Postoperatively, the patient is maintained on limited activity for the first 24 hours. Steroid drops are started 4 hours postoperatively and instilled every hour until bedtime to the operated eye. A full regimen of tolerated glaucoma medications is continued. The patient is discharged home the next day, but if considerable fresh bleeding is noted on the first postoperative day, the patient is kept in-hospital for an additional day or two until the eye appears stable. Some glaucoma medications are gradually withdrawn as the tension stabilizes postoperatively. However, the operated eye is maintained on phospholine iodide 0.25 percent BID indefinitely. Our experience supports that of other observers[4,5,15,27] that a strong miotic is important in maintaining a functional cleft. When miotic ther-

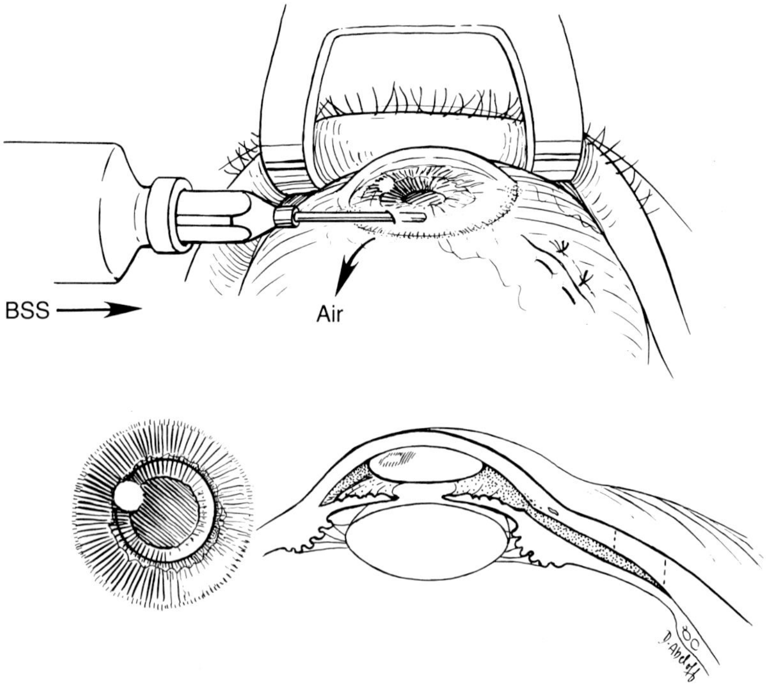

Fig. 31-5. Balanced salt solution (BSS) partially replaces air. (Inset) Air bubble in the anterior chamber (AC).

apy is discontinued, closure of the cleft is a dramatic and frequently observed complication.[64]

RESULTS

In order to tabulate and analyze the results, we have established certain clinically useful categories. Clinical improvement is defined here as a nonphthisical lowering of pressure either with or without glaucoma medications to 22 mmHg or less, with clinical evidence of prevention of further field loss or disc damage. Many of the eyes in this group had pressures within the 40- to 60-mmHg range preoperatively, were aphakic with extensive glaucomatous disc damage and field loss, and had some disease in which conventional therapy was unlikely to succeed, and in which multiple previous glaucoma operations had failed. A reduction in pressure to 22 mmHg or less is clinically significant when it results in the absence of further field loss and disc damage. This is in contrast to many cases of chronic open-angle glaucoma that have persisted for years with chronic, advancing cupping and gradual visual-field loss. Frequently the final pressure does not tell the entire story, we have therefore tabulated the amount of pressure reduction as a percentage reduction of the original pressure to indicate the amount of improvement obtained, as well as the final pressure level, which will be more useful in predicting the ultimate fate of the eye.

In this study, it was necessary to distinguish hypotony from phthisis, since clinically eyes with very soft pressure often had a very different prognosis, outcome, and visual function from those with phthisis. Some eyes attained pressures at 5 mmHg or less yet retained their useful visual function and stability. These eyes were defined as hypotonous. Other eyes, however, followed the typical course of phthisis; that is, the pressure decreased to progressively lower levels (often to 0), corneas thickened, anterior chambers became obliterated, and eyes shrunk with vision progressing to blindness or bare light perception and frequently with pain. These eyes we considered phthisical, a different and worse course from those that appeared to retain useful visual acuity in spite of pressures in the hypotonous range ($\leq$5 mmHg).

This series analyzes 96 operations performed on

Table 31-1. Results

Ocular Status	Patients	No. of Eyes	No. of Operations	M:F	OD:OS	Avg. Age (years)	Avg. Follow-up Time (months)
Phakic	13	14	15	7:6	8:5	36.8 yr (9 mo–80 yr)	33.6 mo (6–87)
Aphakic	66	72	81	29:37	31:35	62.8 yr (10–90 yr)	50.4 mo (3–146)
Total	78[a]	86	96	36:43[a]	39:40[a]	59.2 yr	46.2 mo

[a] One patient with one phakic and one aphakic eye.

86 eyes of 78 patients (Table 31-1). The total population was then subdivided into an aphakic and phakic group. The aphakic group consisted of 66 patients in whom 81 cyclodialysis operations were performed on 72 eyes. In the phakic group, there were 13 patients with 15 cyclodialyses on 14 eyes. The discrepancy in the total number of patients results from one patient who had one phakic eye and one aphakic eye, both of which were treated with cyclodialysis. We first present our findings on the aphakic group.

Table 31-1 shows that a total of 66 aphakic patients had 81 operations on 72 eyes. The average age of this group was 62.8 years (range 10 to 90 years). The average follow up time of all 66 patients was 50.4 months (6 to 146 months). There were 29 males and 37 females with a distribution of 31 right eyes and 35 left eyes. All the other patients in this study had a minimum follow-up of 6 months.

In the phakic patients, 15 operations were performed on 14 eyes of 13 patients. The average age of this group was 36.8 years (range 9 months to 80 years). The average follow-up time was 33.6 months (range 6 to 87 months). There were seven males and six females with a total of eight right eyes and five left eyes.

Table 31-2 shows the distribution of patients according to the type of glaucoma.

In analyzing the data, we used two approaches to our definition of improvement: (1) a final pressure of 21 mmHg or less was considered satisfactory, since many of these patients had preoperative pressures in the 40 to 60-mmHg range and a pressure of 21 mmHg represented a significant improvement; and (2) when the final IOP was expressed as a percentage of the preoperative tension, the extent of clinical improvement was better appreciated. Improvement was defined as postoperative IOP control of 21 mmHg or less with or without medication; 32 of 66 eyes of aphakic patients (49 percent) demonstrated improved tension: The final postoperative IOP was 5 mmHg or less in 3 patients, 6 to 15 mmHg in 10 patients, 11 to 15 mmHg in 7 patients, and 16 to 22 mmHg in 12 patients.

Three other patients had IOPs of 23, 25, and 28 mmHg, respectively, but were not included in this analysis. However, these patients did have a significant decrease in tension from their preoperative values and actually did have clinical improvement (56, 37, and 44 percent, respectively).

When the improvement in IOP was calculated as a percentage of preoperative pressure, 35 of 66 eyes (53 percent) showed clinically significant improvement: The final postoperative IOP (percentage decrease in preoperative tension) was at least 75 percent in 11 patients, 50 to 74 percent in 15 patients, 25 to 49 percent in 9 patients, and less than 25 percent in 1 patient.

The effect of other factors on the success rate was examined.

In Table 31-3, bleeding at the time of, or within

Table 31-2. Glaucoma Types in Phakic and Aphakic Eyes

	Primary			ACG Secondary						
Ocular Status	OAG	ACG	CONG	Uveitis	Pup. Block with PAS	Secondary Scleral Buckle	Post-Cat Flat AC	Malignant Glaucoma	Iris Cyst	Angle Recession
Phakic	5	2	7	—	—	—	—	—	—	—
Aphakic	31	10	—	6	14	2	4	3	1	1
Total Eyes[a]	36	12	7	6	14	2	4	3	1	1

[a] Total: 86 eyes.

Table 31-3. Bleeding at Time of Surgery: Aphakic Patients

Complications at Surgery	Improved		Unimproved		Total Patients	
	N	%	N	%	N	%
Bleed	22	55	18	45	40	61
No bleed	17	65	9	35	26	39
Total	39	59	27	41	66	

[a] $\chi^2 = 0.38$, not significant.

Table 31-4. Glaucoma Type: Aphakic Patients

Glaucoma Type	Improved		Unimproved		Total	
	N	%	N	%	N	%
Primary	15	43	20	57	35	100
Secondary	22	71	9	29	31	100
Total	37		29		66	

[a] $\chi^2 = 5.27$; $P < 0.05$, significant.

the first week of, surgery was found to have no significant influence on the eventual prognosis for improvement in pressure. In Table 31-4, our findings strongly suggest that the secondary glaucomas, with angle closure from peripheral anterior synechiae, show a higher success rate from cyclodialysis than do the primary glaucomas. Further analysis of the data suggests that the presence and extent of angle closure by peripheral synechiae appear to have no significant effect on the eventual outcome of surgery.

In Table 31-5, secondary glaucoma was analyzed in greater detail, and the results were consistent with our findings that secondary glaucoma tended to respond well to cyclodialysis. Of special interest are the three cases of malignant glaucoma in which none of the patients improved with cyclodialysis, all had previous surgery (two patients had two previous operations, and one patient had one previous operation), all patients had preoperative visual

Table 31-5. Types of Secondary Glaucoma: Aphakic Patients[a]

Diagnosis	Improved		Unimproved		Total	
	N	%	N	%	N	%
Secondary to uveitis	4	67	2	33	6	100
Aphakia with pupillary block (secondary closure by PAS)	12	86	2	14	14	100
ACG secondary to scleral buckle	2	100	0		2	100
ACG with PAS secondary to flat AC post-cat. extraction	4	100	0		4	100
Epithelial iris cyst, secondary trauma	0		1		1	
Malignant glaucoma	0		3	100	3	100
Secondary to angle recession	1	100	0		1	

[a] Total: 31 patients.

Table 31-6. Previous Glaucoma Surgery in Aphakic and Phakic Patients

Ocular Status	No. of Previous Glaucoma Operations								Total Patients with Previous Surgery	
	0	1	2	3	4	5	6	7	N	%
Aphakic	21	23	11	6	4	0	0	1	45/66	68
Phakic	4	2	2	2	1	0	2	0	9/13	69

Table 31-7. Influence of Previous Glaucoma Surgery on Success of Cyclodialysis[a]

Ocular Status	Previous Glaucoma Surgery	Improved		Unimproved		Total	
		N	%	N	%		
Aphakic	Yes	21	45	23	52	44	100
Aphakic	No	16	73	5	27	21	100

[a] $\chi^2 = 4.70$; $P < 0.05$, significant.

Table 31-8. Age of Aphakic Patients[a]

Age (years)	No. of Improved Patients		No. of Unimproved Patients		Total Patients	
	N	%	*N*	%	*N*	%
61+	28	65	15	35	43	100
60−	9	39	14	61	23	100

[a] $\chi^2 = 4.11$; $P < 0.05$, significant.

acuity of counting fingers, and all patients showed failure of IOP control with an actual worsening of pressures noted within 1 month or less postoperatively. However, no valid conclusions can be drawn because of the small series.

In Table 31-6, 45 of 66 (68 percent) of the aphakic and 9 of 13 (69 percent) of the phakic patients had previous glaucoma surgery. In Table 31-7, analysis of our data shows that in the aphakic eye, previous glaucoma surgery appears to decrease the chances of clinical improvement from cyclodialysis significantly.

As shown in Table 31-8, our findings are consistent with those of other studies, demonstrating that older patients tend to respond in a more favorable manner to cyclodialysis. This is not unexpected, since younger patients respond poorly to most forms of glaucoma surgery. In our series of patients, the position of the cleft does not have a significant effect on the successful outcome of surgery (Table 31-9), unlike other series,[42] in which the upper quadrants were most successful. However, when cyclodialysis is combined with cataract extraction, the location of the cleft superiorly appears to result in a significantly higher success rate.[65]

In this series, most of the eyes that showed failure of IOP control with cyclodialysis did so within the first 5 months, and none of the eyes that showed improvement has thus far demonstrated loss of glaucoma control after 2 years. In this group, IOP control failed postoperatively in 16 patients after 1 month, in 13 patients after 2 to 5 months, in 2 patients after 6 months to 1 year, and in 1 patient between 1 and 2 years.

Table 31-9. Location of Cleft in Aphakic Patients[a,b]

Location of Cleft	No. of Improved Eyes		No. of Unimproved Eyes		Total	
	N	%	*N*	%	*N*	%
Superior	14	56	11	44	25	100
Inferior	22	54	19	46	41	100

[a] Total patients: 66.
[b] $\chi^2 = 0.03$, not significant.

COMPLICATIONS

Complications are numerous, as with any surgical procedure[66-69] with phthisis frequently cited as a dreaded complication. Our experience with this procedure has been favorable when one considers that these are difficult eyes in which conventional surgery would likely have failed.

Complications Encountered

Bleeding

The most frequent complication encountered in this series was bleeding into the anterior chamber either at surgery or within the first week postoperatively. Of the aphakic eyes, 40 of 66 (60 percent) had operative bleeding. Most of these had a slight ooze of blood into the anterior chamber at the time of surgery. Analysis showed no significance in the surgical success rate in the eyes that showed no bleeding or a small amount of blood. Of the eight eyes with moderate bleeding into the anterior chamber at surgery, four improved, three were unimproved, and one progressed to phthisis. The latter occurred in one eye of a 14-year-old girl with uveitis and secondary glaucoma that was unimproved after several surgical glaucoma procedures. Seven eyes bled considerably at surgery, with three of the seven bleeding into the vitreous. Five of these seven eyes improved, and two were unimproved. Both eyes had three previous failed operations each. Finally, six eyes showed no bleeding at the time of surgery but developed moderate anterior chamber hyphema 3 to 4 days postoperatively. Of these, two improved and four were unimproved. These four eyes each had two to four previous unsuccessful glaucoma operations.

There is no evidence from our results to suggest that the bleeding that occurs at surgery adversely affects the success rate of the procedure, with 50 percent of patients experiencing moderate bleeding and 70 percent of these with large hyphemas at surgery showing clinically significant improvement. The only group in which improvement was poor were those eyes that had late hyphemas (only two of six improved). However, all the unimproved eyes had at least two previous unsuccessful glaucoma surgeries.

Inflammation

Inflammation is no greater than with other procedures and is generally less than that seen with cyclocryotherapy.

Visual Loss

Visual loss is frequently cited as a complication of cyclodialysis. In our series, of the aphakic patients with a successful result, defined either as a 25 percent or greater decrease from preoperative tension (32 of 66) or postoperative tension of 22 mmHg or less (36 of 66), only one patient in the hypotony group (≤5 mmHg) showed visual decrease due to macular edema; the others retained the preoperative level of vision or showed improved acuity.

In phakic eyes in this study, 4 of 14 (29 percent) showed improvement in glaucoma control. Of these, all patients retained preoperative vision, although one eye had bleeding and vitreous loss at the time of surgery. Of the 10 phakic eyes that did not improve with cyclodialysis, visual acuity was unknown in three eyes (all these infants under 14 months of age), three eyes retained preoperative vision, and the other four progressed to phthisis.

Phthisis

Phthisis is a dreaded complication that has possibly fostered the greatest fear of cyclodialysis. In the desperate glaucomatous eye that has failed to show clinical improvement after previous glaucoma operations, any additional surgical procedure carries a real and significant risk of phthisis. This is not exclusive to cyclodialysis; in our series of patients, all the eyes that proceeded to phthisis were complicated cases. In our series of 86 eyes (78 patients), three of 14 phakic eyes (21 percent) and three of 72 aphakic eyes (4 percent) progressed to phthisis.

Closure of the Cleft

Closure of the cleft usually presents as a sudden marked increase in IOP in an eye that has maintained stable tension after cyclodialysis.[64] The symptoms are reminiscent of an angle-closure glaucoma attack. Attempts to reopen the cleft include miotic therapy with strong miotics, such as phospholine iodide and laser to the cleft.[49] In our series, seven eyes showed this complication. Three of seven (42 percent) patients were reversed with medical and/or laser therapy. Two patients had bilateral closure 8 weeks postoperatively; one 4 weeks postoperatively, with the patient discontinuing miotic therapy; the other two occurred at 3 months and 21 months postoperatively. The bilateral cases were unresponsive to miotics or laser, miotics restored tension control in the patient who discontinued treatment, and the other two patients improved following laser to the cleft.

CONCLUSIONS

1. In the aphakic complicated eye, cyclodialysis is a valuable procedure that should be retained as an option in the surgical armamentarium for uncontrolled glaucoma. If success is defined as a clinically significant improvement in IOP, 22 mmHg or less or a decrease of greater than 25 percent from the preoperative tension, then 50 percent of the aphakic eyes in our series, showed a successful result from cyclodialysis.
2. In the phakic eye in this series, the success rate was approximately 30 percent. However, this is still a valuable option in these desperate eyes, in which numerous other procedures have been tried and have failed.
3. The secondary glaucomas appear to respond more favorably (71 percent) than do the primary (43 percent) forms to cyclodialysis; this operation may be considered an early surgical option in aphakic eyes with secondary glaucoma.
4. The eyes with malignant glaucoma in our series showed a consistently poor result. However, the number of cases is too small to form any statistical conclusion.

5. The complications of bleeding and inflammation do not affect the outcome of surgery significantly and are generally not as severe as often quoted.
6. In aphakes, postoperative visual loss secondary to hypotony is infrequent (approximately 3 percent). In phakic eyes with improvement, visual loss was not a complication.
7. Phthisis and subsequent visual loss was seen in 3 of 72 (4 percent) of aphakic eyes and in 3 of 14 (21 percent) of phakic eyes. However, all these cases were complicated, and most had several previous glaucoma operations which had failed.
8. Previous glaucoma surgery appears to decrease the success of surgery significantly. This undoubtedly had some influence on the success rates noted here.
9. One interesting fact was noted in this series: in the seven pairs of eyes with bilateral cyclodialysis, the result of surgery in one eye was a consistent indicator of potential for success in the fellow eye. This has been shown for other types of glaucoma surgery and has been the impression of other investigators but to our knowledge has not previously been confirmed for cyclodialysis. This is therefore not entirely unexpected but would suggest that if cyclodialysis has failed in the first eye, the surgeon should consider other available options for the second eye. However, if the first eye is improved with cyclodialysis, the likelihood for success in the second eye is good. In a similar pattern, seven eyes showed closure of the cleft; two of these eyes showed improvement with laser to the cleft, and one eye improved and remained stable following initiation of miotic therapy. However, in two patients, the closure was irreversible bilaterally, suggesting the need for close observation of the second eye in the patient with bilateral cyclodialysis in whom one eye has had cleft closure.

ACKNOWLEDGMENTS

We wish to thank Sam Douglas for his assistance and patience in the gathering of information, Julie Slattery, Gail Johnson, Lisa Marini, and Linda Terry for their invaluable help in the compilation of this work; and Dr. Paul A. Chandler for providing the benefit of his knowledge and experience.

REFERENCES

1. Gradle HS: Cyclodialysis. Am J Ophthalmol 3:41, 1920
2. Grosz E: Indikation Zur Zyklodialyse. Ber Dtsch Ophthalmol Ges 44:151, 1924
3. Hausmann G: Zur Kenntnis der Dauerresultate der Zyklodialyse. Z Augenheilkd 92:139, 1937
4. Gorin G: Action of Di-isopropyl-florophosphate on cyclodialysis clefts. Am J Ophthalmol p. 789, 1960
5. Sugar HS: Cyclodialysis: A follow-up study. Am J Ophthalmol 30:843, 1947
6. Simmons RJ, Kimbrough R: A modified cyclodialysis spatula. Ophthalmic Surg 10(2):67, 1979
8. Gills JP Jr: Action of cyclodialysis utilizing an implant studied by manometry in a human eye. Exp Eye Res 6:75, 1967
9. Gills JP Jr: Mode of action of cyclodialysis implants in man. Invest Ophthalmol 6(2):141, 1967
10. Clark ST: Gonioscopic observations in cyclodialysis operation. Am J Ophthalmol 24:1026, 1941
11. Swan KC: A scleral flap for combined cyclodialysis and iridectomy. Arch Ophthalmol 71:166, 1964
12. Alper MG: Ciliary body detachment for control of glaucoma. Am J Ophthalmol 61:1490, 1966
13. Kronfeld PC: Anatomic changes after cyclodialysis. Arch Ophthalmol 15:411, 1936
14. Barkan O, Boyle SF, Maisler S: On the surgery of glaucoma: Mode of action of cyclodialysis. Am J Ophthalmol 19:21, 1936
15. Barkan O: Cyclodialysis, multiple or single with air injection. Am J Ophthalmol 30:1063, 1947
16. Barsky D, Schimek RA: Evaluation of absorbable gelatin film (Gelfilm) in cyclodialysis. Arch Ophthalmol 60:1044, 1958
17. Troncoso MU: Cyclodialysis with insertion of a metal implant in the treatment of glaucoma: A preliminary report. Arch Ophthalmol 233:270, 1940
18. Sugar HS: Experiences with some modifications of cyclodialysis for aphakic glaucoma. Ann Ophthalmol 9:1045, 1977
19. Portney GL: Silicone elastomer implantation cyclodialysis. Ophthalmic Surg 5:30, 1974
20. Pinnas G: Cyclodialysis with Teflon tube implants. Am J Ophthalmol 68:879, 1969

21. Nesterov AP: Implantation of a scleral strip into the supraciliary space and cyclodialysis in glaucoma. Acta Ophthalmol (Copenh) 56:697, 1978
22. Boshoff PH: Use of Troncoso's magnesium implant in cyclodialysis for relief of glaucoma: Observations in two cases. Arch Ophthalmol 33:404, 1945
23. Flieringa HJ: Cyclodialysis combined with posterior trephining. Br J Ophthalmol 36:518, 1952
24. Cusick PL: Cyclodialysis with goniotomy in congenital glaucoma. Am J Ophthalmol 38:712, 1954
25. Cavka V: Non-perforating cyclodiathermy with cyclodialysis circumscripta in glaucoma. Br J Ophthalmol 35:307, 1951
26. Carbajal UM: Cyclodiathermy-dialysis: A tunnelizing procedure for glaucoma. Am J Ophthalmol 48:311, 1959
27. Barkan O: Cyclogoniotomy. Am J Ophthalmol 42:63, 1956
28. Alvis BY: Cyclodialysis with scleral shrinkage for open-angle glaucoma. Trans Am Ophthalmol Soc 56:263, 1958
29. Alvis BY: Cyclodialysis with scleral shrinkage for open-angle glaucoma. Trans Am Ophthalmol Soc 47:795, 1959
30. Wooton HW: Cyclodialysis combined with iridectomy in glaucoma simplex: A preliminary report. Trans Am Ophthalmol Soc 30:64, 1932
31. Wheeler JM: Iridectomy with cyclodialysis for the reduction of ocular tension. Arch Ophthalmol 16:569, 1936
32. Romem M: Peripheral iridectomy and cyclodialysis as simultaneous operation in glaucoma surgery. Acta Ophthalmol (Copenk) 50:26, 1972
33. Shaffer RN: Inverse cyclodialysis. Am J Ophthalmol 30:860, 1947
34. Zehetbauer G: Experimental findings in cyclodialysis for the reduction of ocular tension. Arch Ophthalmol 16(4):569, 1936
35. O'Brien CS: Cyclodialysis. Arch Ophthalmol 42:606, 1949
36. Periera RF: Inverse cyclodialysis of blaskovics. Arch Ophthalmol (Buenos Aires) 14:547, 1939
37. Ascher KW: Some details of the technique of cyclodialysis. Am J Ophthalmol 50:1207, 1960
38. Malbran JL: Submuscular sclerecto-cyclodialysis: A new technique for anti-glaucoma operation. Am J Ophthalmol 36:365, 1953
39. Lee OS: Cyclodialysis. I. A discussion of techniques. Am J Ophthalmol 32:1713, 1949
40. Ivanov SN: Cyclodialysis with posterior sclerectomy. Vestn Oftalmol 11:519, 1937
41. Haisten MW: Cyclodialysis with air injection: Technique and results in 94 consecutive operations. Arch Ophthalmol 59:507, 1958
42. Viikari K: On cyclodialysis surgery in the light of follow-up examinations. Acta Ophthalmol (Copenh) 35:528, 1957
43. Touvinen E: On hypotony following cyclodialysis surgery. Acta Ophthalmol (Copenh) 35:543, 1957
44. Schultz RO, Watzke RC, Sawyer TR: The long-term results from cyclodialysis. Arch Ophthalmol 64:408, 1960
45. DeSaint-Martin: La cyclodialyse, sa technique, son pronostic, ses indications. Bull Soc Fr Ophthalmol 49:157, 1936
46. McPherson SD: Cyclodialysis in the treatment of glaucoma. Am Ophthalmol 29:848, 1946
47. Bellows AR: Cyclocryotherapy: Its role in the treatment of glaucoma. Persp Ophthalmol 4:139, 1980
48. Bailliart JP: La cyclodialyse dans le traitement du glaucome chronique. Bull Soc Paris 47:636, 1935
49. Harbin TS: Treatment of cyclodialysis clefts with argon laser photocoagulation. Ophthalmology 89:1082, 1982
50. Chandler PA, Maumenee AE: A major cause of hypotony. Am J Ophthalmol 24:1026, 1941
51. Kronfeld PC: The fluid exchange in the successfully cyclodialyzed eye. Trans Am Ophthalmol Soc 52:249, 1954
52. Grant WM: Experimental aqueous perfusion in enucleated human eyes. Arch Ophthalmol 69:783, 1963
53. Gills JP: Cyclodialysis studied by manometric techniques in the monkey. Br J Ophthalmol 51:199, 1967
54. Elschinig A: Zur Wirkungsweise der Cyclodialyse. Ber Dtsch Ophthalmol Ges 49:277, 1952
55. Dellaporta A, Obear M: Hyposecretion hypotony: Experimental hypotony through detachment of the uvea. Am J Ophthalmol 58:785, 1964
56. Bill A: The movement of albumin and dextran through the sclera. Arch Ophthalmol 74:248, 1965
57. Bill A: The routes for bulk drainage of aqueous humor in rabbits with and without cyclodialysis. Doc Ophthalmol 20:157, 1966
58. Becker B: Clinical aqueous outflow. Arch Ophthalmol 50:557, 1953
59. Barkan O: Cyclodialysis: Its mode of action. Arch Ophthalmol 43:793, 1950
60. Pederson JE, Gausterland DE, MacLellan HM: Experimental ciliochoroidal detachment: Effect on intraocular pressure and aqueous humor flow. Arch Ophthalmol 97:536, 1979
61. Sugar HS: Some recent advances in the surgery of glaucoma. Am J Ophthalmol 54:917, 1962
62. Shea M: Ciliary body reattachment in ocular hypotony. Arch Ophthalmol 99:278, 1981
63. Saeterren T, Thomassen TL: The escape of aqueous

humor after cyclodialysis. Acta Ophthalmol (Kbh) 35:372, 1957

64. Wagdi SF, Simmons RJ: Acute glaucoma from unrecognized closure of surgical cyclodialysis cleft. Glaucoma 3:287, 1981
65. Shields MB, Simmons RJ: Combined cyclodialysis and cataract extraction. Arch Ophthalmol 81:286, 1976
66. Barasch K: Post-cyclodialysis hypotony. Am J Ophthalmol 68:644, 1969
67. Bjorkenheim B: On hypotony following cyclodialysis and its treatment. Acta Ophthalmol (Copenh) 30:18, 1952
68. Miller SJH: Hypotony following cyclodialysis. Br J Ophthalmol 47:211, 1963
69. Neskerov AP, Batmanov E Jr, Cherkasova IN, Eporov EA: Surgical stimulation of the uveoscleral outflow. Acta Ophthalmol (Copenh) 57:409, 1979
69. Shaffer RN, Weiss DI: Concerning cyclodialysis and hypotony. Arch Ophthalmol 68:25, 1962

Section V

PLASTIC SURGERY

Bartley R. Frueh

Section Editor

Eyelid Anatomy

32

John L. Wobig

The eyelid is separated into five planes: (1) skin and subcutaneous fascia; (2) orbicularis oculi muscles and submuscular fascia; (3) septum orbitale; (4) retractors of the lids; and (5) tarsi and conjunctiva.

SKIN AND SUBCUTANEOUS FASCIA

The skin of the upper and lower lids is possibly the thinnest in the body. It is attached to the underlying orbicularis muscle. Transverse furrows are present that denote certain underlying anatomic structures. The superior palpebral furrow is where the firmly adherent pretarsal skin meets the loosely attached border of the tarsus. The inferior fibers of the levator aponeurosis pass into the overlying pretarsal muscle, at this point superior to the inferior margin of the septum. Superior to the furrow, the inferior margin of the septum orbitale attaches to the aponeurosis of the levator. The less noticeable furrow in the lower lid marks the inferior edge of the tarsus. The retractor of the lower lid and septum attach to the inferior edge of the tarsus. There is almost no fat in the skin of the lids other than a thin subcutaneous fascia.

ORBICULARIS OCULI MUSCLES

The orbicularis oculi muscles (Fig. 32-1) arise in the second branchial arch. They migrate medially, bending around the orbit like a horseshoe, attaching to the medial orbital wall. The muscles divide arbitrarily into three divisions on the basis of underlying structures. The pretarsal muscles are firmly attached to the tarsus. Medially, the pretarsal muscles unite from the upper and lower lid to create the medial canthal tendon. A deep head of the pretarsal muscles inserts on the lacrimal bone behind the posterior lacrimal crest. Laterally, the pretarsal muscles attach to the lateral orbital tubercle via a tendon. The preseptal muscles overlay the septum. The medial end of the muscles give a few fibers to the canthal tendon, but most of the fibers attach to the lacrimal diaphragm. The orbital portions of orbicularis muscles are superior to the preseptal muscles and cover the orbital margin. The corrugator supercilli muscle is composed of fibers from the orbicularis and frontalis muscles in a V-shaped pattern. The denser submuscular fascia is firmly attached to the posterior surface of the muscle. It contains a network of all the efferent facial nerve branches.

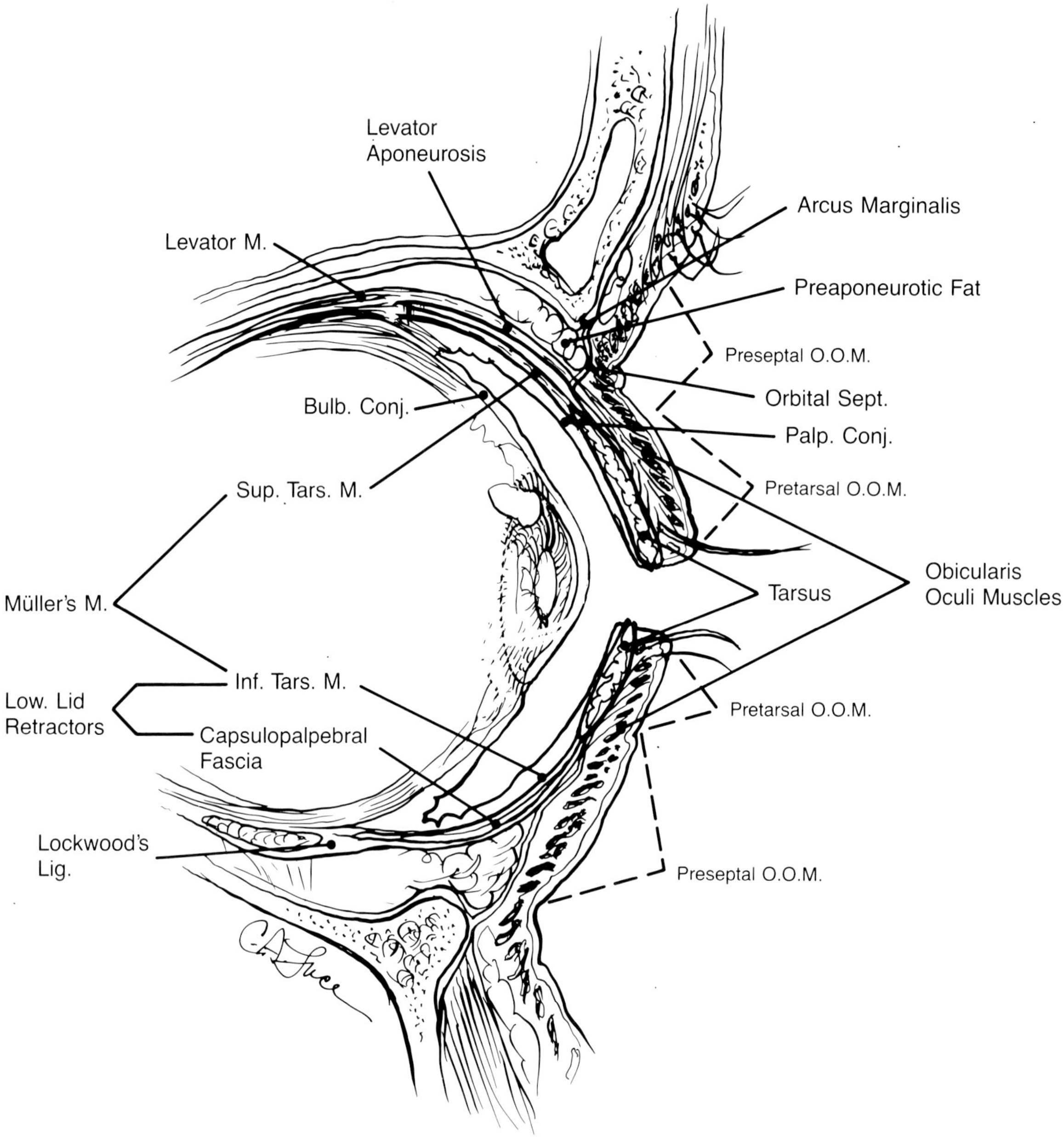

Fig. 32-1. Cross-sectional view of the eyelid anatomy.

SEPTUM ORBITALE

The orbital septum is a thin sheet of fibrous tissue that originates in the periosteum of the orbital margins (Fig. 32-1). A strong band of tissue formed by the junction of the periosteum and periorbita at the orbital margin is called the arcus marginalis. Superiorly, the septum fuses with the levator aponeurosis from 5 mm superior to the tarsus to the upper tarsal margin. In the lower lid, the septum attaches to the tarsus. It acts as a barrier between the orbit and anterior eyelid.

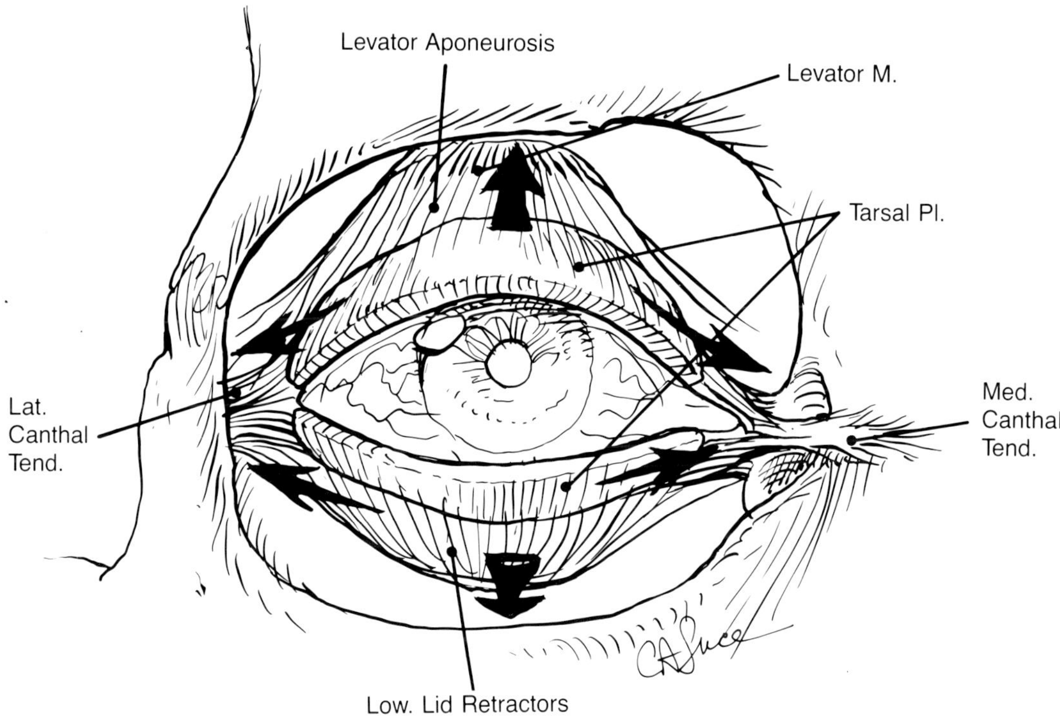

Fig. 32-2. Frontal view of the eyelid anatomy.

RETRACTORS OF THE LIDS

The upper lid retractor is the levator palpebrae superioris (Figs. 32-1 and 32-2). It arises from the apex of the orbit with a tendon fused with a tendon of the superior rectus. The levator progresses anteriorly and divides into two layers at a point where it changes from a horizontal to a more vertical direction. The aponeurosis, the superior layer of the levator, spreads out to form a medial and lateral horn. The superior transverse ligament lies 10 mm above the insertions of the horn, a condensation of fascia from the common sheath. The aponeurosis attaches to the lower one third of the tarsus on its anterior surface and to the pretarsal orbicularis muscle by fibrous bands. Müller's muscle, or superior tarsal muscle (Fig. 32-1), is the deep head of the levator. This smooth muscle attaches to the superior border of the tarsus. An important consideration is the lateral horn of the levator, separating the lacrimal gland into an orbital and palpebral portion. The lower lid retractor is the same as the upper lid retractor, with the exception that it is a continuation of the inferior rectus muscle. The continuation is called the capsulopalpebral fascia; it has three divisions: Tenon's capsule, an inferior tarsal muscle, and the lower lid aponeurosis.

TARSI AND CONJUNCTIVA

The tarsi are the skeletal structures of the eyelid (Fig. 32-2). These firm plates of fibrous tissue contain meibomian glands. The tarsus is approximately 10 mm wide in the upper lid, and 3 to 5 mm wide in the lower lid. The conjunctiva is the internal covering of the lids. The nonkeratinizing squamous epithelium contains goblet cells and the accessory crimal glands of Krause and Wolfring. Preaponeurotic fat separates the septum from the levator. There are usually two fat pads in the upper lid and three in the lower lid continuous with the orbital fat. These act as a cushion to permit movement of the tarsi.

Evaluation of Blepharoptosis

33

Bartley R. Frueh

CLASSIFICATION AND CHARACTERIZATION OF PTOSIS

Blepharoptosis is caused by (1) a defect in the levator or superior tarsal muscle (myogenic); (2) a defect in the transmission of the force of the levator muscle to the lid (aponeurotic); (3) a defect in the nerve supply to either the levator or superior tarsal muscle (neurogenic); or (4) excessive weight on the eyelid pulling it down, inadequate posterior support to the lid, or scar tissue restricting its movement (mechanical), or a combination of these factors.[1] Each of these four types may be present at birth or have its onset some time after birth. Each may be caused by trauma. With the exception of aponeurotic ptosis, each of these groups has various subgroups that must be differentiated. Pseudoptosis may be caused by a hypotropic eye, contralateral upper lid retraction, or dermatochalasis giving the appearance of ptosis.

The two main subgroups of myogenic ptosis deserve special consideration, as they are managed quite differently. J.L. Hargiss (personal communication, 1985) has recommended calling these dysmyogenic ptosis and myopathic ptosis. Dysmyogenic ptosis is the maldevelopment of the levator muscle as it differentiates embryologically. This occurrence is bilateral in 25 percent of cases and unilateral in 75 percent.[2] The levator muscles of these lids have fewer striated fibers than do normal levator muscles. When these abnormal muscles are fully contracted, they shorten less than a normal muscle would. Thus, these patients are characterized by having a reduced levator function, graded by the degree of maldevelopment of the muscle. Myopathic ptosis includes muscular dystrophies, myasthenia gravis, progressive external ophthalmoplegia, and other myopathies. Both the neurogenic and mechanical categories also contain diverse subgroups requiring different treatment but, for conceptual clarity, these two categories are not further subdivided at this point.

Dysmyogenic Ptosis

Most congenital ptoses have maldeveloped levator muscles and therefore fall into this category. The maximum lid excursion in these patients usually varies from 2 to 12 mm. Because of the reduced excursion, the lid, which is ptotic in the primary position and on up gaze, may be higher than the other lid on down gaze. Surgical findings include fibrosis replacing levator muscle in inverse proportion to the amount of levator function.

J.L. Hargiss (personal communication, 1985) describes what he refers to as lipoelastic dysmyogenic ptosis. In these patients, there is very little lid excursion, but no lag on downward gaze. The lid can be passively stretched over the lower lid with little resistance. This is a rare cause of ptosis. At surgery, the levator is found to be a thin, elastic, fatty strip.

Dysmyogenic ptosis is not progressive. It may be associated with superior rectus muscle weakness that is not innervational. Since the superior rectus and levator muscles develop from the same primordium, it is not surprising that maldevelopment of one should be associated with maldevelopment of the other. Successful surgical treatment, which is aimed at placing the lid in an acceptable position when the patient is gazing straight ahead, will most certainly leave the lid at a higher level on downward gaze than it was preoperatively and leave the patient with ptosis on upward gaze.

The syndrome of ptosis, blepharophimosis, telecanthus, and epicanthus inversus fits into this category. Additional findings on these patients may include laterally placed and sometimes elongated lacrimal puncti, ectropion due to insufficient lid skin, and hypoplasia of the supraorbital rim.[3] Patients with this dominantly inherited syndrome should have any telecanthus and epicanthus inversus correction done prior to ptosis surgery. A frontalis suspension procedure is usually required to correct the ptosis in these patients, as they rarely have more than 4 mm of levator function.

Myopathic Ptosis

This group includes all myogenic ptoses in whom normal levator muscles develop embryologically: the myopathies, myasthenia gravis, trauma, and perhaps corticosteroid-induced ptosis. The myopathies include oculopharyngeal dystrophy, progressive external ophthalmoplegia, myotonic dystrophy, and other muscular dystrophies. Oculopharyngeal dystrophy is a dominantly inherited disease that usually has its onset in patients in their 40s or later, is always bilateral although sometimes asymmetric, and usually spares the skeletal and ocular movement muscles. Other facial muscles may be weak, including the orbicularis oculi muscles. Although most discussions of this disease report that it is most commonly seen in French-Canadians,[4] that has not been my experience with such cases. The onset of the ptosis is gradual, and its course is usually progressive until eventually there is 4 mm or less of levator function. Difficulty with swallowing is a progressive condition in these patients, and choking may be the cause of death. Beard[2] mentions a form of hereditary ptosis seen in several members of a family tree in the fourth or sixth decade with normal levator function. These may represent elongated aponeuroses rather than true myopathies.

Progressive external ophthalmoplegia[5] is a dystrophy that is generally confined to the extraocular muscles, including the levator, and may have its onset in childhood or adolescence. The orbicularis oculi muscles may be affected by this condition as well. It progresses gradually until the eyes become fixed in a position usually of slight downward gaze and levator function is lost. Although the eyes are usually not aligned late in the disease, these patients rarely experience diplopia. The condition is dominantly inherited in about 50 percent of cases. Myotonic dystrophy and other systemic muscular dystrophies may cause ptosis that is usually mild. When treating any of the ptoses caused by muscular dystrophy, the amount of levator function at the time treatment is required must be considered, as well as the protection the eye can expect to gain from the decreased orbicularis oculi function closing the eye and the decreased or absent Bell's phenomenon. When the orbicularis oculi muscles are weak and the eye does not elevate, undercorrection is the only safe surgical goal; for some patients, this may mean no correction at all. When treating oculopharyngeal dystrophy or progressive external ophthalmoplegia in a patient who still has a significant degree of levator function remaining, the patient must be warned that progression of the disease will probably require further treatment of the ptosis in the future. The silicone rod sling has shown some promise in treating these patients when a frontalis sling is required, since it can be stretched to allow the eye to close if the patient has sufficient orbicularis oculi muscle function.[6]

Myasthenia gravis is caused by an acetylcholine (ACh) deficiency at the neuromuscular junction. Ptosis may be an early sign of the disease. Other extraocular muscles are frequently involved as well. The patient may also have difficulty swallowing and, tend to fatigue easily.[7] Although one would expect the levator function to be reduced in this disease, I have seen a patient with this condition whose levator function was normal both when she had ptosis and when it was absent. Surgical correction is performed only when medical correction is inadequate. As with the muscular dystrophies, undercorrection may be necessary.

The levator muscle may be damaged by sharp trauma, with resulting scarring that may decrease levator function. The ptosis caused by topical corticosteroids, which is often reversible, may be attributable to a local myopathy, although this has not been proved.

Neurogenic Ptosis

Third nerve palsy causes ptosis in proportion to the degree of paresis. It may be congenital or caused by vascular lesions, tumors, neurotoxins, inflammation, demyelinating conditions, systemic disease (diabetes mellitus), and trauma. The site of the lesion may be supranuclear, nuclear, within the cavernous sinus, superior orbital fissure, or within the orbit. Ophthalmoplegic migraine, although rare, does occur. The defect it leaves may be temporary or, after a time, may result in a permanent defect. Horner's syndrome (ipsilateral ptosis, miosis, and anhidrosis) is a neurologic condition affecting the superior and inferior tarsal muscles. The ptosis it produces is therefore usually 2 mm or less with normal levator function. It also has a myriad of causes, making it important to identify the cause.

Synkinetic ptosis is neurogenic in origin and comprises three types. The best known is the jaw-winking phenomenon of Marcus Gunn.[8] It is probably caused by aberrant connections within the central nervous system (CNS) of the levator to the portion of the fifth cranial nerve going to the muscles of mastication. When these latter muscles are contracted, with either chewing or moving the jaw to the contralateral side, the lid elevates. This condition is usually unilateral and nonfamilial and may occur with varying degrees of both ptosis and elevation of the lid with chewing.[9] If the lid elevates to a normal position during chewing, it is fair to assume that there is no embryologic myogenic factor in the ptosis. In some cases, however, both types of ptosis may occur together. Ophthalmic folklore to the contrary, this seems to be a stable condition that does not improve with age. Decisions on management should therefore be made on the basis of what is present, rather than on projection into the future. Elimination of jaw-winking can only be accomplished by ablating the function of the levator. A frontalis suspension is then required to correct the ptosis.

A second type of synkinetic ptosis is aberrant regeneration of the third nerve, which may be congenital, but which may also occur upon recovery from an oculomotor nerve paralysis. When treatment is necessary, it is the same as for jaw-winking.

A third type of synkinetic ptosis is unrelated to the levator. It is caused by aberrant seventh nerve regeneration after a palsy. There is a mass-action effect on many facial muscles when movement of one group of facial muscles is attempted. Inappropriate contraction of the orbicularis oculi muscles causes ptosis.[10] This problem is relatively common following recovery of a seventh nerve palsy. This may be confused with jaw-winking; the eyelid moves up and down as the patient chews with the mouth closed caused by the secondary effects of the intermittent contractions of the orbicularis oris muscles. However, observation of the lid while chewing with the mouth open in these patients will show that the lid is stationary. Furthermore, the lid will become ptotic when the lips are pursed or other facial movements are initiated.

Sophisticated examination and testing, often with the assistance of a neuro-ophthalmologist, neurologist, or internist, are required to diagnose the cause of neurogenic ptosis. Only when the underlying cause is diagnosed and after it has been properly managed should surgical treatment be considered. When spontaneous recovery is possible, at least 6 months must elapse without evidence of improvement before treatment is undertaken. Treatment considerations must include the amount of levator function, orbicularis oculi function, and ocular motility, just as with the nonembryologic myogenic ptoses. The ptosis associated with Horner's syndrome is mild, and the levator function is normal. The lid can usually be elevated adequately with a tuck of the levator aponeurosis or a Fasanella-Servat procedure.

Aponeurotic Ptosis

Defects of the levator aponeurosis are the most recently described cause for ptosis.[11] The aponeurosis may be congenitally weak, as is probably true for the familial cases of ptosis reported by Beard with normal levator function. It may be weak as a change that occurs with aging, it may be dehisced or disinserted by trauma, or it may be stretched by excessive force on the lid as from an eyepatch on an eye that is attempting to open, lid swelling, or other lid mass. Postcataract ptosis is caused by a defect in the levator aponeurosis, although the mechanism for causing this is not understood. Although dysmyogenic ptosis is frequently considered the commonest type of ptosis, aponeurotic ptosis is the most common cause of ptosis among the patients this author has seen.

The clinical hallmarks of aponeurotic ptosis are normal levator function (which precludes lag on downward gaze), an elevated or indistinct lid crease, and sometimes thinning of the lid above the tarsal plate, such that the iris is visible through the lid. The thinned or damaged levator aponeurosis usually has an area of normal aponeurosis just below its origin at the distal end of the levator muscle, permitting repair by attaching this good tissue either to the tarsal plate or to the aponeurosis stump attached to the tarsal plate.

Mechanical Ptosis

There are three causes of mechanical ptosis: excess lid weight, inadequate posterior lid support, and scarring. Excessive lid mass would include any lid tumor or even an orbital tumor pushing forward into the lid, or lid swelling such as occurs after trauma or with blepharochalasis. Eventually, these mechanical problems tend to cause aponeurosis defects. The management of each lid mass depends on its nature. It should be recognized that even after treating the lid mass, repair of an aponeurosis defect may be required. Injection of steroid seems to be the most effective treatment for capillary hemangiomas that are causing sufficient ptosis to be a threat to vision. Neurofibromas may be resected, but the resection must be incomplete and the lesions should be expected to recur.

Inadequate orbital bulk, as seen in the anophthalmic socket, senile fat atrophy, loss of fat from an orbital fracture, microphthalmia, or phthisis bulbi, may deprive the levator apparatus of its posterior support and give the lid a naturally lower position as well as reduce its levator function by reducing the tension in the levator (a shift to the left on the force–length curve). In the absence of a seeing eye, bulk may be built onto the top of a prosthesis to correct the ptosis.[12] In some of these cases and whenever a seeing eye is present, shortening of the levator aponeurosis and sometimes the muscle itself may be necessary to correct the lid position.

Cicatrix between the lid and the globe or between the levator and the orbital roof may cause ptosis. The scar may be a result of mechanical trauma, nonspecific inflammation, or disease such as ocular pemphigoid, Stevens-Johnson syndrome, or severe trachoma. Management must be directed toward correcting the cicatrix.

Pseudoptosis

Pseudoptosis may be attributable to dermatochalasis, contralateral upper lid retraction, or hypotropia. When the skin comes down over the lashes and interferes with the superior field of vision, resection is required for improved visual function. An underlying aponeurotic ptosis may be present, however, either as an age-associated change or caused by the weight of the excess skin; this will become evident if only skin is removed. A high index of suspicion of an aponeurotic defect should be maintained in patients with functional dermatochalasis and ptosis correction undertaken at the time of skin removal, if warranted. Contralateral upper lid retraction, when it is not so marked that there is scleral show, may be difficult to distinguish from ptosis of the ipsilateral upper lid, particularly when the patient's base upper eyelid positions are on the low end of the normal spectrum. Contralateral lid retraction can sometimes be discerned from ptosis only after repeated observations. Hypotropia, with the lid following the eye in an appropriate fashion, may appear as ptosis. To diagnose this, the contralateral eye is covered. The hypotropic eye will then move up and assume fixation, and the lid will come up to the proper non-ptotic position.

Although the cause of most ptosis cases can be defined and neatly assigned to one of the preceding types, some will have more than one cause for their ptosis, such as the patient with mechanical ptosis and secondary aponeurotic ptosis, and still others will have a ptosis we have not yet learned to define. I have recently seen three teenage patients with a mild ptosis said to have been present all their lives. Levator functions were normal and the lid creases were in the normal position. Surgery on the aponeurosis of each of these patients, done under local anesthesia, led to significant undercorrection. Much more shortening of the levator aponeurosis was required to correct these ptotic eyelids than would have been expected for a patient with normal levator function. It is not clear whether they had some form of mild dystrophy of the levator, a defect in the aponeurosis, or a different problem.

EVALUATION OF PTOSIS

History

The age of onset of ptosis should be determined as well as whether it is progressive or stationary. Inquiry into the variability of the ptosis should be made. Inquiry should be made as to whether a ptotic eyelid has suffered episodes of lid edema in the past. The nature of any eyelid trauma and its repair should be ascertained. Except for ptosis associated with Horner's syndrome, most ptotic lids become even lower when the patient is tired. This is presumably because the levator aponeurosis and superior tarsal muscle function in parallel. If the aponeurosis or levator muscle is weak, it puts a greater percentage of the burden of the lid weight on the superior tarsal muscle, which may then fatigue.

Inquiry regarding the presence of ptosis and its type in other family members should be made. In addition, with dysmyogenic ptosis it is wise to inquire whether any family members have had malignant hyperthermia, as these conditions may be associated. It may be determined whether the patient has had previous ptosis surgery; if so, information about the previous surgery should be obtained. If the patient seems to have dysmyogenic ptosis, an inquiry about lid movements when eating or sucking will usually provide sufficient information to decide whether to examine carefully for jaw-winking. Strabismus, amblyopia, and previous need for glasses correction should be asked about.

Patients with neurologic and myopathic ptosis should also be asked questions appropriate to their problem. These should include taking a general health history, inquiry as to whether they know the cause of their ptosis, and determination as to whether they have had diplopia, dysphagia, or anhidrosis. Other queries may be appropriate, depending on the history the patient gives with regard to their ptosis and associated symptoms.

Physical Examination

The key points of the lid examination are the levator function, the position of each lid relative to the center of the pupil, the contour of each lid, and the position of the upper lid crease(s). Levator function is the maximum lid excursion that occurs when the eyes go from either upward to downward gaze or downward to upward gaze, measured with the frontalis muscle essentially inactivated by the examiner's thumb. The mean levator function is about 15.5 mm in normal adults[13] and probably several millimeters less in children. This measurement indicates the amount of shortening of the levator muscle from its relaxed position to maximal contraction. It is best to indicate the lid position both by measurement of the vertical palpebral fissure width measured at the mid-pupil, to use a consistent reference point, and by the distance from the center of the pupil to the upper lid, each measured when the eye is in the primary position. Measurement of the vertical palpebral fissure alone may be misleading if the lower lids are not at the same level. The lid contour should be described by noting which portions of the lid are low, if the contour is abnormal. The position of the upper lid crease(s) on each upper lid should be noted by measuring from the lid margin to the crease in the central lid. Ideally, to produce lid symmetry, the lid crease, as well as the lid position, should be the same on each side. When no lid crease is present, it usually implies very poor levator function if the patient has dysmyogenic ptosis, or it may imply a large aponeurotic defect if the patient has aponeurotic ptosis with normal levator function. In a small child with no lid crease, in whom it is difficult to measure levator function, the lid may be everted. If the lid slips back into normal configuration when the patient looks up, this suggests that some levator function is present. If the lid does not revert to the usual configuration on up gaze, this further suggests the absence of significant levator function. The anterior and posterior surfaces of the lid should be carefully examined to rule out any lid mass or cicatrix. An exophthalmometer reading should be taken if enophthalmos is suspected. In selected patients, examination for jaw-winking and ptosis caused by aberrant seventh nerve regeneration should be performed. In a patient who has had ptosis of the eyelid following trauma, with no levator function, a finger placed in the superior sulcus as the patient looks down to up may demonstrate movement of the detached levator, which would encourage exploration of the lid under local anesthesia to reattach it.

Whenever a frontalis sling is being contemplated, an estimation of the patient's frontalis function and tendency to use the frontalis should be noted. These patients will usually have severe ptosis to begin with and will maximally use their frontalis, if it is helpful to them. In addition, if the patient does not have single binocular vision, it should be determined whether the patient uses the eye for which the sling is contemplated. If not, it is unlikely that the frontalis will be used to lift the lid postoperatively.

A complete ocular examination should be done on each of these patients both for other information that may be relevant to the ptosis problem and to prevent missing an ocular problem that may be important to the patient. The corrected visual acuity should certainly be ascertained. If amblyopia is present, it should be determined whether it is caused by the ptosis, a relatively rare finding,[14] or more commonly by astigmatism with anisometropic amblyopia or some other condition. Examination of ocular motility is also quite important. It may reveal strabismus, which is present in 32 percent of patients with dysmyogenic ptosis,[15] the presence of a third nerve palsy, or the poor motility that may be associated with nonembryologic myogenic ptosis. Hypotropia, a cause of pseudoptosis, may also be detected with this examination. Aberrant third nerve regeneration may also be detected by examining the ocular motility.

Finally, it should be emphasized that at times it is a good idea to step back and get an overall view of the patient when the history and examination findings do not quite fit. Café-au-lait spot may be noted, suggesting neurofibromatosis, frontal bossing may be caused by an osteoma, and muscle wasting may be seen in patients with muscular dystrophy, to mention only a few findings that may be observed.

Other tests may sometimes be indicated in the office, depending on both the history and the physical findings. If Horner's syndrome is suggested, pharmacologic testing with 4 to 10 percent cocaine and 1 percent hydroxyamphetamine will usually delineate the defect. Lacrimal secretory testing, usually the Schirmer's test, as discussed in Chapter 49, should be performed if a dry eye is suspected. Just as blepharoplasty in the presence of secretory deficiency can cause ocular discomfort and even corneal damage, so can correction of ptosis. If myasthenia gravis is suspected, two simple clinical tests may be used. The patient is asked to look up and maintain that ocular position for 30 seconds, while observing the patient for fatigue. A second test is to have the patient look down and then straight ahead. Myasthenia gravis patients will often appear to have the lid overshoot and then drop a small amount.[16] Edrophonium (Tensilon) may be injected intravenously to see whether it relieves either the ptosis or diplopia, or both. Cardiac arrest, although rare, has been known to occur after edrophonium injection. Testing should be performed where such an emergency can be managed. A test dose of 0.1 ml is injected intravenously. If the patient has no adverse reaction to this, the remaining 0.9 ml is injected relatively rapidly. Any effect from this will be seen within a minute. Atropine, 0.5 mg, should be drawn up and ready for injection into the same intravenous needle, should the patient experience an adverse reaction, such as difficulty breathing, abdominal cramping, and diaphoresis from the edrophonium. A single-fiber electromyogram (EMG) is often diagnostic when other tests are equivocal.[17]

If there is anything to suggest that the patient may have neuroparalytic keratitis, the corneal sensitivity should be determined, as elevating the lid will certainly worsen the patient's symptoms. Skull radiographs or computed tomography (CT) scan are not commonly indicated but, when the patient's findings seem unusual, this may be helpful in revealing a mucocele, an osteoma, or a bone fragment in the levator, each of which may cause ptosis. Although arteriography may be indicated because of a pulsatile mass or a suspected carotid cavernous fistula, the need for such a test usually indicates that the patient should seek consultation with an additional specialist.

Although unnecessary for the purpose of treating the patient properly, the patient's ptosis should be documented with photographs showing both eyes in the primary position, up gaze, and down gaze for both insurance and medicolegal purposes; evaluation of the visual fields should be obtained if it is believed that the patient's medical insurance company will require this documentation, as is usually the case when the ptosis is present in an adult.

REFERENCES

1. Frueh BR: Mechanical classification of ptosis. Ophthalmology 87:1019, 1980
2. Beard C: Ptosis. CV Mosby, St Louis, 1981
3. Kohn R, Romano PE: Blepharoptosis, blepharophimosis, epicanthus inversus, and telecanthus-a syncrome with no name. Am J Ophthalmol 72:625, 1971
4. Johnson CC, Kuwabara T: Oculopharyngeal muscular dystrophy. Am J Ophthalmol 7:872, 1974
5. Lind I, Paine G: Chronic progressive exophthalmologic and muscular distrophy. Acta Ophthalmol 41:497, 1963
6. Leoni CR, Shorr JW, Van Gemert JV: Silicone rod frontalis sling for the correction of blepharoptosis. Ophthalmic Surg 12:881, 1981
7. Cogan DC: Current concepts of myasthenia gravis. Arch Ophthalmol 74:1, 1965
8. Bullock JD: Marcus-Gunn jaw-winking ptosis: Classification and surgical management. J Pediatr Ophthalmol Strabismus 17:376, 1980
9. Spaeth EB: The Marcus Gunn phenomenon. Am J Ophthalmol 30:143, 1947
10. Frueh BR: Associated facial contractions after seventh nerve palsy mimicking jaw-winking. Ophthalmology 9:1105, 1983
11. Jones LT, Quickert MH, Wobig JL: A cure of ptosis by aponeurotic repair. Arch Ophthalmol 94:629, 1975
12. Vistnes LN: Mechanism of upper lid ptosis in the anophthalmic orbit. Plast Reconstr Surg 58:539, 1976
13. Frueh BR: Graves eye disease: Orbital compliance and other physical measurements. Trans Am Ophthalmol Soc 82:492, 1984
14. Anderson RL, Baumgartner SA: Amblyopia in ptosis. Arch Ophthalmol 98:1068, 1980
15. Anderson RL, Baumgartner SA: Strabismus in ptosis. Arch Ophthalmol 98:1062, 1980
16. Cogan DG: Myasthenia gravis: A review of the disease and a description of lid twitch as characteristic sign. Arch Ophthalmol 74:217, 1965
17. Sanders DB, Howard JF, Jolins TR: Single-fiber electromyography in myasthenia gravis. Neurology (NY) 29:68, 1979

Surgical Correction of Blepharoptosis

34

James L. Hargiss

When the surgical correction of a drooping eyelid is contemplated, certain decisions must be made and both general and specific principles followed. The decision as to whether to operate includes several considerations. In mild cases of 1 or 2 mm, the decision depends entirely on the patient's or parents' desires and may include consideration of anesthetic risk. If the patient is a child, the parents may be counseled to wait until the patient is old enough to make a decision. Orbicularis paresis, ophthalmoplegia, or neuroparalytic keratitis may preclude full correction or may even contraindicate surgery.

In children, the best time to operate depends on several circumstances. Motility surgery or the correction of the other defects of blepharophimosis should precede ptosis surgery. Since ptosis rarely causes amblyopia, and the remarks of others have little psychological impact before preschool age, surgery before the age of 3 is rarely imperative.

Since about one fourth of dysmyogenic ptoses are bilateral, and usually unequal, undercorrecting the worse eyelid to match the better one may be considered. However, since the better lid tends to develop an unpredictable increase in ptosis after correction of the worse one because of a decrease in reciprocal innervation, this decision may invite problems. In such cases, the patient or parents must be informed of this effect as well as the likelihood of an increase in lid lag or downward gaze and nocturnal lagophthalmos when a dysmyogenic levator is shortened. If the ptosis is progressive and the patient has adequate visual function, surgery may be delayed with the hope of performing a definitive procedure later.

Deciding which ptosis operation to perform in each case depends on the diagnostic evaluation (Chapter 33). Correction of the primary defect, such as aponeurosis repair for aponeurotic ptosis or Müllerectomy for Horner's syndrome, is the ideal course but is commonly not possible. Use of the primary lid elevator, the levator muscle–aponeurosis complex, is the most physiologic procedure but, since there is no surgical means to increase the total excursion of the levator, less anatomic procedures may be necessary. In some cases of severe dysmyogenic ptosis with only 3 or 4 mm excursion, maximum levator resection may be tried first with the understanding that a frontalis procedure may subsequently be necessary. Each procedure should begin not only with a definite plan, but also with alternatives in the event of an unexpected surgical finding, such as an aponeurotic defect in a presumed dysmyogenic case or a lipoelastic levator in a presumed aponeurotic ptosis. The indications for each procedure are discussed in the appropriate sections.

General principles, such as asepsis, hemostasis, atraumatic and minimal dissection, and familiarity with surgical anatomy, are as essential to ptosis procedures as to all surgery.

No aspirin or dipyramidole (Persantine) is to be taken for 10 days preoperatively. Coumadin, if taken, is stopped 4 days preoperatively. Vitamin K may be given if the prothrombin time is too long.

Local anesthesia is preferred when possible, as it not only avoids the risks of general anesthesia but also aids in the identification of structures (as in traumatic or previously operated ptosis), permits more accurate observation of lid height and motion, and appears to produce less bleeding. Lidocaine 1 percent with 1:200,000 epinephrine is made by dilution of the standard 2 percent solution 1:1. Bupivacaine 0.5 percent may be used as the diluent for procedures expected to last over an hour. An injection of 0.5 ml of this solution beneath the planned line of incision, subconjunctivally above the tarsus, or both, depending on the approach to be used, provides adequate, rapid anesthesia for most ptosis procedures, with negligible akinesia. The vasoconstrictive effect of the epinephrine is evident after 5 or 10 minutes.

Surgical preparation includes conjunctival sac irrigation as well as painting the forehead, nose, cheek, temple, and lids with a providone-iodine preparation. The lashes are not trimmed.

An adhesive drape with an aperture is placed. When using local anesthesia, its lower portion is held away from the lower face by fixation to the instrument stand over the patient's chest. Breathing air is supplied through a double nasal catheter.

For conjunctival or buried sutures, I prefer 6-0 plain catgut, but not the dyed variety, which seems brittle. For skin closure, 6-0 monofilament nylon is placed as a running intradermal suture, tied at each end in a slip knot. At the completion of levator resection and frontalis slings, a modified Frost suture is placed: both arms of a double-armed 5-0 silk are passed through the pretarsal skin of the lower lid into the tarsal plate and out the margin at the lower lid; they are then passed into the upper lid margin into the tarsal plate and out through pretarsal skin and fixed to the forehead with tape. Aponeurotic repair and tarso-Müllerectomy cases do not require the corneal protection of the Frost suture, but ice water compresses are applied to the operated lid for 4 or 5 hours postoperatively. Cold compresses help alleviate postoperative discomfort and minimize edema.

The sutures are removed on the third or fourth day. The nylon skin suture, if left longer, tends to form small abscesses at the emerging ends. It slides out easily by cutting one knot and pulling on the other. Artificial tears and an ointment are used as necessary to protect the cornea.

APONEUROSIS REPAIR

Defects of the aponeurosis are the most common cause of ptosis in adults, variously described as senile ptosis, aponeurosis dehiscence, acquired ptosis, and levator disinsertion. This type of ptosis may occur gradually or rapidly in older adults, sometimes in younger adults, following recurrent episodes of eyelid swelling or even without such episodes, and represents up to 5 percent of congenital ptosis. Most cases of ptosis following cataract surgery fall into this category. The ptosis presents in varying degrees and has the distinct clinical characteristics presented in Chapter 33. Superior tarsal muscle (Müller's muscle) is spared, so that instillation of 0.12 percent phenylephrine produces lid elevation, but treatment by tarso-Müllerectomy is not recommended because it may provide only a temporary cure. Aponeurosis repair corrects the specific defect.

My preferred procedure is much like that used by Jones et al.[1] The procedure can be performed in an office operatory when local anesthesia is used. Subcutaneous injection of anesthetic below the supratarsal crease provides sufficient anesthesia for the procedure without levator muscle akinesia.

The skin incision is placed in the desired supratarsal crease. An Agricola speculum is placed to stretch orbicularis vertically. This muscle is carefully parted in an attempt to avoid penetrating the very thin remaining aponeurosis fibers. The landmarks for the posterior fascia of the orbicularis are the vertical nerves and vessels, the visibility of which is enhanced by the stretch of the speculum. The peripheral arterial arcade of superior tarsal muscle may be seen through the thin portion of the remaining aponeurosis fibers; if there is no film of tissue over the arcade, the thinned portion of the aponeurosis has been penetrated or was dehisced, and the aponeurosis must be dissected from the orbicularis above the incision. A disposable hot cautery is used to control any bleeding encountered during the dissection. The dissection is carried upward, between aponeurosis and orbicularis to well above the insertion of the septum onto the aponeurosis. The septum is cut transversely above its insertion. Preaponeurotic fat may be removed by the clamp–cut–cauterize–unclamp technique as indicated. Near the level of the septum insertion, a distinct line will usually be found, above which is found strong white aponeurosis and below it attenuated aponeurosis. A suture of 6-0 plain catgut is placed in the normal aponeurosis, and then into the aponeurosis stump attached to tarsus, seen as fascial tissue posterior to orbicularis at the lower lip of the incision (Fig. 34-1). Traction with forceps on the stump should raise the lid without much stretching of the tissue. If there is stretching with poor lid elevation, it is not aponeurosis stump, which must then be found lower. The suture is tied in a slip knot, the speculum removed, and the height of the lid observed. This height may be compared with that of the opposite lid, if the latter is normal. Although I do not sit the patient up for this observation, many surgeons find this helpful. The suture is adjusted if the height is not satisfactory. An overcorrection of 0.5 to 1 mm is advisable, as the effect of the orbicularis has been temporarily reduced. When the lid height is satisfactory, the suture is tied and four additional sutures placed and tied. Another inspection is made before closing the skin. If the lid margin is unsatisfactory, sutures are replaced or additional sutures placed, as necessary. The skin is closed with a running intradermal suture. No dressing is required, although an occlusive plastic film such as Nu Skin may be applied.

Another type of adult acquired ptosis is sometimes encountered, generally in obese patients. The lids appear thick rather than abnormally thin as in most lids with involutional aponeurosis defects and do not have an abnormally high crease. The aponeurosis is irregularly weblike and infiltrated by large globules of fat. The levator muscle and septum may be degenerated as well. The dissection is more difficult in these patients. Ingenuity may be required to reconstruct the aponeurosis: an implant of sclera or temporalis fascia may be required to bridge from the levator muscle to the aponeurosis stump or tarsal plate.

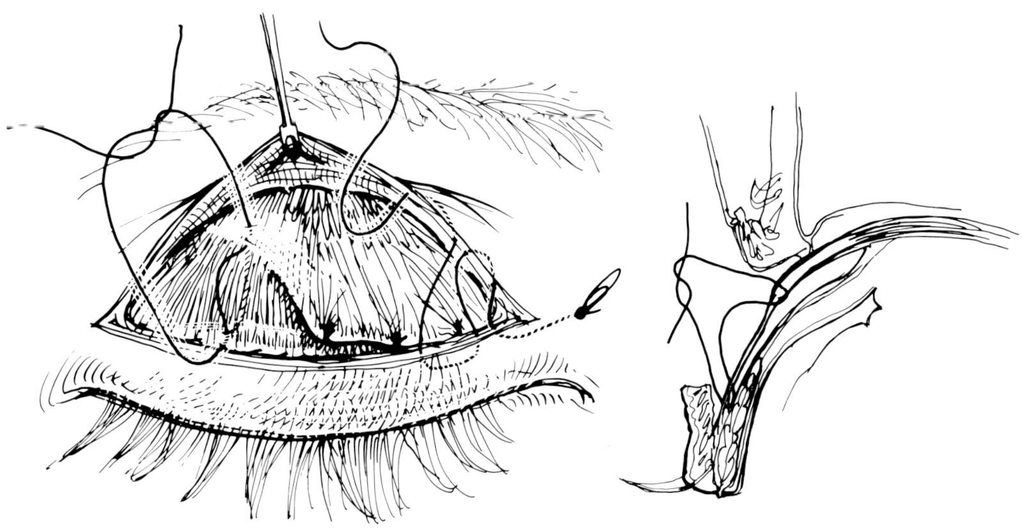

Fig. 34-1. Tucking the levator aponeurosis. The healthy proximal aponeurosis is sutured to the distal stump.

TARSO-MÜLLERECTOMY

Superior tarsal muscle is a sympathetically innervated smooth muscle whose tonic contraction acts in parallel with the aponeurosis. Enhancing its lift will correct up to 1.5 mm of ptosis, which may be present in very mild dysmyogenic ptosis, after undercorrection following levator resection, and in Horner's syndrome. Tarso-Müllerectomy does not consistently correct ptosis when a drop of 0.12 percent phenylephrine fails to provide a satisfactory lift or when the ptosis is caused by an aponeurotic defect.

My preferred technique is similar to the Fasanella–Servat[2] procedure. It may be performed in an office operatory when local anesthesia can be used. The anesthetic is injected subconjunctivally above the top of the tarsus and subcutaneously over the lateral end of the tarsus.

A short horizontal incision is made at the lateral end of the lid through skin and into orbicularis muscle. This incision is placed closer to the lash line than to the supratarsal crease, because the tarsal conjunctival suture will be tied here and higher placement would depress the lateral lid margin into an S curve.

The lid is everted and two curved mosquito hemostats placed (see Fig. 34-2). Because the operation tends to elevate the lid more centrally than

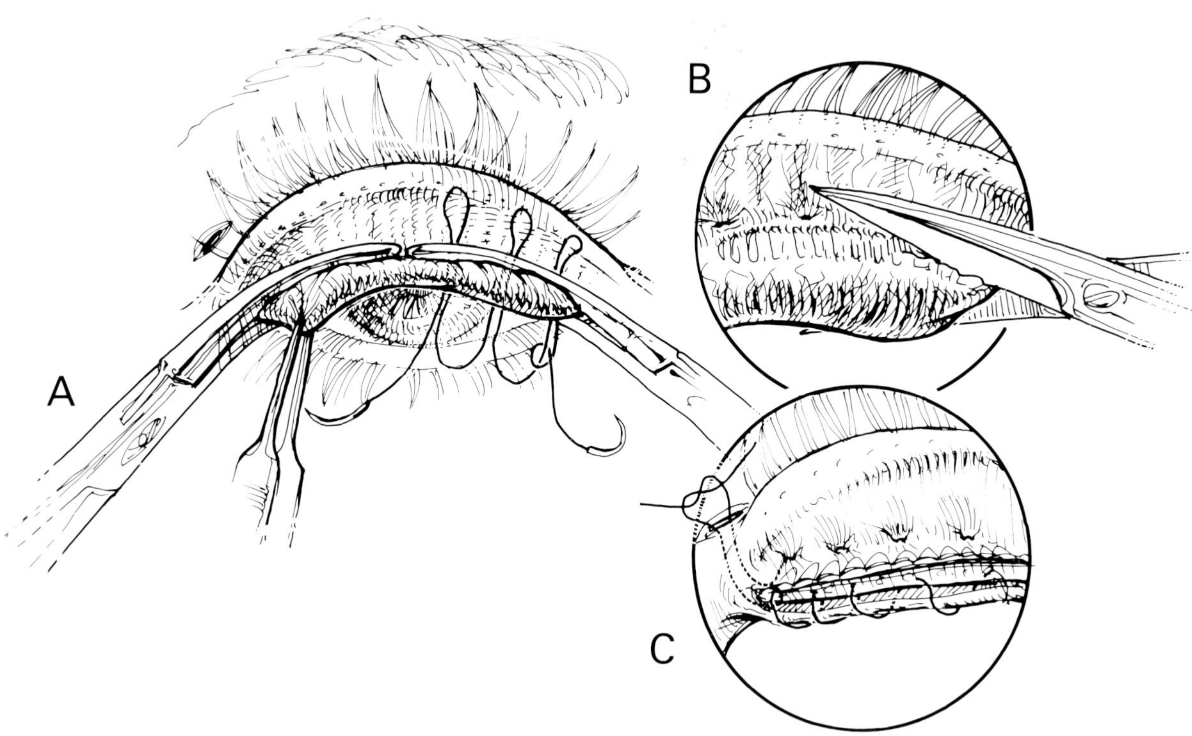

Fig. 34-2. Tarso-Müllerectomy or modified Fasanella–Servat procedure. **(A)** Curved hemostats are placed medially and laterally across tarsal plate, conjunctiva, and superior tarsal muscle with conjunctiva and superior tarsal muscle being pulled farther down for clamping both medially and laterally. A horizontal mattress suture of 6-0 plain catgut is run across the length of the lid. **(B)** After removing the clamp, tissue is excised in the clamped area. **(C)** The other arm of the double-armed suture is passed as a running whip stitch between conjunctiva and tarsal cut edge, catching only the anterior lip of the latter to avoid suture irritation. Both arms of the suture are brought externally through a small skin incision and tied over the orbicularis oculi muscle.

laterally, the clamps are not only placed closer to the lid margin medially and laterally than centrally, but more conjunctiva and superior tarsal muscle are pulled with forceps into each clamp medially and laterally as well. Putterman's clamp requires an assistant for this placement. Since I usually perform the operation alone, and since the curved hemostats require only two hands at a time, I prefer them. After each clamp is placed, the skin at the supratarsal crease is pulled away from it to assure that the levator aponeurosis has not also been clamped. The lacrimal secretory ducts should be identified and avoided.

A double-armed suture of 6-0 plain catgut is placed as a horizontal mattress into the conjunctiva medial to the medial clamp and either tied with a single throw or passed through adjacent conjunctiva to anchor the suture. The first arm is then passed as a running-mattress suture between conjunctiva and tarsus behind the clamps to the lateral extent of the clamped tissue. The suture bites are made far apart on the superior tarsal–conjunctival side but reenter the tarsus at almost the point of exit on the tarsal side and are drawn tightly to umbilicate the tarsus (see Fig. 34-2). This method prevents the tarsal suture loops from irritating the cornea.

The clamps are removed and the fold of tarsus, superior tarsal muscle, and conjunctiva excised along the clamp marks. The cut must be within the clamp marks to avoid cutting the suture, the main intraoperative complication.

The second arm of the suture is passed as a running whipstitch between conjunctiva and tarsal cut edge, catching only the anterior lip of the latter to avoid suture-irritation of the cornea. At the lateral end, again avoiding lacrimal secretory ducts, both arms of the sutures are passed through the lid and tied over the orbicularis muscle exposed by the skin incision. Closure of the skin is usually not necessary. No dressing is required.

With 0.5 to 1.0 mm ptosis and with Horner's syndrome, no tarsus should be included in the resection. The conjunctiva and superior tarsal muscle are loosened from the aponeurosis by forceps manipulation as described by Putterman and Urist,[3] and the clamps are applied above the tarsus after pulling the freed tissue into them with forceps. The remainder of the operation is the same.

LEVATOR RESECTION

As the levator–aponeurosis complex is the primary elevator of the upper lid, shortening of this complex is the most physiologic correction for nonaponeurotic ptosis. It is the preferred procedure for dysmyogenic, myopathic, or neurogenic ptosis when sufficient levator function is present and the ptosis is too great for a lesser procedure such as tarso-Müllerectomy. Since most congenital ptoses are dysmyogenic, it is the most commonly performed procedure in children. The term *levator resection* refers to shortening of the levator aponeurosis and as much of the actual muscle as necessary.

The most critical decision is the length of this complex to resect. Henderson,[4] Beard,[5] and Chimonidou et al.[6] offered general guidelines for the length of levator to resect, but results vary with each surgeon's methods and experience.

Beard[7] finds little or no benefit from resections of 8 mm or less. In my hands, the resection is closer to 10 mm, which is the minimum amount I resect. I preplan the amount to resect on the basis of the amount of ptosis and lid excursion, but I also use Berke's method[8] to determine the upper lid position when using an anterior approach with the patient under general anesthetic. If the two amounts differ, I favor the greater of the two, as I have found myself guilty of undercorrection more often than overcorrection. If the procedure is performed under local anesthesia, the sutures can be adjusted with the patient sitting up on the operating table to attain the best correction.

Table 34-1 presents the author's classification and general guidelines for dysmyogenic ptosis. It must be emphasized that these categories are general only, with no clear divisions between them. For instance, a given case may fall into the moderate category because of the amount of ptosis and excursion, yet have marked lag on downward gaze if the muscle is quite fibrotic. The amount of striated muscle fibers found in the levator for each group is based on the findings of Berke and Wadsworth.[9]

It may be noted that the amount of resection

Table 34-1. Findings in Patients with Dysmyogenic Ptosis, According to Amount of Ptosis

	Degree of Ptosis			
Parameter	Mild (1–2 mm)	Moderate (2–4 mm)	Severe (Fibrotic) (>4 mm)	Severe (Lipoelastic) (>4 mm)
Position of lid margin in primary gaze	From midway between limbus and top of pupil to top of pupil	At or below top of pupil	Below center of pupil	Below center of pupil gaze
Lag on downward gaze	Little or none	Noticeable	Marked; resists passive traction	Little or none; little or no resistance to passive traction
Total lid excursion (levator function)	8–12 mm	5–7 mm	<4 mm	<4 mm
Striated muscle fiber content[9]	Abundant	Significant paucity	Little or none (fibrotic)	None (fatty elastic)
Amount of resection	11–14 mm without advancement	15–18 mm without advancement	19–24 mm with advancement	Heroic (≤27 mm) with advancement
Change in lid height from immediate postoperative in following weeks	Same or slightly higher	Same	Same or lower; marked downward gaze lag	50% or more loss of correction

ranges from a minimum of 11 mm to a maximum of 24 mm, with the exception of a heroic resection of up to 27 mm in the rare cases of lipoelastic ptosis. The latter may be tried in an effort to correct the ptosis with a resection. A good immediate result may be lost in several weeks, necessitating a frontalis suspension.

The levator may be resected through either an anterior or posterior approach. Although the posterior approach can be a very useful one in up to 3 mm of ptosis, I more often use the anterior because it facilitates advancement as well as resection, affords an opportunity to preserve superior tarsal muscle function, and leads to more accurate determination of the amount to resect.

Anterior Approach

My preferred procedure is similar to those used by Johnson,[10] Berke,[11] and Beard,[7] except that the initial isolation of the levator aponeurosis is made with the posterior blade of the ptosis clamp in the postaponeurotic space between aponeurosis and tarsal plate, thus eliminating the need to cut and resuture the superior tarsal muscle–conjunctival layer.

The supratarsal crease is marked to match that of the opposite lid but is marked somewhat shorter than the lid margin. The skin is incised along the mark, and an Agricola speculum is placed to stretch the orbicularis vertically. The muscle is cut with scissors to its posterior fascia, which contains large vertical vessels and nerves. Hemostasis is maintained with a hot disposable cautery throughout the procedure. The speculum is then replaced by an Erhardt clamp.

Scissors dissection is carried upward between aponeurosis and orbicularis until the septum can be identified above its insertion into the aponeurosis by the fat behind it or by its looseness from the aponeurosis when rolling it with a cotton-tipped applicator. The septum is incised transversely across its entire width above its insertion into the aponeurosis; failure to do so will restrict the downward movement of the lid. Strands between fat and aponeurosis are cut as well.

The levator is buttonholed medially and laterally just below the upper edge of the tarsus. The holes need only be about 10 mm apart. The postaponeurotic space between them is bluntly dissected with scissors, between tarsus and aponeurosis. The posterior blade of the ptosis clamp is placed within this tract and the clamp closed with its handle downward. Using the clamp to create downward traction, cuts are extended upward from each buttonhole about 5 mm (Fig. 34-3A). The clamp is loosened, pushed upward to the tops of the cuts, and reclamped. This dissects the aponeurosis from the upper tarsus and from a portion of superior tarsal muscle. The Erhardt clamp is removed. The aponeurosis is cut distal to the clamp (Fig. 34-3B), and cuts are made to free the horns, taking care to spare the lacrimal gland laterally and the superior oblique fascia medially. I do not make an effort to spare the superior transverse ligament.

I believe it is worth the effort to preserve superior tarsal muscle; I dissect it from the posterior surface of the aponeurosis. Medial and lateral sutures of 6-0 plain catgut are locked or tied into the muscle just below its origin from the levator, as in Figure 34-4. Superior tarsal muscle is cut at its origin from the levator. I find this step difficult because the line of origin is indistinct, and bleeding is usually encountered. Upward traction on the clamped levator with gentle downward traction on the superior tarsal muscle sutures aids this dissection. Care is taken to avoid the superior rectus muscle, which is near the origin of superior tarsal muscle. An alternate method, applicable where a large levator resection is planned, is to place sutures at the junction of the levator muscle and its aponeurosis. This junction is preserved, along with its attached superior tarsal muscle, by cutting above and below the sutures when the levator is cut.

With the clamped levator freely mobilized, Berke's method,[8] of setting the upper lid position is used (Fig. 34-5). With the assistant holding the eye in the primary position, the lid margin is lifted to the predetermined position with a needle holder grasping the spatula needle of a 6-0 plain catgut suture, with the point of the needle forward at midtarsus. The height at which the lid is held by the

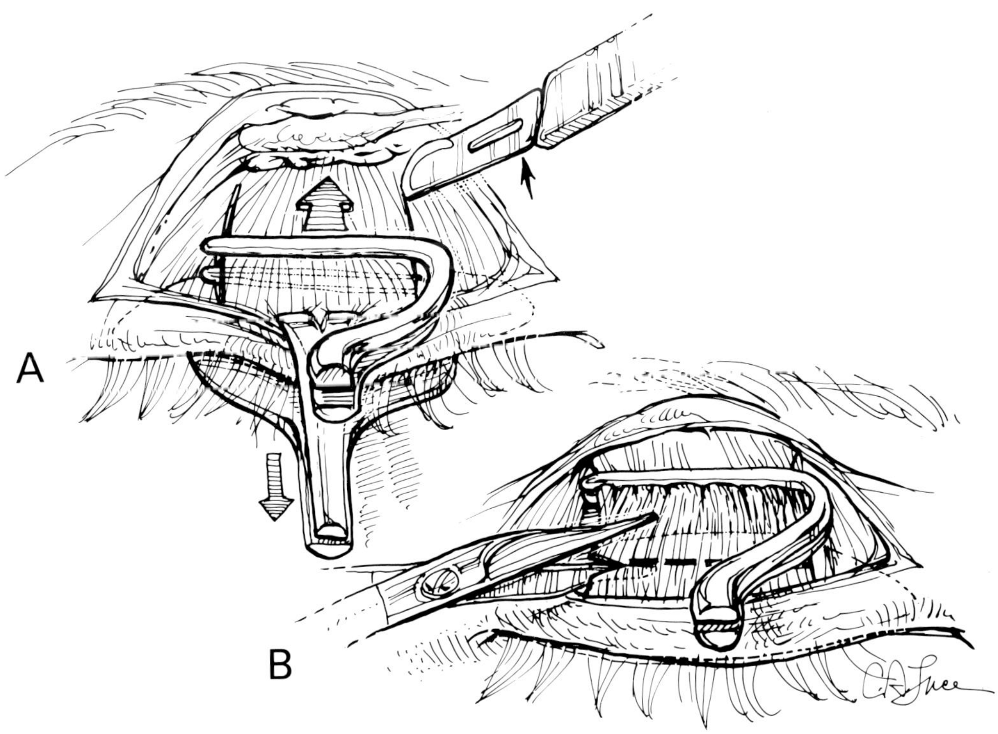

Fig. 34-3. (A) With an anterior levator resection, the ptosis clamp is placed across the aponeurosis over the tarsus, and cuts are made upward through the aponeurosis. **(B)** The clamp is loosened, pushed superiorly and reclamped, and the aponeurosis transected distal to the clamp.

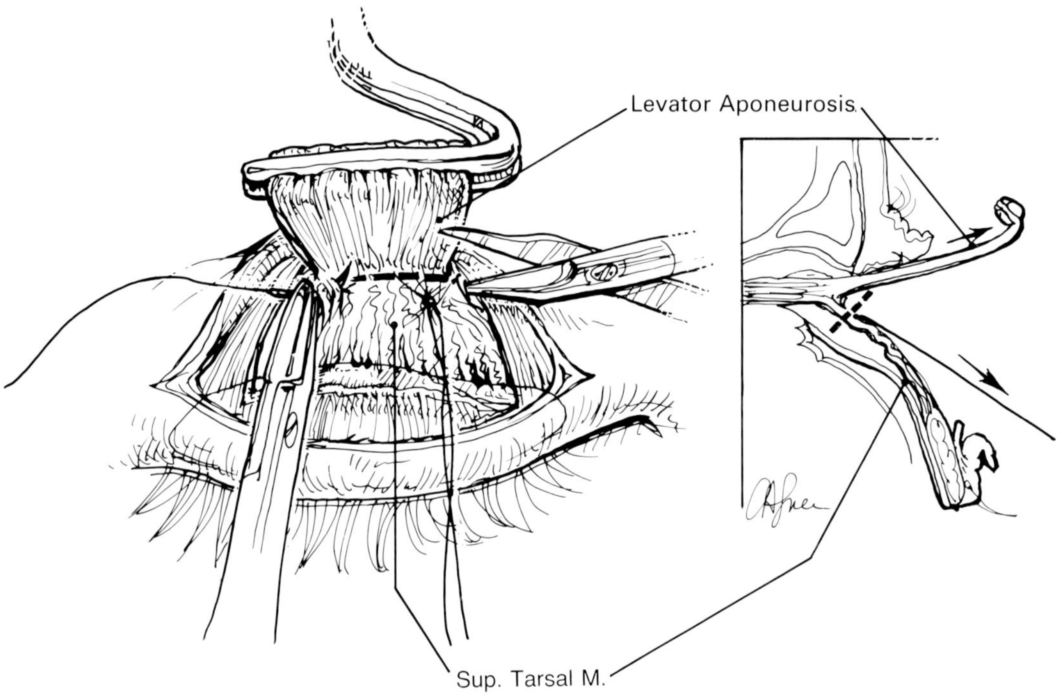

Fig. 34-4. Placement of suture in superior tarsal muscle and transection of it from the levator.

needle holder is graded according to the preoperative levator function (Table 34-2). The levator is then brought downward, maintaining moderate tension with the clamp, and impaled onto the needle. Varying the levator tension slightly seems to cause less than a 1-mm difference in final lid position. The distance from the needle and the cut end of the levator is measured. If this distance is less than the preplanned resection, the needle is reinserted at the predetermined distance from the cut edge. If the distance from the needle to the cut end

Table 34-2. Placement of Upper Eyelid When Correcting Dysmyogenic Ptosis under General Anesthesia, According to Preoperative Eyelid Excursion

Levator Function	
Preoperative Lid Excursion (mm)	Lid Placement at Surgery Relative to Superior Limbus (mm)
2–3	0
4–5	1–2
5–7	2–3
8–9	3–4
10–11	6

of the levator is the same or more than the preplanned distance, the suture is brought through and tied. Three other sutures are then placed at this level, and the levator excised distal to them. If superior tarsal muscle sutures have been placed, they are passed through the levator 12 mm above this level and tied. If muscle–aponeurosis junction sutures were used, the tissue above them is incised and the aponeurosis below them is excised before inserting them into the levator muscle and tying them.

If levator advancement is not felt to be necessary, I prefer to reinsert the resected levator into the aponeurosis stump (Fig. 34-6A). This retains the normal insertions into the lower portion of the tarsus and into pretarsal orbicularis.

If advancement of the levator onto the tarsus is planned, sutures are preplaced in the levator and tied on its posterior surface. They are passed horizontally through the anterior 50 percent of the tarsus at the desired advanced position and then passed back through the levator to be tied over it. It is important to place the sutures above the base of the lash follicles or entropion or loss of lashes may

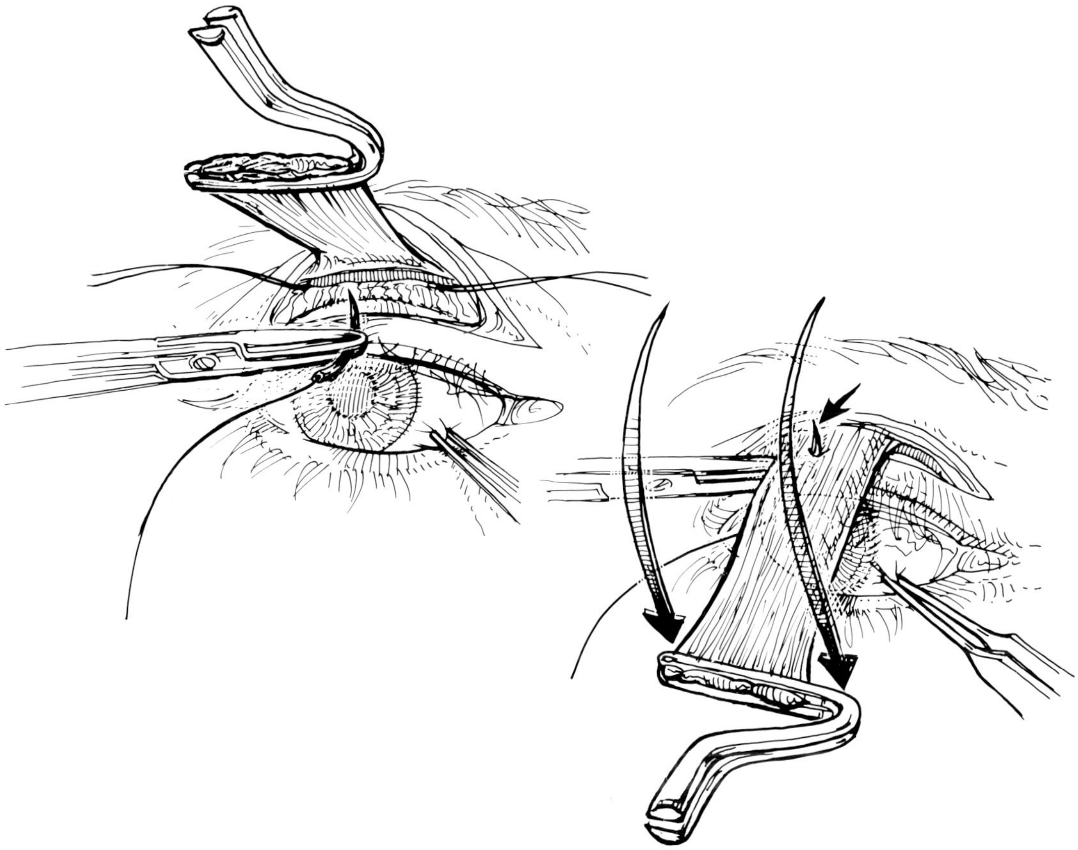

Fig. 34-5. With the upper lid placed at the position predetermined by Berke's table, the levator is pulled down over a needle that is at mid-tarsus, thus determining the amount of levator to be resected.

occur. For large resections, the levator may be split vertically several millimeters to spread the reinsertion to create a satisfactory arch (Fig. 34-6B).

I have not found it necessary to use a procedure to establish a supratarsal crease. In fact, I have been unable to avoid it in orientals who do not wish the occidental fold. The skin is closed with a running intradermal 6-0 monofilament nylon suture.

Posterior Approach

This procedure is useful in up to 3 or 3.5 mm of ptosis. Its main advantage is the easier initial identification of the aponeurosis, since that structure is the first encountered when the tarsus is cut. Disadvantages are that larger resections are more difficult, resection amounts are less easily confirmed, muscle function is sacrificed, and advancement of the levator on the tarsus is difficult.

The procedure I use is every much like the original Blascovics[12] procedure, except that through-the-lid sutures are not used and a strip of tarsus, rather than conjunctival sutures, is used for traction.

The lid is everted on a Desmarres retractor. A horizontal knife incision is made through tarsus, 1 to 2 mm from its upper edge, taking care not to cut deeper, into aponeurosis. Using the superior strip of tarsus for countertraction, the aponeurosis is bluntly dissected from superior tarsal muscle, taking care not to cut the peripheral arterial arcade. The levator is buttonholed at each end of the incision, and a space created from one hole to the other between levator and orbicularis with blunt dissec-

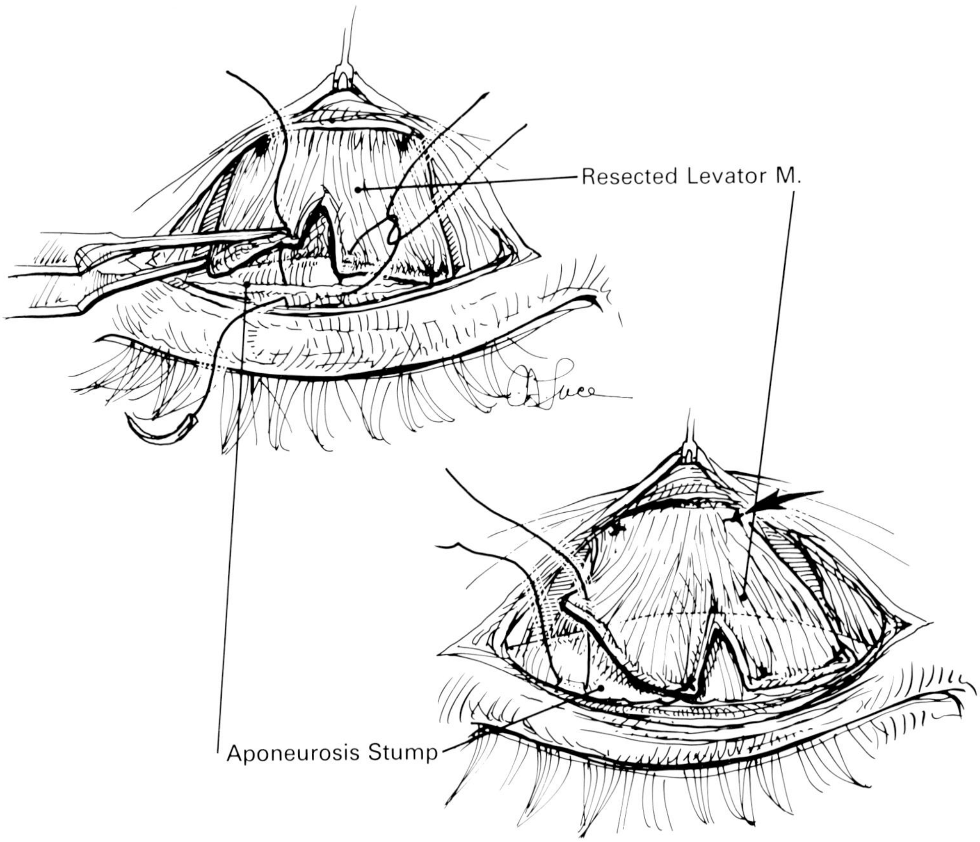

Fig. 34-6. (A) Method of reinsertion of resected levator into aponeurosis stump, the preferred technique when levator advancement is not required. The levator is split to create a satsifactory arch. **(B)** Insertion to tarsal plate.

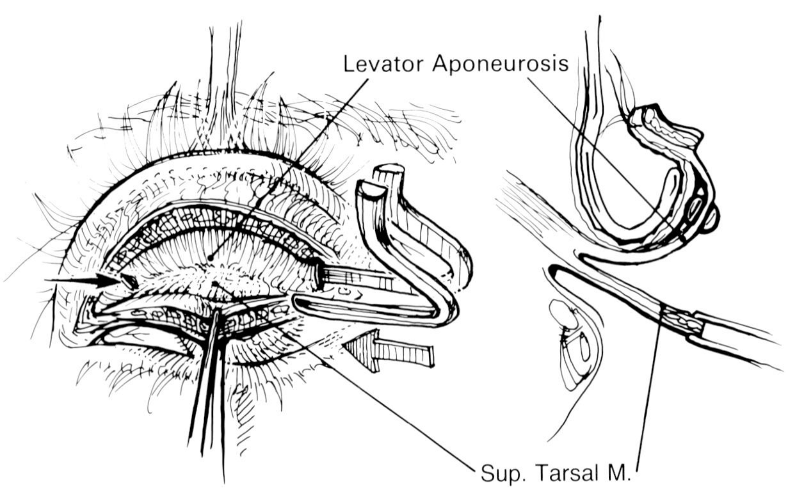

Fig. 34-7. Posterior approach to levator resection. Transection of the tarsus, 1 to 2 mm from its superior border, and a clamp placed across the aponeurosis after it is dissected from the superior tarsal muscle.

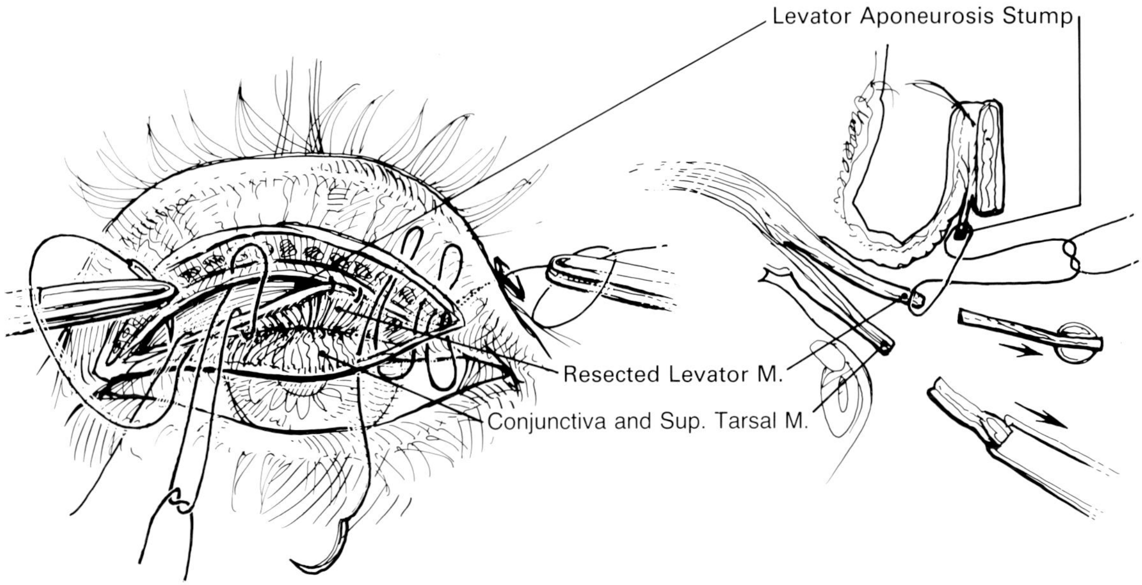

Fig. 34-8. Posterior approach to levator resection. Sutures are placed through the levator at a preplanned level and the distal levator excised. The sutures are inserted into the aponeurosis stump. The conjunctiva is closed by a running buried suture, as in a tarso-Müllerectomy.

tion. A blade of a ptosis clamp is placed through this space and the clamp closed. The Desmarres retractor is removed.

The distal end of the aponeurosis is cut next to the clamp. The levator is freely mobilized by anteriorly separating the septum from the aponeurosis and cutting the horns as needed, and posteriorly, cutting the superior attachments of superior tarsal muscle from the levator (Fig. 34-7). Four sutures of 6-0 plain catgut are tied or locked into the levator muscle at the preplanned level above its cut end. The levator is cut distal to the sutures. Both arms of each suture are then brought through the levator to lie superior to it. One arm of each suture is then passed through the aponeurosis stump from its tarsal side (but not through tarsus) to the orbicularis side and tied to the other arm so that the knot lies between levator and orbicularis (Fig. 34-8). The conjunctiva with the attached tarsal strip is then resected 3 or 4 mm. The new conjunctival edge is sewn to the cut upper tarsal edge in the same fashion as in tarso-Müllerectomy to avoid suture irritation of the cornea. The ends of this suture are brought out through small skin incisions medially and laterally, and tied into orbicularis with reinforced slip knots.

Lid crease-forming sutures are neither necessary nor advisable. Modified Frost sutures are placed, to remain about 4 days. Bland ointment is used as necessary to protect the cornea.

COMBINED RESECTIONS

McCord[13] described full-thickness lid resection for mild ptosis to remove tarsus, levator, orbicularis, and skin at the level of the upper half of the tarsus. In dysmyogenic ptosis, he resects 5 mm more than the amount of ptosis plus 1 mm for every millimeter that the levator excursion is less than 15 mm; in acquired ptosis, McCord resects 3 mm more than the amount of ptosis; and in Horner's syndrome, he resects the amount of ptosis. No more than one half the height of the tarsus should be excised. I find this procedure useful particularly in segmental ptosis, and in severely scarred lids.

Any of the foregoing procedures may be combined with another. Iliff[14] combines levator resection with tarso-Müllerectomy, obtaining greater correction than with levator resection alone. Iliff's approach is that for posterior approach resection, except that he resects tarsus, conjunctiva, and superior tarsal muscle en bloc with the levator aponeurosis complex. Care must be taken not to compromise the upper fornix. Closure is with through-and-through mattress sutures tied above the lash line. Although I do not use this operation, other surgeons use it with success.

FRONTALIS MUSCLE SUSPENSION

The frontalis muscle is not a primary lid elevator. It raises the brow and flattens the preseptal bulge above the tarsal crease to remove these structures from the visual field in upward gaze. It also elevates the upper lid 1 to 2 mm. Its chronic usage to elevate a ptotic upper lid is frequently seen and represents an acquired habit, not an inborn reflex. This habit should be established prior to frontalis suspension, or the patient is unlikely to use brow elevation for correction of the ptosis. The direction of pull on the lid by the frontalis is upward except in deep-set eyes, in which it may even be upward and forward in distinction to the levator's upward and backward pull. However, when a more physiologic lid retractor cannot be used, it is a useful muscle to use for lid elevation. Indications for frontalis muscle suspension include Marcus Gunn jaw-winking, in which the levator action must be sacrificed, congenital fibrosis, progressive external ophthalmoplegia, myotonia, and dysmyogenic ptosis with 4 mm or less of levator function.

Materials appropriate to connect the lid to the frontalis are autologous or preserved fascia lata and silicone rod. Autologous fascia lata is usually preferred because it is well tolerated and maintains its strength. It is sufficiently developed to be harvested by the age of 3. The method of harvesting described by Waller[15] is excellent. With the leg straight, a line is marked between the head of the fibula and the anterior-superior iliac crest. The fascia is then stretched by crossing that thigh over the other. The skin is incised along the mark for 6 or 7 cm, beginning about 4 cm above the lateral condyle. The incision is deepened through fat to the fascia. Fat and circumferential fascial fibers are scraped away with a knife. A mastoid or other self-retaining retractor, hinge upward, provides good exposure of the fascia. The fat is separated from the fascia by blunt scissors dissection for 12 to 15 cm toward the iliac crest. Two vertical parallel cuts are made in the fascia near its lower end, about 8 mm apart. These are extended upward a few centimeters with scissors. The lower ends of these incisions are joined and several centimeters of the strip of fascia separated from the underlying muscle. This strip is then fed into a Crawford fascia stripper. This stripper is preferred because it cuts less muscle or fat, provides a wide strip of fascia, has centimeter marks indicating the length of fascia, and has a sliding blade to cut the upper end of the fascial strip and thereby permit a small skin incision. Two Kocher or Allis clamps hold the lower end of the strip while the stripper is pushed up until 12 to 15 cm of fascia has been cleared. The safety cam is then unlocked and the upper end of the fascia cut. The fascial strip and stripper are slid out together. Hemostasis is secured by pressure. The skin is closed with a running 3-0 silk suture and a pressure dressing applied. The fascia is cleaned and cut into 2-mm strips.

There are many ways of placing the fascia between frontalis and the pretarsal tissues. I believe that at least three points of suspension in the lid facilitate the formation of a satisfactory lid arch. My preference is to use two strips of fascia in rhomboid fashion.

Most surgeons pass the fascia into pretarsal tissues from one of three eyelid incisions to another with the Wright needle. I feel more secure exposing the tarsal plate through a supratarsal crease incision and suturing each facial strip to the tarsus with two 5-0 supramid sutures (Fig. 34-9, inset). Three incisions are made through skin into frontalis muscle, above the eyebrow, the central incision 2 or 3 mm above the medial and lateral ones (Fig. 34-9). The two strips of fascia are drawn from the center of the lid incision to the central brow incision with one pass of a Wright needle. Each pass of the needle from above should engage frontalis muscle and then pass behind the orbital septum and out the lid incision. This is facilitated by manually

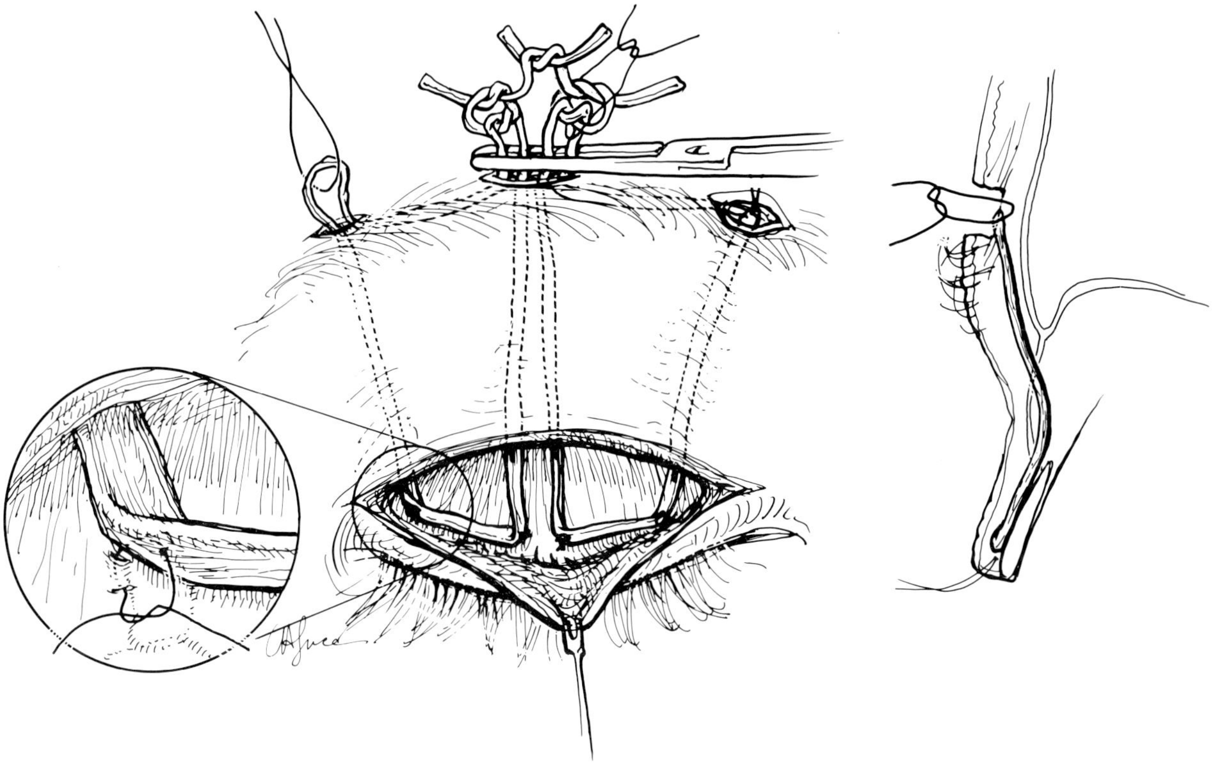

Fig. 34-9. Placement of fascia lata for a frontalis suspension by means of a lid-crease incision and three incisions above the brow. Each strip is fixed to the tarsus in two places with 5-0 sypramid suture (inset). Each strip is tied to itself at the central brow incision; they are then tied to each other.

depressing the brow downward while passing the needle. The other ends of the fascia strips are similarly brought up through either the lateral or medial brow incision. The lid is pulled upward by the strips into an overcorrected position with the desired arch and the strips sutured to frontalis while this traction is maintained. The fascia ends at the medial and lateral brow incisions are then passed to the central brow incision and tied to each other. The knot is secured with Supramid suture. The skin incisions are closed with 6-0 nylon, a modified Frost suture placed, and a pressure dressing applied.

If, as described by Crawford,[16] preserved fascia is used, it should be well soaked. I soak it in neomycin – bacitracin – polymyxin solution diluted 50 percent with saline.

Silicone rod 0.6 to 1.0 mm in diameter is a reasonable substitute if fascia is not available, as in children under 3 years of age or in cases in which the orbicularis is weak, making a distensible connection desirable, or if reversal of the procedure is anticipated, as in the presence of myotonia, dry eye, third cranial nerve paralysis in the elderly, or progressive ophthalmoplegia. I have used the rod as a test procedure before the final use of fascia but have not yet had to replace the rod with fascia.

When this rod is used, sutures are not used to secure it because they cut through the silicone. At the eyelid level, the rod is passed through pretarsal tissues from one of three incisions to another with the Wright needle, as described by Older and Dunne.[17] The lid incisions are made 3 mm above the lash line. The ends of the rod are united with a sleeve commonly used in scleral buckling procedures.

LEVATOR TRANSPLANT

This procedure also transfers the action of the frontalis muscle to the lid, but uses the levator–aponeurosis complex as the suspension material. The need to take fascia lata or to use foreign material is thus eliminated. This procedure is particularly useful in situations in which levator function has been irreversibly lost, as in congenital fibrosis, third nerve paralysis, or severe fibrotic dysmyogenic ptosis, especially when there is severe preoperative lag on downward gaze and when levator function must be sacrificed, as in correction of Marcus Gunn jaw-winking. Lipoelastic dysmyogenic ptosis should not be corrected with this procedure because the levator remnant has insufficient tensile strength.

General anesthesia is preferred, but frontal nerve block well back on the orbital roof may be used. The exposure of the anterior and superior surface of the aponeurosis and levator and separation of the septum is made through a supratarsal lid crease incision as described for aponeurosis repair. One should not dissect below the skin incision. If an

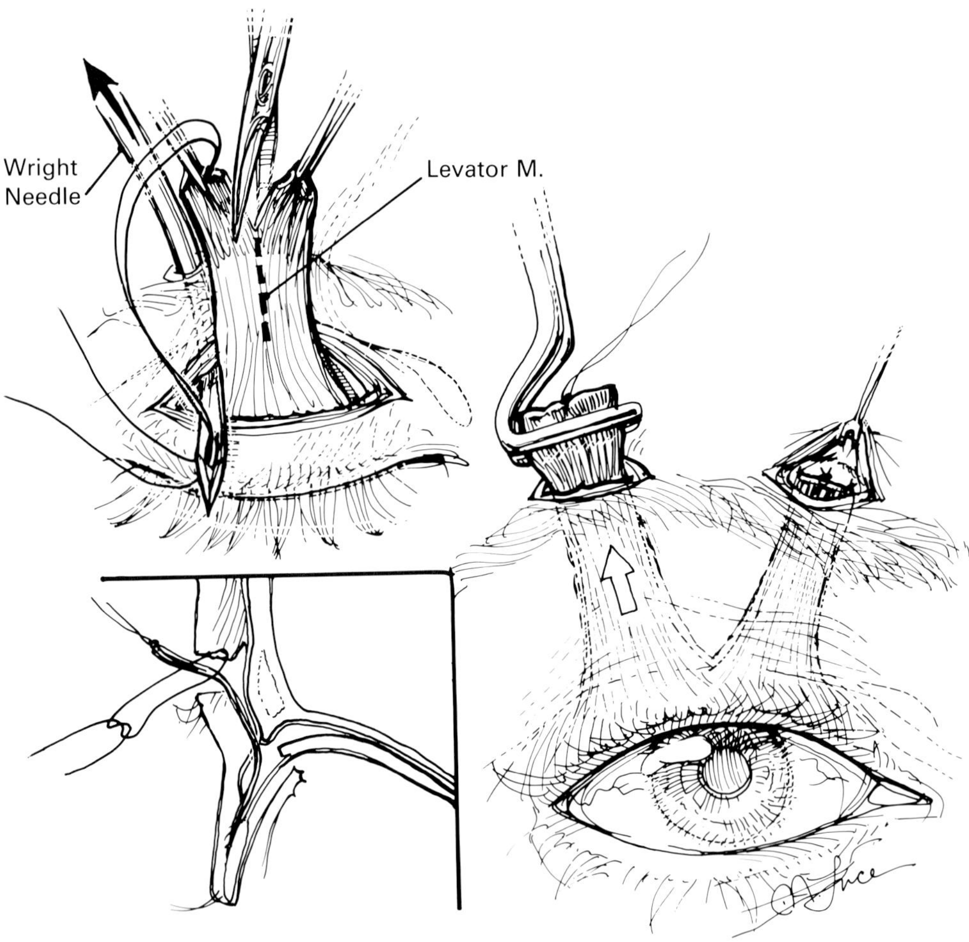

Fig. 34-10. Frontalis suspension using the levator muscle, which has been isolated and split vertically (levator transplant). Each arm of the levator is then tunneled with the aid of a suture placed through its cut end and passed up through a Wright needle. It is then sutured to the frontalis muscle and the distal end excised.

unsubstantial levator muscle is encountered, the planned procedure is aborted, and either a very large levator resection or another frontalis procedure is performed.

A small ptosis clamp is applied to the levator as proximal as possible. The levator muscle is cut distal to the clamp. The distal portion of the levator is folded forward and superior tarsal muscle separated from it.

An attempt to suture superior tarsal muscle to the proximal stump of the levator may be made, although I find this very difficult. This should not be done in jaw-winking cases. In either event, the clamp is removed.

A vertical cut is made from the center of the cut end of the distal levator through muscle into aponeurosis to just below the upper border of the tarsal plate (Fig. 34-10). A 4-0 silk suture is tied tightly around each of the two strips near its cut end.

Two incisions are made above the brow through skin into frontalis muscle. A Wright needle is passed through each brow incision to the lid incision, taking care to place it behind the septum in order to pull the lid in a posterior-superior direction. Each of the two levator strips is then drawn up and out of its respective brow incision by inserting its preplaced silk suture through the needle and withdrawing the needle. The levator strips should be pulled upward slowly and gently, as these strips can be fragile.

With the lid held upward by the levator strips in an overcorrected position and with the desired arch, the strips are sewn to frontalis muscle with 5-0 supramid sutures. All three incisions are closed with running intradermal 6-0 nylon sutures and a modified Frost suture is placed.

PTOSIS IN SPECIAL CIRCUMSTANCES

Several special circumstances with ptosis deserve to be singled out for comment: ptosis after trauma and ptosis in the presence of an anophthalmic socket.

Ptosis following injury may be caused by any of the basic causes of ptosis: an aponeurotic defect, damage to the levator muscle, injury to the third nerve or to the sympathetic chain, scarring, or increased lid bulk. Examination will usually reveal the cause. Immediate surgery is not usually necessary, unless there is an open laceration. Swelling or contusion of nerve or muscle is frequently the cause of ptosis and usually will spontaneously resolve. When there has been no improvement for 6 months, the residual ptosis should be repaired. It is preferable to use local anesthesia so that the patient's gaze change may be used to aid in identification and mobilization of the levator. Also, the adjustment of the lid height and contour are more accurate when judged in the awake patient.

Anophthalmic ptosis may be aponeurotic or mechanical, or a combination of both. It is frequently purely aponeurotic, having the same characteristics as aponeurotic ptosis without anopthalmos, and is treated by aponeurosis repair. It may also be a result of enophthalmos due to fat atrophy and loss of orbital tissue. This moves back the fulcrum of the levator and decreases the tension on the muscle, causing ptosis.

Ptosis in the presence of an anophthalmic socket also may be caused by contraction of conjunctiva and Tenon's capsule, sagging of the prosthetic eye from stretching of the lower lid, or contracted orbital scar. Direct treatment of these causes is usually unsatisfactory, and aponeurosis surgery or levator resection may be required. Procedures that remove conjunctiva or tarsus should usually be avoided, as they may jeopardize prosthesis retention and lid function. Treatment of anophthalmic ptosis is also covered in Chapter 58.

LASH PTOSIS

Lash ptosis may be present prior to surgery or may be induced by dissection of pretarsal skin near the lash follicles. It can be corrected, either segmentally or across the entire lid, whenever there is a lid crease incision exposing the tarsal plate. Multiple mattress sutures are placed in the following fashion: A 6-0 silk suture is passed through the skin 1 mm above the lashes and brought into the pretarsal area at about the same level. It is then passed horizontally through 2 mm of tarsal plate or newly created attachments of the levator, 3 to 4 mm above the initial passage. The suture is then passed back through the pretarsal skin, parallel to the first passage and 2 mm away from it, exiting 1 mm above the lashes. The suture is not tied until all the sutures have been placed. Additional sutures are placed, each starting 2 mm from the previous one, until the entire area of lash ptosis has sutures above it. Each is initially tied with a surgeon's knot, with the tension on each adjusted so that the lashes are lifted into a slightly overcorrected position. When suture adjustment has created uniform overcorrection of the ptotic lashes, 2 more knots are added to each. These sutures are allowed to remain for 2 to 3 weeks, to ensure that sufficient scar will have been created to maintain the lashes in a nonptotic position.

COMPLICATIONS

General complications are those of any surgical procedure, such as hemorrhage, infection, and wound dehiscence. Fortunately, these are all rare after ptosis surgery, except for infection along foreign materials used for frontalis suspension. In these cases, attempts are made to control the infection medically for as long as possible, in the hope that scar will form adjacent to the material and maintain the correction when the material is removed.

Hemorrhage into the orbital fat is potentially blinding. Significant hemorrhage should be treated by widely opening the wound and draining the preaponeurotic space.

Wound dehiscence usually occurs only in short segments, rarely requires resuturing, and does not tend to cause significant permanent scar. Fistulas can occur if through-the-lid sutures are used to establish the lid crease. They also interfere with the normal shearing motion in the subcutaneous and postaponeurotic tissues. For these reasons, such sutures should not be used.

Complications specific to ptosis surgery are undercorrection, overcorrection, poor lid contour, poor lid crease, entropion, ectropion, corneal abrasion, exposure keratopathy, dry eye, lagophthalmos, and lag on downward gaze.

Undercorrection occurs frequently after levator resection for dysmyogenic ptosis, especially in those with poor levator function. If the undercorrection is slight, a tarsomüllerectomy can provide 1 or 2 mm more lift. If moderate or marked, additional levator resection or frontalis suspension is necessary.

Most overcorrections are of aponeurotic ptosis, and are most likely to occur if levator resection rather than aponeurosis repair has been done. Use of local anesthesia with observation of the lid position during surgery minimizes the likelihood of overcorrecting it. If overcorrection is noted during the first few days, one or two sutures may be removed. Downward lid massage will often overcome up to 2 mm of overcorrection. Levator recession with the interposition of a spacer such as preserved sclera or orbital septum is required for treatment of residual overcorrection. A traction suture is always necessary after surgical management of overcorrection.

The lid contour is adjusted at surgery in all cases, and usually remains as it appears at the completion of surgery. A low area of lid margin may be raised by excising a small ellipse of full-thickness eyelid above it. A high area of the arch may require section of the levator above it with interposition of a spacer.

I find loss of the lid crease rare, and it does not occur if the original insertions of the aponeurosis are preserved. A new crease can be formed by incising the skin at the position of the desired crease and placing sutures between levator and posterior orbicularis fascia.

Entropion with trichiasis is caused by advancing the levator too low on the tarsus. This also produces a low lid crease. Correction consists of cutting the insertion and reinserting the levator higher on the tarsus. The levator is sutured to the orbicularis at the desired height of the crease.

Ectropion results when lid crease sutures, either through the lid or from levator to skin, create too much tension on the skin below the sutures. The orbicularis should be surgically freed from the levator.

Corneal abrasion can occur accidentally during ptosis surgery, since a protective contact lens, which interferes with observation of the height of the lid, is not ordinarily used. The abrasion ordinarily heals quickly. However, abrasion caused by sutures placed entirely through tarsus or by posterior exposure of tarso-Müllerectomy sutures will persist until the offending sutures are removed. Abrasion can be prevented by examining the conjunctival surface of the tarsus during surgery.

Persistent exposure keratopathy is peculiarly infrequent in children, tending to resolve within 1 to 2 weeks, even in the presence of severe lagophthalmos. The use of artificial tears while awake and ointment at bedtime for several weeks is usually sufficient to prevent significant symptoms. Lagophthalmos can be a serious problem in adults, especially if keratitis sicca, weak orbicularis, decreased fifth nerve function, or paralysis of upward gaze are present. Artificial tears, ointments, moist chambers, and/or taping the lid closed may help. Uncorrection is advisable in such patients to prevent this potentially severe problem.

Insufficient ocular lubrication can precede but be aggravated by ptosis surgery. Tear production should be evaluated in adults preoperatively. Most ptosis operations spare the lacrimal gland and ducts, but tarso-Müllerectomy always removes many accessory lacrimal glands, and all procedures widen the palpebral fissure, increasing tear loss by evaporation.

Lagophthalmos exists preoperatively in most cases of dysmyogenic ptosis and is increased by the surgery. Most ptosis operations, with the exception of aponeurosis repair, produce some degree of lagophthalmos. Patients should be made aware that the operated eye may appear abnormally wide in downward gaze and that the eye may remain open in sleep.

REFERENCES

1. Jones LT, Quickert MH, Wobig JL: A cure of ptosis by aponeurotic repair. Arch Ophthalmol 94:629, 1975
2. Fansanella RM, Servat J: Levator resection for minimal ptosis: Another simplified operation. Arch Ophthalmol 65:439, 1961
3. Putterman AM, Urist MJ: Mueller's muscle–conjunctiva resection. Arch Ophthalmol 93:619, 1975
4. Henderson JW: Present status of blepharoptosis in surgery. Postgrad Med 33:153, 1963
5. Beard C: The surgical treatment of blepharoptosis: A quantitive approach. Trans Am Ophthalmol Soc 64:401, 1966
6. Chimonidou E, Palimeris G, Iliakis E, et al: The necessary resection of the levator muscles of the upper eyelid in the operation for congenital blepharoptosis. J Pediatr Ophthalmol 14:18, 1977
7. Beard C: Ptosis. 3rd Ed. CV Mosby, St. Louis, 1981
8. Berke RN: Results of resection of the levator muscle through a skin incision in congenital ptosis. Arch Ophthalmol 61: 177, 1959
9. Berke RN, Wadsworth JAC: Histology of levator muscle in congenital and acquired ptosis. Arch Ophthalmol 53:413, 1955
10. Johnson CC: Blepharoptosis: A general consideration of surgical methods with results in 162 operations. Am J Ophthalmol 38:129, 1954
11. Berke RN: Results of the resection of the levator muscle through a skin incision in congenital ptosis. Arch Ophthalmol 61:177, 1959
12. Blascovics L: A New operation for ptosis with shortening of the levator and tarsus. Arch Ophthalmol 52:563, 1923
13. McCord CD Jr: An external minimum ptosis procedure—External tarso-aponeurectomy. Trans Am Acad Ophthal Otolaryngol 79:683, 1975
14. Iliff CE: A simplified ptosis operation. Am J Ophthalmol 37:529, 1954
15. Waller RR: Evaluation and management of the ptosis patient. p.60. In McCord CD Jr (ed): Oculoplastic Surgery. Raven Press, New York, 1981
16. Crawford JS: Repair of ptosis using frontalis muscle and fascia lata: A 20-year review. Ophthalm Surg 8:31, 1977
17. Older JJ, Dunne PB: Silicone slings for correction of ptosis associated with progressive external ophthalmoplegia. Ophthalmol Surg 15:379, 1984

Entropion

35

Ted H. Wojno

Entropion is perhaps the most common lid disorder encountered by ophthalmologists. A multiplicity of corrective surgical procedures have been devised, suggesting that many techniques are initially successful in relieving entropion but that recurrences are not unusual. Ophthalmic surgeons have therefore continued to modify procedures and devise new ones, with the hope of finding a long-lasting physiologic and functional cure.

No one surgical technique will correct all types of entropion. The methods presented in this chapter must be tailored to fit the findings of each patient. Nevertheless, the surgical procedures are derived from widely accepted principles and will be useful in most patients with entropion.

ETIOLOGY OF ENTROPION

Involutional Entropion

Involutional entropion (senile entropion), by definition due to aging changes in the lids and orbital tissues, usually affects patients who are in the sixth decade of life or later. Jones[1] demonstrated that stretching, dehiscence, or disinsertion of the lower lid retractors is of prime importance in the development of involutional entropion. He showed that these changes, each of which produces inferior lid retractor laxity, permit anterior rotation of the lower tarsal border and turning in of the lid margin.

Also important in the causation of entropion is horizontal laxity in the aging eyelid.[2,3] Although the laxity may involve the entire length of the eyelid, it is often most notable at the lateral and medial canthal tendons.

Other factors contributing to the causation of entropion are of lesser importance. With age, a relative enophthalmos develops, presumably due to atrophy of the orbital fat.[1] Thus, the outward pressure exerted by the globe against the lid margin is reduced and causes relative horizontal lid laxity. Other investigators have found the preseptal muscles to become lax and to lose their attachments to the orbital septum.[4] The preseptal muscles then override the pretarsal muscles, allowing the lower border of the tarsus to move outward and the margin to rotate inward. In addition, with age, the tarsus thins and permits it to buckle on itself when subjected to the above-mentioned alterations in lid anatomy.[5]

Involutional entropion is recognized only in the lower lid. Although similar changes take place in the upper lid, they result in ptosis, not entropion. Lash ptosis, a downward tilt to the upper lid lashes, is caused by relaxation of the pretarsal skin and orbicularis oculi muscles. When lash ptosis is severe, the lashes may abrade the cornea. This is not truly an entropion, since the lid margin is not inverted. Its treatment is discussed in Chapter 34.

SPASTIC ENTROPION

Confusion exists with regard to the meaning of the term *spastic entropion*. Earlier workers often did not distinguish this condition from involutional entropion. Orbicularis spasms, although once considered an important cause of entropion, have not been shown to play a major role. Fox[6] showed that injections of local anesthetic into the orbicularis oculi muscle will not cure entropion, making this explanation unlikely. In actuality, most cases of what was previously called spastic entropion would now be classified as involutional entropion.

Spastic entropion, a relatively rare condition, is one that develops acutely from squeezing the lids shut in the presence of ocular irritation, as occurs after cataract surgery or with keratitis. Removal of the inciting cause or instillation of topical anesthetic should therefore relieve the entropion and serve to distinguish spastic from involutional entropion. However, spastic entropion may eventually stretch the inferior lid retractors, or a defect in them may predispose the patient to develop entropion with ocular irritation. Thus, involutional entropion should be suspected and the lid assessed for findings of it.

Cicatricial Entropion

Cicatricial entropion is caused by contracture of either the conjunctiva or the tarsus, or both, thereby shortening the posterior lamella of the lid. It may be secondary to alkali burns or other chemical trauma, ocular pemphigoid, Stevens-Johnson syndrome, mechanical trauma, trachoma, and various other disorders. The shortened posterior lamella buckles the lid, pulling the margin and lashes posteriorly where they may abrade the cornea. Scarring may cause lashes to exit the lid aberrantly and irritate the globe even when the position of the margin is corrected. Involutional horizontal laxity may additionally be present in an older patient. Cicatricial entropion occurs in both the upper and lower lids.

RELATED DISORDERS

Congenital entropion, trichiasis, and distichiasis are discussed in Chapters 37 and 42.

EVALUATION OF ENTROPION

The examiner should determine the length of time the entropion has been present and whether it is constant or intermittent. The patient should be questioned about previous lid injury or surgery and conjunctival disease such as pemphigoid, Stevens-Johnson syndrome, and keratoconjunctivitis sicca. The severity of the symptoms should be ascertained.

During the examination, the position of the lid margin and lashes should be noted. In true entropion, the lid margin will be inverted, and the meibomian orifices will not be visible. In simple trichiasis, the lashes are misdirected against the globe, but the lid margin is in its normal position, and the meibomian orifices are visible.

The lid pathology and degree of the changes present are determined. There are a number of techniques to differentiate involutional from cicatricial entropion.

The examiner places an index finger on the lower lid and draws it laterally against the orbital rim, in effect shortening the lid horizontally. An involutional entropion will usually be temporarily eliminated by this maneuver, while cicatricial entropion usually remains or is only slightly improved. The movement of the lower punctum is noted during the lid-tightening maneuver. Normally, the punctum will move only 1 to 2 mm laterally. With medial canthal tendon laxity, it may be displaced to the medial limbus or further, signaling the need for correction of medial canthal tendon laxity during the entropion repair.

The lower lid is then pulled inferiorly with the index finger. In cicatricial entropion and normal patients, the tarsus will assume a position roughly parallel to the orbital floor. In involutional entropion with lower lid retractor laxity, although the lid pulls away from the globe, the tarsus often maintains its vertical position.[7]

Evaluation of the palpebral conjunctiva and cul-de-sac is also helpful. Normally the palpebral conjunctiva inferior to the tarsus is white because of the color of the underlying lower lid retractors. When the retractors are dehisced or markedly thinned, the palpebral conjunctiva inferior to the tarsus is pink because the orbicularis muscles can be seen through it.[7] In cicatricial entropion, scarring, symblepharon, or a shallow inferior cul-de-sac may be detected.

The degree of horizontal laxity of the lid with involutional entropion should be determined. In the distraction test, the examiner grasps the lower lid between the index finger and thumb and pulls it away from the globe. The median distraction found in people over age 50 is 8 mm.[8] In many cases, the displacement will be greater than 10 mm.[3] Usually a lid with distraction of greater than 8 mm will require repair; sometimes a lid with less than 8 mm of distraction will require repair if the lid does not snap back against the globe when it is released.

The examiner should still assess the lid for laxity in the presence or obvious cicatricial changes because it may occur secondarily. This horizontal laxity may have to be corrected, possibly as a second procedure, to obtain a satisfactory result, despite the fact that the main problem is cicatrix.

The findings with cicatricial entropion of the upper lid may also include conjunctival–tarsal scarring, symblepharon, foreshortening of the superior fornix, and tarsal thickening. An additional sign is difficulty everting the upper lid, even though the patient is not squeezing the lids.

DECISION TO OPERATE

Entropion should be corrected without excessive delay. Corneal abrasion from the lashes with subsequent corneal ulceration is a serious complication of neglected entropion.

In early, mild, or intermittent involutional entropion, the surgeon may be able to delay definitive correction by taping the lower lid up and laterally. The entropion will eventually become more frequent, however, and require surgical correction.

Ideally, repair of cicatricial entropion is delayed until the active cicatricial phase of the disease or injury has passed. However, significant corneal complications may necessitate repair of an inflamed eyelid. Both the patient and surgeon should then be aware that additional procedures may be required once the disease is quiescent.

SURGICAL CORRECTION

Involutional Entropion

Techniques for repair of involutional entropion can be divided into four categories: (1) shortening or reattachment of the lower lid retractors, (2) horizontally shortening the lid, (3) increasing the horizontal tension of the orbicularis along the inferior border of the tarsus to evert the lid, and (4) creation of a scar barrier between the preseptal and pretarsal orbicularis to prevent the former from overriding the latter.

The preferred procedures for involutional entropion correct any excess vertical and horizontal laxity, the two most significant pathologic alterations in the lid. The lower lid retractors are thus tucked or reattached to the tarsus, and/or a portion of the lid is functionally shortened horizontally.

Lower lid retractor tuck procedures were originated by Jones[1] (Fig. 35-1). A skin incision is made in the lateral two thirds of the lid at approximately the lower tarsal border and is extended slightly

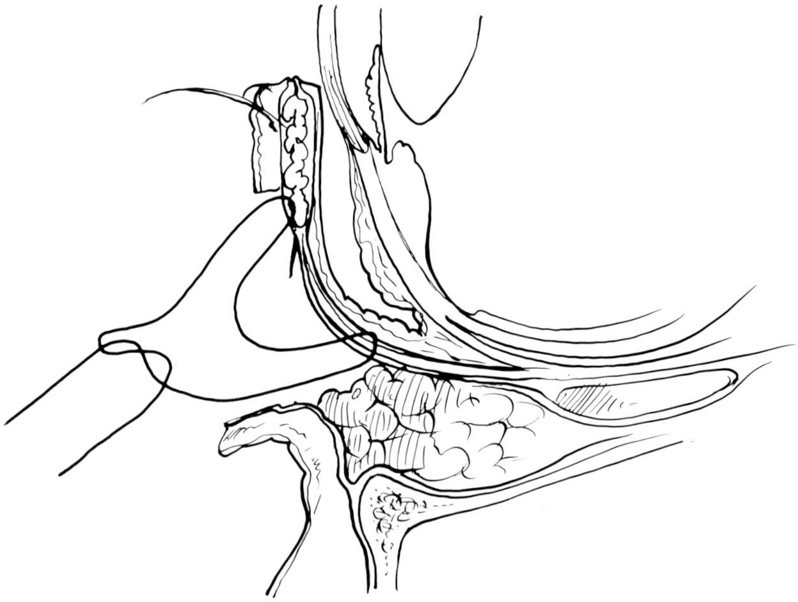

Fig. 35-1. Lower lid retractor tuck for involutional entropion. The skin, orbicularis, and orbital septum have been opened, exposing the lower lid retractors. Absorbable 6-0 sutures are passed first through the retractors and then through the lower tarsal border and tied. The skin is closed with a running 6-0 monofilament suture.

beyond the lateral canthus. The orbicularis muscle is incised and elevated from the lower tarsal border and orbital septum. The septum is opened transversely at the lower tarsal border. Redundant fat may be excised. The lower lid retractors are identified, and three or four absorbable 6-0 or 7-0 sutures are passed through the retractors. The sutures are then passed through the lower tarsal border and tied, effectively tucking the retractors. The skin is closed with a running 6-0 monofilament suture. Skin sutures are removed in 5 to 7 days. The main complication is lower lid retraction from excessive tucking of the retractors.

In approximately 25 percent of lids with involutional entropion, an excessively lax medial canthal tendon will have to be shortened during the repair. If this laxity is not corrected, the lid shortening will pull the punctum laterally out of the lacrimal lake and possibly compromise its function. The medial canthal tendon tuck should precede any other lid-shortening procedure, or an adequate tuck of the medial canthal tendon will not be possible.

A 1-cm horizontal skin incision is made over the medial canthal tendon, approximately 2 mm below the lid margin (Fig. 35-2). This incision begins 3 to 4 mm lateral to the punctum and continues just medial to the medial canthus. The skin above the incision is sharply dissected from the underlying orbicularis and inferior crus of the medial canthal tendon, for a distance of approximately 2 mm. A double-armed permanent 6-0 suture is used to tuck the tendon. The first bite is placed vertically, lateral to the punctum through approximately 2 to 3 mm of tarsus. The same needle is then passed back through the orbicularis only, in the opposite direction. The needle is once more passed through the tarsus. These three passages of the needle ensure that the suture will not cheesewire through the tissue. Both arms are then passed medially through the canthal tendon, approximately where the tendon overlies the lacrimal sac. Each arm is then passed back through the tendon. The suture is tied with sufficient tension to secure the punctum in its appropriate position. This suture should not be overly tight, or the punctum will be too medial and canaliculus kinked. If this procedure is combined with a vertical lid retractor shortening, the skin incisions may be joined and both closed with the same skin suture. Possible complications are suture granulomas and cheesewiring of the suture through the tendon and tarsus. A slightly different technique of tucking the medial canthal tendon is presented in Chapter 36.

To shorten a lid horizontally, I prefer the procedure performed by Dr. Richard R. Tenzel (personal communication) (Fig. 35-3). A 5-mm skin incision

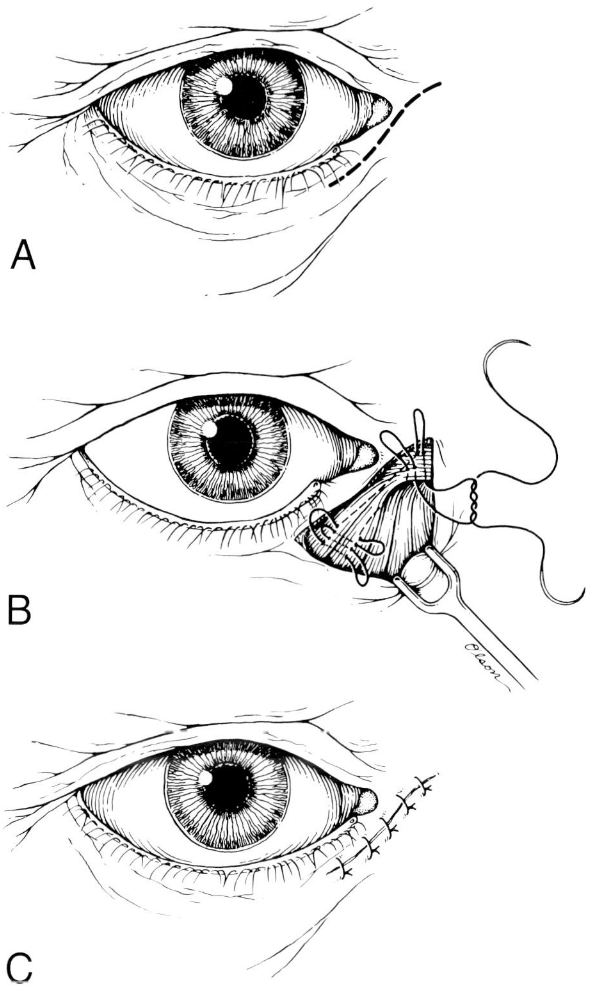

Fig. 35-2. Medial canthal tendon tuck. **(A)** The skin is incised over the medial canthal tendon. **(B)** One arm of a double-armed 6-0 permanent suture takes three bites through the tissue down to the tarsus. Each arm is then passed medially through the tendon to emerge in the medial canthus. Each arm takes one additional bite through the substance of the tendon and is then tied. **(C)** The skin is closed with a 7-0 silk suture.

starts 2 mm lateral to the lateral canthus, angled slightly downward away from the eye in a laugh line. While the lower skin edge is tented up with forceps, sharp-tipped scissors buttonhole the orbicularis. Blunt-tipped scissors inserted into the buttonhole dissect a pocket deep to the orbicularis for the entire length of the lower lid. The skin incision is then extended with scissors in an infraciliary line to the lower punctum, creating a skin–muscle flap. The orbital septum is opened transversely to gain access to the lower lid retractors. Fat may be removed. A 2-mm lateral canthotomy and an inferior crus cantholysis are performed with scissors. The cut edges of the lid are overlapped to determine the amount of redundancy, and this excess is excised. The inferior crus of the canthal tendon is reconstituted with three sutures, that is, 6-0 or 7-0 synthetic absorbable sutures (Vicryl), placed through the cut edge of the tarsus and the cut edge of the canthal tendon. Two or three buried sutures of 7-0 Vicryl close the overlying orbicularis. If the lateral canthal tendon is extremely lax or a more secure closure is desired, a lateral canthal sling may be used to shorten the lid, as described in Chapter 36.

At this point, the lower lid retractors may be tucked as previously described. Since the lid margin was shortened, some redundancy in the skin beneath the incision line may now be present, and this may be excised. Caution is advised when removing such excess skin, since an overzealous excision may cause ectropion. The subciliary portion of the wound is loosely closed with a running 6-0 monofilament suture with widely spaced bites. This ensures that any postoperative hemorrhage will leak anteriorly out of the incision rather than dissect posteriorly into the retrobulbar space. The suture is converted to a running vertical mattress at the lateral canthus to close both the muscle and skin adequately. If desired, the muscle laterally can be closed with interrupted absorbable sutures. Skin sutures are removed on the fifth to seventh postoperative day. The major complication of horizontal shortening is a rounded appearance of the lateral canthus when the canthotomy is made too large.

Another procedure that is rapid and effective is that described by Fox[9] (Fig. 35-4). The technique is based on horizontally shortening the lid at the lower border of the tarsus. It is useful in patients who require bedside surgery or in those who can spend only a minimal amount of time in the operating room for reasons of poor health or cooperation.

After anesthetizing the lower lid, it is everted with a chalazion clamp applied to the middle third of the eyelid. A triangle is outlined, with the base at the lower tarsal border and 7 to 10 mm long, de-

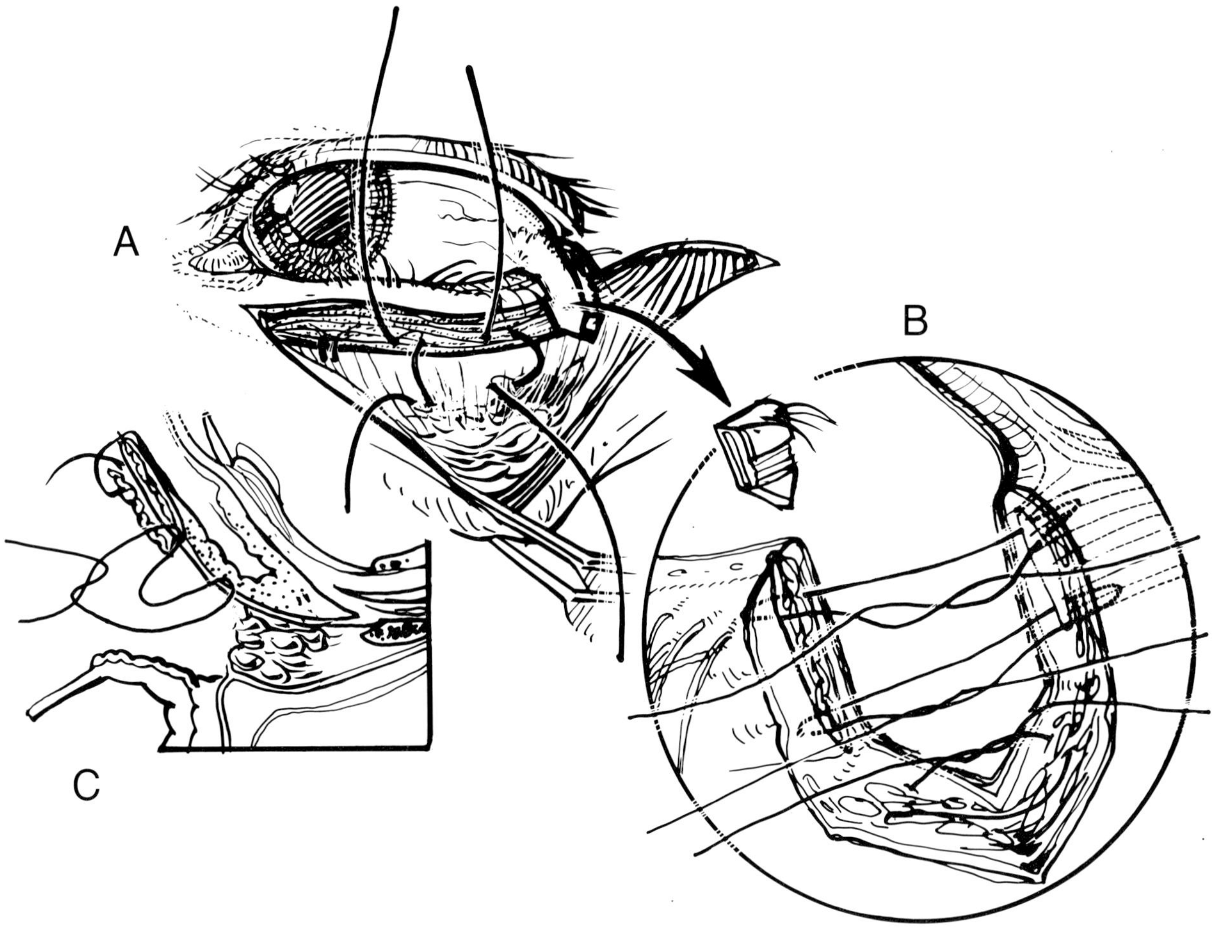

Fig. 35-3. Horizontal lower lid shortening. **(A)** A skin–muscle flap has been dissected and retracted and the orbital septum opened, exposing the lower lid retractors. The redundant portion of the lower eyelid is excised at the lateral canthus. **(B)** The tarsus is sewn to the cut edge of the lateral canthal tendon with interrupted 6-0 Vicryl sutures, while the overlying muscle is closed with buried 7-0 Vicryl sutures. **(C)** The lower lid retractors may be tucked as outlined in Figure 35-1. The skin is closed with a running 6-0 monofilament suture.

pending on the degree of laxity. The apex of the triangle is at least 1 mm away from the lid margin to prevent postoperative notching. The conjunctiva and tarsus are incised with a razor knife, and the triangle is excised with scissors. The chalazion clamp is slowly loosened, exposing the bleeding vessels, which are then cauterized. Buried 6-0 Vicryl sutures are placed through the cut edges of tarsus, starting at the apex. A base-up triangle of skin and muscle may be excised lateral to the lateral canthus to tighten the anterior lamella of the lid, but this is not necessary for the success of the procedure. If properly performed, the lid margin will be tented outward at the completion of the procedure, but this will even out in approximately 1 month. Complications include lid margin notch, chalazion, ectropion, and corneal abrasion. Recurrences should be treated as a new case of entropion by a lid shortening and retractor tuck.

Another procedure that may be performed at the bedside or in the office is the placement of Snellen–Quickert sutures[10] (Fig. 35-5). This tech-

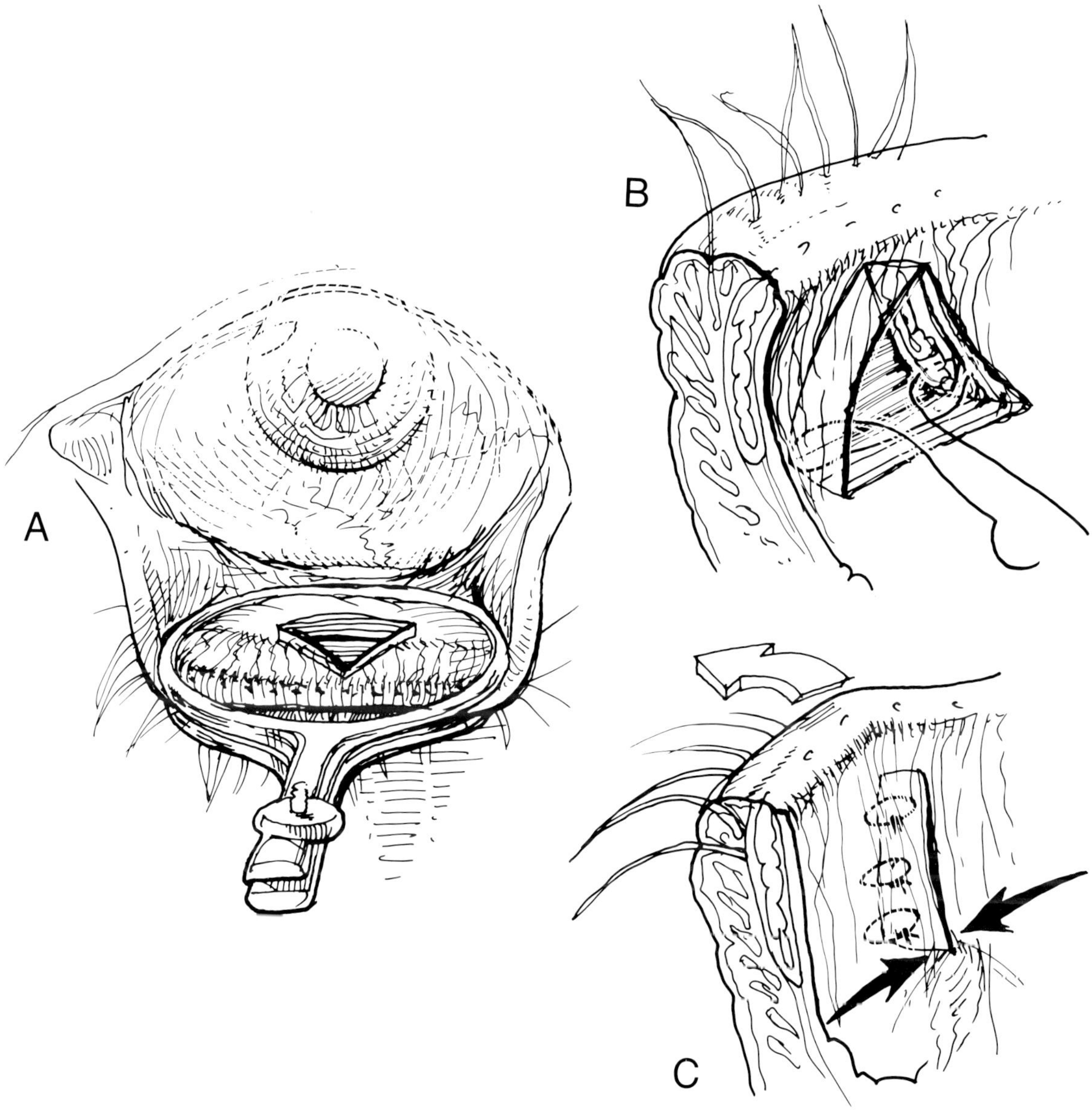

Fig. 35-4. Fox procedure for involutional entropion. **(A)** Base-down triangle of tarsus and conjunctiva excised from the center of the eyelid. **(B)** Buried 6-0 Vicryl sutures passed through the cut edges of the tarsus and tied. **(C)** Lid margin will be tilted outward slightly — a temporary effect.

nique indirectly tucks the lower lid retractors and creates a scar barrier between the preseptal and pretarsal orbicularis. The first needle of a double-armed 4-0 silk or chromic suture is passed vertically from deep in the lower fornix through the conjunctiva and lower lid retractors, travels anterior to the tarsus, and exits the skin 2 mm below the lashes. The second arm is passed parallel to, and 3 mm from, the first arm. Two or three additional sutures are placed in a like manner. All sutures are tied so that the lid is mildly overcorrected. The sutures are removed 2 or 3 weeks postoperatively.

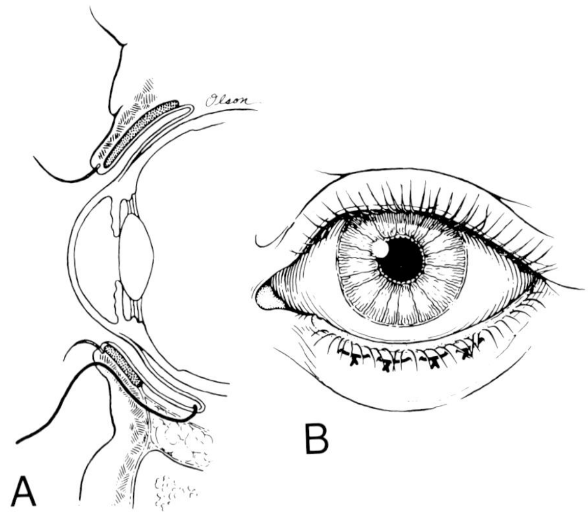

Fig. 35-5. Snellen-Quickert suture repair of entropion. **(A)** Double-armed 4-0 silk or chromic sutures are passed from the lower fornix through the lower lid retractors and exit the skin 2 mm below the lashes. **(B)** Sutures are tied.

Cicatricial Entropion

Surgical repair of cicatricial entropion is accomplished by outward rotation of the lid margin and/or lengthening the posterior lamella, which may require excision of scar tissue first. The Wies procedure[11] and its modifications are most commonly used for marginal rotation, while grafts to the posterior lamella of the lid are used for lengthening.

Although developed for spastic entropion, the Wies procedure is very effective for cicatricial entropion (Fig. 35-6). This transverse blepharotomy with marginal rotation redirects the forces on the anterior lamella so that the lid margin is turned outward. It may be employed on the upper and lower lids.

A horizontal incision is made through skin and orbicularis 3 mm from the lid margin. If the entropion involves only a portion of the lid, the incision should extend 2 mm medial and lateral to this seg-

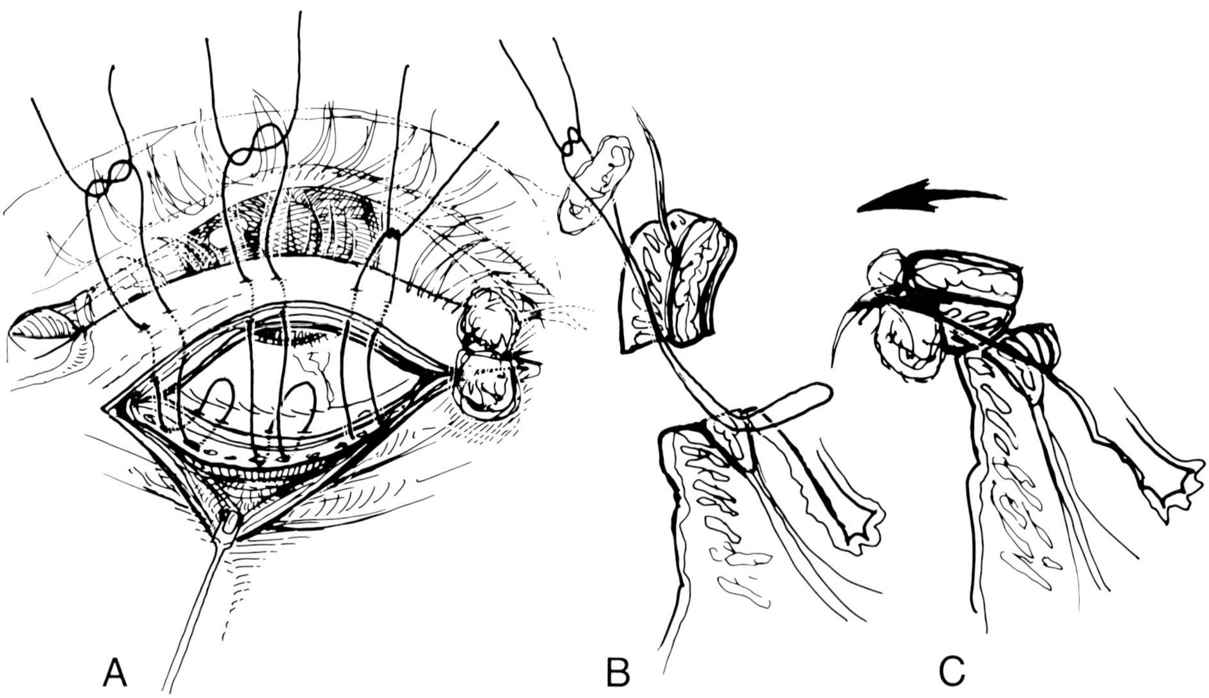

Fig. 35-6. Wies procedure for cicatricial entropion. **(A)** Full-thickness transverse blepharotomy performed 3 mm from the lid margin. Double armed 4-0 silk sutures are passed through the conjunctiva and tarsus on the lower edge of the incision and then through the subcutaneous tissues of the upper edge of the incision. **(B)** Cross-sectional view of suture placement. **(C)** Sutures tied (over a bolster if desired) and the tension adjusted for moderate overcorrection of the lid.

ment (but never medial to the punctum). When, as often occurs, the entire length of the lid is affected, the incision then extends across the entire lid. The lid is then everted and an incision is made through tarsus and conjunctiva, again 3 mm from the lid margin. This full-thickness blepharotomy is done in two steps to ensure that the incision is made perpendicular to the plane of the lid in both the anterior and posterior lamellae. Any strands of uncut tissue remaining in the incision can be cut with scissors. Four double-armed 4-0 silk sutures are passed through the conjunctiva and tarsus, 1 mm from the cut edge of the proximal segment, exiting on the anterior surface of the tarsus. When the procedure is performed on the upper lid, the suture should enter the tarsus through the cut edge, not through the conjunctiva, to avoid exposing suture on the conjunctival surface that could abrade the cornea. These sutures are then passed into the subcutaneous tissue of the distal segment and exit on the skin 1 to 2 mm from the lash margin. The sutures are then tied and the tension is adjusted to place the lid into a position of mild eversion. This overcorrection gradually resolves over the ensuing one to two months. The sutures are removed 10 to 14 days postoperatively. Complications include pyogenic granuloma, necrosis of the bridge flap, and ectropion.

A little more correction may be obtained with this procedure by splitting the lid margin at the gray line to a depth of 2 mm. This will provide slightly greater eversion of the lashes. For lower lid cicatricial entropion with a significant component of horizontal laxity, Quickert's modification may be useful.[12] This incorporates a full-thickness horizontal eyelid resection with a Wies procedure.

When the upper lid tarsus is thickened (as from scar formation), resection of a horizontal anterior wedge of tarsus may be useful[13,14] (Fig. 35-7). An incision is made in the upper lid crease down to the anterior tarsal surface. The tarsus is exposed by blunt dissection to just above the lash buds. A

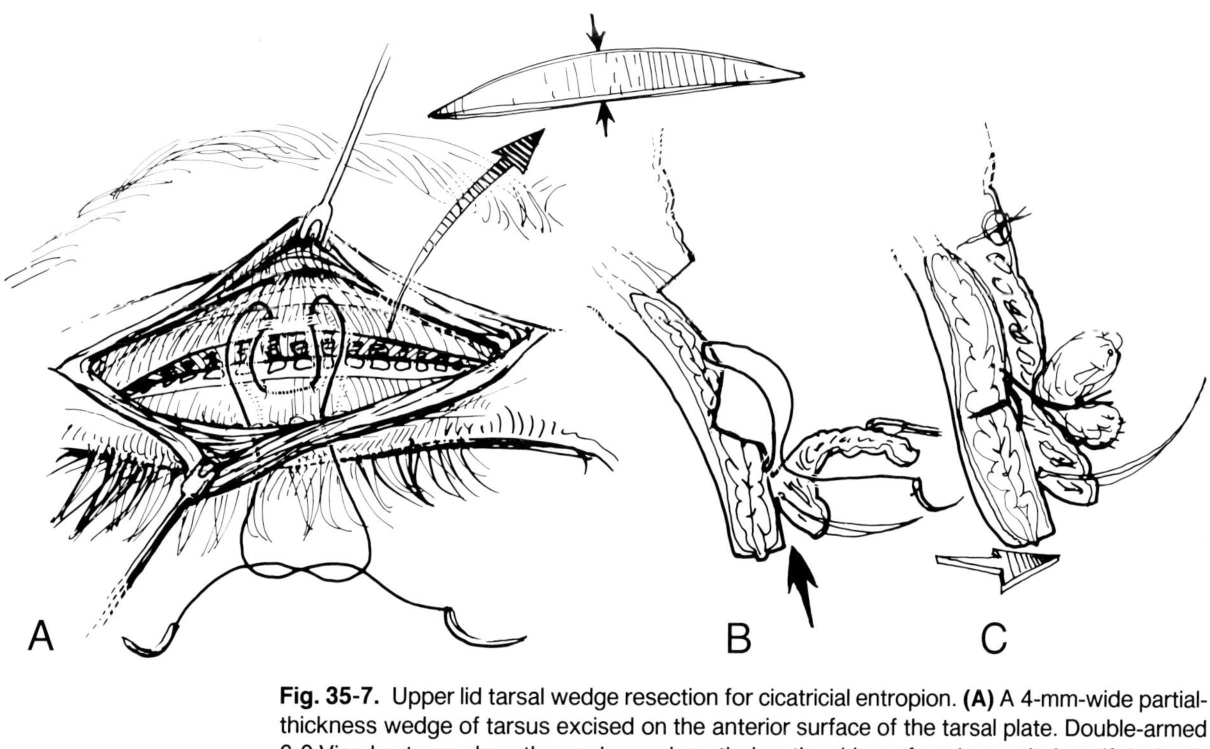

Fig. 35-7. Upper lid tarsal wedge resection for cicatricial entropion. **(A)** A 4-mm-wide partial-thickness wedge of tarsus excised on the anterior surface of the tarsal plate. Double-armed 6-0 Vicryl sutures close the wedge and are tied on the skin surface (over a bolster if desired). **(B)** Cross section showing the suture placement and gray line incision, which allows recession of the lashes superiorly on the tarsus. **(C)** Final result.

4-mm-wide partial-thickness horizontal wedge of tarsus is excised with a knife, usually starting 3 to 4 mm above the lid margin. The distance of the wedge excision from the lid margin can be varied, depending on the amount of curl in the lid and the site of this curl. This trough is continued medially and laterally the full width of the tarsus. Another incision is made in the gray line to a depth of 2 mm, again, the full length of the tarsus. The tarsal wedge is closed with four double-armed 6-0 Vicryl sutures by passing a needle horizontally into the tarsus just below the wedge. Each needle of the double-armed suture takes a bite of tarsus just above the wedge. Both needles are then passed through the skin just above the lashes, 2 mm apart, and tied. Sutures are removed in 10 days. The gray line incision permits recession of the lashes superiorly on the tarsus, while the tarsal wedge excision permits eversion of the lid margin and lashes.

For severe cicatricial entropion with marked contracture of tarsus and conjunctiva, a graft must be placed in the conjunctival surface to lengthen the posterior lamella. A variety of materials have been used as spacers, including nasal septal cartilage, upper lateral nasal cartilage, sclera, ear cartilage, buccal mucosa, bulbar conjunctiva, and cadaver tarsus. Sclera is most commonly employed because of its availability and ease of handling. When performing posterior lamella lengthening procedures on the upper lid it is important that no suture material be exposed on the conjunctiva surface to avoid corneal irritation and even abrasion.[14]

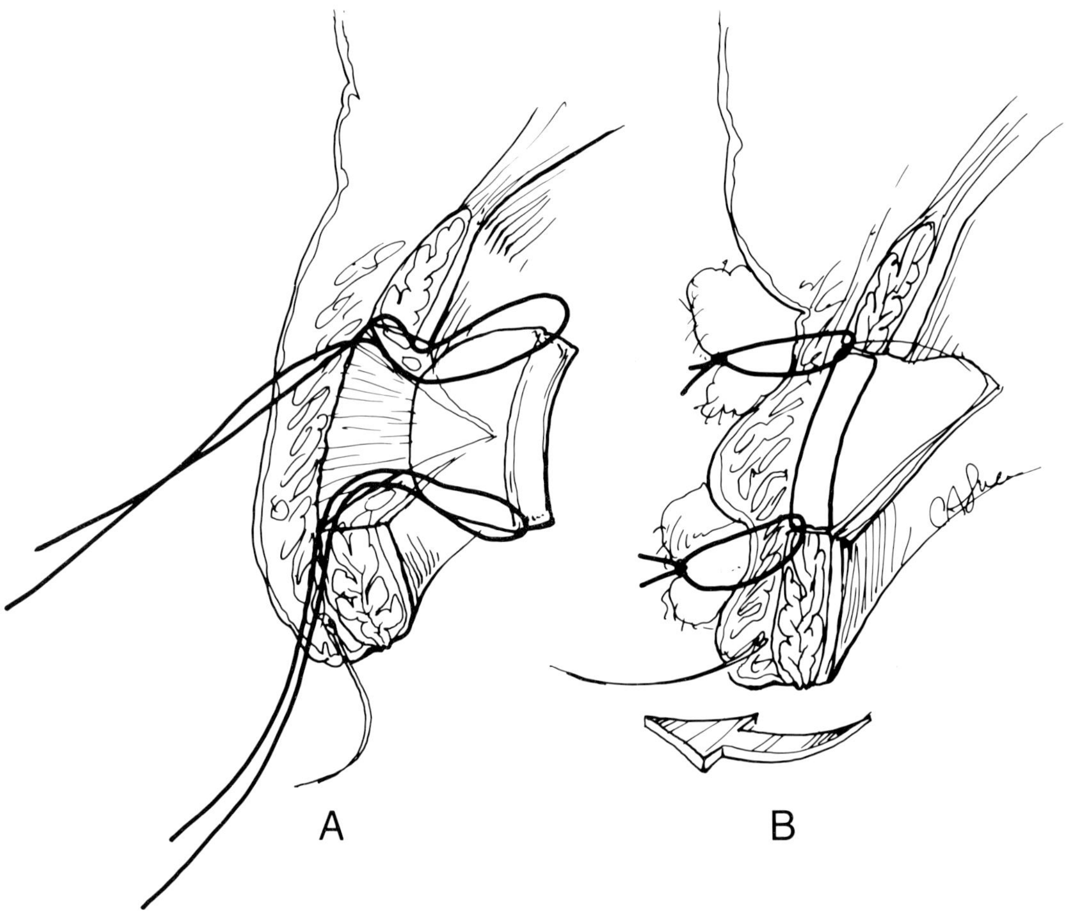

Fig. 35-8. Posterior lamella graft for cicatricial entropion. **(A)** Conjunctiva and tarsus incised 5 mm above the lid margin and a scleral graft cut to fit the defect; 6-0 monofilament suture is passed through the lid and graft as shown (see details in text). **(B)** Sutures are tied over bolsters and the tension adjusted so as to evert the upper eyelid minimally.

The lid is everted on a Desmarres retractor, and a knife incision is made 5 mm above the lid margin through conjunctiva and tarsus (Fig. 35-8). The length of the incision should cover the portion of the lid involved by the scar, which is usually the entire lid. The fibers of the levator aponeurosis will be exposed on the upper lid; these are cut to facilitate vertical expansion of the posterior lamella. This will not cause ptosis, since the levator remains attached to the tarsus above the incision. A pocket is dissected anterior to the lower tarsal segment down to the lash follicles. A graft is cut to fit the posterior lamella defect, and sutures of 6-0 prolene are passed as follows. The needle is inserted just above the lashes and exits in the pocket dissected between tarsus and orbicularis. The needle is passed into the anterior surface of the lower tarsal segment, 1 mm from the cut edge, and exits through the cut edge. It is then passed into the cut edge of the graft and exits its anterior surface. The suture returns parallel to the initial passage and exits the skin 2 to 3 mm from it. The upper border of the graft is secured in a similar manner except that the sutures enter the skin 5 mm above the lash line. The sutures are tied over small cotton bolsters with sufficient tension to place the lids into a position of minimal eversion. They are removed in 12 to 14 days. If a marked overcorrection is noted, some of the sutures may be removed as early as the fifth postoperative day. When sclera is used as the spacer, it will epithelialize with conjunctiva in 4 to 6 weeks. The patient will be more comfortable if kept on a lubricating antibiotic ointment until epithelialization of the graft occurs.

This technique of scleral grafting[15] is advocated because no sutures are exposed to the cornea, minimizing the danger of keratitis. In addition, the direction of the sutures allows eversion of the lid margin to be adjusted by tightening, loosening, and even removing sutures. Revising early overcorrections by removing individual sutures is not possible when a running suture has been used.

Spastic Entropion

When entropion occurs in relationship to ocular irritation, such as after cataract or corneal surgery, the lids should be evaluated. If no involutional changes are present, the patient has spastic entropion. This can be managed by the injection of absolute alcohol. The lower lid and the lateral canthal area are injected with local anesthetic. Then 0.3 to 0.5 ml of absolute alcohol is injected into the pretarsal orbicularis near the lateral canthus. Pain, edema, and skin slough are possible complications of this procedure.[16] However, most of these cases will show involutional changes of increased horizontal or vertical laxity, or both. Repairs should be in accordance with the principles for management of involutional entropion.

REFERENCES

1. Jones LT: The anatomy of the lower eyelid and its relation to the cause and cure of entropion. Am J Ophthalmol 49:29, 1960
2. Bick MW: Surgical management of orbital tarsal disparity. Arch Ophthalmol 75:386, 1966
3. Reeh MJ: Pathophysiology and surgery of involutional entropion. p. 110. In Aston SJ, Hornblass A, Meltzer M, Rees TD (eds): Third International Symposium of Plastic and Reconstructive Surgery of the Eye and Adnexa. Williams & Wilkins, Baltimore, 1982
4. Dalgleish R, Smith JLS: Mechanics and histology of senile entropion. Br J Ophthalmol 50:79, 1966
5. Sisler HA, Laboy GR, Finlay JR: Senile ectropion and entropion: A comparative histopathological study. Ann Ophthalmol 8:319, 1976
6. Fox SA: Etiology of senile entropion. Am J Ophthalmol 48:607, 1959
7. Dryden RM, Leibsohn J, Wobig J: Senile entropion. Pathogenesis and treatment. Arch Ophthalmol 96:1883, 1978
8. Hill JC: An analysis of senile changes in the palpebral fissure. Can J Ophthalmol 10:32, 1975
9. Fox SA: Repair of senile entropion. Arch Ophthalmol 72:501, 1964
10. Quickert MH, Rathbun E: Suture repair of entropion. Arch Ophthalmol 85:304, 1971
11. Wies FA: Spastic entropion. Trans Am Acad Ophthalmol Otolaryngol 59:503, 1955
12. Quickert MH: Malpositions of the eyelid. p. 941. In Sorsby A (ed): Modern Ophthalmology. Vol. 4. Butterworth, London, 1972

13. Tenzel RR: Repair of entropion of upper lid. Arch Ophthalmol 77:675, 1967
14. Collin JRO: Entropion and trichiasis. p. 18. In Collin JRO (ed): A Manual of Systematic Eyelid Surgery. Churchill Livingstone, New York, 1982
15. Tenzel RR, Miller GR, Rubenzik R: Cicatricial upper lid entropion treated with banked scleral graft. Arch Ophthalmol 93:999, 1975
16. Soll, DB: Entropion and ectropion. p. 137. In Soll DB (ed): Management of Complications in Ophthalmic Plastic Surgery. Aesculapius, Birmingham, AL, 1976

Ectropion

36

Douglas P. Felt
Bartley R. Frueh

Ectropion is the outward turning of any portion of the eyelid margin away from the globe. It may involve upper or lower lids, but more commonly the lower. Ectropion is classified as congenital, involutional (senile), paralytic, cicatricial, mechanical, or allergic. Since treatment is based on the lid pathology, it is important to take a careful history and perform a thorough examination.

HISTORY

The history should include onset, duration, and symptoms. If the ectropion is mild, there may be no symptoms at all. When the eyelids no longer perform their normal functions of protecting and lubricating the globe and draining tears, the corneal surface dries out, and the patient experiences burning, foreign body sensation, and reflex tearing. With the puncti everted out of the lacrimal lake, epiphora results, which is not only annoying but may also be associated with irritation and maceration of eyelid skin. If the tear film and corneal epithelium are sufficiently disrupted, visual acuity may be decreased. These symptoms are the same regardless of the etiology of the ectropion.

Etiologic factors may be elicited in the history. Congenital ectropion is discussed in Chapter 37. Involutional ectropion is usually seen in patients over age 60, who have a general tendency toward laxity of tissues. They may also have a history of chronic rubbing of the eyelids, with stretching of tissues.

Paralytic ectropion results from facial nerve paresis of any cause. The history should cover the possibilities of Bell's palsy, of trauma including surgery near the pathway of the seventh nerve, of parotid disease, and of associated localizing findings, such as nerve deafness, loss of taste, or decreased salivary secretion.

A history of trauma to the eyelids may indicate cicatricial ectropion. Burns or lacerations can result in vertical shortening of the lid skin from loss of tissue or scar tissue contraction. Gradual cicatricial changes occur following prolonged ultraviolet exposure; an occupational history of lifelong exposure to sunlight may therefore contribute to the diagnosis. The most common cause of vertical tightness of the skin is skin shrinkage secondary to chronic involutional ectropion alone.

Previous eyelid surgery is a common cause of

cicatricial changes in the lids. Ectropion, usually of the lower lid, is the most common complication following blepharoplasty. It is usually caused by excessive skin removal but may also result from tucking of the orbital septum when suturing or by subcutaneous scarring.[1] Surgical overcorrection of entropion can lead to ectropion.

Ectropion is associated with cicatrizing dermatologic conditions. These include scleroderma,[2] porphyria cutanea tarda,[3] ichthyosis,[4-6] epidermolysis bullosa,[7] mycosis fungoides, herpes zoster ophthalmicus,[8] and chickenpox.[9]

Mechanical factors causing ectropion may be elicited in the history. Tumors or cysts on the cutaneous aspect of the lower lid can pull the lid down and away from the globe or, if on the conjunctival side of either upper or lower lid, may push the lid away from the globe. Exogenous factors may also play a role. Large eyeglass frames that rest on the lower lid or upper aspect of the cheek can push the lower lid downward.[10] A careful history may reveal that the patient is only symptomatic when wearing eyeglasses.

A history of allergies or the use of topical medications or makeup should be determined to avoid unnecessary surgery in the patient with allergic ectropion. Allergic ectropion is secondary to a contact dermatitis, and stopping the offending agent will be curative unless scarring has occurred.

EXAMINATION

The physical examination will confirm the etiology, which may now be suspected from the history. Often more than one factor is involved in causing the ectropion.[11] If each contributing factor is not identified and treated, the results following surgery may not be satisfactory. The examination will pinpoint the area(s) of lid pathology and thus aid in planning treatment.

Seven elements of lid pathology may be present in various combinations in an ectropic eyelid:

1. Horizontal tarsal laxity
2. Lateral canthal tendon laxity
3. Medial canthal tendon laxity
4. Punctal malposition
5. Inferior lid retractor laxity or disinsertion
6. Orbicularis oculi paresis
7. Vertical tightness of the skin
8. Excess bulk

Horizontal laxity is assessed by measuring the amount of lid distraction. The lid is grasped centrally and pulled away from the globe as far as possible without causing discomfort. The maximum separation from the globe centrally is normally less than 10 mm. When greater than 10 mm, horizontal lid laxity is present. The amount of laxity still present after correction of medial canthal tendon laxity is the horizontal tarsal laxity and lateral canthal tendon laxity. Horizontal tarsal laxity and lateral canthal tendon laxity may be lumped together when examining the patient and correcting by the methods we recommend. Early horizontal laxity is sometimes manifested as sagging of the lid with inferior scleral show, which may precede frank ectropion. The lid should snap back into position when pulled away from the globe. When the lid returns slowly or incompletely, this is also an indication of horizontal laxity.

Medial canthal tendon laxity is assessed by noting the excursion of the punctum as the lid is pulled laterally. When the punctum is observed to move out of the lacrimal lake and approaches the medial limbus, medial canthal tendon laxity is present.

The puncta are best assessed at the slit lamp. Patency and size of the puncta are noted. Puncta that appear stenotic can be treated at the time of surgery with dilatation or a simple one-snip procedure. The puncta should be noted in relationship to the lacrimal lake and the lid margin. If they are wholly or partially everted out of the lake, the lid should be pulled up either laterally, or in both directions, to see whether surgical treatment of medial or generalized horizontal laxity will correct the punctal ectropion. The punctum may be rotated anteriorly relative to the posterior lid margin. Correction of punctal malposition is more difficult when the punctum has rotated forward from the posterior lid margin.

Inferior lid retractor laxity, dehiscence, or disinsertion is perhaps the most difficult element of lid pathology in ectropion to diagnose. If there is little or no horizontal laxity, the entire tarsal plate everts at its base. Fox[12] used the term *tarsal ectropion* to describe this condition. The tarsus can be rotated back into proper position manually but when released rolls outward again. Slit-lamp examination may reveal a separation between the red inferior tarsal border and the gray capsulopalpebral fascia beneath the palpebral conjunctiva. On downward gaze, the fascia is seen to move with movement of the inferior rectus to which it is connected, but the force is not transmitted to the base of the tarsus. This is similar to the condition of senile entropion with lid retractor dehiscence, except that in one the other lid forces rotate the lid margin outward, while in the other they rotate the margin inward. If horizontal laxity is present, inferior lid retractor dehiscence is even more difficult to diagnose. Failure to correct the dehiscence when correcting the horizontal laxity may precipitate or exacerbate tarsal ectropion.[13,14]

Orbicularis oculi paresis may be associated with an obvious facial nerve palsy or may be isolated and subtle. The palpebral fissure is examined with gentle closure of the lids to look for lagophthalmos, and then with forced closure while the examiner attempts to push the lids apart to reveal a more subtle paresis. In an effort to find other indications of paralysis, the examiner also observes the function of the other muscles innervated by the facial nerve, looking for decreased definition of the forehead furrows and nasolabial fold, brow droop with poor brow elevation, and decreased ability to wrinkle the nose, elevate the upper lip, and purse the lips. An incomplete blink may be present, although the blink frequency is normal if the paralysis is incomplete. Ectropion occurs with orbicularis oculi paresis only when there is concomitant horizontal lid laxity.

Vertical tightness of the skin is evaluated by drawing the lid up into the normal position against the globe and observing the skin wrinkles. Fine horizontal wrinkles indicate no significant vertical tightness. Smooth skin with loss of the horizontal wrinkles indicates some vertical shortening of the skin. If this is not corrected at the time of surgery, the surgical results may not be satisfactory or permanent. Vertical tension lines indicate even more severe vertical shortening of the skin.

Excess bulk may be dermatochalasis, adding to the downward gravitational pull on the lid margin, a lid tumor pulling or pushing the lid away from the globe, inflammatory swelling, or edema. Allergic ectropion is characterized by swelling or edema and by inflamed, wrinkled skin. The lids should be inspected, palpated, and everted to examine for masses.

In addition to examination of the eyelids, careful biomicroscopic examination of the corneal surface should be performed to determine the presence and extent of exposure keratopathy. When the palpebral conjunctiva becomes inflamed from chronic exposure, it may become keratinized. Exposure keratitis may leave the eye more susceptible to ocular infection; temporizing measures to protect it are sometimes necessary until surgery can be performed.

MANAGEMENT

Keratopathy secondary to ectropion is treated with topical lubricants until the ectropion is surgically corrected. Another temporary measure is to tape the lower lid to the skin overlying the lateral orbital rim so as to pull the lid margin upward and laterally. This also gives some indication of how beneficial a lid-shortening operation would be. Except for allergic ectropion, which is corrected by eliminating the offending agent, surgery is required to effect a permanent cure for ectropion.

Any ectropion may be predominantly one type but contain elements of any other type. For this reason we advocate treating each element of the involved lid pathology rather than just using a standard procedure for each class of ectropion. Once the lids have been carefully examined and the degree of pathology of each of the seven elements determined, a surgical plan can be made to treat each element (Table 36-1). When more than one element is involved, the order for performing each procedure is important and will be discussed at the end of the chapter. All the procedures described can be done under local anesthesia.

Table 36-1. Surgical Approach to the Patient with Ectropion

Classification	Lid Pathology	Procedure
Involutional	Horizontal tarsal laxity and lateral canthal tendon laxity	Horizontal lid shortening (lateral)[a] Horizontal lid shortening (central) (Kuhnt–Szymanowski–Smith modification) Rotational lid sutures
	Medial canthal tendon laxity	Medical canthal tendon plication (tuck)[a]
	Punctal malposition	Fusiform resection of conjunctiva and lid retractors below the punctum[a] One snip[a] Thermal cautery Lazy-T
	Inferior lid retractor laxity or disinsertion	Inferior lid retractor tuck or reinsertion[a]
Paralytic	Orbicularis oculi paresis	Lateral canthal sling[a] Medial canthoplasty[a] Tarsorrhaphy (medial and lateral) Fascia lata sling Temporalis muscle transfer
Cicatricial	Vertical tightness of the skin	Skin grafts[a] Transposition flaps (Z-plasty)
Mechanical	Excess bulk	Excision of lesion[a]
Allergic		Discontinuation of offending agent[a]

[a] Preferred method.

HORIZONTAL TARSAL LAXITY AND LATERAL CANTHAL LAXITY

Horizontal Eyelid Shortening

The lid is shortened laterally with a pentagonal wedge resection or a lateral canthal sling. To perform the former, a vertical incision is made at the lateral canthus, dividing lower lid from lateral canthal tendon. The incision is carried sufficiently inferiorly to sever all attachments to the lateral canthal tendon. The lid is grasped with a forceps and pulled gently laterally (Fig. 36-1). The amount of lid extending beyond the lateral canthus is the amount of lid to be excised. The medial aspect of the overlapped lid is marked at the lid margin, and another vertical incision is made at this mark through full-thickness lid and through the entire tarsal plate. Below the tarsus, the two vertical incisions are connected with a V to remove a pentagonal wedge of lower lid (Fig. 36-1).

The lid is reattached laterally by placing a 5-0 polyglycolic acid suture through the inferior edge of the exposed end of tarsus, through the body of the tarsus, and out the upper edge of the cut tarsus (Fig. 36-1). The suture is then passed down through the cut lateral canthal tendon or the periosteum of the rim. If a more posterior position of the lateral end of the lid is required for it to conform to the globe, the tarsus should be sutured to the periosteum of the lateral orbital tubercle. If the suture is properly placed in the tendon or periosteum, tension on both arms of the suture will meet firm resistance as though the suture were through bone. The suture is tied, and a second suture is placed just anterior to the first. A 7-0 chromic suture can be placed, if needed, in the lid margin to secure the lid margin to the lateral canthus. The skin is closed with 6-0 nylon or silk.

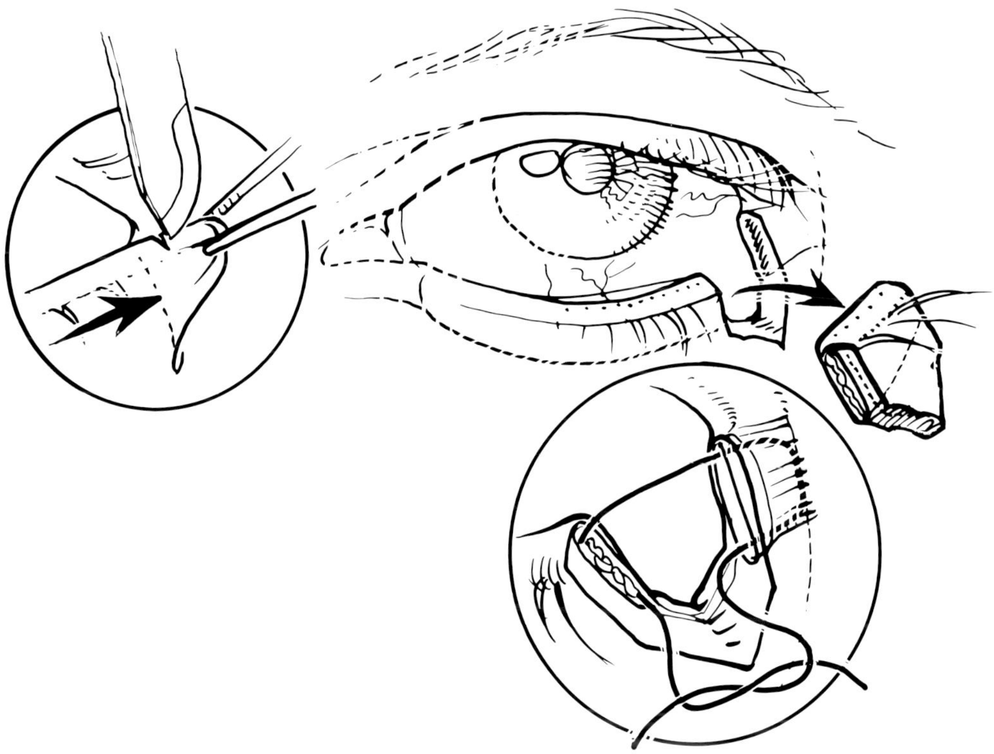

Fig. 36-1. Horizontal lid shortening by excision of a pentagonal wedge. A vertical cut is made through full-thickness lid at the lateral canthus to below the lower edge of tarsus, severing the attachments of the lateral canthal tendon. The length of lid to excise is determined by then pulling the lid laterally (upper inset). The lid is closed with a suture passed wholly within the tarsal plate and through the lateral canthal tendon or zygomatic periostem.

Horizontal Eyelid Shortening and Blepharoplasty: Kuhnt–Szymanowski–Smith Modification

The classic Kuhnt–Szymanowski procedure[15] for ectropion involved splitting the eyelid at the gray line and should not be used because of a high incidence of trichiasis.[16,17] Smith's modification[18] of the technique is still used by many, but carries the added risks of lid notching and of creating a cicatricial ectropion by excising too much skin. Removal of extra skin is not required for ectropion correction and is of cosmetic benefit only.

A subciliary incision is made 2 mm below the lashes and is extended about 6 mm inferolaterally beyond the lateral canthus following a skin crease, as with a lower lid blepharoplasty incision. Skin is dissected from orbicularis oculi muscle, and a pentagonal wedge of lid is resected about 5 mm from the lateral canthus. The vertical cuts through the tarsal plate should extend the entire height of the tarsus before angling the incisions toward each other in a V to form the pentagonal wedge. If the angled V incisions are made while still in the tarsal plate, the lid margin will be notched, not straight, when the edges are brought together.

The lid margin is reapproximated by passing a 5-0 polyglycolic acid suture entirely within the tarsus from the inferior to the superior cut edge, coming out just below the lid margin. It is then passed through the other side of the cut tarsal edge in a superior-to-inferior direction, entering and exiting the tarsus at the same levels as the first bite. When the suture is tied, the lid margin should be well approximated; if it is not, the suture should be replaced. Interrupted 7-0 chromic sutures are

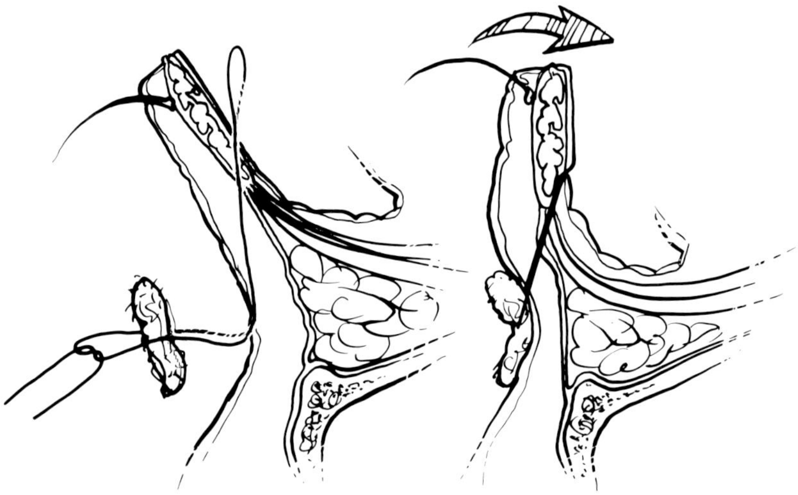

Fig. 36-2. Suture correction of ectropion. Sutures should be placed higher posteriorly than anteriorly to rotate the lid margin toward the globe.

placed at the anterior lid margin, at the gray line and, if needed, at the posterior lid margin. The ends are left long and are tied to the knot of a skin closure suture to maintain them away from the cornea. The skin is pulled laterally and a triangle excised if there is excessive skin. In most cases, no skin need be excised. The skin is closed with 6-0 nylon in a running or interrupted fashion.

Rotational Lid Margin Sutures

Mild degrees of ectropion can be corrected with rotational sutures in the office or at the bedside, but the effect is often only temporary. The lid margin can be rotated by approximating two vertically different points. In treating ectropion with rotational sutures, the goal is to approximate a point high on the posterior lamellae with one lower on the anterior lamellae of the lower lid (Fig. 36-2). This is done using two or more 4-0 silk or chromic gut horizontal mattress sutures exiting the lid posteriorly just below the lid margin (or inferior border of tarsus) and anteriorly near the orbital rim. The amount of rotation is controlled by adjusting the tension on the sutures tied over a cotton bolster on the skin (Fig. 36-2). Care should be taken to avoid overcorrection with resultant entropion. The scar along the suture tracks helps hold the lid in position when the sutures are removed 2 to 3 weeks later.

MEDIAL CANTHAL TENDON LAXITY

Medial Canthal Tendon Plication (Tuck)

Medial canthal tendon laxity is corrected by tucking the medial canthal tendon. This is done by making a skin incision at each end of the tendon. The first is a 5-mm curvilinear incision made vertically over the medial aspect of the tendon. The tendon can be seen or palpated as it inserts into periosteum. Dissection is carried out bluntly above and below to isolate the tendon. The second skin incision is made horizontally 4 mm below the lid margin and 4 to 5 mm long, over the medial aspect of the tarsus (Fig. 36-3). With blunt dissection through orbicularis muscle, the inferomedial border of the tarsus is identified. A 6-0 polyester fiber or polypropylene suture is passed through the tendon in the medial incision, tunneled beneath orbicularis oculi muscle, and brought out the lower lid incision. If the suture is not tunneled beneath the orbicularis muscle, the suture may be visible and may even erode through the skin postoperatively. The suture is then passed through the inferior portion of the tarsal plate taking care to avoid the canaliculus, tunneled back beneath orbicularis, brought out the medial incision, and tied (Fig. 36-3). Only sufficient tension should be placed on

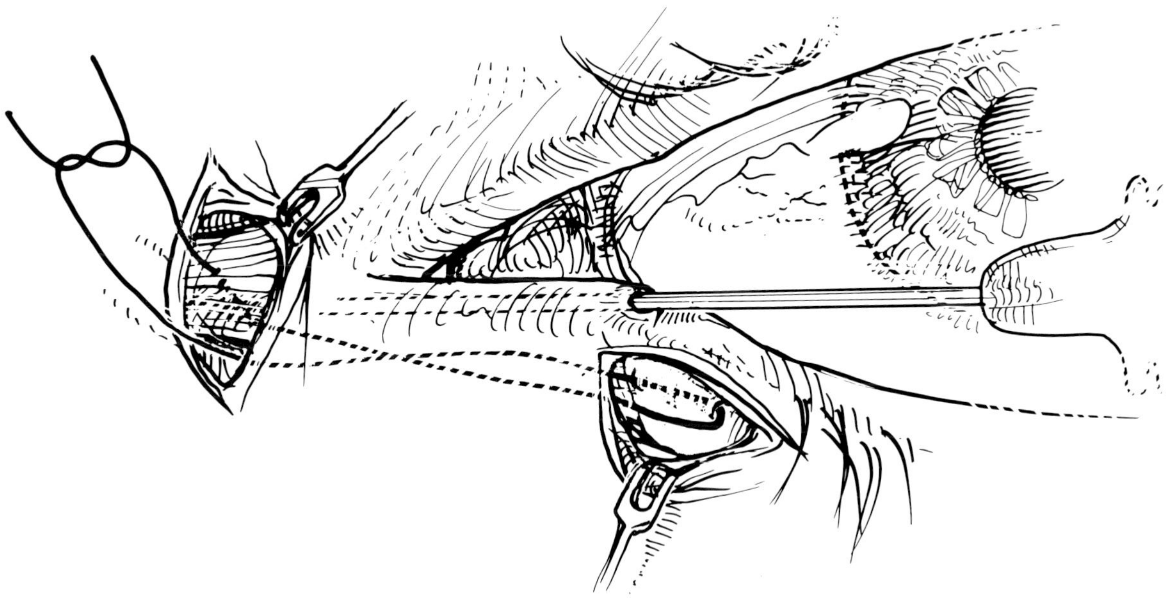

Fig. 36-3. Medial canthal tendon tucking is performed by inserting a permanent suture placed through the tendon and tunneled under orbicularis oculi muscle before passing it through the tarsal plate and back under the orbicularis muscle to the medial incision. The suture is tied with sufficient tension to place the punctum at its proper position and prevent lateral displacement. Overcorrection is undesirable.

the suture to bring the lower punctum back into proper position beneath the upper punctum or just lateral to it. If the suture is too tight, the inferior punctum will be too medial and out of the lacrimal lake. If the tension is correct, the punctum will not move from its proper position when the lid is gently pulled laterally. Both skin incisions are closed with interrupted sutures. Another method of medial canthal tendon plication is described in Chapter 35.

PUNCTAL MALPOSITION

Fusiform Resection of Conjunctiva and Eyelid Retractors below the Punctum

If the punctum does not come back into proper position with tightening of the medial canthal tendon and horizontal shortening of the lid, further rotation of the medial aspect of the lid can be accomplished with a vertical shortening of the posterior lamellae of the lid medially. This is done by excising a fusiform or diamond-shaped wedge of conjunctiva and lid retractors at the lower margin of the tarsus beneath the punctum. Care should be taken to avoid the canaliculus. A lacrimal probe can be left in the canaliculus during the procedure to make cutting the canaliculus less likely and to facilitate its identification and repair if it is cut. The excised wedge is usually 4 to 6 mm horizontally and 3 to 5 mm vertically; the exact size depends on the degree of punctal ectropion. The wound is closed with three or four 7-0 chromic gut buried sutures passed through lid retractors and conjunctiva inferiorly and through conjunctiva and lower tarsal edge superiorly. If the lid retractors are not included in the closure, the rotational force desired will be lost.

If further support of the medial canthus is needed, particularly in paralytic ectropion, a medial canthoplasty is done in addition to the above to bring both the upper and lower puncti in apposition against the globe. This is described in the section on orbicularis oculi paresis.

One-Snip Procedure

If minimal punctal ectropion is present or if the punctum is stenotic, the punctum can be opened to the lacrimal lake with a Jones one-snip procedure. The initial portion of the canaliculus is 2 mm and is nearly vertical. The punctum, either topically or locally anesthetized, is dilated with a sterile safety pin or punctal dilator. Sharp scissors are then used to cut the vertical canaliculus on the conjuntival side. If a larger opening is desired, a triangular wedge can be excised base up from the vertical canaliculus with a snip on each side of a forcep placed in the punctum. The horizontal portion of the canaliculus should not be incised.

Thermal Cautery

Thermal cautery has been used to treat mild medial ectropion using a very hot cautery in several spots below the tarsus through the posterior aspect of the lid to cause cicatrization. The procedure is more destructive and not as well controlled as other available procedures. We therefore do not recommend it.

Lazy-T

The lazy-T procedure described by Smith[19] is another method of providing horizontal shortening of the lid and posterior vertical shortening medially for medial or punctal ectropion. With a probe in the canaliculus, an ellipse of conjunctiva and lid retractors is excised as described previously. At the lateral edge of the ellipse, the lid is transected vertically thus forming a T-shaped incision with the shank of the T horizontal and its top vertical (i.e., lazy-T). A pentagonal wedge of full-thickness lid is excised and the wounds closed as previously described. The major complication with this procedure is a central lid notch. We therefore recommend doing the pentagonal wedge resection at the lateral canthus.

INFERIOR LID RETRACTOR LAXITY OR DISINSERTION

Inferior Lid Retractor Tuck or Reinsertion

Dehiscence of the lid retractors in the upper lid causes ptosis; in the lower lid, it causes either entropion or ectropion. Repair is analogous to repairing an aponeurotic ptosis of the upper lid by reattaching or tucking the lid retractors. When the laxity or dehiscence causes ectropion, the repair is best done transconjunctivally so that any vertical shortening from the repair will be only in the posterior lamellae and aid in resolving the ectropion. The anterior approach to lid retractor tuck described in Chapter 35 is appropriate for entropion.

The conjunctiva is incised along the inferior border of the tarsal plate, and dissection is carried inferiorly just beneath conjunctiva until the lid retractors, that is, lower lid Müller's muscle and capsulopalpebral fascia, are identified. The lid retractors are grasped with a forcep and the patient is asked to look down. If the lid retractors are properly identified, a strong downward pull on the forcep will be felt. When sturdy mobile tissue is isolated, it is sutured to the inferior tarsal border with interrupted 5-0 polyglycolic acid sutures (Fig. 36-4). The conjunctiva is closed with interrupted 7-0 chromic gut sutures.

The keratinized palpebral conjunctiva from chronic tarsal ectropion will revert to normal with time once the lid position is corrected and requires no additional treatment.

ORBICULARIS OCULI PARESIS

Lateral Canthal Sling

The lateral canthal sling described by Tenzel[20,21] will effectively shorten the lid horizontally and elevate it laterally. It is the procedure of choice for

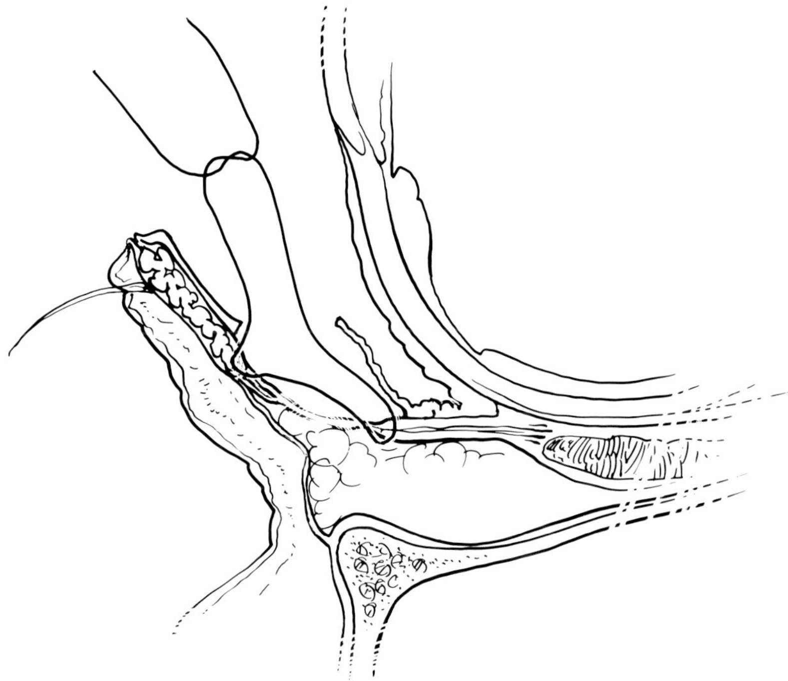

Fig. 36-4. Inferior lid retractor tuck by a posterior approach. The dehisced lid retractors are located and sutured to the lower edge of the tarsal plate.

shortening a paralytic lid or the lid of an anophthalmic socket, but it may be used for any horizontal lid shortening.

A lateral canthotomy is made, and the lower crus of the lateral canthal tendon is severed from all attachments to the periosteum by pulling the lower lid medially, feeling connections to periosteum with the scissors blade, and cutting them. When all attachments are severed, the lateral lid should be freely mobile. With the lid pulled laterally, a cut is made to mark the point at which the lid crosses the lateral canthus (Fig. 36-5). This segment of excess lid is then denuded to the tarsal plate by removing the lid margin, including lash follicles, the skin anteriorly, the conjunctiva posteriorly, and lid retractors inferiorly. Blunt dissection is used to expose the periosteum of the lateral orbital rim above the superior crus of the lateral canthal tendon. A 6-0 polypropylene or a 5-0 polyglycolic acid suture is placed through the periosteum. Lack of distensibility when both ends of the suture are pulled ensures proper placement. A tunnel is created through the superior crus with blunt dissection, and the denuded tarsal segment is brought through the tunnel and secured with the periosteal suture in a mattress fashion (Fig. 36-5). Another suture can be used through the denuded tarsus and the superior crus to secure the sling.

The skin is closed with interrupted 6-0 nylon or polypropylene sutures. A vertical mattress suture can be placed, if needed, at the lateral canthus through the lid margins to sharpen the lateral canthal angle and avoid the rounded appearance that tends to occur otherwise after this procedure. If a more posterior position of the lateral end of the lid is required for it to conform to the globe, the tarsal strip should be sutured to the periosteum of the lateral orbital tubercle.

Medial Canthoplasty

With orbicularis oculi paresis, a medial canthoplasty is often needed in conjunction with a lateral canthal sling for vertical support of the lower lid medially and to help invert the lower punctum. With lacrimal probes in the upper and lower canaliculi, the mucocutaneous junction is incised from just medial to the lower punctum around the medial canthus to just medial to the upper punctum. The surrounding skin is undermined. A triangle of skin with the base at the original incision is excised

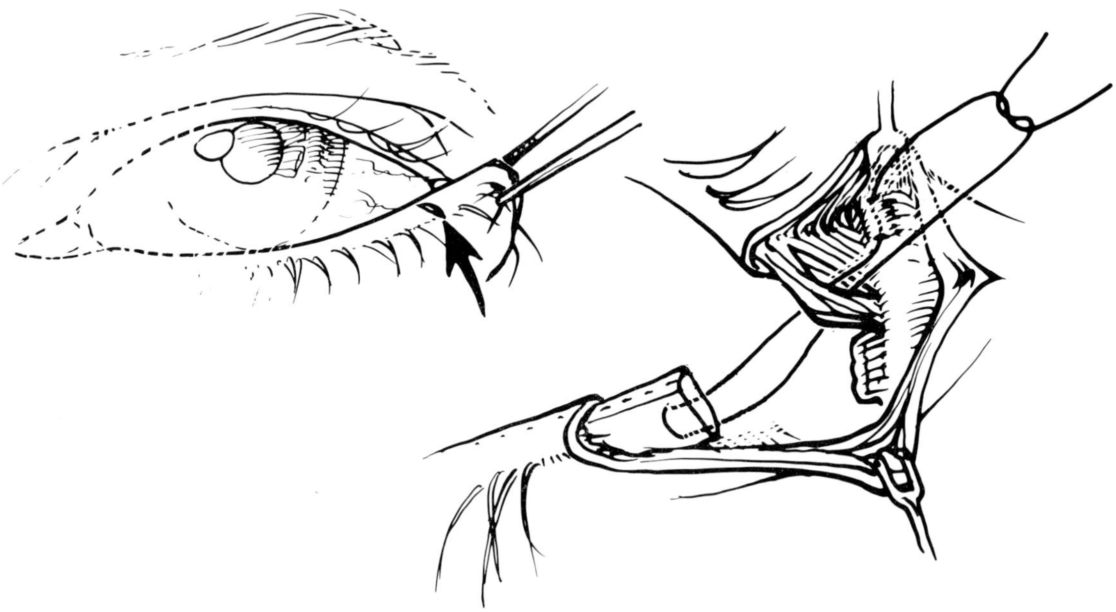

Fig. 36-5. Lateral canthal sling for horizontal lid shortening. After a lateral canthotomy and lysis of the lower lid attachments to the lateral orbital rim, the lid is stretched laterally to determine the effective shortening required (upper left). That portion of tarsal plate is denuded, passed through the upper crus of the lateral canthal tendon, and sutured to the zygomatic periosteum.

from the upper lid medial to the punctum, and a corresponding skin flap is fashioned from the lower lid. Conjunctiva with medial canthal tendon from the upper lid is sutured to that of the lower lid with interrupted 6-0 or 7-0 chromic gut sutures. The triangular transposition skin flap from the lower lid is then sutured in place in the upper lid with interrupted 6-0 silk or nylon sutures. Other methods that are useful in supporting the paretic lower lid, including tarsorrhaphy, fascia lata sling, and temporalis muscle transfer, are discussed in Chapter 45.

VERTICAL TIGHTNESS OF THE SKIN

Skin Grafts

If there is generalized vertical tightness across the lower or upper lid, more skin will have to be added with a skin graft or transposition flap. If only localized tightness is present, the ectropion may be treated with single or multiple Z-plasties. Eyelid skin is the thinnest skin of the body. The best color and texture match for the lower lid is retroauricular skin; for the upper lid, contralateral upper lid skin is used, although either can be used for upper or lower lid. Alternative sources are the inner aspect of the upper arm and the supraclavicular area.

The bed for the skin graft is prepared by making an incision 3 mm below the lashes and parallel to the lid margin in the lower lid or at the desired lid crease in the upper lid, extending several millimeters beyond the area of vertical tightness. The incision is carried to sufficient depth, usually through the orbicularis oculi muscle, until all vertical tension is released, and the lid margin rests in normal position. The skin graft should be 15 to 25 percent larger vertically than the defect measures to allow for postoperative shrinkage. An ellipse of the proper size is drawn at the donor site.

For a retroauricular graft, the vertical retroauricular crease is first marked with the ear in its resting position to delineate the center of the graft. The ear is pulled forward, and the graft is sketched with an equal amount of skin on each side of the central mark. The vertical dimension on the ear will become the horizontal dimension on the lid. The retroauricular wound is closed with interrupted 4-0 silk sutures without undermining and dressed with fluffs and a gauze head wrap. The dressing can be removed on the first postoperative day and the sutures on the tenth day.

If the upper lid is used as the donor site, the lower border of the graft will be at the lid crease. No more skin should be removed than can be pinched between a forceps without causing the upper lid margin to elevate. `Otherwise, lagophthalmos may develop.

The skin to be grafted is thinned with scissors placed flat against the undersurface, with all subcutaneous tissue removed until the dermal pegs are well defined. The graft is kept moist in saline-soaked gauze until required.

One or two traction sutures are placed in the lid margin by going through the gray line, out the skin, over a cotton stent, back though skin, and out the gray line. These are taped to the forehead if doing the lower lid or to the cheek if doing the upper lid to put vertical traction on the lid. Alternatively, a suture tarsorrhaphy may be performed.

The skin graft is sutured in place with interrupted 6-0 silk sutures, leaving one end of each suture long. Some surgeons place two or three stab wounds 2 mm in length in the graft to allow for possible serosanguineous drainage. We have found this unnecessary if good hemostasis is obtained and the graft firmly stented. The long ends are then tied somewhat loosely over compressed cellulose sponges, which when moistened swell to push the graft firmly against the host bed. The sutures and stent are removed 8 to 10 days postoperatively after thoroughly soaking the stent.

Transposition Flaps (Z-Plasty)

A Z-plasty, a transposition flap that alters the direction of contracture by 90 degrees, will correct a localized band of vertical shortening of the lid. In the case of cicatricial ectropion, the goal is to change the shortening from vertical to horizontal. The middle segment of the Z is made vertically, directly over the contracture band. The other two segments are made 60 degrees to this line, one at each end, forming a Z. All three incisions are of equal length. The surrounding tissue is undermined and scar tissue is excised. The V-shaped skin flaps are transposed and sutured in place with interrupted 6-0 nylon sutures. Lid margin traction sutures as described above are used postoperatively to put the lid on stretch. Multiple Z-plasties are done if the scar is very long.

A large flap of skin can be transposed from the upper lid to the lower lid if either medial or lateral cicatricial ectropion is present.[22,23] A pedicle flap from the upper lid based just medial to the medial canthus or just lateral to the lateral canthus is created and rotated to the lower lid to a bed prepared as described for a skin graft.

Excess Bulk

The treatment for mechanical ectropion is to eliminate the underlying problem. A tumor is excised, edema is treated medically, and a hematoma unless organized is evacuated with a syringe. Edema from allergic contact dermatitis resolves when contact with the offending agent is stopped.

SUGGESTED TECHNIQUE

Our preferred method of correcting horizontal lid laxity is with a medial canthal tendon tuck if needed and a full thickness pentagonal wedge resection at the lateral canthus. Taking the wedge resection at the lateral canthus avoids the complication of a lid notch or of corneal irritation from sutures or misdirected lashes. If the lid is atonic, it is better elevated laterally with a lateral canthal sling and medially with a medial canthoplasty to counteract the unopposed forces of the lid retractors and the weight of the lid. These procedures are also useful with the anophthalmic socket to counteract the weight of the prosthesis. We prefer the fusiform resection of conjunctiva and lid retractors below the punctum for punctal ectropion. A one-snip procedure of the punctum may be added. If there is tarsal ectropion with generalized lid retractor laxity, we recommend the conjunctival approach for tucking lid retractors. For cicatricial ectropion, full-thickness skin grafts are cosmetically more acceptable with less shrinkage than split-thickness grafts. Split-thickness grafts should be used only when a suitable donor site for a full-thickness graft is not available.

The sequence of performing each procedure is important when more than one element of lid pathology needs correcting. The vertical forces holding the lid out of position are released first. Lax lid elements are corrected next. The punctum should be brought into proper position with medial canthal tendon plication and/or lid rotation before horizontal shortening is completed to avoid pulling of the punctum laterally. A skin graft, if needed, is sutured in place last. The sequence of procedures for ectropion repair is as follows:

1. Prepare the bed for a skin graft by releasing vertical contracture.
2. Tuck the medial canthal tendon.
3. Excise a pentagonal wedge or dissect for a lateral canthal sling.
4. Tuck the inferior lid retractors or resect a wedge of conjunctiva and lid retractors.
5. Complete the horizontal shortening procedure from step 3.
6. Suture the skin graft in place.

REFERENCES

1. Levine MR, Boynton J, Tenzel RR, Miller GR: Complications of blepharoplasty. Ophthalmic Surg 6(2):53, 1975
2. Nancarrow JD, Jawad SMA: A rare case of severe bilateral ectropion from scleroderma. Plast Reconstr Surg 67(3):352, 1981
3. Sober AJ, Grove AR, Muhlbauer JE: Cicatricial ectropion and lacrimal obstruction associated with the sclerodermoid variant of porphyria cutanea tarda. Am J Ophthalmol 91:396, 1981
4. Katowitz JA, Yolles EA, Yanoff M: Ichthyosis congenita. Arch Ophthalmol 91:208, 1974
5. Shindle RD, Leone CR: Cicatricial ectropion associated with lamellar ichthyosis. Arch Ophthalmol 89:62, 1973
6. Leung PC, Ma GFY: Ectropion of all four eyelids associated with severe ichthyosis congenita: A case report. Br J Plast Surg 34:302, 1981
7. Hill JC, Rodrigue D: Cicatricial ectropion in epidermolysis bullosa and in congenital ichthyosis: Its plastic repair. Can J Ophthalmol 6:89, 1971
8. Smith JP, Lavine DM: Cicatricial ectropion of the upper lid secondary to herpes zoster ophthalmicus. Ann Ophthalmol 13(5):579, 1981
9. Guibor P: Surgical correction of severe cicatricial ectropion caused by chicken pox. Arch Ophthalmol 92:307, 1974
10. Chalfin J, Putterman AM: Ectropion produced by eyeglass frames. Arch Ophthalmol 97:306, 1979
11. Frueh BR, Schoengarth LD: Evaluation and treatment of the patient with ectropion. Ophthalmology 89:1049, 1982
12. Fox SA: Marginal (tarsal) ectropion. Arch Ophthalmol 63:660, 1960
13. Putterman AM: Ectropion of the lower eyelid secondary to Mueller's muscle-capsulopalpebral fascia detachment. Am. J Ophthalmol 85:814, 1978
14. Wesley RE: Tarsal ectropion from detachment of the lower eyelid retractors. Am J Ophthalmol 93:491, 1982
15. Kuhnt H: Ueber die Behandlung hock gradiger Formen des Blepharitis-ektropium. Z Augenh 20:143, 1908
16. Soll DB: Management of Complications in Ophthalmic Plastic Surgery. Aesculapius, Birmingham, AL, 1976
17. McCord CD: Oculoplastic Surgery. Raven Press, New York, 1981
18. Smith B, Cherubini T: Oculoplastic Surgery. CV Mosby, St. Louis, 1970
19. Smith B: The "lazy-T" correction of ectropion of the lower punctum. Arch Ophthalmol 94:1149, 1976
20. Tenzel RR: Treatment of lagophthalmos of the lower lid. Arch Ophthalmol 81:366, 1969
21. Tenzel RR, Buffam FV, Miller GR: The use of the "lateral canthal sling" in ectropion repair. Can J Ophthalmol 12:199, 1977
22. Leone CR: Repair of cicatricial ectropion by horizontal shortening and pedicle flap. Ophthalmic Surg 6(2):47, 1975
23. Anderson RL: Medial ectropion. Arch Ophthalmol 97:521, 1979

Congenital Eyelid Anomalies

37

John A. Burns
Kenneth V. Cahill

Congenital lid anomalies are a heterogeneous group of defects linked by their presentation at birth. They can be unilateral or bilateral, sporadic or inherited, isolated or associated with other ocular and systemic anomalies. Ptosis, one of the more common congenital eyelid anomalies, is discussed in Chapters 33 and 34.

The primary consideration in the evaluation of congenital lid anomalies is the functional integrity of the lids. This is of particular importance in terms of protecting the corneal surface and maintaining a normal visual axis. Corneal exposure or pupillary axis occlusion demand immediate action. If conservative management is unsuccessful, surgery is required as soon as possible. If, however, the lid deformity is well tolerated, it is best to defer surgery until the child is older. The benefits of observation include the advantages of later surgery on more mature lid tissues and the fact that some defects regress spontaneously. The effect of lid anomalies on social interaction and emotional development of a child are also important considerations. Correction of defects prior to grade school enrollment is strongly recommended since this is known to decrease psychological problems.

Since congenital lid defects can be associated with other ocular and systemic anomalies, a complete ophthalmologic and general physical examination should be performed. Genetic family counseling is important so that the risk of involvement of potential future siblings or offspring of the patient with the deformity is fully understood.

Many surgical techniques used for the correction of congenital lid anomalies are identical to those used in patients with acquired lid defects. These are covered in other chapters. The procedures unique to congenital lid defects are described in this chapter.

EPICANTHAL FOLDS

Epicanthal folds are curved vertical skin folds that pass around the medial canthal region with their concave curvature directed laterally. They are consistently found in the Oriental race. They are rarely seen at birth. During the first 2 years of life they increase in frequency and eventually affect 20 percent of all children. Thereafter, epicanthal folds begin to diminish as the brow and bridge of the nose develop. Four distinct variations

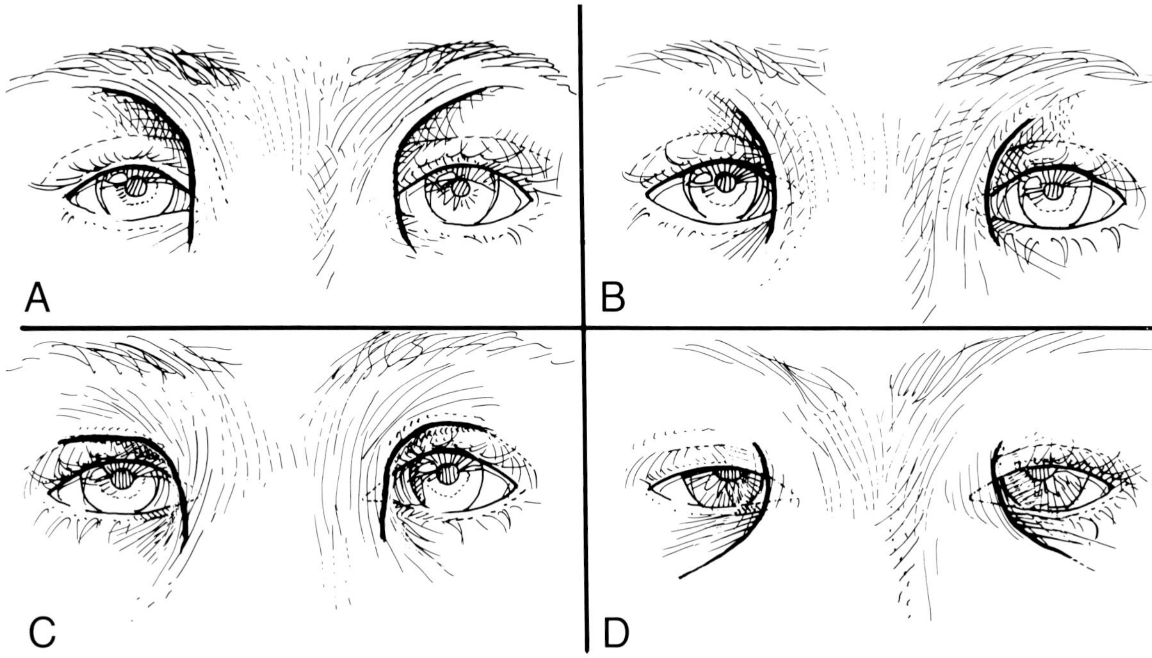

Fig. 37-1. Epicanthal folds. **(A)** Epicanthus superciliaris. **(B)** Epicanthus palpebralis. **(C)** Epicanthus tarsalis. **(D)** Epicanthus inversus.

occur, differing by the precise location of the curved skin fold (Fig. 37-1). In epicanthus superciliaris, the fold arises along the brow and runs down the side of the nose toward the lacrimal sac region or the nostril. Epicanthus palpebralis is the most common form. This fold involves the upper lid above the tarsus, runs vertically over the medial canthal region, and extends inferiorly over the lower orbital margin. In epicanthus tarsalis, a prominent fold arises over the superior tarsus and there is less lower lid involvement. These three types often follow no genetic pattern. Epicanthus inversus exhibits a fold originating over the lower lid with minimal superior lid folding. This form of epicanthus is commonly associated with the autosomal dominant blepharophimosis syndrome, which includes ptosis and telecanthus. Unlike the other three forms it has little tendency to regress with growth.

Epicanthal folds cause no functional problems but are of cosmetic concern. They are a frequent cause of pseudostrabismus. Since the folds usually

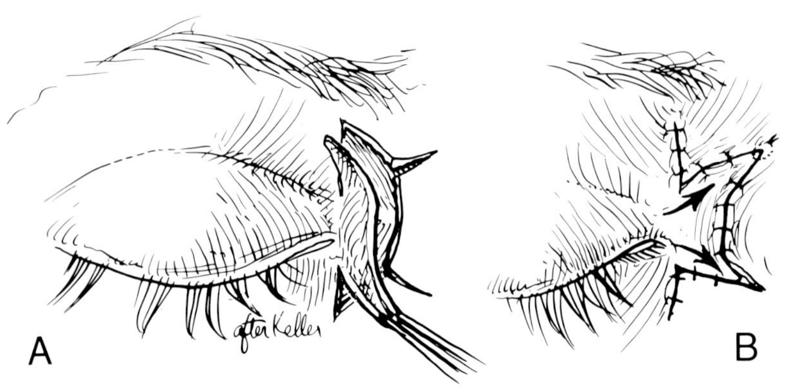

Fig. 37-2. Epicanthal repair by the Spaeth technique. The undermined skin flap **(A)** is gently draped medially to determine the location for its transposition **(B)**. The skin surrounding incision B is undermined to create a bed for flap A.

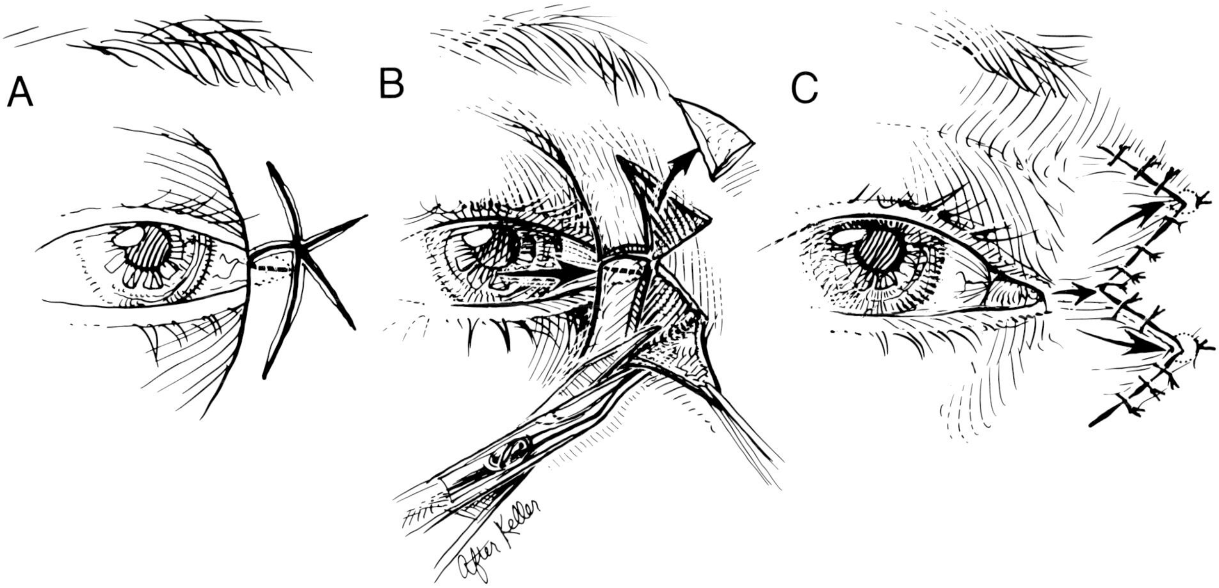

Fig. 37-3. Epicanthal repair by the Roveda technique. **(A)** Initial skin marks. **(B)** Minimal skin excision in preparation for skin undermining and transposition. **(C)** Final appearance.

regress spontaneously, very few patients will have enough residual by the early grade school years to warrant surgery.

The raised fold of skin represents a vertical shortage of skin combined with a relative horizontal skin redundancy. The goal of surgical therapy is to redistribute skin to alleviate these discrepancies.

In all epicanthus repairs, wide subcutaneous undermining must be performed so that the transposed flaps will lay down flat. Subcutaneous tissue and orbicularis muscle are excised to produce a natural concave contour. Meticulous care in handling and suturing of the skin (particularly the flap points) is necessary to minimize postoperative scarring. Even with good technique, obvious scars may result. This must be considered before deciding to operate.

The Spaeth technique is used for moderate cases when the fold is vertically oriented and limited to the medial canthal area (Fig. 37-2). For more severe cases the Roveda technique produces greater amounts of correction (Fig. 37-3) and is usually the procedure of choice in blepharophimosis syndrome.[1] The lengths of the upper and lower incision lines are tailored to the extent of the upper and lower lid epicanthal folds. Since there is a medially directed sliding skin flap involved, this procedure is useful when an epicanthus repair is combined with a medial canthal tendon shortening procedure for telecanthus.

EPIBLEPHARON

Epiblepharon is characterized by a prominent horizontal fold of skin adjacent to the lid margin in the upper and lower eyelids. This skin may press eyelashes inward and cause them to touch the globe, but must be distinguished from entropion with an actual inturning of the lid margin. Epiblepharon may be familial and can be associated with epicanthal folds. The condition is usually bilateral and is most frequent in Orientals. Spontaneous resolution is common, especially in the lower lid. However, surgical correction is indicated if corneal irritation is uncontrolled by ocular emollients or persists past age 3 or 4. Rarely, surgical correction for cosmesis may be desirable, when the deformity persists until the child is of school age. Surgical

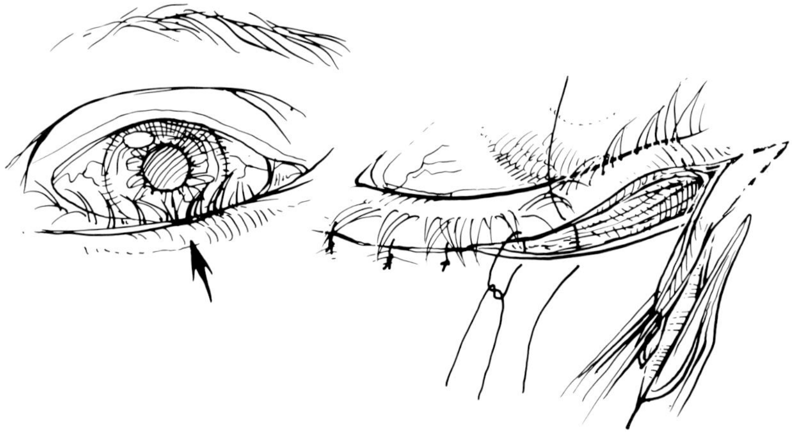

Fig. 37-4. Epiblepharon repair. A spindle-shaped strip of redundant skin is excised, followed by simple closure.

correction of epiblepharon usually involves only the excision of a spindle of excess skin (Fig. 37-4). Primary closure alone may suffice, but frequently it is helpful to secure the skin edges to the underlying tarsus.

ENTROPION

Congenital entropion involves the lower lids more frequently than the upper lids. The inward rotation of the lid margin is usually accompanied by a bulge of pretarsal skin and orbicularis muscle. Lower lid retractor aponeurosis disinsertions have also been documented in several cases.[2] In rare instances, inadequate tarsal rigidity is a pathologic component. Congenital entropion may be familial and can be associated with epicanthal folds. It usually does not regress with facial growth. Surgical correction can be achieved using the Celsus procedure (Fig. 37-5). A horizontal strip of skin and orbicularis muscle is excised from the involved area. This defect is closed with interrupted sutures that incorporate tarsus as well as skin and muscle so that the lid margin is mechanically rotated outward. Lower lid retractor aponeurosis disinsertion repair has also proved successful when performed through an infraciliary incision combined with resection of excess pretarsal orbicularis muscle and skin.

An extreme form of congenital entropion is horizontal tarsal kink. This rare condition results in corneal complications and can be repaired during infancy with a tarsal-splitting procedure.[3]

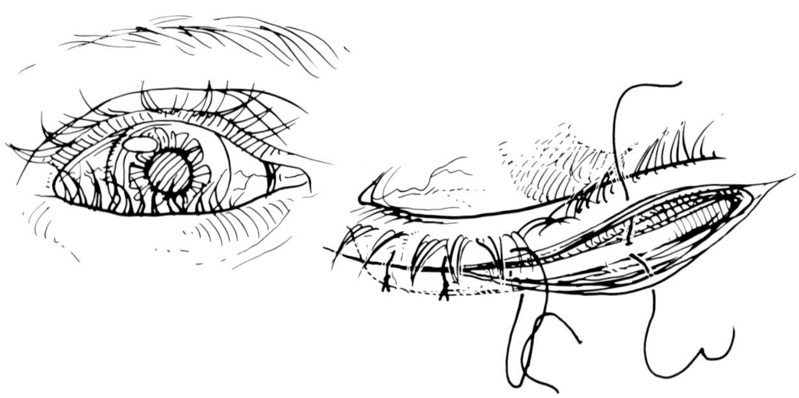

Fig. 37-5. Congenital entropion repair. A strip of pretarsal orbicularis muscle is excised along with skin, and the cut skin edges are closed with fixation to the tarsal plate.

ECTROPION

Excessive horizontal length of upper or lower eyelids can produce congenital ectropion. This may be associated with Down's syndrome. If the lid laxity is minimal and ectropion is only present temporally, a small lateral tarsorrhaphy will usually be sufficient. If greater laxity is present, a full-thickness pentagonal wedge should be excised to shorten the lids horizontally. Congenital upper eyelid eversion should be distinguished from ectropion.[4,5] Both upper eyelids are everted and markedly edematous at the time of birth. The precise mechanism responsible is not known. These infants do, however, exhibit horizontal laxity of the upper eyelids. Conservative management to maintain conjunctival and corneal hydration is indicated and the lids usually assume a normal position in a few days or weeks.

Inadequate vertical height of lid skin and orbital septum can also produce ectropion. The tarsal size and rigidity may be decreased as well. This is usually most marked temporally in the lower eyelid and is the form of ectropion associated with blepharophimosis syndrome. Its correction usually requires a full-thickness retroauricular skin graft to the involved eyelids after releasing the orbital septum sufficiently to allow the lid to assume the proper position. Intermarginal sutures tied over rubber bumpers are utilized to keep the grafted lids stretched for 3 weeks postoperatively.

COLOBOMAS

Lid colobomas are congenital full-thickness lid-margin clefts resulting from the absence of fusion between two growing edges during embryologic development. They may be associated with other ocular anomalies such as orbital dermoid cysts, limbal dermoids, skin or conjunctival adhesions to the globe, corneal opacities, microphthalmos, conical cornea, correctopia, iris coloboma, and persistent pupillary membrane.[6] Upper lid colobomas are most often found at the junction of the medial and middle thirds of one or both lids. Colobomas in this location are usually sporadic. They are a frequent finding in patients exhibiting Goldenhar's syndrome (oculoauriculovertebral dysplasia), which is not hereditary. True colobomas at the junction of the lateral and middle thirds of the lower lid may occur, but more frequently there are intact lid margins which are hypoplastic and are retracted inferiorly over hypoplastic maxillary bones. These are usually associated with the Treacher Collins-Franceschetti Syndrome, which is transmitted as an autosomal dominant trait with weak penetrance.

Colobomas may lead to problems of corneal exposure, although infants generally tolerate this surprisingly well. Corneal epithelial drying should be treated with frequent instillation of ointment during the day plus covering the eye with a sheet of plastic food wrap to create a moist chamber. If these conservative measures do not control the problem, surgery to correct the defect can be performed at any age. Repair of small asymptomatic defects may be deferred until 3 or 4 years of age.

Small colobomas involving up to one fourth of a lid can be repaired by direct closure after trimming the edges to expose parallel tarsal surfaces perpendicular to the lid margin. The closure technique is the same as for a transmarginal lid laceration. For larger defects, direct closure may require a lateral cantholysis or even a Tenzel semicircular rotational skin flap (see Chapter 39). If more than half of the lid is missing, a sliding or transpositional flap is used. Lid-sharing procedures should be avoided in children in order to avoid occlusion amblyopia. In older patients, however, the Hughes procedure is useful for lower lid reconstruction and the Cutler–Beard technique is recommended for upper lid reconstruction. Both procedures require bridge-flap occlusion of the visual axis of approximately 2 months in children and must not be used unless all other potential treatment techniques have been tried and corneal integrity continues to deteriorate. Since other anomalies may coexist, the patient should undergo thorough systemic and ophthalmologic examinations before planning surgery.

Lower lid colobomas may be associated with antimongoloid palpebral fissure slant, hypoplasia of the inferior orbital rim, and a vertical deficiency of skin over the cheek and lower lid. Raising the lateral canthus and grafting bone and skin are often required in addition to closure of the coloboma to achieve a desirable result.[7]

ANKYLOBLEPHARON

Fusion of a portion of the lid margin produces a shortened horizontal fissure. This occurs as a sporadic or irregular autosomal dominant trait, usually occurs bilaterally, and is associated with an increased incidence of microphthalmos, clinical anophthalmos, or phthisis bulbi. The adhesion most commonly involves the lateral canthus and this is referred to as external ankyloblepharon. A lateral canthoplasty can be performed before school age to widen the fissures and eliminate pseudoexotropia. In this procedure, a single horizontal cut is made extending the lateral canthal angle to attain the desired fissure widening (Fig. 37-6A,B). A 1.0- to 1.5-mm strip of skin is excised along each edge of this opening so that conjunctiva can be wrapped over the newly created lid margin and sutured to skin. This prevents reclosure of the lateral canthal angle and helps maintain a temporal fornix.

In internal ankyloblepharon, the adhesion is at the medial canthus. The puncta, canaliculi, plica semilunaris, and caruncle may be abnormal or absent. Any surgical correction for cosmesis is best deferred until the age of 4 years. The adhesion is cut and the skin edges are resected minimally so that conjunctiva can be wrapped over the new lid margin and sutured to the skin. Lacrimal probes should be placed in the canaliculi to prevent damage to them during the procedure. Lacrimal anomalies can be present and may necessitate additional surgical management.

If the lids are joined by single or multiple short bands rather than by direct fusion at a canthus, the condition is termed ankyloblepharon filiforme ad-

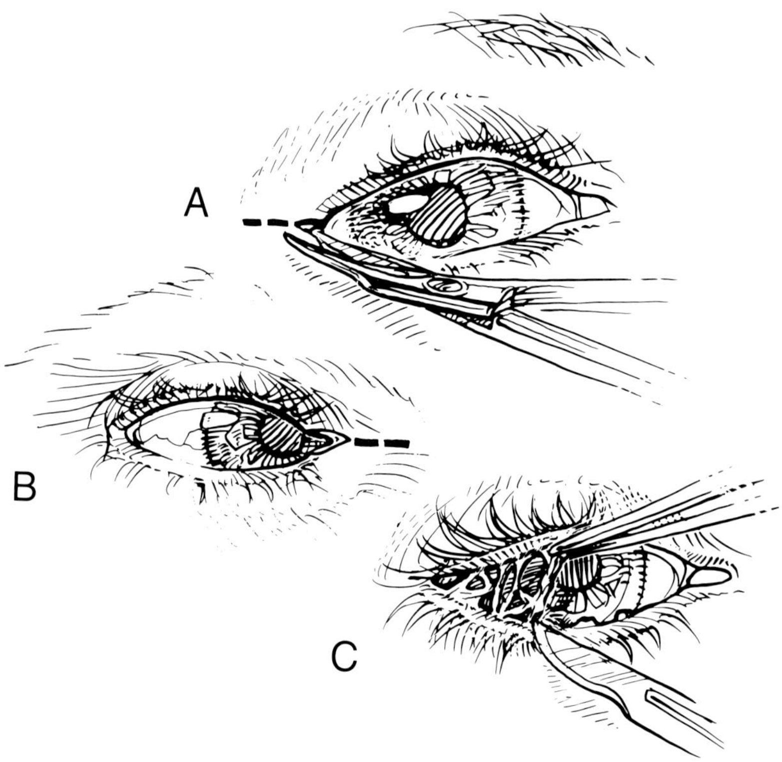

Fig. 37-6. Ankyloblepharon repair. **(A)** External ankyloblepharon. **(B)** Internal ankyloblepharon. **(C)** Ankyloblepharon filiforme adnatum.

natum (Fig. 37-6C). The bands are attached to the lid margin between the lashes and the meibomian gland orifices. Very fine threadlike bands can be ruptured with a muscle hook at any age, leaving the remnants to regress. Larger bands may contain vascular elements. These bands should be shaved from the lid margin, with mild cautery applied for hemostatic control.

DISTICHIASIS

Distichiasis refers to the presence of a second, posteriorly positioned row of eyelashes emerging from meibomian gland orifices.[8] This can occur as an autosomal dominant trait and may be associated with congenital ectropion. The abnormal lashes can range from very fine to better formed and stiffer cilia. They can occur in both upper and lower lids and may represent an aberrent differentiation of meibomian glands. Meibomian glands actually are rudimentary or absent where distichiasis lashes are present. From one to approximately 25 lashes can arise in the abnormal posterior row. Distichiasis can be asymptomatic if the abnormal lashes are directed anteriorly or if they are particularly fine. In such instances, no treatment is necessary. If, however, the lashes continually abraid the cornea, scarring and neovascularization will occur and vision may be decreased. Early treatment is mandatory in such instances. If only a few lashes are involved, electrolysis may be used to ablate their follicles.[9] If more lashes are present, surgical correction must be undertaken. One method is to remove a 2-mm-high horizontal strip of tarsal plate containing the distichiasis lash follicles from the involved lid. This defect is then filled with a graft of full thickness buccal mucosa from the lower lip[10] (Fig. 37-7). An alternative technique involves splitting the lid along the gray line to develop anterior and posterior lid lamellae.[11,12] The abnormal lashes of the posterior lamella are then treated with cryosurgery and the lamellae are rejoined. The lid splitting eliminates skin depigmentation and loss of normal lashes from the cryosurgery and decreases the rounding and atrophy of the lid margin inherent in full-thickness lid cryosurgery.

TELECANTHUS

Congenital telecanthus is a bilateral condition in which the medial canthal tendons are abnormally long, increasing the distance between the medial canthi. This is to be differentiated from hypertelorism, in which there is an increased distance be-

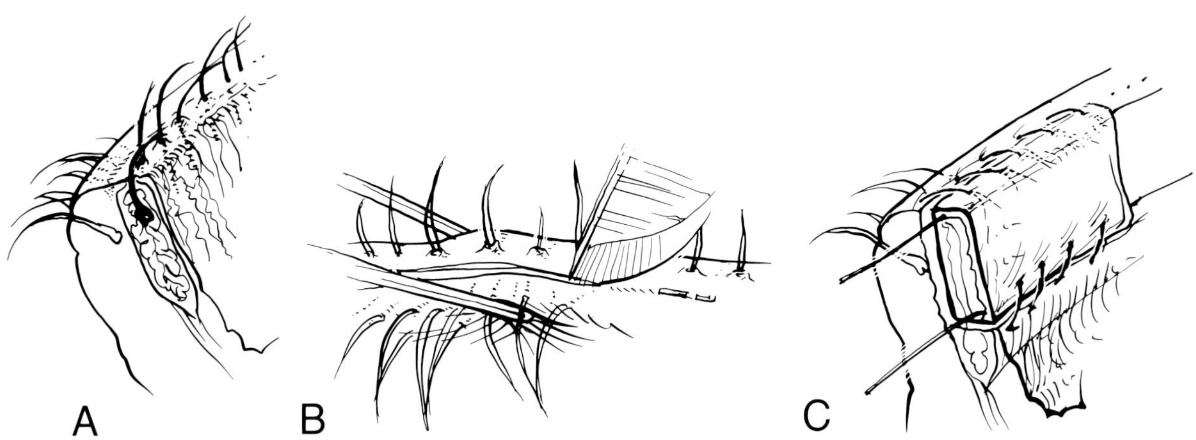

Fig. 37-7. (A) Distichiasis. **(B)** Splitting the lid along the gray line. **(C)** Excision of tarsus severely involved by distichiasis with replacement using autogenous buccal mucosa.

tween the medial walls of the two orbits. Telecanthus is most frequently found in the blepharophimosis syndrome in association with ptosis, epicanthus inversus, and lower lid ectropion. Telecanthus does not decrease with age or bony growth, so surgery is necessary if correction is desired for cosmesis. Shortening of the medial canthal tendons by transnasal wiring is the preferred treatment. This induces horizontal skin redundancy over the medial canthal region. Therefore, an epicanthal fold skin transposition must be performed along with the wiring to produce a normal concave skin contour between the canthal angle and the bridge of the nose. If there are no preexisting epicanthal folds, vertical incisions are made 4 mm medial to the medial canthus, and tapered spindles of skin are excised. If there are preexistent epicanthal folds, they must be managed as described in the prior section, but with an increased amount of skin transposition to correct for the additional folding that is created by the transnasal wiring. Sliding Y–V skin flaps or the Roveda technique (see Fig. 37-3) are used in these cases.

The surgical procedure for transnasal wiring begins with the appropriate skin incision and wide undermining of skin with excision of excess subcutaneous tissue.[13] Lacrimal probes are placed in the

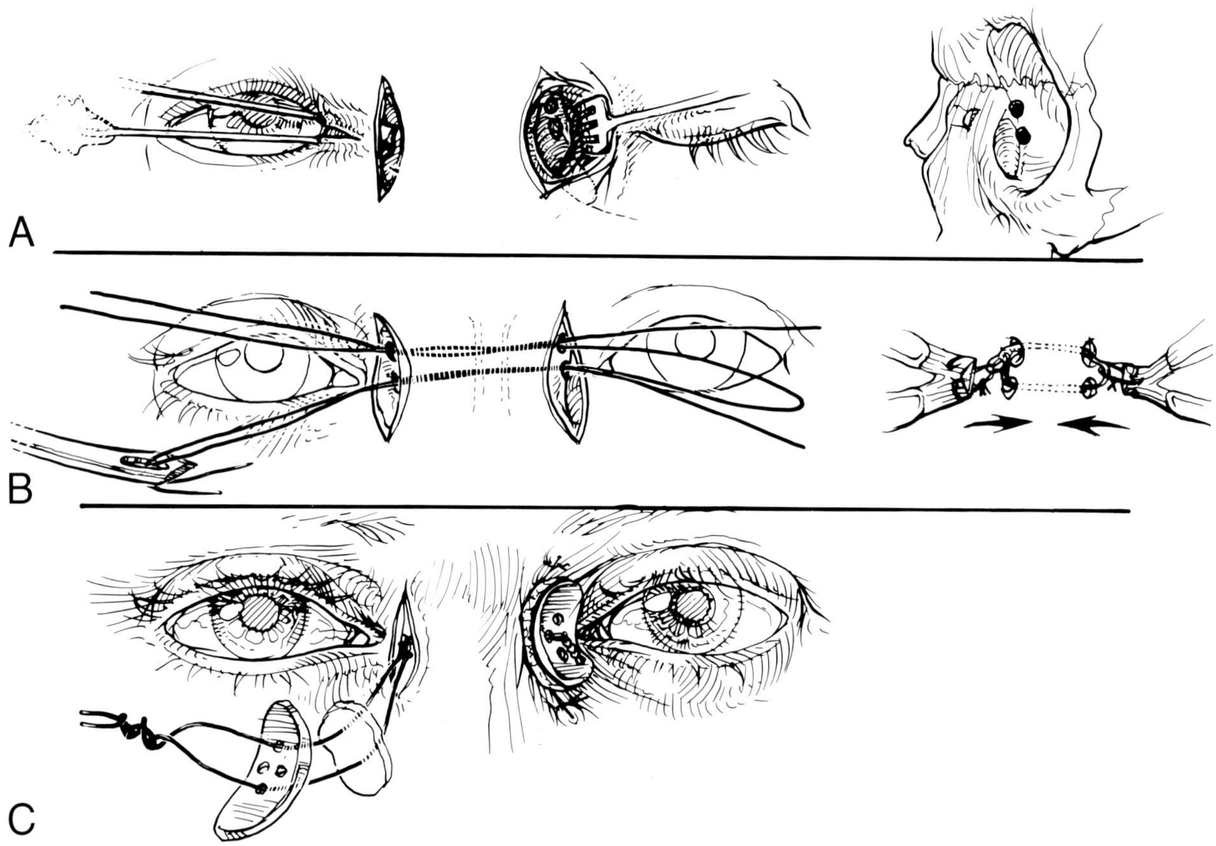

Fig. 37-8. Telecanthus. **(A)** Excision of excess skin and subcutaneous tissue. Placement of lacrimal probes in canaliculi. Gentle lacrimal sac retraction. Formation of bony ostia. **(B)** Passage of transnasal wire. Attachment of medial canthal tendons to a closed wire loop. **(C)** The skin incision is sutured. Canthoplasty buttons and Telfa gauze are secured with the remaining two transnasal wires.

canaliculi to avoid damage to the lacrimal system. The medial canthal tendons are isolated and transected. The medial orbital wall is frequently thickened and must be planed down with an instrument such as a Hall drill to produce the best results. Two 3-mm holes are drilled through each medial orbital wall superior and posterior to the original attachments of the medial canthal tendons (Fig. 37-8A).

The lacrimal sacs may need to be retracted laterally during this step. A Mustarde awl with a suture eye is then passed from right to left through one set of the bone ostia piercing the nasal septum. Two 25-gauge wires are drawn back through these holes. The awl is then passed from right to left across the nasal cavity through the second set of corresponding bone ostia. A third wire plus one end of one of the two wires passed through the other ostia are pulled back across the nasal cavity. The left medial canthal tendon is secured to the U-shaped loop of wire with 5-0 prolene suture. The two free ends of this U wire are then twisted together on the right side to form a loop. The right medial canthal tendon is attached to the loop with prolene sutures. The loop should be twisted tight, excess wire is cut off, and the twisted ends are buried in one of the ostia (Fig. 37-8B). The remaining two wires are brought around the tendons and through the skin. The skin incision is closed with absorbable subcuticular sutures and 7-0 nylon skin sutures. Canthoplasty buttons are secured with the exteriorized wires to keep the skin flat in the medial canthal concavity and to take some of the tension off of the canthal tendon wires (Fig. 37-8C). The buttons, exteriorized wires, and skin sutures are removed after 10 days. The canthal tendon wires are left in place indefinitely.

BLEPHAROPHIMOSIS

Blepharophimosis syndrome refers to bilateral diminution of the eyelid fissure dimensions. It includes numerous eyelid and facial anomalies. This is inherited as an autosomal dominant trait with strong penetrance. The face exhibits a mongoloid contour with fairly flat brows and nasal bridge. The eyelid fissures, however, often have an antimongoloid slant. A moderate to severe bilateral upper lid ptosis is present with shallow superior sulci and minimal or absent creases. The medial canthal tendons are long, producing telecanthus. The lateral canthal tendons may also be elongated and poorly developed. The lower puncta are frequently displaced laterally and form horizontal slits. The brow hair is frequently thickened in a vertical distribution, and the two brows may join at the midline. The presence of other features has led to the classification of blepharophimosis syndrome as three distinct types. In type 1, ptosis and telecanthus are associated with prominent epicanthus inversus (Fig. 37-9A). Type 2 is characterized by ptosis, telecanthus, and lower lid ectropion. The ectropion is most prominent temporally with a vertical skin deficiency, as well as poor lateral canthal tendon fixation (Fig. 37-9B). Type 3 is similar to type 2 except that there may be a more pronounced skin deficiency of all four lids, and there is increased intraorbital distance with hypertelorism.

Although the typing of blepharophimosis syndrome simplifies the discussion of evaluation and management, it must be remembered that there is considerable overlap among the three types. Each patient must be examined for all the possible anomalies. The extent of each defect is considered before a treatment plan is devised.

Multiple operations over several years may be necessary to achieve optimal correction. Nevertheless, even the best results are unlikely to produce a fully normal appearance. In type 1, ptosis is usually the most prominent defect. It is corrected during the preschool years with levator resection and advancement or frontalis suspension as described in Chapter 34. If the horizontal fissure is short temporally, a von Ammon canthoplasty is performed at the same time. This procedure is explained in the section of this chapter on lateral ankyloblepharon.

If the telecanthus and epicanthus remain a bothersome cosmetic defect they can be repaired one or more years later. The growth of the bridge of the nose frequently reduces the prominence of the widely spread medial canthi as does spectacle cor-

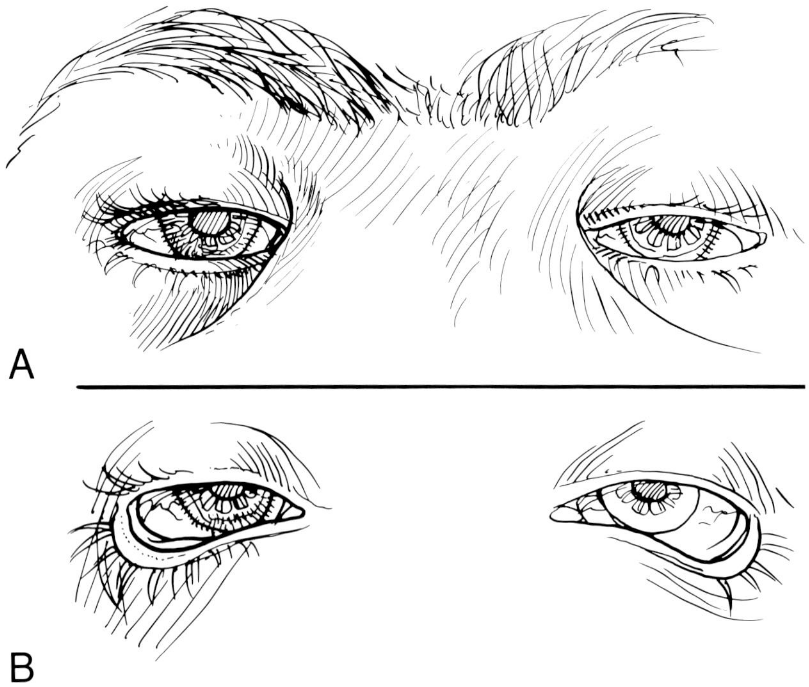

Fig. 37-9. Blepharophimosis syndrome. **(A)** Type 1. **(B)** Type 2.

rection of refractive errors. The selection of surgical procedures for the repair of epicanthus and telecanthus has already been discussed.

In the management of type 2 blepharophimosis, the ptosis is best corrected during the preschool years. At a later time, the lower lid ectropion can be alleviated by releasing the inferior orbital septum and placing retroauricular full-thickness free skin grafts in both lower eyelids as described for congenital ectropion. If the telecanthus warrants surgery, it can be corrected at the same time as the ectropion. Since there are no epicanthal folds, transpositional skin flaps are not necessary in the medial canthal region. The excision of spindle-shaped sections of skin along with the vertical medial canthal incision compensates for the relocation of the medial canthi.

Type 3 blepharophimosis is the most unusual form. A detailed craniofacial evaluation should be performed if it is anticipated that the therapy recommended for type 2 would provide insufficient correction. A multispecialty surgical approach is necessary if the increased interorbital distance requires correction.

EURYBLEPHARON

Euryblepharon is a symmetric enlargement of the palpebral apertures. The lateral canthi are displaced temporally and often downward. The lower lids are usually ectropic temporally. The condition may be familial or associated with craniofacial anomalies. It should be distinguished from secondary enlargement of the palpebral apertures due to buphthalmos, staphylomas, axial myopia, and proptosis.

No correction is indicated for mild cases. With more prominent involvement, however, permanent lateral tarsorrhaphies will suffice as long as the lateral canthi are not markedly depressed and ectropion is absent. For more severe cases, the superior and inferior arms of the lateral canthal tendons must be isolated and transected. They are then reattached to the desired position on the periostium just inside of the lateral orbital wall. Permanent lateral tarsorrhaphies are then performed. There is often an inadequate vertical anterior lamellar height of the lower lids. In such instances, full-thickness retroauricular skin grafts must be placed in the lower lids to provide adequate vertical skin dimensions.

REFERENCES

1. Callahan MA, Callahan A: Ophthalmic Plastic and Reconstructive Surgery. Aesculapius, Birmingham, AL, 1979
2. Tse DT, Anderson RL, Fratkin JD: Aponeurosis disinsertion in congenital entropion. Arch Ophthalmol 101:436, 1983
3. Biglan AW, Buerger GF: Congenital horizontal tarsal kink. Am J Ophthalmol 89:522, 1980
4. Stern EN, Campbell CH, Faulkner HW: Conservative management of congenital eversion of the eyelids. Am J Ophthalmol 75:319, 1973
5. Gilbert HD, Smith RE, Mahlon HB, et al: Congenital upper eyelid eversion and Down's syndrome. Am J Ophthalmol 75:469, 1973
6. Guibor P: Surgical repair of congenital colobomas. Trans Am Acad Ophthalmol Otol 79:671, 1975
7. Tessier P, Rougier J, Hervouet F: Plastic Surgery of the Orbit and Eyelids. Masson, New York, 1981
8. Fox SA: Distichiasis. Am J Ophthalmol 53:14, 1962
9. Scheie HG, Albert DM: Distichiasis and trichiasis: Origin and management. Am J Ophthalmol 61:718, 1966
10. White JH: Correction of distichiasis by tarsal resection and mucous membrane grafting. Am J Ophthalmol 80:507, 1975
11. Fein W: Surgical repair for distichiasis, trichiasis, and entropion. Arch Ophthalmol 94:809, 1976
12. Anderson RL, Harvey JT: Lid splitting and posterior lamella cryosurgery for congenital and acquired distichiasis. Arch Ophthalmol 99:631, 1981
13. Reeh, MJ, Beyer CK, Shannon GM: Practical Ophthalmic Plastic and Reconstructive Surgery. Lea & Febiger, Philadelphia, 1976

Blepharoplasty and Brow Elevation

38

J. Earl Rathbun

As the number of older persons in our population increases and the emphasis on preservation of youthful characteristics continues, there is increasing interest in reversing the visible effects of aging. People are very aware of facial aging changes, with the eyelids being a focal point of concern. While some seek eyelid surgery to improve the cosmetic appearance, more older people are desiring surgical correction of upper lid tissue excess and correction of brow ptosis for functional improvement of visual-field compromise and for relief of eyelid and brow fatigue. With the increasing coverage by the lay press, patients have become more sophisticated in selecting a surgeon and expect perfection in the postoperative result.

PREOPERATIVE EVALUATION

When examining a candidate for eyelid or brow surgery, it must be remembered that the patient has arrived at the present status through the normal process of individual aging. Surgery will change this "normal" state. One must determine the patient's motivation, social and cultural background, and psychological state.[1,2] It must also be determined whether the expectations from surgery are realistic and whether the patient can be satisfied with the results. If there is uncertainty about any of these areas, the patient should be seen again before any surgical decisions are made. Unless both the surgeon and the patient are comfortable with the proposed procedures, the probable results, and the possible complications, surgery is best avoided.

Initially the patient's complaints should be determined. I prefer to give patients a mirror to enable them to point to specific problems. On a number of occasions, patients have requested excision of skin that they erroneously expected to correct blepharoptosis.

The evaluation must include a thorough history of present and past medical problems. One should inquire about diabetes, thyroid disease, renal compromise, cardiovascular disease, and other chronic diseases. These conditions should be under stable control, and an inquiry to the patient's general physician may be needed. A history of present medications should be elicited with specific questions as to anticoagulants and antimetabolites. Although aspirin is frequently not thought of as a medication, it increases operative and postoperative bleeding significantly, which can be cata-

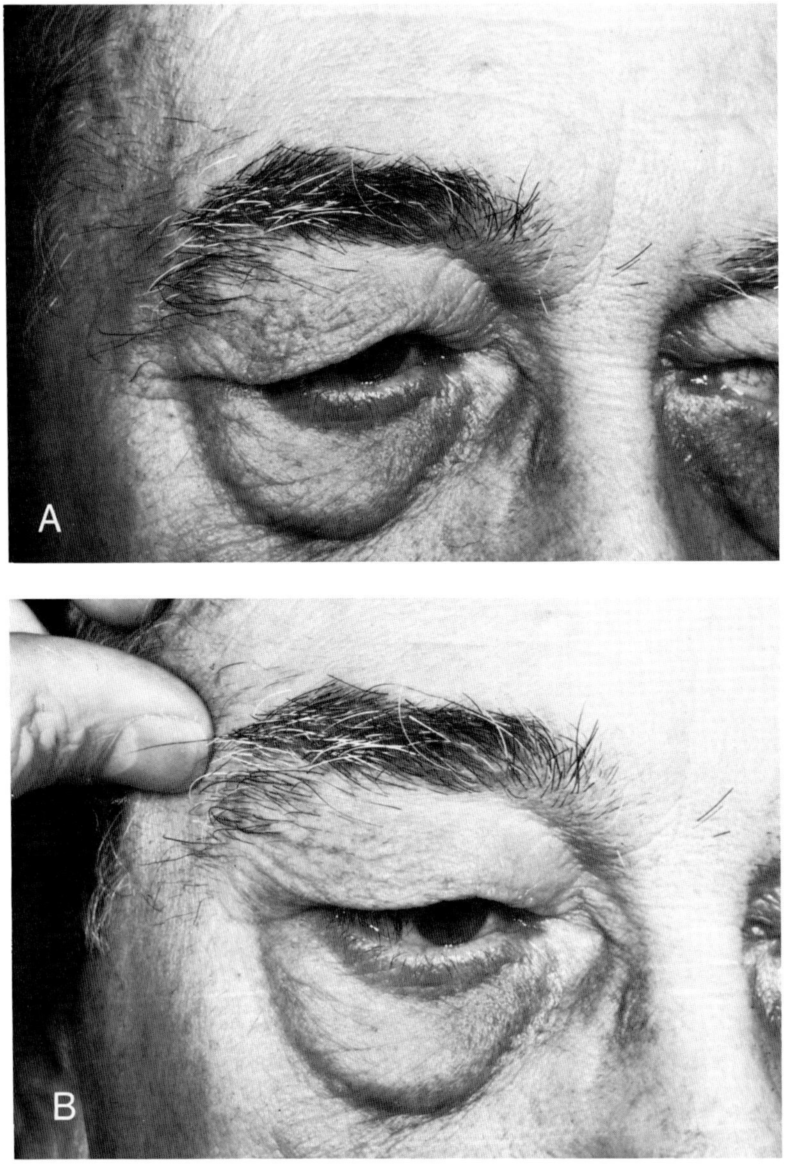

Fig. 38-1. (A) Preoperative photograph of patient with brow ptosis and excess eyelid tissue. **(B)** Effect of temporal brow elevation. *(Figure continued.)*

strophic; aspirin should be discontinued 10 days before surgery, if possible. Other anticoagulants should be discontinued and monitored with appropriate bleeding times, with the realization that hypercoagulation can result. These medications usually can be resumed 1 week postoperatively. An allergic history with particular emphasis on local anesthetics is obtained. Systemic edema problems result in eyelid edema, especially when the patient is supine. The patient must be informed that excision of excess eyelid tissue will not eliminate the edema but will only improve the effect by decreasing the amount of tissue that swells.

An eye examination to determine the visual acuity of each eye, strabismus, adequacy of tear secretion, conjunctival and corneal health, and the status of known ocular disease is essential. A basic secretion test[3] with topical anesthetic and Schirmer test paper (S.M.P. Division of Cooper Laboratories, Inc., San German, Puerto Rico 00753) should be done if there is any question as to the adequacy of tears upon biomicroscopy.

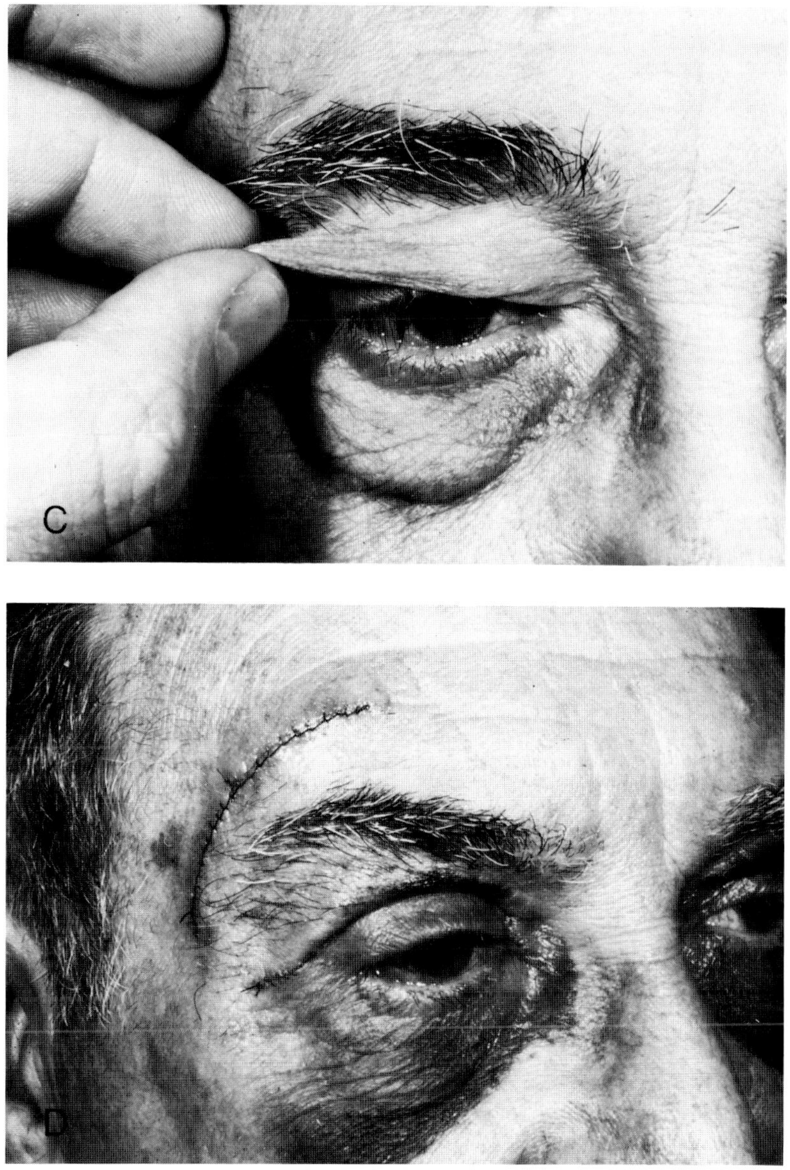

Fig. 38-1 *(Continued).* **(C)** Evaluation of amount of excess eyelid tissue with brow manually elevated. **(D)** Immediate postoperative appearance with temporal brow lift and upper lid blepharoplasty.

BROW PTOSIS EVALUATION

The examination of all patients who are candidates for eyelid or brow elevation surgery begins with evaluation of all the facial characteristics. The position of the hairline is noted. The extent of general facial laxity as well as any facial paresis or asymmetry are noted. The actual eyebrow location without cosmetics or plucking of hairs is determined. The amount of eyebrow ptosis is measured medially, centrally, and laterally, as the amount of ptosis may vary. This is measured by holding a millimeter ruler vertically at the superior border of the relaxed eyebrow and then manually, lifting the eyebrow to the desired nonptotic location. The difference is measured and recorded. Frequently the lateral brow is most ptotic, and significant improvement can be obtained with a temporal brow lift (Fig. 38-1). The presence and location of brow furrows both centrally and temporally influence the choice of procedure.

UPPER EYELID EVALUATION

The general characteristics of the eyelid are noted before the amount of excess tissue is measured. The presence of lid edema and erythema suggests chronic fluid problems or inflammatory processes. Ptosis is often present in the older patient and must be pointed out. The amount of levator muscle function and the adequacy of lid closure are noted. The symmetry or asymmetry of the eyelid creases and the presence of any hollowing of the lid due to fat atrophy are noted and brought to the patient's attention (Fig. 38-2A,B). The amount of excess skin is noted medially, centrally, and laterally. If brow elevation is being considered, these observations should be made with the brow in the desired elevated position (Fig. 38-1C). The presence of protruding fat that can be accentuated and better observed with gentle pressure on the closed lower eyelid is noted. The medial fat pads frequently require attention. The central preaponeurotic fat should be treated less vigorously so as to avoid a hollow appearance, as the orbital fat atrophies with the normal process of aging. Temporally, fat is occasionally removed, but one must be aware of and avoid the lacrimal gland, which may be prolapsed anteriorly and inferiorly. Webbing in the medial canthus may be accentuated by removal of upper eyelid skin. A tendency for webbing can be observed by pulling the upper lid skin up and laterally (Fig. 38-3). If significant webbing occurs, a medial Z-plasty[4] or Y–V-plasty[5] may be required.

LOWER EYELID EVALUATION

More complications occur with lower than with upper eyelid blepharoplasty. Most will be avoided by a careful preoperative evaluation and choice of

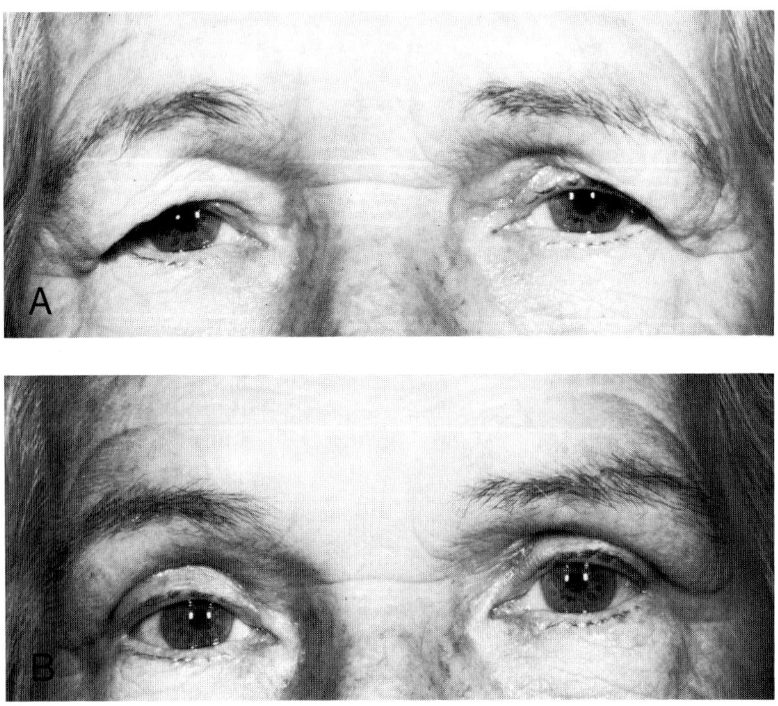

Fig. 38-2. (A) Preoperative crease asymmetry and hollow left upper sulcus. **(B)** After blepharoplasty improvement but with remaining asymmetry.

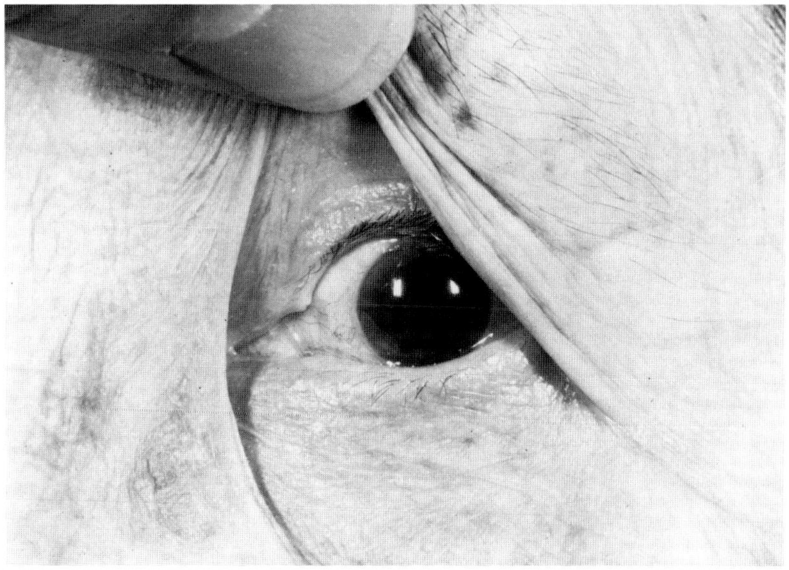

Fig. 38-3. Medial canthal webbing with elevation of excess tissue.

appropriate procedure. Lower eyelid tone is evaluated by pulling the lid down and observing how briskly it snaps back into place. The position of the eyelid in relationship to the inferior limbus is noted. Scleral show especially in the younger patient should be pointed out. Some consider scleral show attractive, while others believe it produces a stare effect. The presence of mild ectropion or excessive laxity due to medial and/or lateral canthal tendon stretching may require additional procedures to prevent gross postoperative ectropion. The eyelid skin considered in excess should be elevated while observing the cheek. If the cheek is elevated, the entire amount of skin being grasped cannot be excised, as the cheek will pull the eyelid down. The position of the inferior punctum and its relationship to the lacrimal lake are noted. The presence of prominent lower eyelid fat pads is observed and can be accentuated by finger pressure on the closed upper eyelid. The bags-on-bags phenomenon with the edematous fold of skin over the maxilla (Fig. 38-4) is not correctable with the usual lower eyelid blepharoplasty and requires additional procedures. The characteristics of the lower eyelid skin should be noted, as they influence the result. For example, deep lines in thick, ruddy skin will not be removed with surgery. Very thin skin is likely to become darker due to blood staining and exposure of the underlying muscle. Fine, crinkly wrinkles will also persist. Crow's-feet or laugh lines

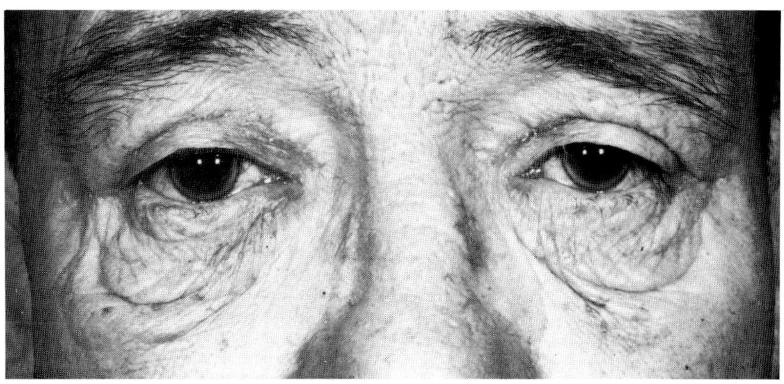

Fig. 38-4. Bags-on-bags phenomenon.

at the lateral canthus may be improved but will not be eliminated with the usual blepharoplasty procedures.

In all cases in which eyelid or brow procedures are being considered, preoperative photographs in the upright position are essential. During the postoperative period, the patient and surgeon may forget the preoperative appearance. A photograph accurately depicts the preoperative state and serves as a useful reference. Photographs as well as visual fields are frequently requested by insurance companies to prove functional compromise.

At the conclusion of the evaluation, the findings should be summarized for the patient and specific defects and areas of concern again brought to attention. A determination can usually be made as to whether the proposed procedures are functional or cosmetic. With four-lid blepharoplasty, the upper eyelids may be functional, while the lower eyelids, which almost never cause visual compromise, are cosmetic. These factors may determine which procedures the patient elects to have done.

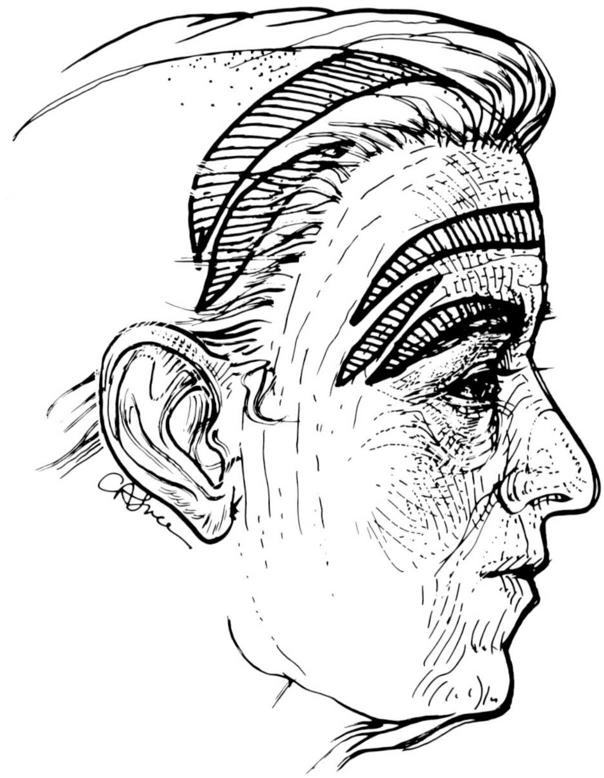

Fig. 38-5. Illustration showing possible locations for brow elevation with selection depending on patient's characteristics.

BROW ELEVATION

If both upper eyelid tissue excision and brow elevation are to be done, the brow elevation should be done first, as this will reduce the amount of excess upper eyelid tissue that can be excised. The most desirable location of tissue excision will vary with each patient[6] (Fig. 38-5).

Direct Brow Elevation

If the eyebrow is equally ptotic medially to laterally and the central tissue between the brows is not in great excess, excision of the tissue immediately above each brow is effective (Fig. 38-6). The inferior incision is placed at the upper edge of the brow hairs and extends from the medial aspect of the brow to the lateral aspect. The fusiform figure to be excised is outlined with a marking pen after sterile preparation and draping. One percent lidocaine with 1 : 100,000 or 1 : 200,000 epinephrine is infiltrated subcutaneously. The skin is then incised with the scalpel blade. If the eyebrow hairs come obliquely from the skin from a superior direction, the incision should be beveled in the direction of the hairs to avoid hair loss. The skin and underlying orbicularis muscle are then excised with sharp scissors dissection. Care must be taken not to carry the tissue plane of excision deep, as anesthesia of the forehead may result due to severing the branches of the superior orbital nerve. The dissection may be carried into the interbrow tissue in an attempt to reduce glabellar creases, by separating skin from the corrugator and procerus muscles.[7,8] Copious bleeding frequently results from brow incisions and must be meticulously treated. Since forehead skin is thick and scars more than eyelid skin, and gravity gives a downward pull on the wound, a meticulous three-layer closure is advised. The subcutaneous tissue is closed with multiple interrupted 5-0 chromic gut sutures. A subcuticular 6-0 nylon

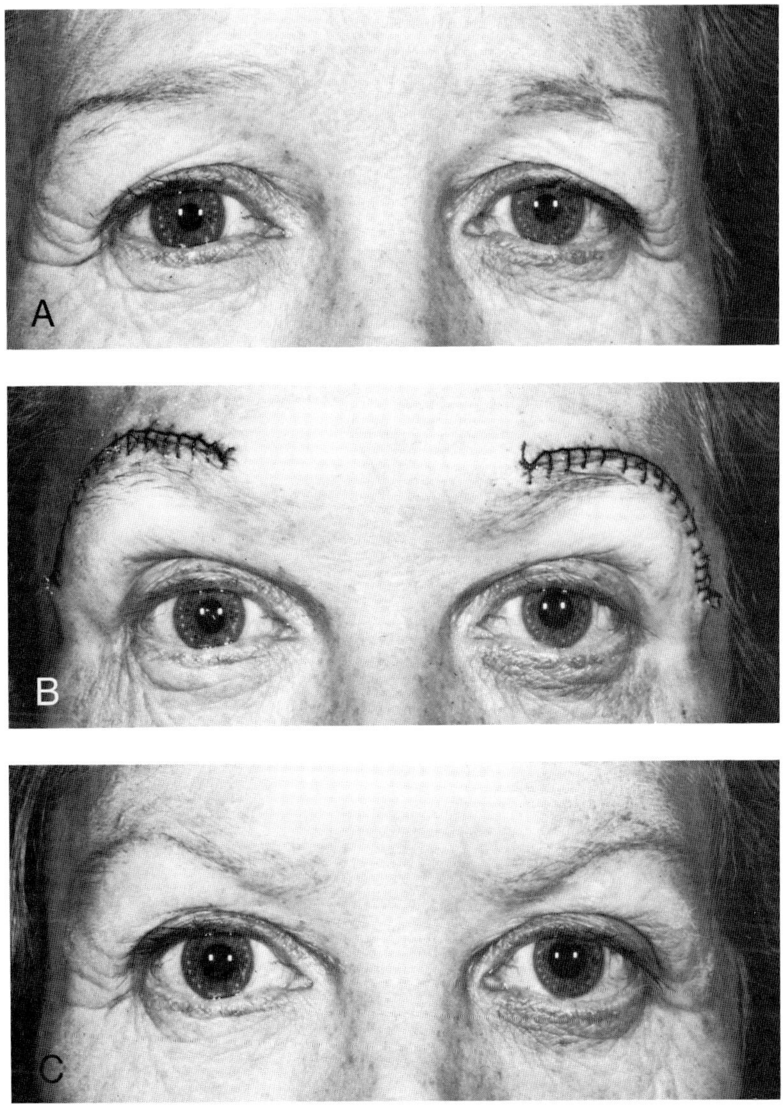

Fig. 38-6. (A) Preoperative, **(B)** immediate postoperative, and **(C)** result from direct brow elevation without eyelid surgery.

suture is next placed to relieve tension on the line of skin closure and to allow for the use of finer sutures in the final skin closure. This 6-0 nylon suture is externalized medially and laterally as well as in the central portion of the incision to allow for later pullout. This subcuticular suture should leave the skin edges well approximated and allow for a final skin closure without tension. The third layer of closure is with 6-0 silk placed in a narrow-running interlocking fashion. This silk suture is removed within 5 to 7 days, while the nylon subcuticular suture is left approximately 14 days. Thus the wound remains reinforced while the fine scars from the skin closure are essentially eliminated.

Temporal Brow Lift

The lateral eyebrow is frequently found to droop, while the medial portion remains in good position (Fig. 38-1A). Excision of a portion of the lateral forehead can be done in one of several locations. A fusiform figure of skin can be removed by combining skin creases with the lower incision being 1 to 3 cm superior and lateral to the lateral portion of the eyebrow. Manual elevation of the ptotic brow preoperatively with the patient in the sitting position will determine the location and extent of skin excision. Frequently the incisions can be made in forehead creases, so that the result is to combine two creases. A scar in the direction of the normal forehead creases minimizes the attention of the observer. The incision can also be made at the hairline, a location that is advantageous in a woman with a high hairline who does not wish further elevation or in a patient who wears the hair down over the forehead. The third location is 2 cm above the hairline, a location at which the scar is hidden unless the hairline recedes. This is a good location in women but is questionable in men. The closure for the three locations is as described for the direct brow lift. The temporal brow lift results in a superior and lateral elevation whereas the direct brow lift gives mainly a superior elevation. Dissection into the area of the lateral canthus at the time of temporal brow lift may reduce the prominence and number of crow's-feet or laugh lines.

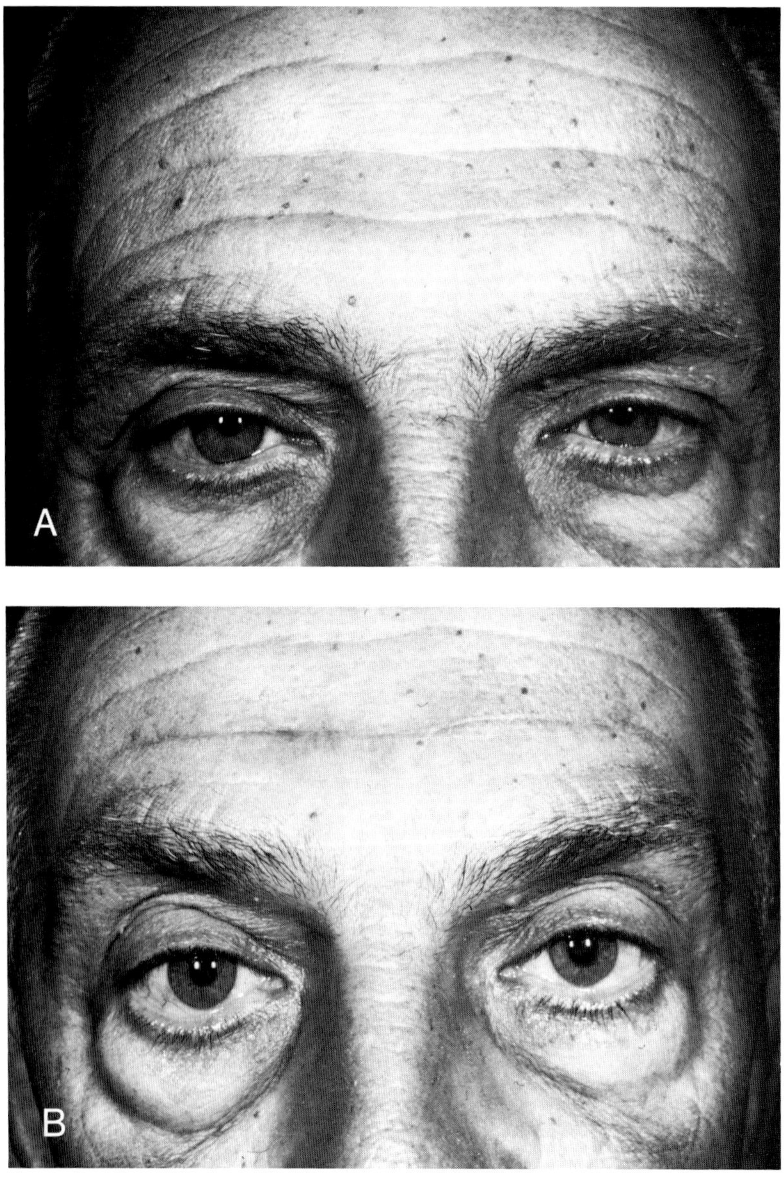

Fig. 38-7. Excision of mid-forehead strip of tissue combining two brow furrows **(A)** preoperatively and **(B)** postoperatively.

Mid-forehead Brow Lift

In a man with a receded hairline and with a lax forehead and brow ptosis, there is no inconspicuous place to hide a scar. When elevation of both brows and the central area between the brows is desired, tissue resection of the mid-forehead area is effective. Frequently two skin creases can be combined effectively to disguise the scar (Fig. 38-7). The incision can be brought inferiorly at the lateral aspect to give lateral pull to the lateral portions of the brows. With the previously described three-layer closure, the scar is usually minimal. Nevertheless, with any brow or forehead scar, 6 to 12 months may be required before the redness fades as the scar matures. Cosmetics will camouflage nicely if the patient is willing to use them.

Coronal Brow Elevation

The resection of scalp tissue above the hairline[9,10] with dissection inferiorly in the supraperiosteal plane to a level below the superior orbital rims allows for a general forehead and brow lift. The corrugator and procerus muscles may be excised to relieve the central frown lines. Excision of horizontal strips of frontalis muscle can make mid-forehead creases less apparent. This procedure does raise the hairline, a result that some patients have considered objectionable. This change in the hairline must be pointed out preoperatively. Care must also be taken in men, as the hairline may recede, leaving a visible scar.

UPPER EYELID BLEPHAROPLASTY

The location and amount of ptotic upper eyelid tissue vary in each patient (Figs. 38-8 and 38-9). Thus one cannot use a standard configuration for tissue excision but must measure the amount of excess in several places from the medial canthus to beyond the lateral canthus. Examination should take place with the patient in the upright position and an estimate made of the amount of tissue to be excised in each portion of the lid as well as how far laterally the excision should extend. Also, any

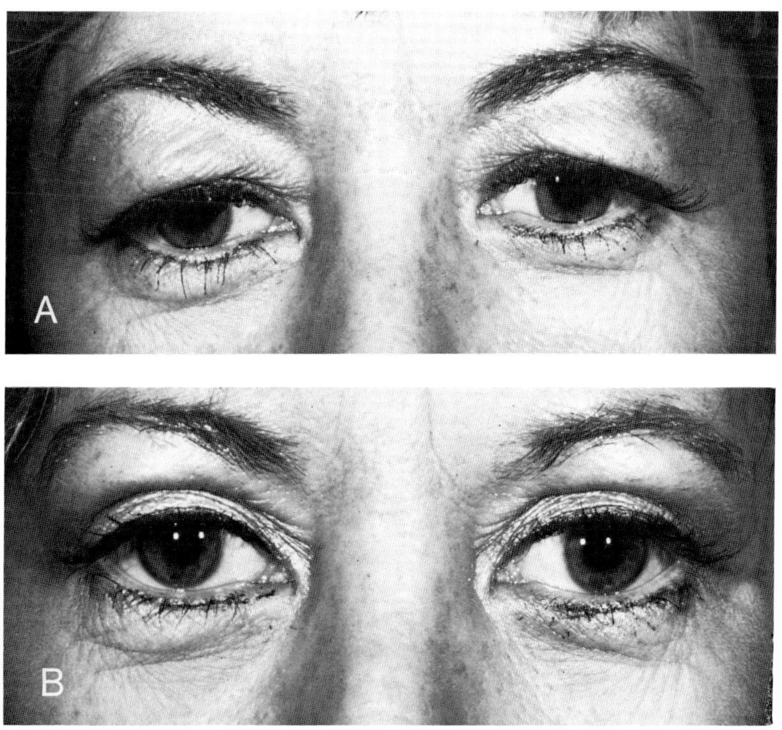

Fig. 38-8. Upper lid blepharoplasty in a 46-year-old patient **(A)** preoperatively and **(B)** postoperatively.

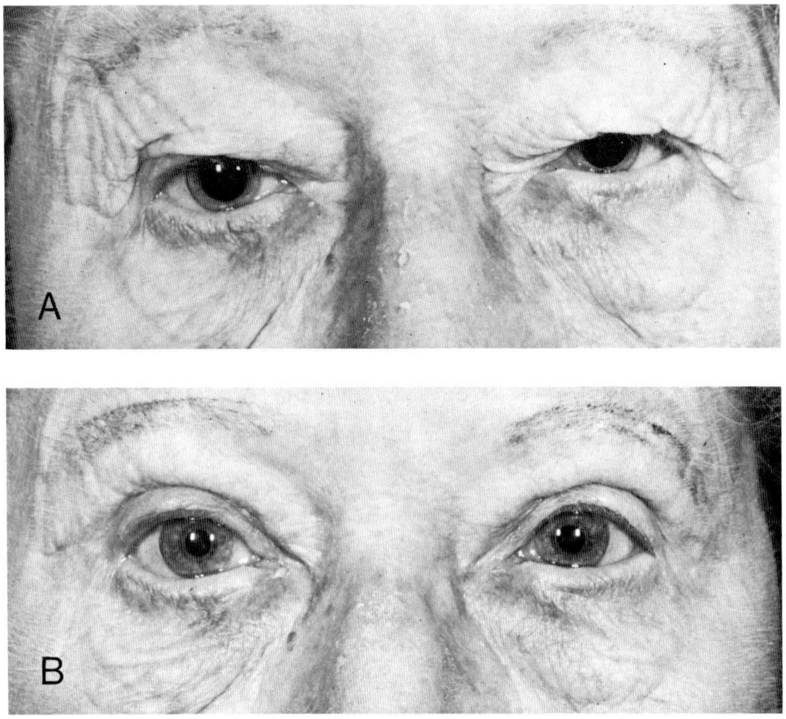

Fig. 38-9. Upper lid blepharoplasty in a 75-year-old patient **(A)** preoperatively and **(B)** postoperatively.

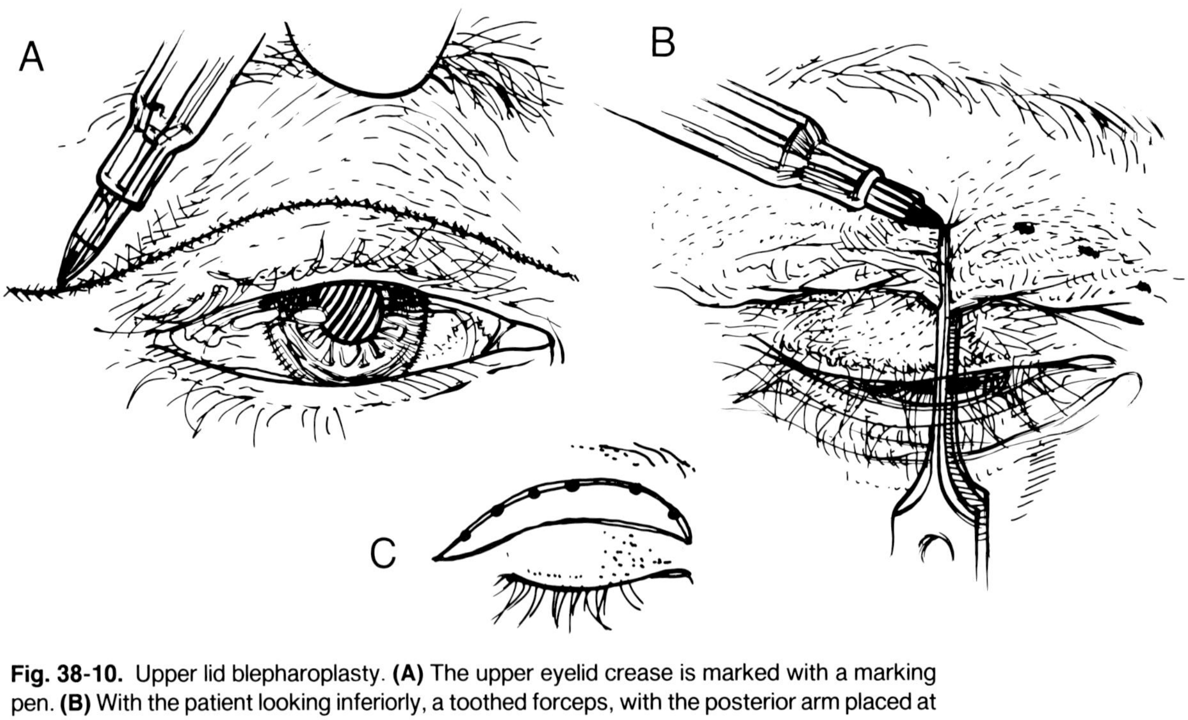

Fig. 38-10. Upper lid blepharoplasty. **(A)** The upper eyelid crease is marked with a marking pen. **(B)** With the patient looking inferiorly, a toothed forceps, with the posterior arm placed at the lid crease, is used to grasp the excess tissue. **(C)** Outline of skin to be excised prior to injection of local anesthetic.

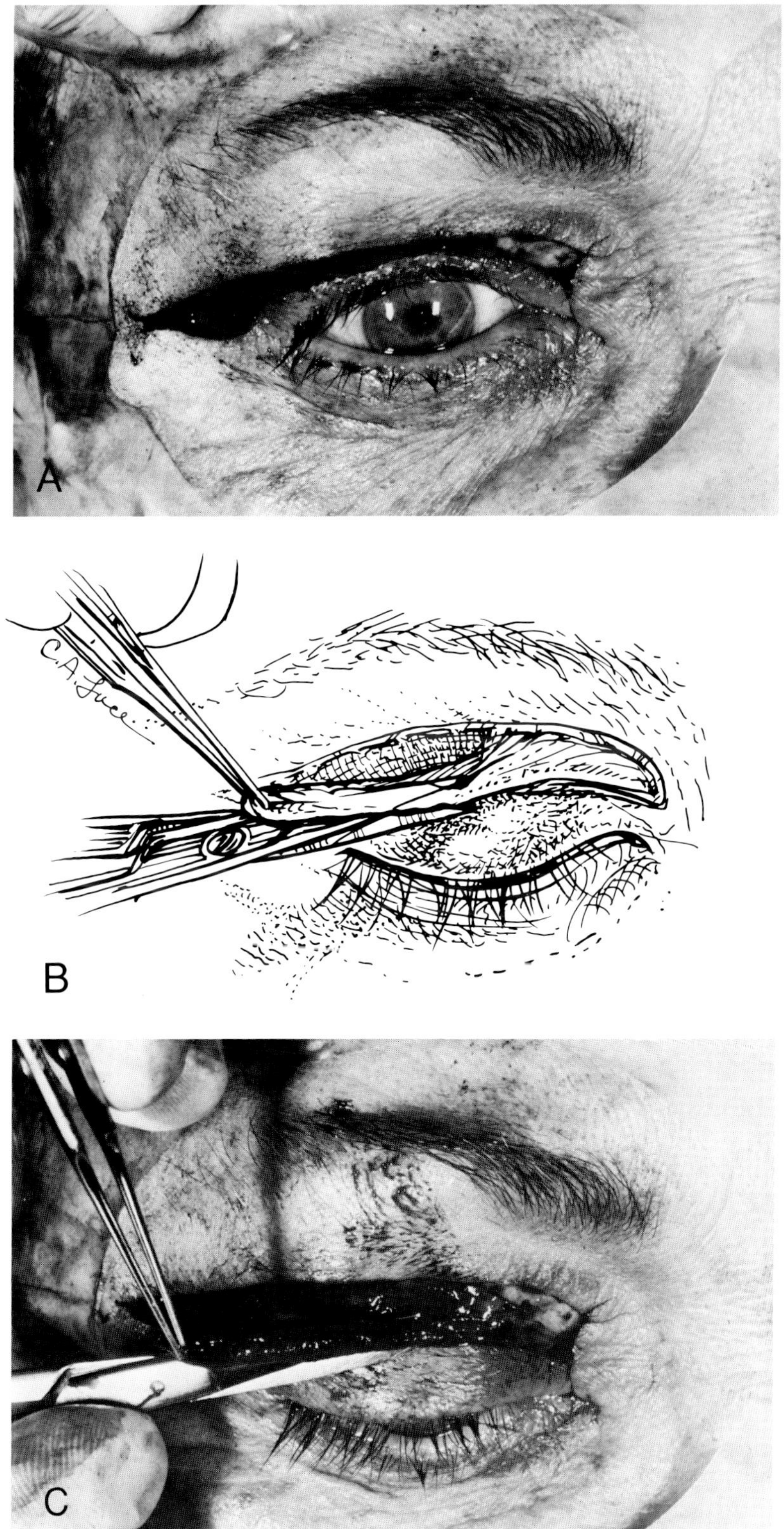

Fig. 38-11. (A) Fold of excess orbicularis muscle following skin excision. **(B,C)** Excision of strip of orbicularis muscle.

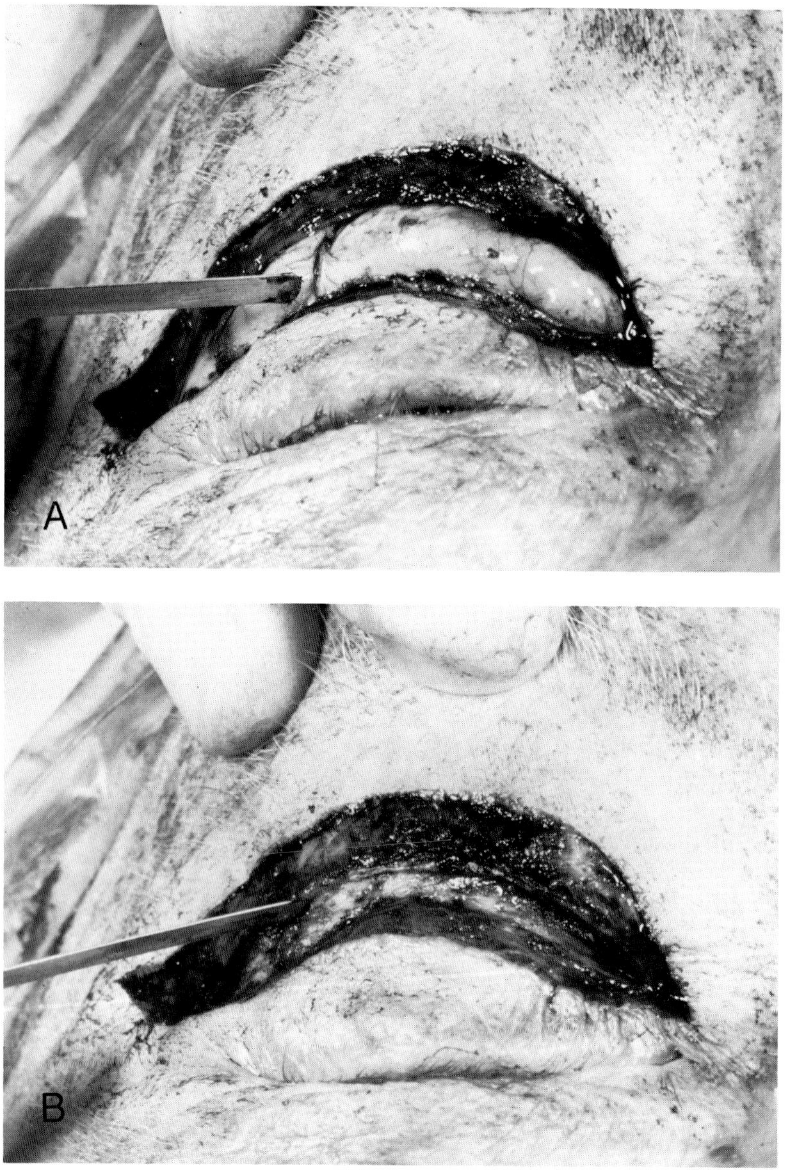

Fig. 38-12. (A) Orbital septum before application of a grid of cautery. **(B)** Immediately after grid of cautery to the orbital septum.

asymmetry of lid creases, upper sulci, or brows should be noted. After the periorbital areas are sterile and draped, the upper eyelid creases are marked with a marking pen. This inferior incision line is then carried superolaterally beyond the lateral canthus, the distance being determined by the amount of lateral tissue excess. The markings for the lid crease incisions should be symmetric, even when preoperative lid asymmetry is noted. With the patient looking inferiorly (not with the eyes closed), one arm of a toothed forceps held vertically in the plane of the eyelid is placed at the lid crease (Fig. 38-10A,B). The excess tissue is then rolled inferiorly with the brows in a relaxed position, and the amount that can be excised with slight eversion of the lashes is marked. This is done in at least five positions across the eyelid and beyond the lateral canthus. The marks are then connected, outlining the upper incision line (Fig. 38-10C). The two upper eyelids are measured separately and then compared as to symmetry. If preoperative evaluation showed asymmetry, the amount of excess marked should reflect this difference. If there is a question, remeasuring should be done, as no changes should be made after the injection of local anesthesia, which distorts the tissue and compromises eyelid function. Local anesthesia is preferred, as this allows for tissue measurement and marking in the awake patient immediately before the procedure. Approximately 4 ml 1 percent lidocaine with 1 : 100,000 or 1 : 200,000 epinephrine is infiltrated subcutaneously. Skin incision is done with a scalpel and skin excision with sharp scissors dissection. The orbicularis muscle is left exposed, and the multiple areas of bleeding are cauterized with fine point cautery. With the patient looking in the primary gaze, one will observe a fold of orbicularis muscle similar to the previously observed skinfold (Fig. 38-11A). This fold of orbicularis muscle is tented up with forceps with the eye closed and a 6-mm strip of muscle is excised with scissors from the lateral end of the incision to the medial end (Fig. 38-11B,C). If the muscle is held tented up with the forceps, injury to the levator aponeurosis will not occur. Hemostasis is again obtained. The inferior portion of the orbital septum with its attachment to the anterior levator sheath is now exposed. Gentle pressure on the lower eyelid with the eye closed will accentuate the upper fat pad protrusion. If the fat pads are mildly or moderately protruding, I prefer to apply cautery to the lax orbital septum to contract and thicken the septum and correct the laxity, thus avoiding the excision of fat. Cautery is placed in a 2-mm grid in four or five vertical rows medially to laterally (Figs. 38-12 and 38-13). This results in an immediate shrinkage of the septum. Cautery is also placed in a line along the anterior levator sheath in the line of the lid crease. This leads to horizontal shortening and accentuates the crease.

If one elects to excise fat, which is a more common practice than orbital septum cautery, the orbital septum is tented over the area of fat prominence with forceps and is then incised with scissors (Fig. 38-14A,B). Pressure on the closed lids results in fat herniation (Fig. 38-14C). Reaching into the orbit to extract fat is a practice to be avoided. The herniated fat is clamped in a fine hemostat. I prefer to excise the fat along the anterior aspect of the

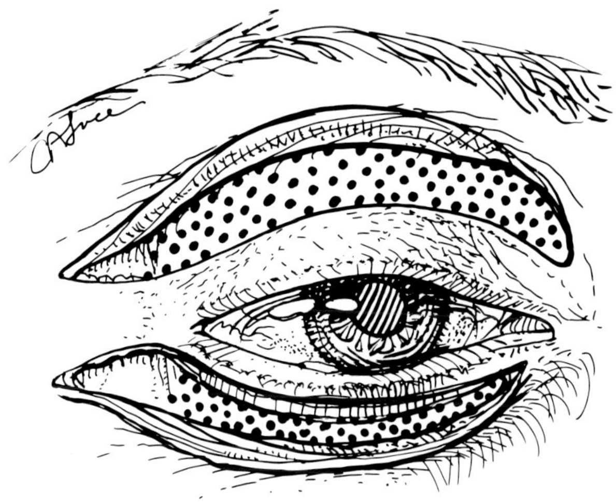

Fig. 38-13. Distribution of cautery to superior and inferior orbital septum.

clamp with scissors (Fig. 38-14D), leaving a small amount of fat to cauterize directly (Fig. 38-14E) rather than shave the fat smooth to the clamp with a scalpel, thus depending on indirect cautery to the hemostat to seal vessels. The clamp is then released slowly with the fat grasped in forceps. The fat is observed for bleeding and then allowed to retract back into the orbit. The process is then repeated starting with pressure on the lids until the desired amount of fat has been excised. The orbital septum does not require suture closure.

The initial placement of interrupted sutures serves to establish the lid crease as well as to outline the pattern of skin closure. Three to five 7-0 silk sutures are placed, dividing the lid horizontally (Fig. 38-15). Each is placed through inferior skin edge, orbicularis muscle, cauterized aponeurotic sheath, orbicularis muscle, and superior skin edge. With these sutures in place, the patient is asked to open the eye, and the contours of the eyelid crease and the eyelid margin are checked. Symmetry with the other side is evaluated as well. Final skin closure is done with running 7-0 silk from the medial to the lateral canthus. Interrupted 7-0 silk sutures are used laterally to the lateral canthal angle. Other fine skin or subcuticular sutures of mild chromic gut or nylon may be used as long as attention is given to accurate skin closure.

Postoperatively antibiotic ointment may be ap-

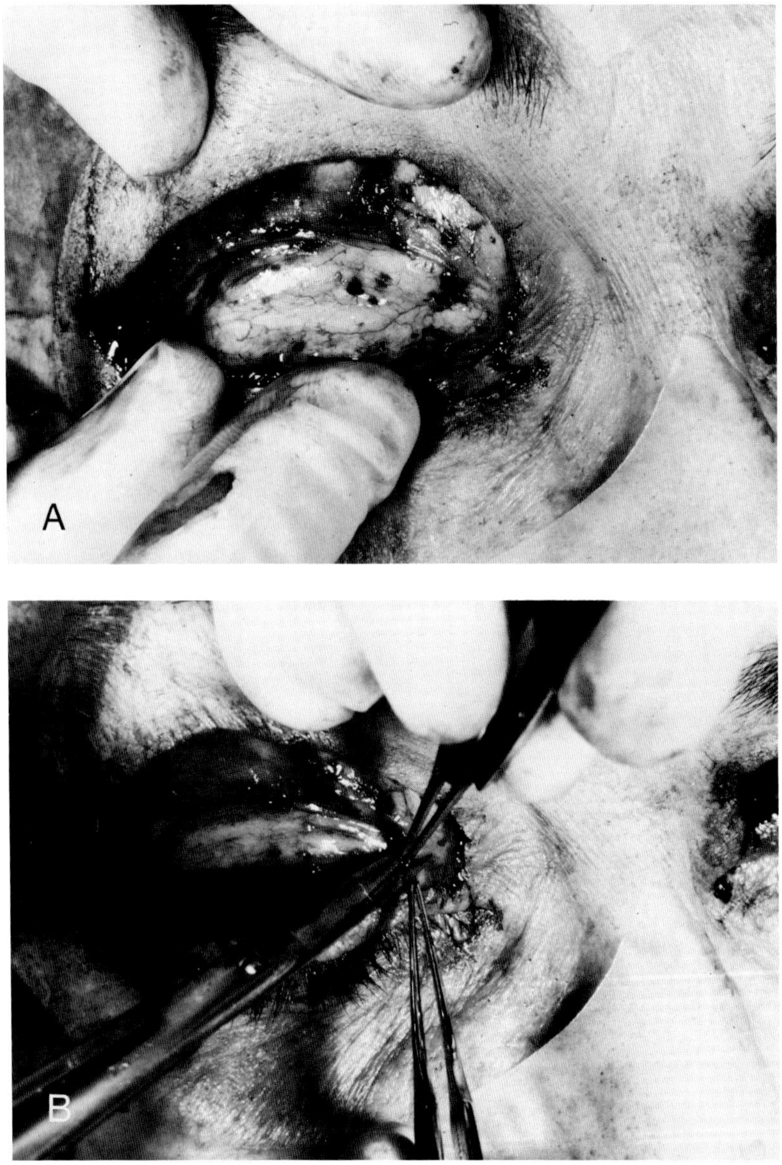

Fig. 38-14. **(A)** Pressure is applied to the closed lids enhancing fat pads. **(B)** The orbital septum is tented with forceps and incised with scissors. *(Figure continued.)*

plied. No dressing is necessary, although I prefer to use half-patch dressings over the incision line to collect the small amount of ooze that results. In no event should a pressure dressing or a full eyepad be used, as both obscure evaluation of bleeding and vision. The patient should be instructed to check for visual changes as well as for excessive bleeding and to call immediately if either occurs. The patient is instructed to apply ice packs as much as tolerated, to remain in a position so that the head is above the heart, and not to use aspirin or aspirin-containing compounds. I provide each patient with acetaminophen or acetaminophen with 30 mg codeine to use for discomfort. The patient is personally examined the next day. The sutures are removed 5 to 7 days later. Massage of lateral scars is started 2 weeks postoperatively if thickening occurs. The skin excised is retained in saline gauze in the refrigerator if there is any question as to the adequacy of lid closure. This may be used up to 3 weeks postoperatively to correct excessive skin removal.

Fig. 38-14 *(Continued)*. **(C)** Pressure is applied to the closed lids, causing fat herniation. **(D)** After the herniated fat is clamped, it is excised, leaving a small amount of fat **(E),** which is directly cauterized.

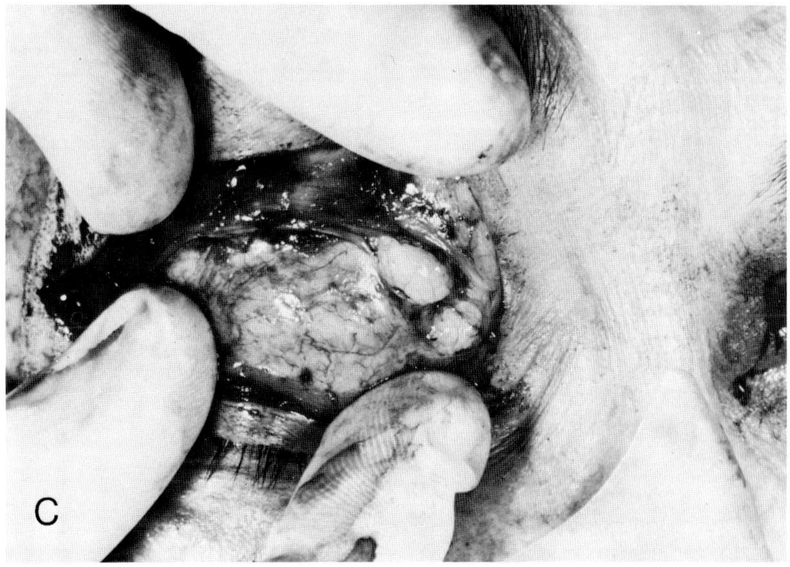

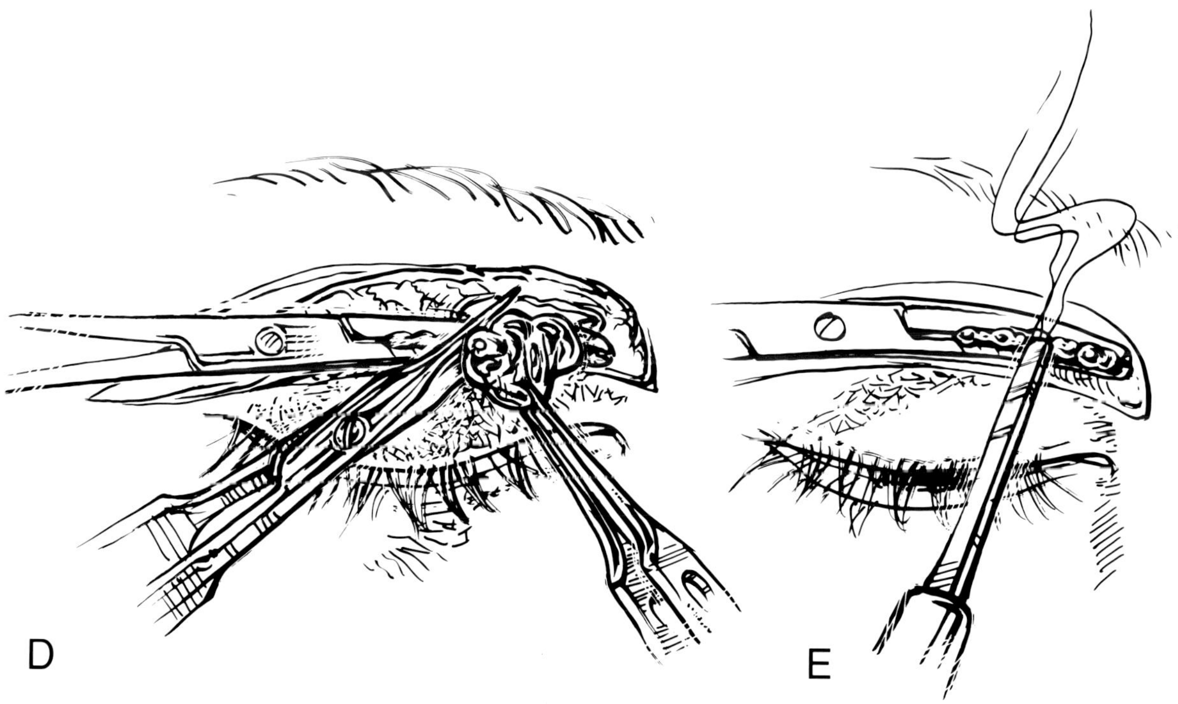

Variations in Upper Blepharoplasty Technique

The most important prerequisite for successful blepharoplasty is to individualize the procedure to the patient. The surgeon contemplating a blepharoplasty procedure should be familiar with variations of the technique. Excess medial eyelid skin superior to the incision may require specific attention to prevent bunching with closure. In the W-plasty technique, the upper and lower skin incisions are designed to end at separate points rather than at a single point. A triangular segment of skin is left to protrude laterally between the two points,

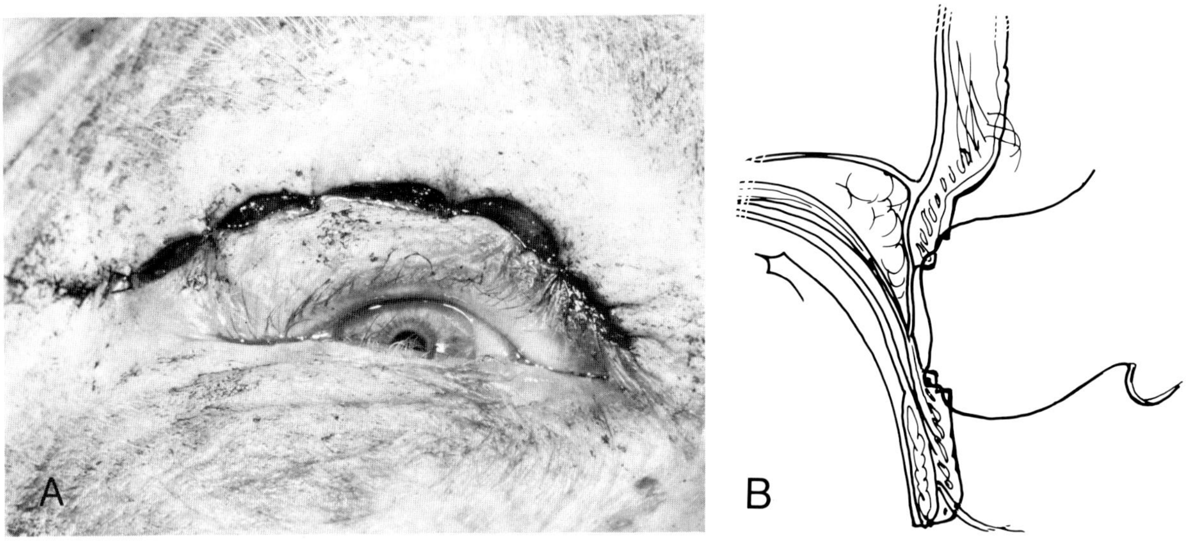

Fig. 38-15. (A) Lid crease sutures in place. **(B)** Cross section of lid crease suture placement.

giving the configuration of a horizontal W, with its base directed medially (Fig. 38-16). Thus the medial skin excess is shortened vertically.

Another technique is to shorten the skin horizontally by excision of a superomedially directed triangle with the base on the superior incision line. The initial skin incision is made approximately 1 cm lateral to the medial point of joining of the superior and inferior skin incisions and is directed superomedially. The skin medial to this incision is undermined, overlapped to determine the amount of excess, and the excess excised in the form of a triangle. The resulting vertical defect is then closed horizontally with interrupted 7-0 silk sutures. A separate V–Y-plasty[5] or Z-plasty[4] of the medial canthal skin may be required to correct severe

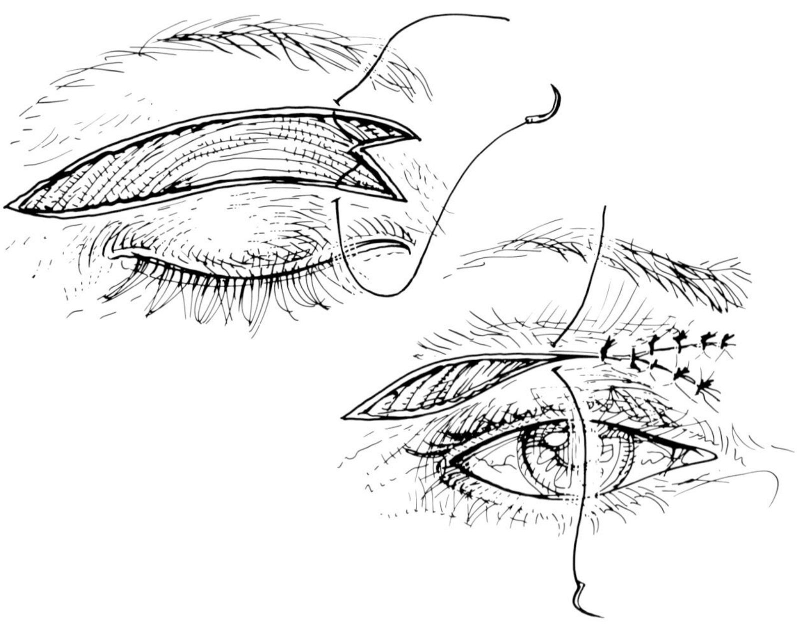

Fig. 38-16. The W-plasty incision for excess medial eyelid skin and its closure.

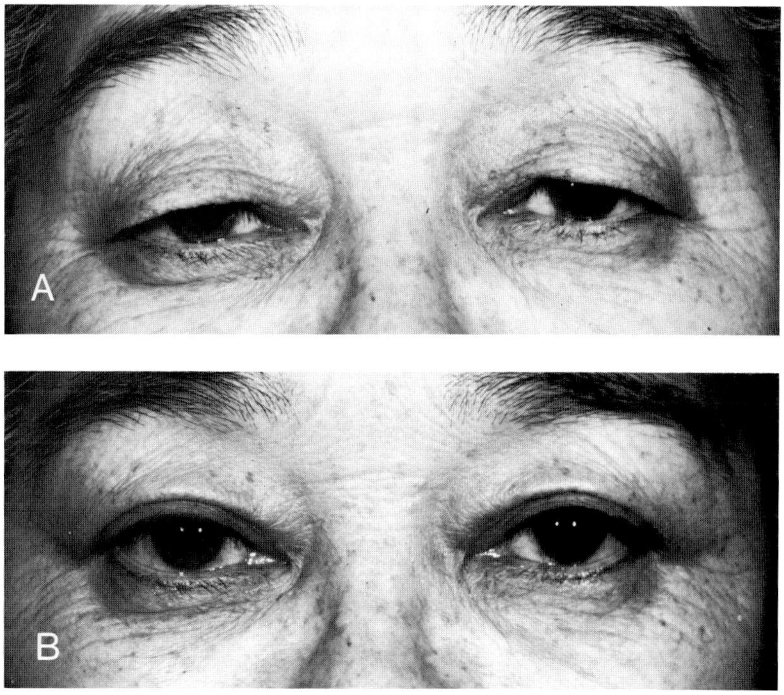

Fig. 38-17. (A) Preoperative upper eyelid blepharoplasty in an Oriental patient. **(B)** Postoperative upper eyelid blepharoplasty in an Oriental patient maintaining low eyelid crease.

webbing. In the Y–V plasty, an incision is made in the form of a horizontal Y, with the arms of the Y either in the web or parallel to the upper and lower lid margins and the tail of the Y directed medially. The incision is closed in the configuration of a V with the point of joining of the arms sutured to the base of the tail.

An alternative method is to use multiple Z-plasties with the incisions along the web line. The points are transposed and closed with 7-0 silk sutures. The eyelid crease can be augmented by supratarsal fixation using buried nonabsorbable sutures to fix orbicularis muscle to levator aponeurosis and/or to the superior tarsal border.[11,12] Full-thickness 5-0 chromic gut sutures can also be used to create a full-thickness scar, thereby augmenting the eyelid crease.[13] The plan to create a prominent upper eyelid crease should be discussed with the patient preoperatively, as some equate a high crease with an undesirable stare appearance.

The Oriental patient can either be given a high upper lid crease using one of the above techniques or be left with the normal low crease just above the lash line. The Oriental eyelid characteristic may be preserved by making a low skin excision in the previous crease and leaving a small excess of skin to provide a fold (Fig. 38-17A,B). The full appearance of the lid is thus preserved. No fixation to the tarsus or to the levator aponeurosis should be done. If acquired blepharoptosis is present, a levator disinsertion or dehisence may be identified and repaired with attachment to the superior tarsal border at the time of blepharoplasty.[14]

LOWER EYELID BLEPHAROPLASTY

As with upper eyelid blepharoplasty, the lower eyelid blepharoplasty patient should be reexamined in the sitting position immediately prior to surgery, noting the lower eyelid position, lid tone, amount of excess skin, asymmetry, and the degree of protruding fat pads. In patients with good lid tone, minimal skin excess, and prominent fat pads, usually falling into the younger age group, I prefer the skin–muscle flap technique, while in patients with skin excess, with relatively decreased lid tone, and with or without protruding fat, I prefer a skin flap with excision of a strip of preseptal orbicularis muscle, if necessary. Thus, the pretarsal orbicularis muscle is left to aid in lid tone.

Skin – Muscle Flap Technique

After skin preparation and subcutaneous injection with 1 percent lidocaine with epinephrine, an incision is made just inferior to the lash line from inferior to the punctum to inferior to the lateral canthal angle[15] (Fig. 38-18A,B). The incision is extended laterally beyond the lateral canthus, being curved slightly inferiorly in a laugh line, the distance increasing with the amount of skin to be excised. A traction suture of 4-0 silk is placed in the central lid and the lid pulled superiorly. The incision is carried through the orbicularis muscle to the anterior surface of the tarsus, where it is directed inferiorly along the anterior surface of the orbital septum to the inferior orbital rim. The areas of prominence of orbital fat protrusion are then determined by pressure on the closed eyelids. Two or three incisions are made in the orbital septum with scissors and the fat allowed to herniate without reaching into the orbit. The fat is then clamped, excised, and cauterized as described for the upper eyelids. It must be remembered that the inferior oblique tendon divides the larger temporal fat pad, and care should be taken to avoid it. Fat excision is repeated until the desired result is obtained. The skin – orbicularis muscle flap is then drawn superiorly and laterally and the excess tissue of the flap determined with the patient looking superiorly (Fig. 38-19A – C). One must remember that the flap that bulged forward preoperatively may need to conform to the resulting concave configuration of the lid postoperatively. Thus the flap should be allowed to conform to the concave contour rather than bridge over in a taut fashion when determining the amount of excess so as to avoid excessive tissue excision. After the excess skin – muscle flap is excised, the incision is closed with a running 7-0 silk or other fine suture from the medial lid to the lateral canthal angle (Fig. 38-19D). Interrupted sutures are used on the thicker lateral skin.

Cautery can be used on the orbital septum either in place of fat excision or in conjunction with fat removal (Fig. 38-13). Logically, it seems that thickening of the orbital septum with the fibrosis of

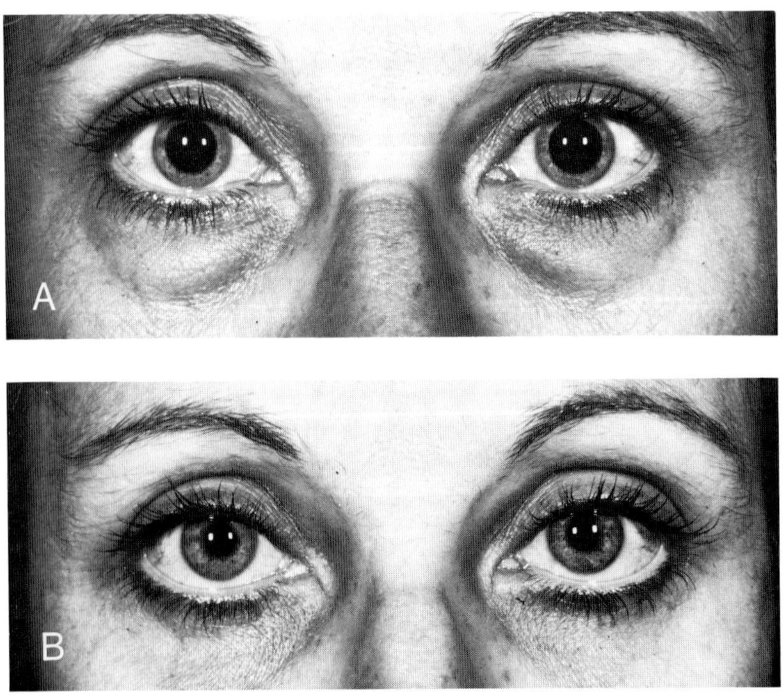

Fig. 38-18. (A) Preoperative lower eyelid blepharoplasty. **(B)** Postoperative lower eyelid blepharoplasty using skin – muscle flap technique.

cautery would reduce later stretching of the weak orbital septum. Cautery has not been used long enough, however, to draw a conclusion though the results to date indicate that cautery to the orbital septum is an excellent technique.

Skin-Flap Technique

In patients with considerable skin excess, I prefer the skin flap technique, thus avoiding the excision of a large amount of pretarsal and preseptal orbicularis muscle (Fig. 38-20). After skin preparation and draping, with care to leave the lower lid skin undistorted, a subcutaneous injection of local anesthetic is given. An incision through the skin is made just inferior to the lash line, starting medially inferior to the punctum and extending laterally to the lateral canthal angle. The incision is then extended laterally and curved slightly inferiorly in a natural crease line. The skin is dissected from the anterior surface of the orbicularis muscle down to the level of the inferior orbital rim.

If fat is to be excised, digital pressure on the closed eyelids will demonstrate the areas of prominence.[16] Using forceps to tent the tissue, a scissors incision is made through orbicularis muscle and orbital septum in two or three locations, depending on the configuration of the fat pads. The fat is allowed to prolapse with pressure on the closed lids. It is then clamped, excised, cauterized, and observed for bleeding as it retracts. After sufficient fat has been excised, the skin is drawn superiorly and laterally.

If there is redundant or hypertrophied orbicularis muscle, a strip of preseptal orbicularis is excised from medial to lateral and the resulting defect closed with several 6-0 plain gut sutures. The excess skin is then excised in two steps. The strip of excess skin over the lash line is excised first, and the lateral triangle from the lateral canthus outward is excised second.

In judging the amount of skin to excise, it is helpful to have the patient open the mouth to see whether there is downward pull on the lid margin and also to have the patient sit upright to observe the effects of gravity on the lax facial tissues. The skin is then closed with a running 7-0 silk or other fine suture medially to laterally, using interrupted sutures in the thicker skin lateral to the lateral canthus. Half-patch mild pressure dressings are used. Postoperative care is as with the upper eyelid blepharoplasty.

VARIATIONS IN LOWER EYELID BLEPHAROPLASTY

Frequently the older patient has considerable eyelid laxity due to elongation of the medial and lateral canthal tendons as well as the tarsus. If the lateral canthal tendon is lax, allowing the lateral canthal angle to migrate medially when the eyelid is pulled medially, fixation of the tendon by reattachment, imbricating, or shortening is necessary. If the lateral canthal tendon is firmly in place or if fixation does not completely correct the lid laxity, horizontal full-thickness shortening, as with ectropion repair, is necessary. If the lid laxity is primarily medial, a medial ectropion procedure or shortening of the medial canthal tendon should be done at the time of blepharoplasty. (See Chapter 36 for details of these procedures.)

Orbital fat may be removed using the conjunctival approach. This technique should be used only by those thoroughly familiar with the lower eyelid retractors and by those with sufficient surgical volume to master the technique.

COMPLICATIONS OF BROW ELEVATION AND BLEPHAROPLASTY

As with any surgical procedure, complications may occur during the operation, during the early postoperative period or the late postoperative period. A thorough preoperative evaluation, proper selection of procedure, meticulous surgical technique, and close postoperative observation will minimize the incidence and severity of complications.

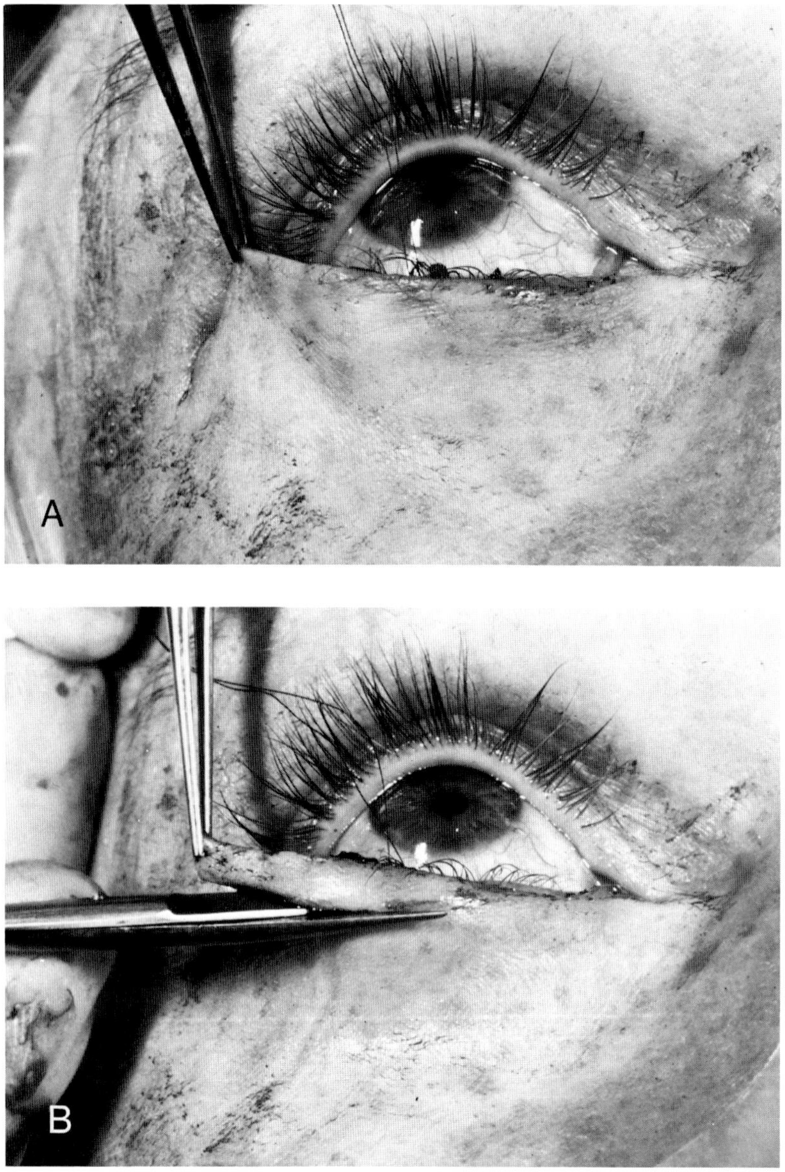

Fig. 38-19. (A) Skin–muscle flap is pulled superiorly and laterally. **(B)** Excess skin and muscle is excised with patient looking superiorly. *(Figure continued.)*

Operative Complications

Anesthetic complications can occur with local or general anesthetics. Problems with specific drug reactions, airway compromise, or cardiac arrhythmias should be anticipated and treated early and appropriately. Bleeding must be meticulously controlled so as to prevent hematomas or orbital hemorrhage. Surgical technique must be precise, avoiding damage to adjacent structures or the globe.

Early Postoperative Complications

The most serious complication of blepharoplasty is visual loss due to optic nerve compromise.[17] In almost all cases, this tragic event has occurred following lower eyelid fat excision with bleeding considered the etiologic factor. Prevention of bleeding by avoiding traction on the orbital fat, meticulous hemostasis, and avoidance of aspirin is imperative. All blepharoplasty patients should be instructed to assess vision during the early postoperative period

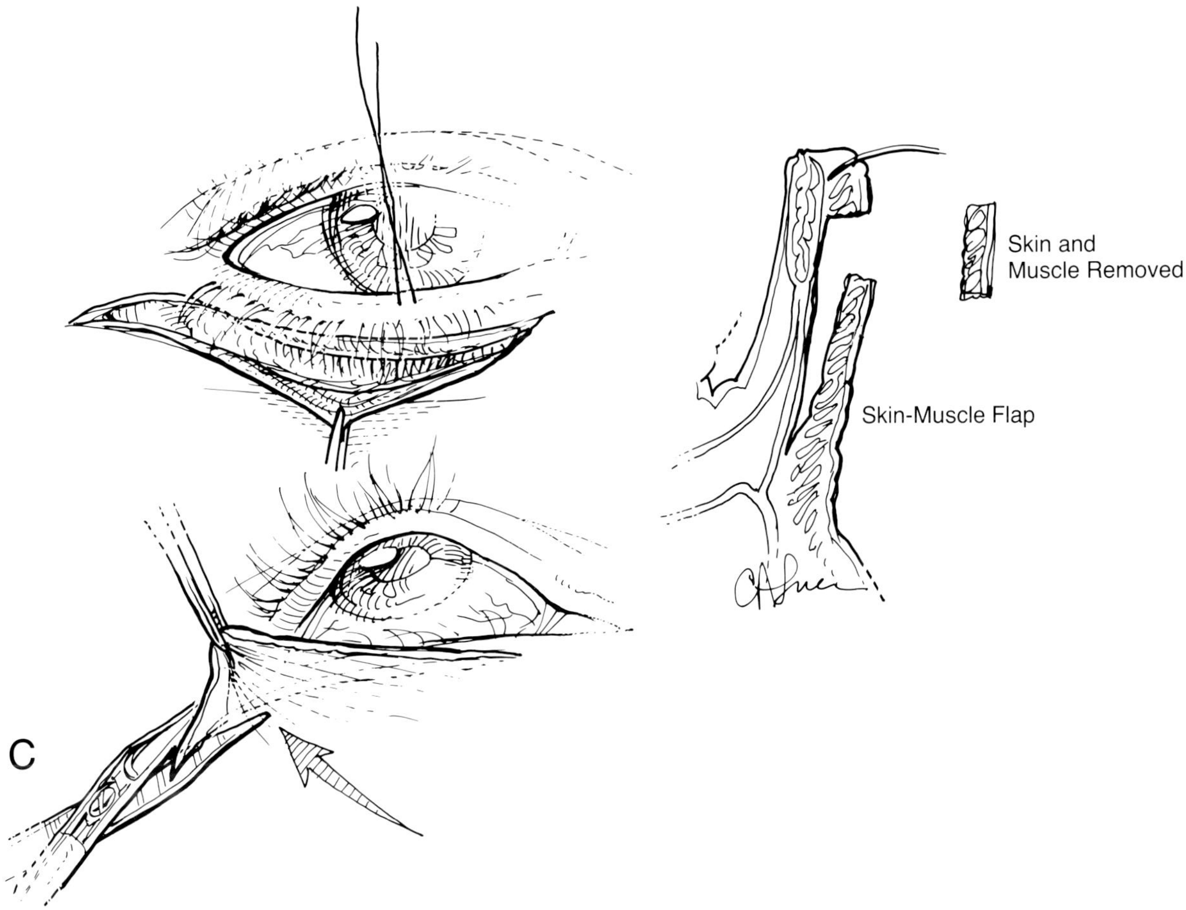

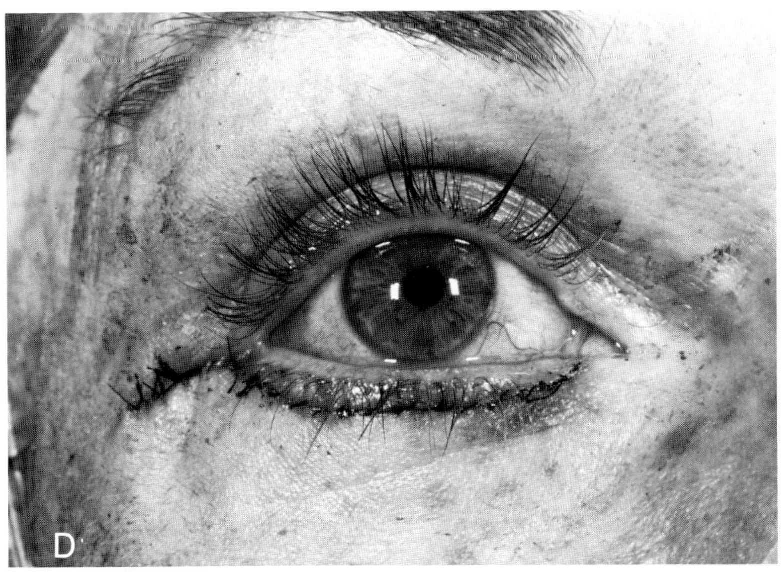

Fig. 38-19 *(Continued)*. **(C)** With patient looking superiorly, excess skin–muscle flap is excised. **(D)** Final closure.

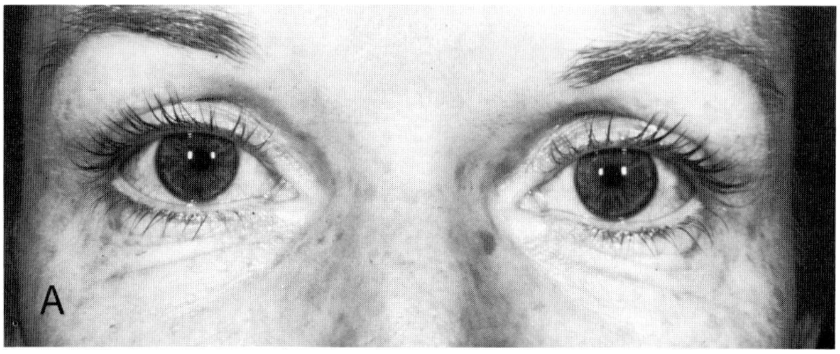

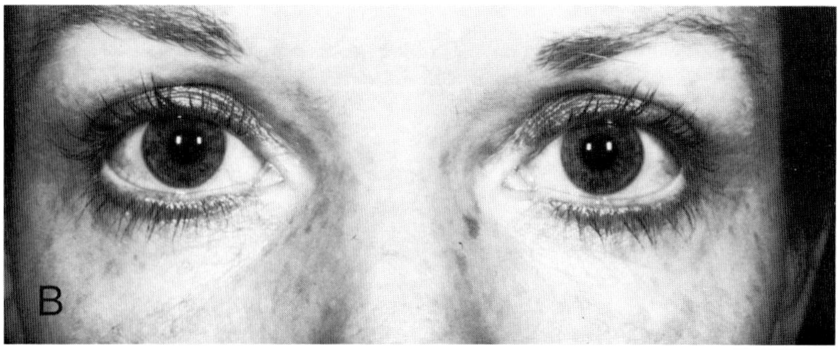

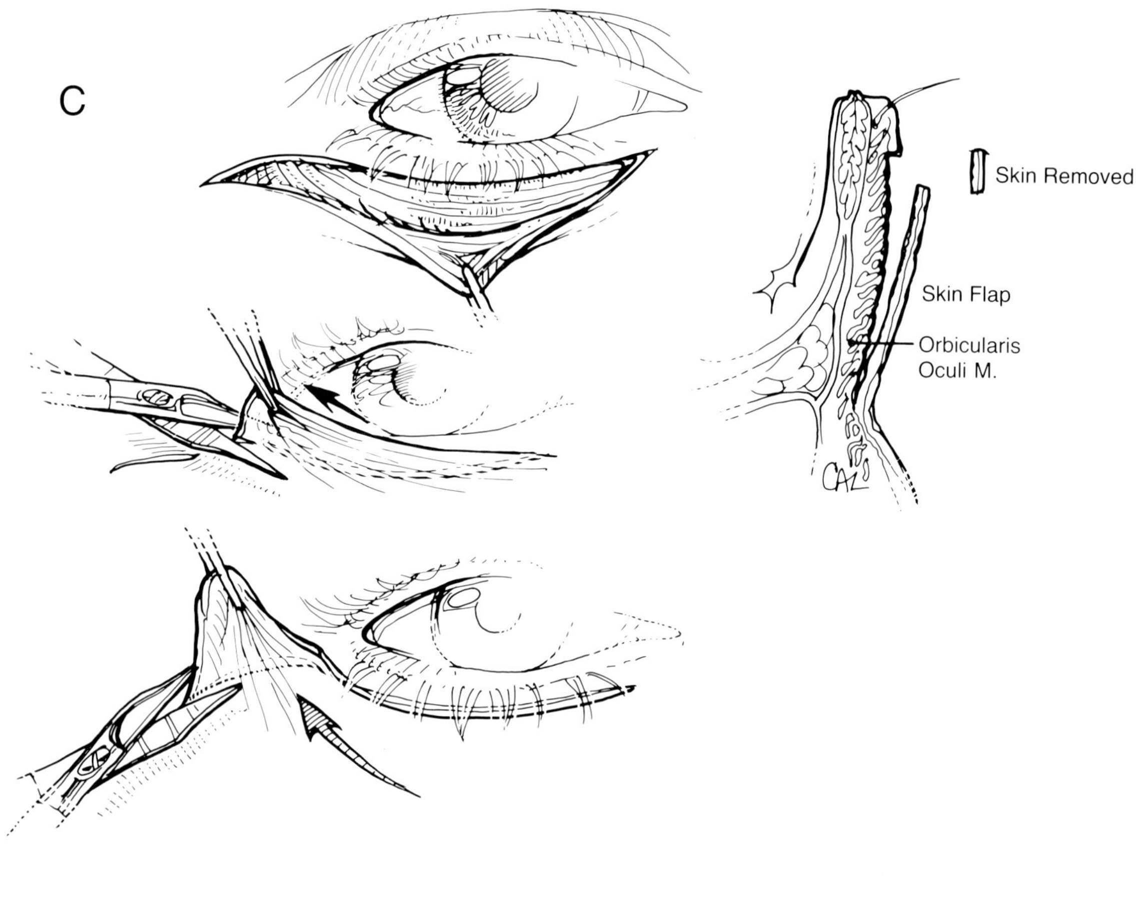

Fig. 38-20. (A) Preoperative lower lid blepharoplasty. **(B)** Postoperative lower lid blepharoplasty using skin-flap technique. **(C)** With patient looking superiorly, excess skin flap is excised.

and to call immediately if there is significant change. Early detection of visual loss with aggressive treatment has prevented permanent visual loss.[18] The treatment is prompt takedown of the wound and opening of the orbital septum incisions to permit drainage. Any site of bleeding should be treated and a drain placed. Indirect treatment such as lateral canthoplasty, anterior chamber decompression, and systemic medication to lower intraocular pressure is less effective and wastes valuable time.

Subcutaneous hematomas may occur and should be drained, if significant, to prevent fibrosis, tissue distortion, or skin-flap necrosis.

Late Postoperative Complications

Late complications are frequently related to the surgical technique and are best prevented by careful preoperative assessment and precise surgical technique. Excessive removal of eyelid skin may result in inadequate eyelid closure with corneal exposure, eyelid retraction, or lower eyelid ectropion. A less serious problem, but one that also makes a patient unhappy is insufficient removal of skin, leaving redundancy of tissue in either upper or lower eyelids. Crease asymmetry, wound breakdown, epicanthal folds or medial webbing, hypertrophic scars, suture cysts, residual fat pad protrusion, epiphora, blepharitis, and levator aponeurosis disinsertion are among the problems that may occur. Treatment of the particular patient is individualized for the nature and degree of the problem.

REFERENCES

1. Shulman BH: Psychiatric issues in cosmetic blepharoplasty. p. 46. In Putterman A (ed): Cosmetic Oculoplastic Surgery. Grune & Stratton, New York, 1982
2. Lubkin V: Psychological aspects of ophthalmic plastic surgery. p. 43. In Silver B (ed): Ophthalmic Plastic Surgery. 3rd Ed. American Academy of Ophthalmology and Otolaryngology, Rochester, MN, 1977
3. Jones LT, Wobig JL: Surgery of the Eyelids and Lacrimal System. Aesculapius, Birmingham, AL, 1976
4. Mustarde JC: The treatment of ptosis and epicanthal folds. Br J Plast Surg 12:252, 1959
5. Hughes WL: Surgical treatment of congenital palpebral phimosis: The Y–V operation. Arch Ophthalmol 54:586, 1955
6. Webster RC, Fanous N, Smith RC: Blepharoplasty: When to combine it with brow, temple, or coronal lift. J Otolaryngol 8:339, 1979
7. Castanares S: Forehead wrinkles, glabellar frown and ptosis of the eyebrows. Plast Reconstr Surg 34:406, 1964
8. Rafaty FM: Elimination of glabellar frown lines. Arch Otolaryngol 107:428, 1981
9. Kaye BL: The forehead lift. Plast Reconstr Surg 60:161, 1977
10. Pitanguy I: Indications for and treatment of frontal and glabellar wrinkles in an analysis of 3404 consecutive cases of rhytidectomy. Plast Reconstr Surg 67:157, 1981
11. Sheen JH: Supratarsal fixation in blepharoplasty. Plast Reconstr Surg 54:424, 1974
12. Sheen JH: A change in the technique of supratarsal fixation in upper blepharoplasty. Plast Reconstr Surg 59:831, 1977
13. Pang HG: Surgical formation of the upper lid fold. Arch Ophthalmol 65:783, 1961
14. Dryden RM, Leibsohn J: The levator aponeurosis in blepharoplasty. Trans Am Acad Ophthalmol Otolaryngol 85:718, 1978
15. Beare R: Surgical treatment of senile changes in the eyelid: The McIndoe-Beare technique. p. 362. In Smith B, Converse JM (eds): Proceedings of the Second International Symposium on Plastic and Reconstructive Surgery of the Eye and Adnexa. CV Mosby, St. Louis, 1967
16. Castanares S: Blepharoplasty for herniated intraorbital fat; anatomical basis for a new approach. Plast Reconstr Surg 8:46, 1951
17. Waller RR: Is blindness a realistic complication of blepharoplasty procedures? Trans Am Acad Ophthalmol Otolaryngol 85:730, 1978
18. Putterman AM: Temporary blindness after cosmetic blepharoplasty. Am J Ophthalmol 80:1081, 1975

Eyelid Margin Reconstruction

39

George F. Buerger, Jr.

CLINICAL CONSIDERATIONS

When a patient presents with a lesion involving the eyelid margin, the lesion must be diagnosed and characterized in terms of the degree of apparent involvement and a determination made as to whether the lesion borders are well defined or indeterminate. In planning excision, consideration should be given to repairing the defect.

The most frequently occurring malignant skin lesion is a basal cell carcinoma. This lesion may be sharply demarcated, or its borders may be indistinct. It may appear as a classic basal cell, or it may make one think of basal cell. The only way to know for sure what the lesion is is to perform a biopsy. A simple shave biopsy of a lesion involving the lid margin should furnish the pathologist with sufficient tissue for adequate study.[1] If the lesion is benign, the biopsy itself may be adequate treatment. The shave biopsy is truly an incisional biopsy (as compared with an excisional biopsy); therefore, if the lesion is found to be malignant, further surgery is necessary. It must be stressed that whereas the clinical basal cell lesion may seem unmistakable, even the most experienced surgeon may be fooled, so a biopsy is essential before proceeding to radical excision.

Recurrent chalazia may not necessarily be chalazia. The lesion may represent a sebaceous carcinoma; sometimes the only way to make the diagnosis is with a full-thickness biopsy of the lid/margin. If the lesion is small, a transmarginal wedge resection will serve as a full-thickness biopsy as well as the definitive mode of treatment. In addition to a shave or slice biopsy, a biopsy may also be performed with a needle-punch technique. The simple shave technique, however, is simple to perform, requires no specialized equipment, and is easily adapted to lesions in all locations. Biopsy of a suspected basal cell carcinoma should be from the heaped-up border, rather than from the central crater.

Once the lesion is definitively excised, one should insist on frozen-section examination of the borders of the lesion. This will give the best assurance that the lesion has been totally excised.[2] A morpheaform basal cell carcinoma, most commonly seen in the medial canthal area, is the most likely to recur because of small fingers of tumor that can be missed if the complete margin is not checked. When this diagnosis is suspected or biopsy-proven, I prefer to perform the excision via the Mohs fresh tissue technique, followed by appropriate reconstruction.[3]

Other types of therapy, in addition to surgery, must be mentioned. Radiation therapy can be undertaken, with the dosage and treatment regimen determined by an experienced radiotherapist. Arguments invariably arise between the ophthalmic surgeon and the radiotherapist as to which offers the better chance of eradication. Dr. Arthur Goldstein, of the Manhattan Eye, Ear, and Throat Hospital, reports excellent results that are frequently disputed by the ophthalmic surgeon, (Goldstein A: Lid Lesion Course, Manhattan EET Hospital, February 1984). He points out, however, that he is very selective in choosing those cases he will treat: only the smallest, most superficial lesion, known by his experience to respond very favorably.

Cryotherapy has been advocated by Fraunfelder and associates,[4–6] who believe this modality offers less morbidity to the patient while giving excellent results. When using cryotherapy, a thermocouple is an absolute must in order to be sure that the tissue temperature has reached $-35°C$. If the temperature is not monitored, the probability of recurrence is significant.

Statistics from the best published results for radiation therapy, cryosurgery, and Mohs surgery illustrate that the latter is better for both basal cell and squamous cell carcinoma of the eyelid.[6–8] However, when the margin of excision is not controlled to ensure absence of tumor in the margin, surgical excision loses its advantage over radiation and cryosurgery.[9] Recurrent lesions and morpheaform basal cell carcinoma should be treated surgically, preferably with Mohs surgery or a variant because of their predilection to recur when not completely treated.[10]

This chapter discusses the surgical management of lid malignancies. There are several schools of thought regarding reconstruction of the defects created, that is, the Hughes tarsoconjunctival techniques and modifications versus the Mustarde rotation-type flaps. I am of the Hughes school, but I do perform other techniques too.

The preoperative evaluation of the lid on which a lesion is located should include assessment of the degree of lid laxity present. In general, the older the patient, the more laxity present in the lid. The laxity is considered when formulating reconstruction alternatives. However, one must be prepared to perform a variety of procedures, based on the defect created in the process of eradicating the cancer.

ANESTHESIA FOR EYELID SURGERY

After the appropriate procedure is decided on, the type of anesthesia necessary to carry out the planned surgery is considered. A general anesthetic may be the anesthesia of choice, depending on the anxiety level of the patient and the needs and requirements of the surgeon or the procedure.

Local infiltration of the anesthetic agent of choice into the involved tissues is assumed to be known by all readers of this text. If one uses 1 : 100,000 or 1 : 200,000 epinephrine in the anesthetic agent, it should be given adequate time to work (usually about 10 to 12 minutes). If the cut is made immediately after the injection, the advantage of the epinephrine is negated. The main problem with local infiltration anesthesia is the distortion of normal anatomy from the induced tissue edema. For this reason, I employ regional block anesthesia whenever possible.

The most commonly used local anesthetic agents are lidocaine (Xylocaine) and mepivocaine (Carbocaine). They are comparable in potency and are used as 1 or 2 percent solutions. Their action is prolonged with the addition of 1 : 200,000 dilution of epinephrine. The maximum amount of drug used should be 500 mg (50 ml of a 1 percent solution or 25 ml of a 2 percent solution); otherwise, the patient may develop signs of overdosage (hypotension or convulsions).[11]

Bupivacaine (Marcaine) is a homologue of mepivacaine and is chemically related to lidocaine. When used for retrobulbar block, a 0.75 percent solution is used. For nerve block, either 0.25 percent or 0.50 percent is used, while only 0.25 percent is recommended for local infiltration. It is used alone or with epinephrine in the ratio of 1 : 200,000. The main advantage of bupivacaine is its longer duration of action, often up to 7 hours, and occasionally longer, often diminishing postoperative requirements for analgesic drugs. However, the onset of action is slower than when lidocaine or mepivacaine is used.

The single dose should not exceed 225 mg with epinephrine 1 : 200,000 and 175 mg without epinephrine. Total daily doses should not exceed 400 mg. Although some workers mix bupivacaine and lidocaine 1 : 1, Breon Laboratories, Inc., recommends against the prior or intercurrent use of any other local anesthetic with bupivacaine.[12]

Knowledge of the anatomic distribution of the sensory nerves supplying the lids and adnexa is essential before attempting regional block anesthesia.[11]

Frontal Nerve Block

The frontal nerve divides into the supraorbital and supratrochlear branches along the orbital roof posterior to the superior orbital rim. Posteriorly, the frontal nerve lies in close proximity to the lacrimal nerve. An injection of the anesthetic agent into this area, about 4 cm behind the superior orbital rim, will give a sensory block to the upper lid and forehead area except for the most nasal portion of the lid. A 23-gauge 4-cm needle is passed through the skin just below the superior orbital rim, at or just lateral to the center of the orbital rim. The needle is walked along the roof in stepwise fashion until the desired position along the roof on the orbital side of the periosteum is reached. The volume of anesthetic solution injected should not exceed 0.5 ml. The properly placed injection will be effective within several minutes.

Infratrochlear Nerve Block

To block the most nasal portion of the upper lid, as well as the lacrimal sac and roof of the nose, the infratrochlear nerve block is used. It is blocked by an injection of 0.5 ml anesthetic about 1 cm from the rim along the medial orbital wall, just below the trochlea. If the needle goes deeper than 1 cm, it may penetrate the anterior ethmoidal artery, causing significant hemorrhage in the retrobulbar space and necessitate cancellation of the surgery.

Infraorbital Nerve Block

The infraorbital nerve supplies conjunctiva and skin of the lower lid, except for the most medial and lateral portions. The nerve emerges on the face through the infraorbital foramen, located about 1 cm lateral to the nasal ala on a line dropped from the supraorbital notch, although there is some anatomic variability. The needle is directed into or at the foramen, angling the needle upward. Although difficulty may be encountered in locating the foramen, infiltration of the general area is usually adequate to block the emerging nerve.

Lacrimal and Zygomaticofacial Nerve Block

The most lateral portion of the lower lid can be blocked with a pure lacrimal nerve block. An injection is made about 1 cm deep to the lateral orbital rim, just above the lateral canthal tendon. The zygomaticofacial nerve block gives a larger area of sensory loss in the lateral canthal area but the nerve's foramen is often difficult to locate. However, infiltration along the zygoma about 1 cm below the inferior angle of the orbit is often sufficient to give adequate sensory loss.

While a properly placed regional nerve block should give adequate sensory loss, local subcutaneous infiltration can be used when necessary to supplement the regional block. Except for the frontal nerve, there will be blood vessels in the immediate area of the nerves. Therefore, aspiration is necessary prior to injecting the anesthetic agent.

SURGICAL TECHNIQUE

Transmarginal Wedge Resection

The transmarginal wedge resection[13–15] can be performed on either the upper or the lower lid (Fig. 39-1). A marking pencil is used to indicate the borders of the proposed resection. If the lesion is a basal cell carcinoma, I leave about 2 mm on each side of the lesion borders. When the Mohs technique is used, a smaller free zone is left. A vertical mark, perpendicular to the lid margin, is made on each side of the lesion from the lid margin to the

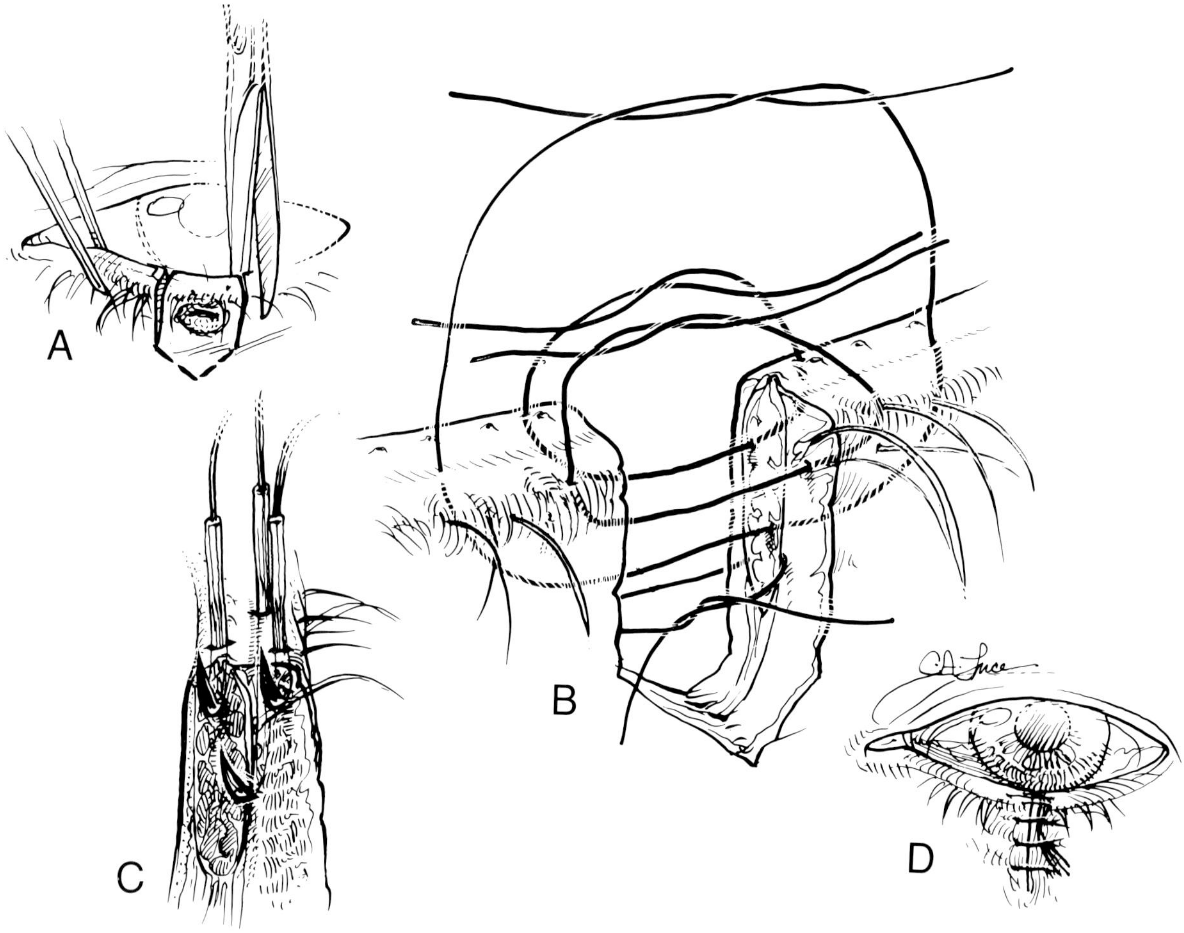

Fig. 39-1. Transmarginal wedge resection with primary closure. (**A**) Full-thickness pentagonal excision of lid is performed with scissors. (**B**) Three-suture closure of lid margin using 6-0 silk in lash line, gray line, and posterior margin. Tarsus edges are closed with a 6-0 polyglycolic acid suture. (**C**) Cross-section of lid showing the three marginal sutures. (**D**) Appearance with sutures tied.

tarsal border. Here the two lines are brought together to form the pentagonal or house-shaped resection. One can use either a sharp blade or heavy scissors to make the cuts through the full thickness of the lids. I prefer heavy scissors.

While some advocate corn-crib-shaped or angulated vertical lines, I feel very strongly that this is not only unnecessary but inadvisable. The tarsus is a firm tissue. When two straight edges, perpendicular to the lid margin, are brought together, no lid notch will be created. Angulating these lines should only increase the chances of a notch or hump.

Care must be taken that each vertical cut goes through the entire vertical height of the tarsus, before angling toward the other. Light cautery can be used to stop any bleeding.

A transmarginal wedge resection with primary closure can be used to remove at least one fourth of a lid margin, regardless of the patient's age. The greater the lid laxity, which usually increases with patient age, the wider the resection that can be performed and still closed primarily. The ability to close a resected area is determined after the lesion has been excised. Sufficient tissue must be excised to permit adequate removal of the lesion, without stopping prematurely to facilitate closure. One should excise first, then determine the type of closure, yet have alternative game plans in mind at the start of the procedure.

The closure of the wedge resection is carried out via a two-layer closure: conjunctiva–tarsus and skin–muscle. Traditionally, three sutures are placed on the lid margin. The gray-line suture is placed about 3 to 3.5 mm from the cut edge and is angled backward slightly so as to include some tarsus in this bite. The anterior lid margin–lash line suture is placed about 2 mm from the cut edge, as is the posterior margin suture. These two sutures will ensure excellent margin alignment. While some surgeons have a distinct preference for one or the other, I have no personal preference as to which suture is placed first. A 6-0 black silk suture is used for the margin closure; these sutures are left in place for 10 to 14 days, the longer period for the older patient or a tight lid. The gray-line and posterior margin sutures ends are held forward by the knot of the lash-line suture.

The tarsus and its tightly adherent conjunctiva are closed as one layer. Either 5-0 or 6-0 polyglycolic acid sutures are used. One can remain entirely within the tarsus, not exiting on the conjunctival surface; for a more solid bite of tissue, or surgery by a less experienced surgeon, one can go through tarsus and conjunctiva on each side of the excised area. Such a suture exiting through the conjunctival surface does not usually cause any significant symptoms if the knot is buried. Symptoms are more likely with upper lid reconstructions but are still infrequent. Perfectly placed tarsal and marginal sutures ensure a perfect lid margin.

If there is a slight excess of tension in the lid, a deep orbicularis muscle suture of 6-0 polyglycolic acid can be used to relieve it. The routine use of this suture is unnecessary. The skin and superficial orbicularis are closed with any of several interrupted sutures: 6-0 silk, 6-0 prolene or Surgilene, Surgilon, or the new Ethicon 1916G 6-0 mild gut suture. If nonabsorbable sutures are used, they are removed between the fourth and sixth postoperative days. I use an antibiotic ointment on the wound area twice a day for 1 week, then once a day for another 4 to 7 days. An antibiotic drop is used three or four times a day until the margin sutures are removed.

Transmarginal Wedge Resection with Cantholysis

After the lesion has been excised with a transmarginal wedge resection, if the two edges of the resection margin lack approximation by less than 5 mm, a lateral canthotomy with lysis of the inferior branch of the lateral canthal tendon[13–15] is needed (Fig. 39-2). This procedure is occasionally performed during cataract surgery if the lids are tight.

A horizontal cut is made directly through the lateral canthal angle for a distance of 5 to 7 mm. With medial traction on the lateral portion of the lid, the tight lateral canthal tendon is palpable. Adjacent conjunctiva and skin are cut from the inferior branch of the lateral canthal tendon. A vertical cut through the tendon allows the lateral lid segment to move medially to close the wound. No sutures in the lateral canthus may be necessary when the skin incision is short. If the skin incision is more than 7 mm, an absorbable 6-0 or 7-0 suture may be used to close the cut edges of the skin. Cantholysis will permit 5 to 6 mm of medial advancement of the lateral lid segment.

Transmarginal Wedge Resection with Lateral Cantholysis and Tenzel Semicircular or Minirotation Flap

When more than 5 to 6 mm remains to be closed with the margin on tension following a wedge resection, as when about one third or more of the lid margin has been excised, lateral cantholysis is insufficient. Tenzel[16] designed a minirotation semicircular or advancement flap that arches upward, starting immediately at the lateral canthal angle, which is excellent for repairing up to 60 percent loss of lid length (Fig. 39-3). If one were to place the upper half of a quarter at the lateral canthal angle, this would give the direction and size of the intended flap. Decision to use a lateral flap must be made prior to making a lateral canthotomy, because the lateral skin incision is different than with a simple cantholysis.

The semicircular incision is made through skin and orbicularis and undermined adequately. The inferior branch of the lateral canthal tendon is lo-

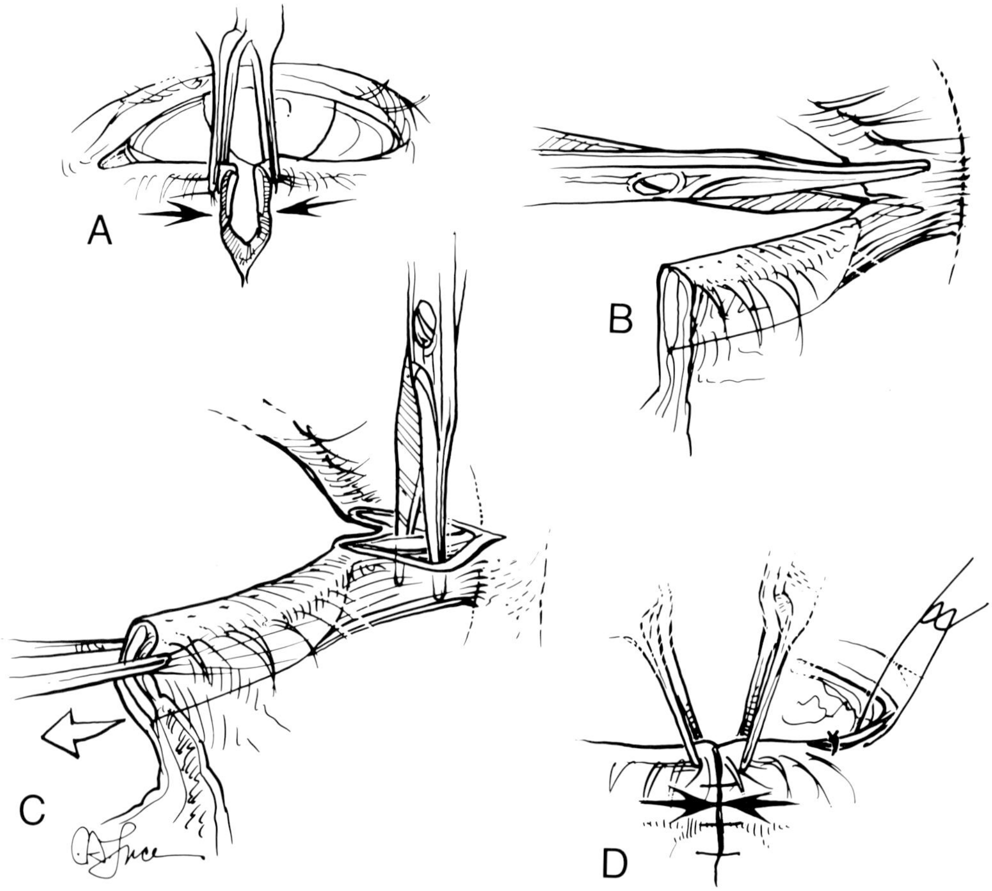

Fig. 39-2. Transmarginal wedge resection with lateral cantholysis. (**A**) Inability to close the wedge resection primarily. (**B**) Horizontal incision of skin and conjunctiva at lateral canthal angle. (**C**) Vertical incision of the inferior branch of the lateral canthal tendon. (**D**) Closure of the wedge resection area is performed as described in Figure 39-1. Conjunctiva is sutured to skin near the lateral canthus with several interrupted 7-0 polyglycolic acid sutures.

calized and cut, permitting medial movement of the flap and lateral lid segment. If additional medial movement of the lid is required to close the lid defect, more undermining can be done, even to the point of cutting some of the lateral attachment of the orbital septum from the lateral aspect of the inferior orbital rim. Hemostasis is secured with cautery.

Closure of the wedge resection is performed immediately lateral to the old lateral canthal angle with fine absorbable sutures (7-0 or 8-0 polyglycolic acid), taking small bites of each. I frequently remove these sutures after several weeks, but they can be allowed to absorb. Using a 4-0 Dexon suture with a small half-curve (P-1) needle, several deep bites of orbicularis are taken and sutured to the periosteum just lateral to where the new lateral canthal angle will be formed. This prevents lateral sagging of this flap. The skin is closed with the preferred skin closure material.

I frequently put in an intermarginal suture of 5-0 or 6-0 prolene or Surgilene, going in and out of the gray line of each lid, including the reconstructed margin area if necessary. The suture is tied to approximate the lids, producing a suture tarsorrhaphy. This relieves downward traction. I remove the tarsorraphy suture by the sixth postoperative day.

The postoperative care routine I use consists of

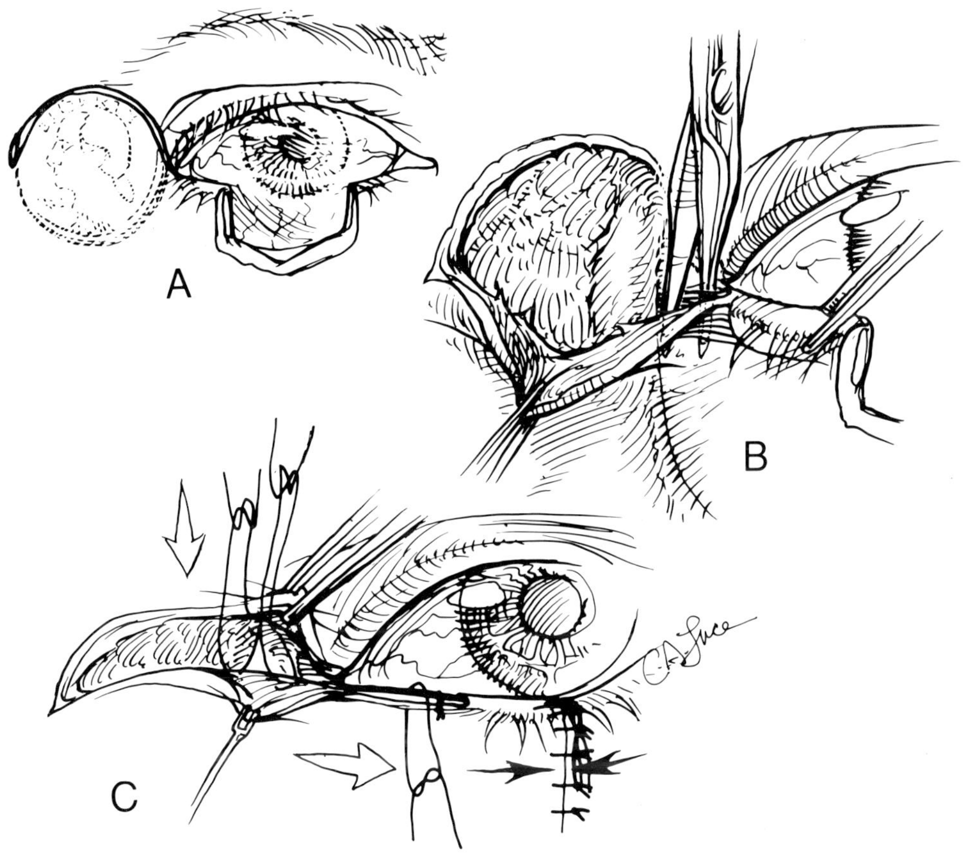

Fig. 39-3. Transmarginal wedge resection with lateral cantholysis and semi-circular rotation flap of Tenzel. (**A**) Visualize a quarter sitting at the lateral canthus; outline the upper half of the coin for the proposed skin and subcutaneous incision. (**B**) The inferior branch of the lateral canthal tendon is cut and the skin, subcutaneous tissue and orbicularis muscle are undermined. (**C**) Closure of the wedge resection area is performed as described in Fig. 39-1. Skin may be closed to available conjunctiva using 7-0 polyglycolic acid suture. At the lateral orbital rim area, deep bites of orbicularis oculi muscle are sutured to periosteum with 4-0 polyglycolic acid suture. Additional bites of subcutaneous tissue are closed with interrupted 6-0 polyglycolic acid suture. Skin is closed with either interrupted or continuous sutures.

instilling an antibiotic ointment on the globe and lid area and applying a patch over the lid with a sterile Telfa pad and eye pad with mild pressure. This is removed the following morning, and the lid is cleaned with moistened cotton balls. Ointment is applied sparingly to the incision area twice a day, and antibiotic drops are used four times a day. This daily regimen is continued by the patient until seen in the office on the sixth postoperative day, when the nonabsorbable skin sutures are removed. An alternative to the use of topical antibiotics is to put an occlusive plastic film such as Nu Skin over the skin sutures. The 6-0 silk lid margin sutures are removed between days 10 and 14, depending on the patient's age and the appearance of the wound.

The main advantage of the Tenzel semicircular flap for resections of up to 60 percent of the lid margin is that it is a one-stage repair. This is a particularly important consideration if the involved lid is over the patient's only seeing eye. Also, the cosmetic result is usually quite good. This technique avoids the use of a skin graft.

Full-Thickness Composite Graft

Another reconstruction technique that can be used when one fourth to one half the lid margin has been resected from either the upper or lower lid is a full-thickness composite graft taken from the contralateral lid, that is, upper lid for upper lid, lower lid for lower lid.[1] The graft is one fourth or less of the donor lid, so the donor site is closed as described for the wedge resection. The composite graft is closed on each side in a similar fashion. Some surgeons excise the skin and orbicularis muscle from the donor graft, then slide adjacent skin and orbicularis onto the graft to bring in a better blood supply to it. While this maneuver is theoretically beneficial, I do not find it a necessary or practical maneuver. The patient should be advised that the graft may not retain its lashes.

A composite graft shrinks slightly during its healing phase. To compensate, the graft should be offset about 0.5 mm into the palpebral fissure from the adjacent lid margin. This will help prevent a dip in the lid margin at the graft. This procedure has the advantage that it can be performed in a patient with only one seeing eye as a one-stage surgical procedure. The postoperative care is essentially the same as already discussed, with *gentle* the byword.

The preceding methods for transmarginal wedge resection followed by lateral cantholysis or a Tenzel semicircular flap are suitable for either the upper or lower lids. I will now discuss various repairs that are applicable to only lower lids and others applicable to only upper lids.

LOWER LID RECONSTRUCTION TECHNIQUES

Hughes Tarsoconjunctival Flap Technique

A useful technique when the excision removes more than 60 percent of the lid margin, or as an alternative to the Tenzel semicircular flap, is the time-honored two-stage Hughes repair.[13,17] With this technique, a tarsoconjunctival flap from the upper lid forms the posterior lamella of the resected area of the lower lid (Fig. 39-4). The anterior lamella is either a full-thickness skin graft or advancement skin flap.

To determine the width necessary for the tarsoconjunctival flap, each resected edge is grasped with forceps or a skin hook and pulled toward the other. The residual defect is the necessary flap width. The reconstructed lid must be sufficiently tight against the globe; if laxity remains, the reconstructed lid will develop ectropion. Now is the time to prevent this problem. At least one fourth of the lid margin length can be lost and need not be replaced. After the flap width is determined, the upper lid is everted and stabilized. I use a shortened Erhardt clamp; the shortened clamp facilitates eversion of the lid. If the full tarsal height of the lower lid has been excised, about 4 to 5 mm of tarsus must be brought into the lower lid. If some tarsus remains in the lower lid, the amount brought down is correspondingly reduced. Assuming the upper tarsus to be about 10 mm high, we will be using at most the upper half of the upper lid tarsus. A cut is made through conjunctiva–tarsus for the desired flap width. Vertical cuts are then made from each end of the flap through conjunctiva–tarsus until the upper tarsal border is reached. The vertical cut is continued toward the upper cul-de-sac area through conjunctiva only. Müller's muscle (superior tarsal muscle) is dissected free of the conjunctival flap. If the conjunctival flap seems tight vertically, additional separation from the superior tarsal muscle and extension of the vertical cuts must be made until the tarsus may be easily brought into the lower lid defect.

If a protective corneal–scleral lens is used, it is important to remember to remove it before suturing the tarsoconjunctival flap. A colored lens is a useful reminder. I have known of the necessity of tearing down a reconstructed lid to remove a clear lens!

Interrupted 5-0 or 6-0 polyglycolic acid sutures fix the two vertical sides of the tarsus to the edges of the tarsus of the lid. Inferiorly, the tarsoconjunctival flap is sutured to the conjunctiva. It has been recommended that these sutures go through only the anterior two thirds of the tarsus and not emerge through the conjunctival surface. However, this

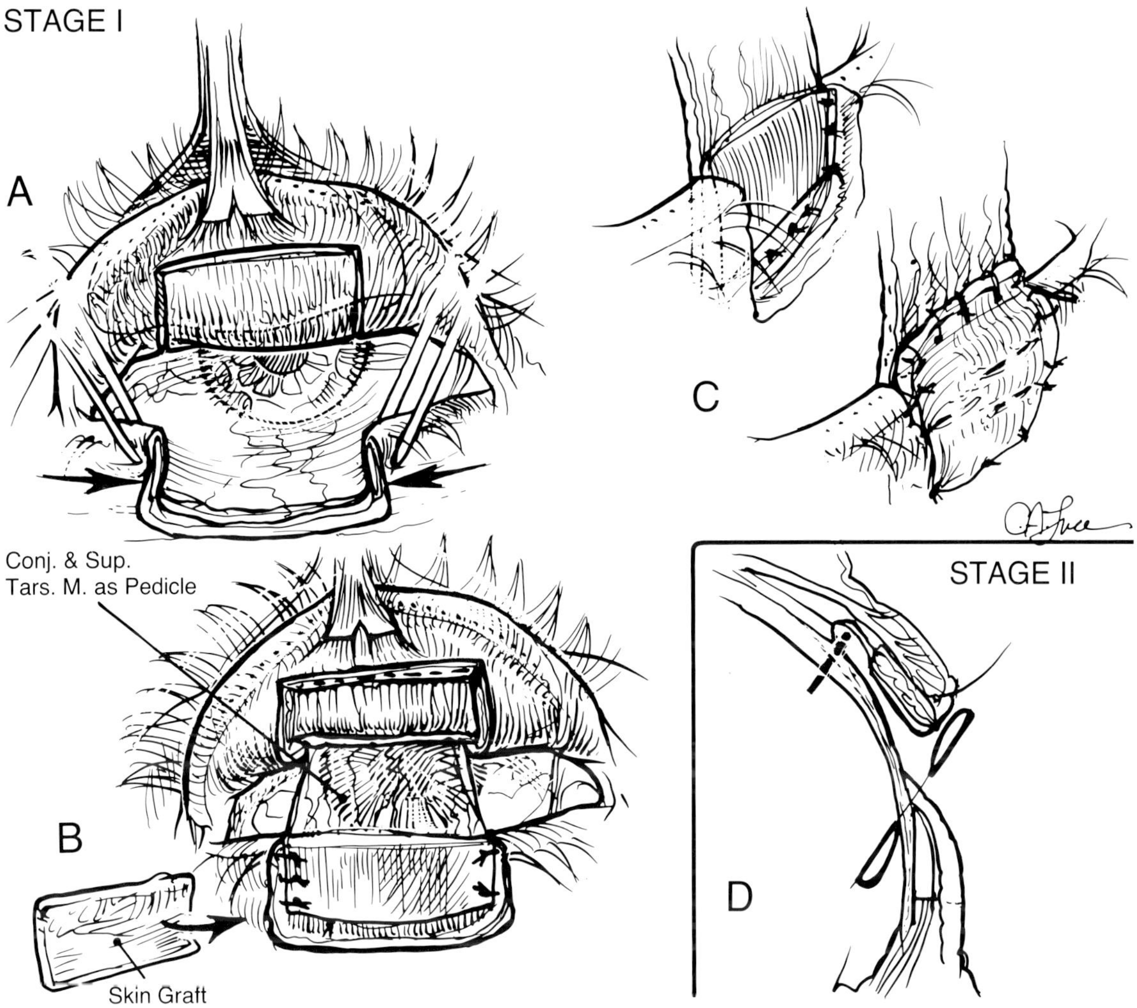

Fig. 39-4. Hughes staged reconstruction of lower lid defect. Stage I: (**A**) With the edges of the lower lid defect pulled toward one another, the lid defect is measured. A cut is made through the conjunctiva and tarsal plate, parallel to the lid margin and 5 mm above it, for the length of the defect as just measured. At the upper tarsal border, the superior tarsal muscle is transected and pushed bluntly off the conjunctiva. (**B**) The tarso-conjunctival flap is advanced downward into the lower lid defect. The tarsus of the tarso-conjunctival flap is sutured to the lower lid tarsus with 6-0 polyglycolic acid sutures. The lower border of the advanced tarsus is sutured to conjunctiva of the inferior cul-de-sac with interrupted sutures. (**C**) The lower lid is *not* split; direct end-to-end suturing of the tarsus of flap to tarsus of lower lid is performed. A full-thickness skin graft is sutured onto the cutaneous defect with interrupted or continuous sutures. Stage II: (**D**) Note angle of the scissor blades for severing of the tarso-conjunctival flap. The upper incision removes the unneeded area of conjunctiva.

rule can be violated without creating problems of a suture-induced keratitis.

Full-thickness passage through the adjacent edges of conjunctiva and tarsus provides a firmer bite. For the less experienced surgeon, this could be the preferable technique. While a running suture could be used, I prefer interrupted sutures, especially when closing the vertical edges. Particular attention must be paid to the suture closest to the lid margin at each vertical end of the flap. To help prevent a notch, this suture should be as close as possible to the upper tarsal border of the flap and the margin of the host lid. The older technique of splitting the vertical edges of the host lid and imbricating the tarsoconjunctival flap between the anterior and posterior lamella causes excessive scarring and is unnecessary. Full-thickness bites with the suture will ensure a tight lid.

The donor sites for the full-thickness skin graft can include the opposite upper lid, postauricular area, subclavicular area, or the inside of the upper arm. My preference for lower lid reconstruction is postauricular skin. Although slightly thicker than the lower lid skin, it is cosmetically superior to the thinner upper lid skin. Since I do not routinely form an advancement or apron of orbicularis muscle to cover the tarsal flap, I find the slightly increased thickness of the postauricular skin satisfactory. A full-thickness skin graft need not exceed the size of the defect it is to cover, as is necessary with split-thickness skin grafts. However, I do have the piece of skin extend about 2 mm higher than the adjacent lid margin onto the conjunctiva of the flap. This will compensate for possible vertical contraction of skin. Any excess skin on the conjunctival flap is easily resected during the second stage of the reconstruction. The two vertical edges and lower horizontal edge of the skin graft are sutured to the adjacent lid skin with skin closure suture (silk, prolene, Surgilene, or nylon). I personally prefer Ethicon 1916G mild gut, as no sutures need to be removed. The upper edge of the skin graft is sutured to the conjunctival flap with fine bites of 7-0 or 8-0 absorbable suture on a fine needle.

The dressing for the reconstructed lid consists of a light application of antibiotic ointment of choice to the skin graft and under the upper lid, followed by placing several pieces of Telfa over the skin graft for extra pressure to the graft, then dressing the lids with another Telfa pad. Eye pads are taped with mild pressure. The dressing is left in place for 3 or 4 days. On the initial dressing change, the Telfa overlying the graft must be left in place for another several days. One must avoid lifting off the graft from its base. Starting on the fourth to sixth postoperative day, the conjunctival flap must be carefully separated from the inside of the upper lid. Such an adherence can cause the upper lid to be retracted after the second stage has been completed. Separating the flap from the lid with gentle pressure of a Q-tip during the first several postoperative weeks will allow the flap to remain free and make the second stage procedure easier. Antibiotic drops are used from the sixth postoperative day for the next several weeks.

The second stage of the Hughes reconstruction can be performed anytime after 2 weeks, usually before the sixth week. The conjunctival flap is excised from its uppermost point of attachment on the upper lid to the level desired on the reconstruction lower lid. The cuts are made with scissors, with the lower cut made with them tilted slightly, so as to allow a slightly higher level of skin than conjunctiva. This allows the skin to have a head start on epithelializing the lid margin. If the conjunctiva achieves this first, the reconstructed lid margin will remain more erythematous than if skin has covered most of the new margin. If skin occupies the new posterior lid margin, however, it may cause keratitis. Experience teaches the exact amount of scissor-tilting necessary to achieve the ideal result.

Postoperatively, antibiotic drops are instilled into the eye then the area dressed with a Telfa pad plus an eye pad. This is left in place for 1 day, then discarded. Antibiotic drops are used three or four times a day for 7 to 10 days.

Hewes–Beard Technique

When the lower lid lesion involves the lateral portion of the lid, and the defect created by the excision extends to the lateral canthal angle, and the consideration of a one-stage procedure is important, the Hewes–Beard procedure[18] (or as some of us call it, the "other Hughes procedure") can be used (Fig. 39-5). A laterally based horizontal tarsoconjunctival flap from the upper lid is rotated into the lower lid defect. The length of the laterally based flap is determined by the width of the remaining defect after pulling the medial remnant of the lower lid laterally with moderate tension.

The upper lid is everted over an Erhardt clamp. The flap is outlined on the under surface of the

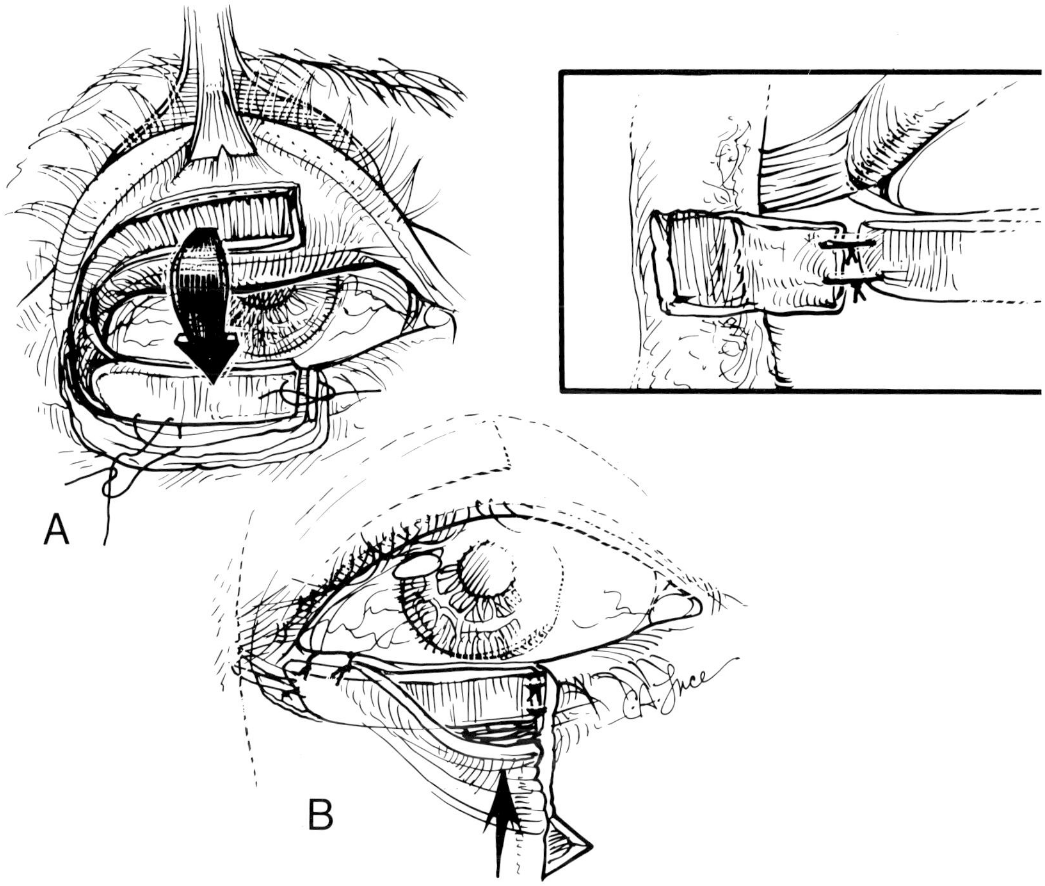

Fig. 39-5. Laterally based Hewes–Beard tarso-conjunctival flap rotated into the laterally located lower lid defect. (**A**) The laterally based tarso-conjunctival flap is sutured end-to-end to the lower lid tarsus using interrupted 6-0 polyglycolic acid sutures. (**B**) A vertical advancement skin flap is created, undermining only skin. It is sutured to the upper edge of the tarso-conjunctival flap with 7-0 polyglycolic acid sutures. A Burrow's triangle is excised to allow for redundancy of skin as the flap is advanced upward. Inset: If maximum tarsus is obtained horizontally from the upper lid but a defect remains, a medial-based periosteal flap is created, so that it is based on the inside of the lateral orbital rim.

upper lid, starting at the lateral end of the tarsal plate just below the upper tarsal border. Its vertical dimension should be about 5 mm. It is better to make the flap slightly longer than was determined necessary, as excess length can be excised before suturing the medial vertical edge. The Hewes–Beard flap is sutured to the conjunctiva of the lower lid/cul-de-sac area with 5-0 or 6-0 polyglycolic acid sutures, as in the Hughes procedure. When this flap is sutured in place, the lower lid should be snugly against the globe, or there will be postoperative ectropion. Now is the time to prevent this!

The anterior lamella can be either a full-thickness skin graft or an advancement skin flap. I have found the latter to usually be quite acceptable, since there is laxity of the skin in this area. Adequate undermining of the skin is performed. Medially, a vertical cut is made at the prior medial resection edge so that the skin can be advanced to the reconstructed lid margin. A small Burow's triangle will have to be excised medially to allow for the advancement. Skin is sutured to the upper edge of the tarsus with small bites of 7-0 or 8-0 polyglycolic acid suture, forming the new lid margin. A protective corneal–scleral lens can be left in place until completion of this procedure.

The area is dressed with a small amount of antibiotic ointment or drops, a Telfa pad, followed by a moderate pressure dressing. I leave this in place for several days, depending on the visual status of the remaining eye. A useful trick I use at the conclusion of the skin suturing is a 6-0 prolene/Surgilene intermarginal suture medial to the reconstructed lid margin. This forms an intermarginal suture tarsorrhaphy as previously described, and provides support to the reconstructed lid during the first few postoperative days. If the patient has vision in the remaining eye, this suture can be left in place for 6 days; if the patient has vision in only one eye, the suture is removed at the time of the initial dressing change or on the second postoperative day. One must remember to remove the Telfa pad carefully from the skin flap to avoid pulling the skin from the underlying tarsus. Antibiotic drops are used three or four times a day for 10 to 14 days.

Medial Lower Lid/Medial Canthal Reconstruction

Whatever type of repair is used, for a lesion involving the medial portion of the lower lid or extending into the medial canthus, the tarsus replacement must be attached medially in the area of the normal attachment of the medial canthal tendon. That the lower canaliculus might have been excised is of no real concern, especially if the upper canaliculus is patent. If the Tenzel semicircular flap is being used, the medial advancement of the lower lid tissue is carried to the bone at the medial canthal tendon area. Using either absorbable 4-0 Dexon on a PR-1 half-curved needle or nonabsorbable 4-0 Mersilene on an S-2 half-curved needle one bite is taken through the medial border of the tarsus and is then carried through the residual tissue of the deep head of the medial canthal tendon. The byword here is: high enough and deep enough. Additional sutures attach the lower tarsal edge and deep orbicularis muscle to corresponding areas medially. This will reform the medial canthal angle area. If a large amount of medial advancement is required, it may be necessary to cut the orbital septal attachment from the lateral aspect of the inferior orbital rim. If a large amount of skin has been excised from the medial canthal area, a full-thickness skin graft in this area may also be needed.

The morpheaform-type of basal cell carcinoma is frequently seen in the medial canthal area. This can necessitate a wide area of resection. In this situation, the Mohs fresh tissue technique clearly provides the best opportunity for adequate excision.

Lateral Lower Lid/Lateral Canthal Reconstruction

When the lesion is located laterally and a Hughes tarsoconjunctival flap is used, it must be wide enough to permit attachment of the lateral border of the tarsus of the flap to the area of attachment of the lateral canthal tendon just inside the lateral orbital rim.

When the horizontal extent of the lower lid defect is such that it uses the maximum width of a Hughes tarsoconjunctival flap, yet is still unable to be attached laterally, rotation of zygomatic periosteal flap will permit this attachment. With sharp and blunt dissection, tissue overlying the periosteum at and lateral to the lateral orbital rim in the area of the tendon attachment is separated from it. A 6- to 7-mm-wide medially based periosteal flap is cut with a scalpel. The periosteum is carefully lifted from the bone to the orbital rim. This periosteal flap is sutured to the lateral border of the tarsoconjunctival flap with two interrupted 4-0 polyglycolic acid sutures. The reconstructed lower lid must be taut. The anterior lamella is closed by an advancement or rotational skin flap, if adequate skin is available, or with a full-thickness skin graft.

Other procedures described for lower lid reconstruction include the Mustarde method, reverse Cutler–Beard method, and advancement of adjacent lower lid tarsus. For the occasional or less-experienced surgeon, the techniques described will usually suffice.

UPPER LID RECONSTRUCTION TECHNIQUES

The wedge resection without or with a lateral cantholysis or Tenzel semicircular flap described earlier is suitable for the upper lid as well as the lower. Lesions involving the medial or lateral canthus and adjacent upper lids are reconstructed as described for the lower lid/canthal areas.

When the lesion involves mainly the lid margin and less than 4 to 5 mm of lid height (skin or tarsus), it is not excised in a pentagonal transmarginal wedge resection as described for the lower lid, as this approach would require removal of another 5 mm of tarsus above the area. Instead, a rectangular area of tissue is excised. By leaving tarsus, a Hughes-type tarsoconjunctival flap can be fashioned superiorly but advanced only to the lid margin area, rather than into the lower lid. The advanced flap will be made narrower than the width of the excised lesion, since one fourth of the lid need not be replaced, to create the necessary tautness of the lid. The medial and lateral borders of the advanced tarsoconjunctival flap are sutured to the corresponding medial and lateral borders of the resected area as in the Hughes procedure. The anterior lamella is best closed with a full-thickness skin graft from the opposite upper lid or, as a second choice, from the postauricular area. The skin is sutured to adjacent skin on the medial, upper, and lateral borders with the skin suture material of choice (again, I prefer Ethicon 1916G mild gut, so there are no sutures to remove). The skin is attached to the lower border of the advanced tarsoconjunctival flap with several 7-0 or 8-0 polyglycolic acid sutures. The wound is dressed as previously described. This procedure can be performed for a very wide lid margin lesion involving the medial or lateral canthal areas, with the appropriate border sutured to the canthal tendon. This procedure has two advantages: the reconstructed lid margin contains at least 4 to 5 mm vertical height of the tarsus, giving better stability to the reconstructed lid, and it is a one-stage procedure.

When the upper lid defect is about one half the lid length but includes a full height of the tarsus, a sliding flap of adjacent tarsus and conjunctiva may be used to fill the defect (Stephenson CM, LaJolla CA: personal communication, 1983), another variation of the Hughes repair. The width of the flap is determined by pulling the medial and lateral resection edges together. The adjacent tarsus is incised horizontally the distance of the predetermined flap width, beginning 4 to 5 mm above the lid margin. The tarsus is incised vertically at the end of the horizontal incision through the upper border. The conjunctival base of the flap is dissected toward the upper fornix from the superior tarsal muscle, thereby creating a pure tarsoconjunctival flap, as in the Hughes procedure. The tarsoconjunctival flap is advanced into the defect and secured to the adjacent lid with 6-0 polyglycolic acid sutures. The anterior lamella is formed with either a full-thickness skin graft or, if adequate skin laxity is present, a flap from adjacent skin.

If the lid defect is central and there is insufficient tarsus on either side to close the defect adequately, smaller flaps with a total width equaling that needed to fill the defect can be dissected from each side of the defect.[17] The only difference in closure is that the two flaps of tarsus must be sutured together.

Cutler–Beard Procedure

The Cutler–Beard procedure[13,19,20] is a time honored technique useful for repairing large upper lid defects, particularly when the full height of the tarsus has been excised (Fig. 39-6). After the width of the flap to be used to repair the upper lid defect has been determined by pulling the two cut edges toward each other with moderate tension, the proposed flap is outlined on the lower lid skin. A horizontal mark is made about 3.5 mm below the lash line, parallel to the lid margin; and vertical marks are made at the medial and lateral aspects of the line, creating the predetermined width.

The flap is cut with a full-thickness horizontal incision. I find this easiest with an Erhardt clamp on the lower lid, cutting through the entire lid onto the clamp with a #15 Bard–Parker blade. Care must be taken to ensure that this cut is perpendicu-

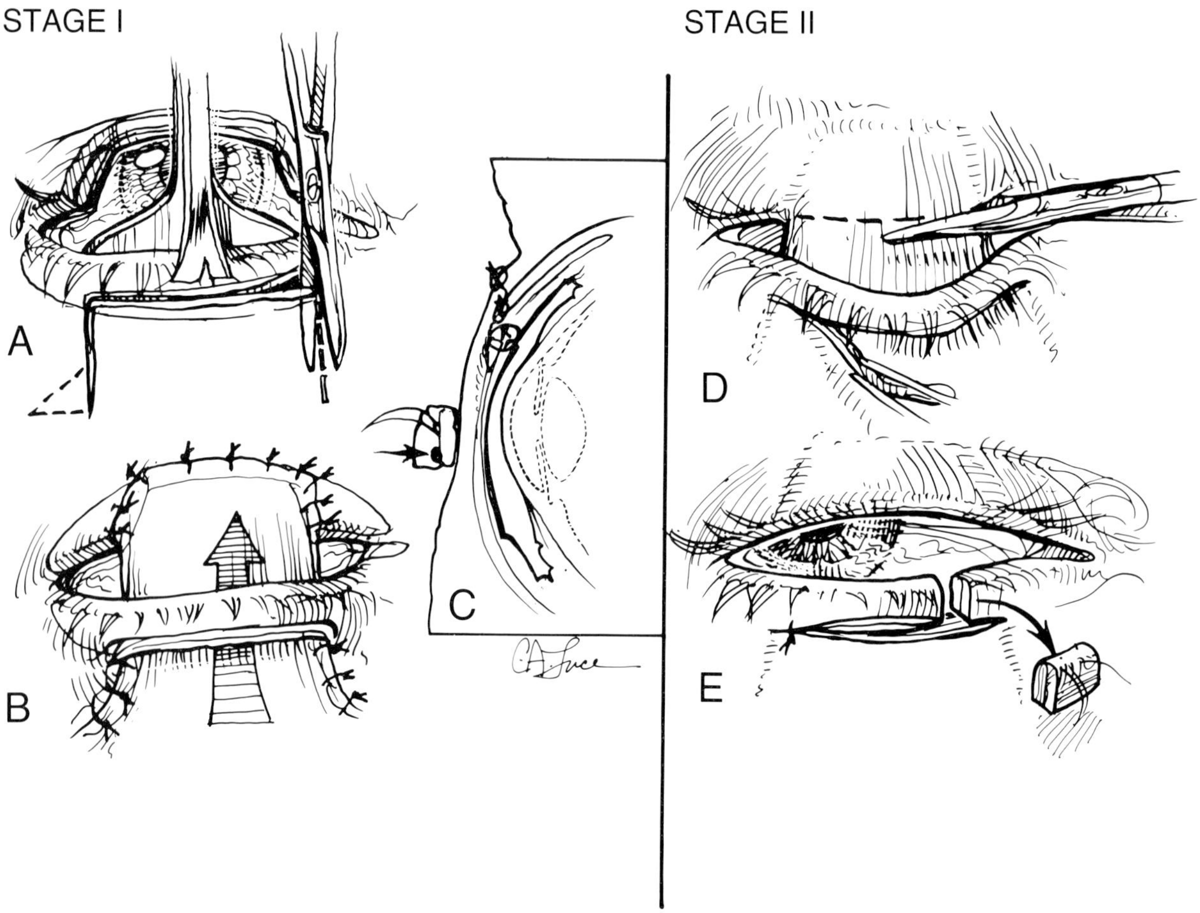

Fig. 39-6. Cutler–Beard full-thickness lower lid advancement flap for upper lid defect. Stage I: (**A**) Full-thickness incisions through lower lid are made about 3.5 mm below and parallel to the lower lid margin. Vertical full-thickness cuts are made from the first incision to the inferior cul-de-sac. A Burrow's triangle is excised from each side of the vertical incision. (**B**) The full-thickness flap is passed underneath the lower lid margin (bridge flap) and elevated into the upper lid defect. A layered closure is done: conjunctiva to conjunctiva, levator aponeurosis to deep orbicularis, skin to skin. (**C**) Cross section demonstrating the above layered closure. Stage II: (**D**) The flap is taken down after 4 to 8 weeks by cutting the advanced full-thickness lower lid flap at the appropriate level to create an upper lid margin. (**E**) The lower edge of the marginal bridge flap is freshened and, when necessary, the marginal bridge flap is shortened via a transmarginal wedge resection. The lower lid defects are then closed.

lar to the skin and not angled upward toward either the lid margin or the lower tarsal border. Heavy scissors are used to make the medial and lateral vertical cuts. These extend into the depth of the inferior cul-de-sac to allow for adequate mobilization of the flap. The lower lid flap is elevated posterior to the lower lid margin bridge into the upper lid. If not at this point, then as soon as possible, the corneal–scleral protective lens should be removed.

The conjunctiva with the 1 mm of tarsus of the advanced full-thickness lower lid flap is sutured to the conjunctiva of the upper cul-de-sac and to the medial and lateral borders of the corresponding tarsus of the upper lid with interrupted or continuous 6-0 polyglycolic acid sutures. The levator aponeurosis of the upper lid is then attached to the orbicularis muscle layer of the flap with interrupted 6-0 polyglycolic acid sutures. The skin edges are closed with the skin suture of choice, down to the residual lid margin, both medially and laterally. A Burow's triangle is excised at the lower end of both the medial and lateral flap incisions of the lower lid. The vertical edges of skin inferior to the lower lid margin bridge are closed. Nothing is done with the raw lower surface of the margin bridge.

When dressing the lid, care must be taken not to compromise the blood supply of the bridge flap by pressure. Several thicknesses of Telfa pads are placed on both the upper and lower sides of the bridge flap in order to build up the height of each adjacent area equal to the bridge height. After the third or fourth day, the initial dressing change is made. Antibiotic ointment is placed along the raw surface of the bridge flap and drops placed at the medial or lateral canthal opening and continued for 10 to 14 days.

The interval to the second stage can vary from 4 weeks to several months. When edema has subsided in the portion of the advancement flap above the lid margin bridge, the second stage can be performed.

The second stage consists of cutting through the full-thickness advancement flap at the level of the upper lid margin, shortening the bridge of the lower lid, and repositioning the remainder of the flap into the lower lid. The lower lid margin bridge is gently retracted inferiorly to expose the upper lid margin and flap. Using slightly curved scissors, a full-thickness flap is cut to create the new upper lid margin. The scissors' blade is angled (as was done earlier for the second stage of the lower lid Hughes repair) to permit slightly more skin than conjunctiva to remain. Small bites of skin and conjunctiva are united with 7-0 or 8-0 polyglycolic acid suture.

Because the lower lid bridge has stretched, a wedge of the margin bridge is resected. The width to be excised is determined by overlapping the edges after the initial cut. That incision line is closed as described for primary closure of the lower lid margin defect. The reepithelialized inferior border, which was left raw at the conclusion of the first stage, is freshened by excising its epithelialized edge. The upper edge of the advancement flap is sutured onto the lower lid in a two-layered clo-

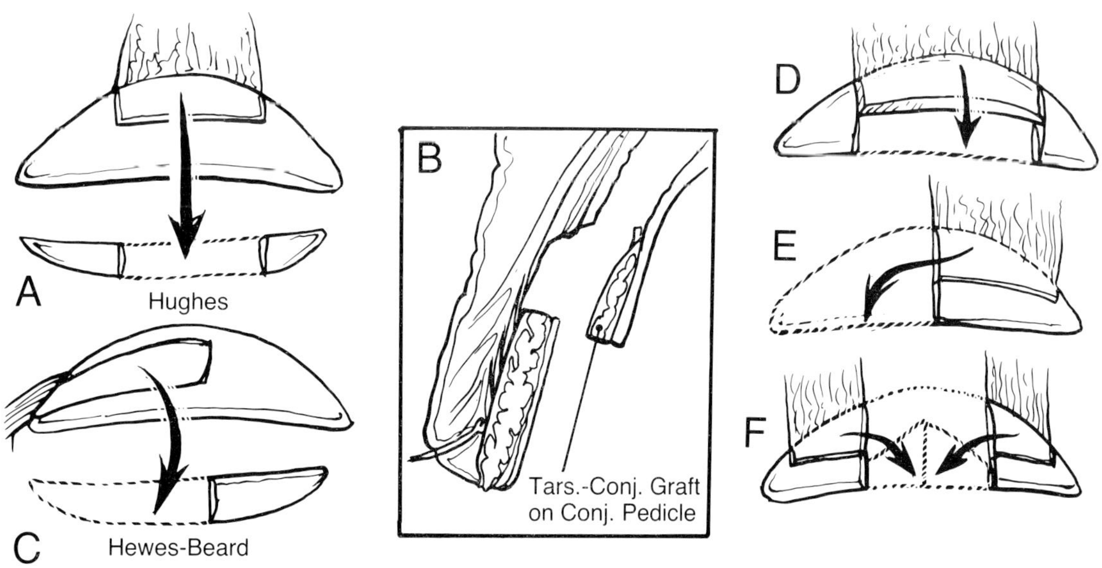

Fig. 39-7. Overview of the various lid reconstruction methods utilizing tarso-conjunctival flaps: **(A)**, **(B)** Hughes flap. **(C)** Hewes–Beard flap. **(D)** Superior tarso-conjunctival flap to same lid. **(E)** Sliding tarso-conjunctival flap from adjacent portions of the same lid. **(F)** Double sliding tarso-conjunctival flap.

sure: tarsus–conjunctiva and skin. The wound is treated as with any postwedge lid. If the wedge resection is not performed as part of the second stage, the lower lid will likely remain lax and ectropion will occur. Since other texts frequently do not mention this, I urge the reader's attention to this detail.

Callahan and Callahan[13] modified the Cutler–Beard technique by advancing only the posterior lamella of the lower lid into the upper lid and upper fornix. Figure 39-7 shows the various lid reconstruction methods that use tarsoconjunctival flaps.

COMPLICATIONS IN EYELID MARGIN RECONSTRUCTION

Adherence to details when surgically reconstructing an eyelid will prevent many complications. Although I speak of specific details of a procedure, there are probably as many subtle variations as there are surgeons performing surgical procedures. It is certainly much easier to prevent complications than to correct them. As with any surgery, techniques may sound easy when read, but there is no substitute for observing the performance of a procedure. There is no blood covering the text of a book, but in real life, bleeding, until controlled, may obliterate the anatomy.

Knowledge of the facial and lid anatomy and the experience to recognize it are essential before surgical reconstruction of a lid is undertaken. Local infiltration of an anesthetic agent into the lid structures may sufficiently distort the normal anatomic picture that one might get lost. For this reason, I prefer regional block anesthesia.

Scarring is a most unpredictable complication that may or may not be preventable with good surgical technique. If the surgeon is uncomfortable using a flap or a skin graft, and therefore closes a lower lid defect primarily, the resultant cicatricial ectropion is not a result of adverse scarring, but poor surgical judgment.

In any postoperative situation, bleeding or infection can cause problems. Light cautery at the time of surgery minimizes early postoperative bleeding problems. Bleeding during the early postoperative period can cause separation of a skin graft from its base and lead to death of the graft. The patient should be instructed to keep activities to a minimum—not to do heavy or dirty work, not to lift more than 2 pounds, and not to bend over such that the head is below the waist. If this advice is followed, it helps prevent problems for both the patient and the surgeon.

If a postoperative infection causes a graft to sluff, restraint should be exercised, rather than surgical intervention. The area should be kept as clean as possible with hydrogen peroxide or moist dressings and local and/or systemic antibiotics used, letting nature take its course. The surgeon may be pleasantly surprised at how well the lid ultimately looks and functions. Certainly patience is a virtue at this time!

Tumor recurrence may in fact not be recurrence at all, but rather residual tumor left behind by a surgeon who perhaps might not have known how to close a large defect; consequently, the tumor excision was defined to limit the defect to one the surgeon knew how to close. This is a preventable complication. Again, it is important to have a game plan preoperatively but to be prepared to do more, depending on the findings at the time of surgery. The surgeon who undertakes excision of a lid lesion should be prepared to excise until the lid is free of tumor and to reconstruct with whatever technique seems best. If the defect is larger than the surgeon feels comfortable closing, it is best to have done the excision and then pack the lid with a moist dressing and refer the patient for closure.

REFERENCES

1. Smith BC, Nesi FA: Practical Techniques in Ophthalmic Plastic Surgery. CV Mosby, St. Louis, 1981
2. Karcioglu ZA, Caldwell DR: Frozen section diagnosis in ophthalmic surgery. Surv Ophthalmol 28:323, 1984
3. Mohs FE: Chemosurgery for the microscopically controlled excision of cutaneous cancer. Head Neck Surg 1:150, 1978
4. Fraunfelder FT, Wallace TR, Farris HE, et al: The

role of cryosurgery in external ocular and periocular disease. Trans Am Acad Ophthalmol Otolaryngol 83:713, 1977
5. Fraunfelder FT, Zacarion SA, Limmer BL, et al: Cryosurgery for malignancies of the eyelid. Ophthalmology 87:461, 1980
6. Fraunfelder FT, Zacarion SA, Wingfield DL, et al: Results of cryotherapy for eyelid malignancies. Am J Ophthalmol 97:184, 1984
7. Mohs FE: Chemosurgery: Microscopically Controlled Surgery for Skin Cancer. Charles C Thomas, Springfield, IL, 1978
8. Cobb GM, Thompson GA, Allt WEC: Treatment of basal cell carcinoma of the eyelids by radiotherapy. Can Med Assoc J 91:743, 1964
9. Doxanas MT, Green WR, Iliff CE: Factors in the successful surgical management of basal cell carcinoma of the eyelids. Am J Ophthalmol 91:726, 1981
10. Swanson NA: Mohs surgery: Technique, indications, applications, and the future. Arch Dermatol 119:761, 1983
11. Felts JA, Silver B: Anesthesia. p. 32. In Stewart WB (ed): Ophthalmic Plastic and Reconstructive Surgery. American Academy of Ophthalmology, San Francisco, 1984
12. Breon Laboratories, Inc., drug insert for Marcaine
13. Callahan MA, Callahan A: Ophthalmic Plastic and Orbital Surgery. Aesculpius, Birmingham, AL, 1979
14. Flanagan JC: Lower eyelid reconstruction. p. 258. In Stewart WB (ed): Ophthalmic Plastic and Reconstructive Surgery. American Academy of Ophthalmology, San Francisco, 1984
15. Frueh BR: Upper eyelid reconstruction. p. 258. In Stewart WB (ed): Ophthalmic Plastic and Reconstructive Surgery. American Academy of Ophthalmology, San Francisco, 1984
16. Tenzel RR: Reconstruction of the control one half of an eyelid. Arch Ophthalmol 93:125,1975
17. Hughes WL: Reconstruction of the Lids. CV Mosby, St. Louis, 1958
18. Hewes EH, Sullivan JH, Beard C: Lower eyelid reconstruction by tarsal transposition. Am J Ophthalmol 81:512, 1976
19. Cutler NL, Beard C: A method for partial and total upper lid reconstruction. Am J Ophthalmol 39:1, 1955
20. Smith B, Conway S: Surgical treatment of upper lid tumors. p. 84. In Hornblass A (ed): Tumors of the Ocular Adnexa and Orbit. CV Mosby, St. Louis, 1979

Eyelid and Canthal Defects Not Involving the Eyelid Margin

40

Charles M. Stephenson, Sr.

HISTORICAL BACKGROUND

Daviel, in 1755, first proposed that cancer of the eyelid area be treated by surgical excision, but he made no attempt to repair the defect after the tumor was excised. The development of techniques for reconstructing this region was greatly stimulated by von Graefe's monograph, which described the reintroduction of the cheek advancement flap of Celsus (1818)[1] and by Fricke's description of the transposition flap and a primitive form of Z-plasty (1829).[2] Other basic reconstructive procedures were described by Dieffenbach,[3] Blasius,[4] and others.[5,6] Modern oculoplastic surgery largely consists of refinements of nineteenth century innovations made possible by our access to better anesthesia, instrumentation, and suture materials.

GENERAL CONSIDERATIONS

The eyelids and canthi have certain special attributes that should be factored into any plan for managing defects in them. An excellent blood supply greatly facilitates the survival of flaps and grafts and decreases the incidence of infection. The plethoric blood supply also makes possible and desirable the conservative debridement of wounds and the preservation of all possible damaged eyelid tissue. Eyelid skin has good elasticity, is loosely attached to underlying tissue, and, in adults, is frequently in surplus. This also facilitates the development of flaps and grafts.

The special characteristic most likely to cause a complication is the tendency for the lower eyelid to retract or evert if vertical tension is placed on it or develops within it. This problem is especially likely to occur when there is preexisting horizontal lid laxity. It is frequently prudent, therefore, to tighten the lower lid by means of a tarsal sling,[7] contemporaneously with the repair of a defect in it.

REPAIR OF DEFECTS REQUIRING MINIMAL TISSUE MOBILIZATION

A small linear skin incision or laceration may only require support with a sterile adhesive strip, especially if it parallels the natural skin lines.[8] If this does not provide secure closure, interrupted 7-0 silk sutures should be used for 2 or 3 days. When a wound divides the orbicularis muscle parallel with its fibers, only skin sutures are generally required. When the muscle fibers are transversely divided, they should usually be reapproximated with 7-0 or 6-0 synthetic absorbable sutures, such as Vicryl (Ethicon) or Dexon (Davis & Geck), and the skin is closed separately with fine silk or nylon.

When a small round or oval skin lesion is removed, a narrow ellipse of tissue should be excised around it so that a linear closure can be made, if possible. The most inconspicuous scar results from a closure that parallels the natural skin lines. These lines can usually be followed in the closure of small- to medium-sized skin ellipses in the upper lid and in canthi. The horizontally oriented skin patterns in the lower lid must be followed with caution, however, as the associated vertical mobilization of skin may cause an ectropion.

Burow's Triangle

The closure of a wide oval defect or of any defect involving much mobilization of tissue tends to leave an elevated cone at the ends of the incision. This problem can be minimized by placing skin hooks at each end of the wound as it is being closed to help equalize the length of the defect sides. Suturing begins in the middle of the wound (Fig. 40-1A). As the closure reaches the end of the incision, if a "dog ear" develops, a skin hook is used to draw it to one side of the incision line (Fig. 40-1B). The redundant tissue is marked off and excised

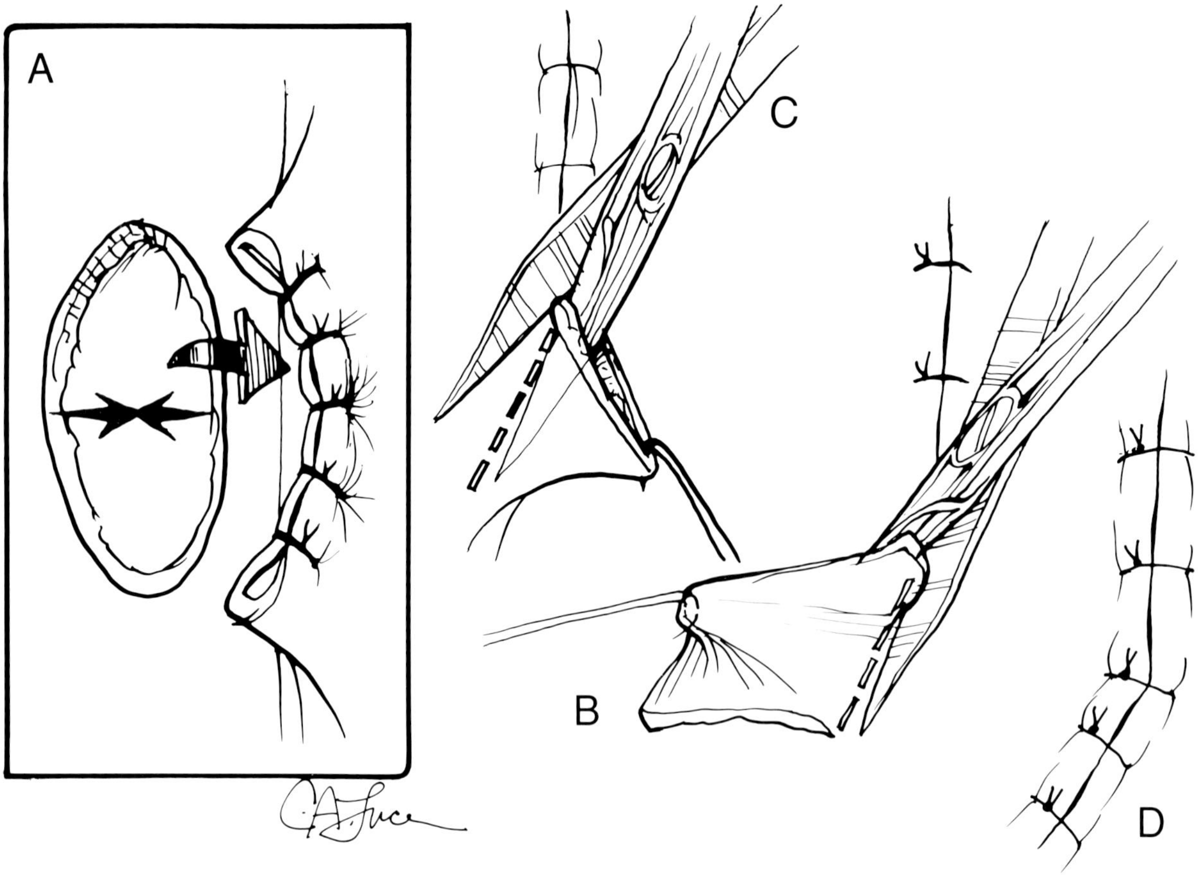

Fig. 40-1. Eliminating "dog ear" in wound closure. **(A)** Closure begins centrally. **(B)** Elevated cone pulled to one side. **(C)** Burow's triangle excised. **(D)** Terminus of closure forms angle.

(Fig. 40-1C). The final terminus of the incision will now be at an angle to the original closure line (Fig. 40-1D). Carl Burow (1855), a German surgeon and ophthalmologist, was the first to advocate this maneuver as a means of improving flap mobility and cosmesis.[9]

RECONSTRUCTION WITH FLAPS

A wound that cannot otherwise be closed by primary approximation is reconstructed by means of a flap or a graft, except for special circumstances in which healing by granulation is permitted. A flap remains partially attached to surrounding tissue by a pedicle through which it is nourished. (An exception is the microvascular free flap.[10,11]) A graft is completely detached and transferred to a host bed, from which it acquires a new blood supply. If a local flap can be readily developed, it has some advantages compared with a graft. It requires less postoperative immobilization and usually provides the optimal match of skin texture and color. It also supplies more bulk than a graft does, although there are situations in which this is not desirable. Frequently, the effectiveness of a reconstruction by flaps is enhanced by combining elements from more than one type of flap.

Advancement Flap

The advancement flap moves tissue in a straight line. Because skin and muscle in the eyelid area tend to be elastic and loosely attached, the advancement flap is more effective here than in many other parts of the body. The key to its successful development is in orienting the flap so that tissue is mobilized in the proper direction and in extensively undermining the flap area. An eyelid advancement flap is usually composed of skin and muscle. An eyelid flap may be formed of only the skin, however, when skin is all that is required and an ample supply is available. A lengthy skin flap is actually primarily nourished from the recipient bed as a free graft.

All flaps should be carefully planned and the proposed incisions dye marked on the skin. Advancement flaps in the eyelids can safely be devised of much greater length to width ratio than the maximum of 1 : 1 recommended for other parts of the body.[12] Advancement flaps involving the lower eyelids should be horizontally oriented and are usually temporally based. Upper lid flaps may be oriented either horizontally or vertically.

To minimize bleeding, the surgical site should be injected with a solution containing epinephrine 10 minutes prior to the incision. The principal releasing incisions are made approximately parallel to each other, extending from each corner of the defect to the base of the flap (Fig. 40-2A). The flap is then thoroughly undermined with scissors and advanced into position. Sutures are placed between the sides of the flap and the adjacent tissue in a slightly oblique direction that augments advancement of the flap. After the flap has been sutured into position, it is usually necessary to make angled cuts at either side of the pedicle base to remove elevated cones of tissue, that is, Burow's triangles (Fig. 40-2B). If the defect cannot be closed as the flap was initially designed, mobility can be increased by lengthening the flap, by developing a rotation flap at the pedicle base, or by converting the skin to an island flap.

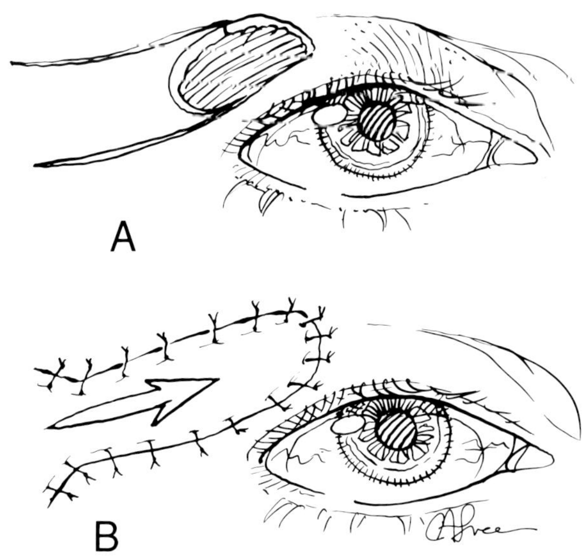

Fig. 40-2. Closure with advancement flaps. **(A)** Releasing incisions. **(B)** Flap advanced into position.

It has been traditionally taught that a flap must be constructed such that it is under no significant tension when placed in its new location.[13] This concept should be modified somewhat, at least regarding well-vascularized flaps.[14] Eyelid flaps actually do quite well when closed on a moderate stretch, if temporary traction sutures are used to prevent tension on the healing wound surfaces. The flap must also be designed such that the tension will not retract the eyelid. A 5-0 or 6-0 prolene near-far–far-near suture[15] or a horizontal mattress suture is used for 7 to 10 days to prevent wound tension (see Fig. 41-2G).

Laboratory experiments have demonstrated that skin elongates rapidly,[16,17] developing increased vascularity when stretched.[18] This concept has recently been applied in the placement of inflatable implants to stretch tissue preparatory to the development of flaps in the head, hand, chest, and elsewhere.[19–21]

Rotation Flap

A rotation flap reconstructs a defect by swinging tissue about a pivot point and is most commonly based in the lateral canthal or cheek area when used for eyelid reconstruction. The small temporal rotation flap of Tenzel[22] and the large cheek-rotation flap of Mustarde,[23] were introduced for the reconstruction of defects involving the eyelid margins. They are also applicable, however, for the repair of nonmarginal eyelid defects.

Transposition Flap

While a rotation flap swings tissue about an axis, a transposition flap moves tissue horizontally. A bipedicle transposition flap from the upper eyelid can be used to repair a defect in the central part of the lower lid (Fig. 40-3A,B); single-pedicle trans-

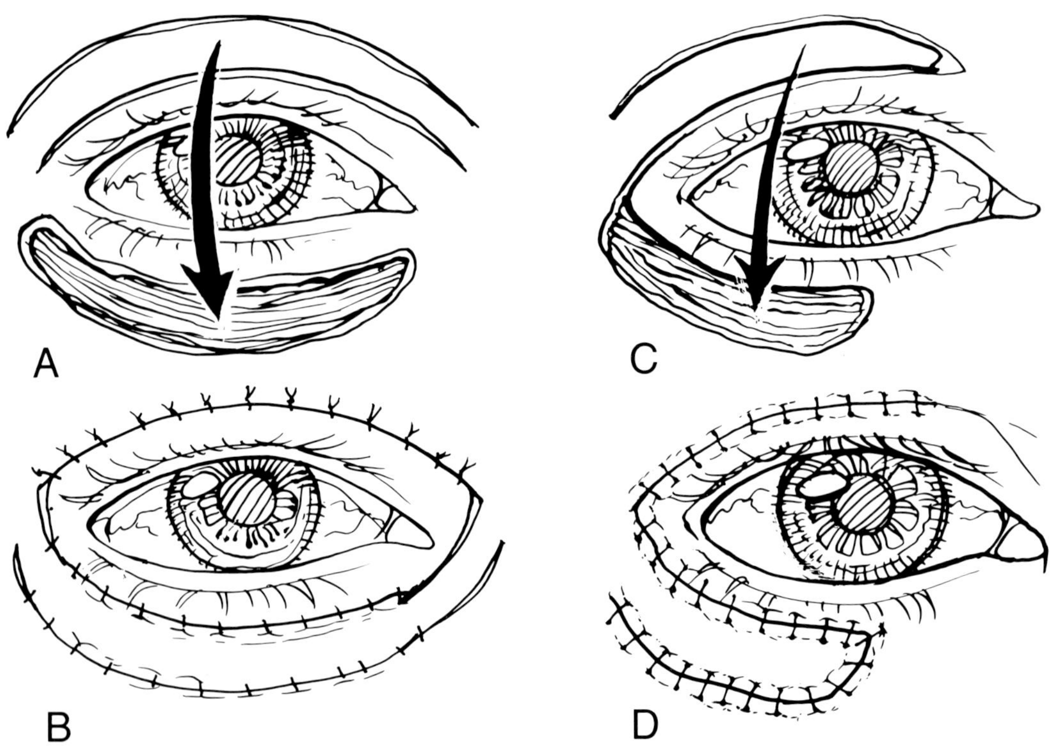

Fig. 40-3. Closure with transposition flaps. **(A,B)** Bipedicle flap. **(C,D)** Single pedicle flap.

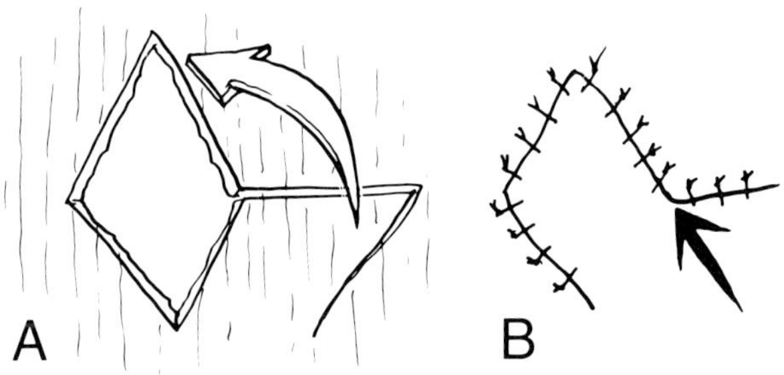

Fig. 40-4. Closure with rhombic flap. **(A)** Flap preferentially oriented with lines of election. **(B)** Transposition completed.

position flaps can be used to repair medial and lateral lower lid defects[23] (Fig. 40-3C,D). A minor operation is required later to revise the pedicle base. I seldom use this technique but prefer reconstructing these areas with an advancement flap, a rotation flap, an island flap, or a free skin graft.

Rhombic Flap* of Limberg/ Dufourmentel

This specialized transposition flap is particularly useful for the repair of cutaneous defects that are located peripheral to the eyelids proper.[24] In general, the rhombus should be planned such that its longest diagonal is in the direction of the relaxed skin tension lines (Fig. 40-4A). The flap was originally described for the excision of eliptical lesions when the resultant defect could be transformed into a rhombus of 60- and 120-degree angles.[25]

When the adjacent flap is designed to be this same size and shape, it can be transposed to cover the defect exactly (Fig. 40-4B). When there is some tissue laxity, the precise size and shape of the transposed flap are not as critical. A circular defect, for example, may be best reconstructed by means of a rhombic flap with 90-degree angles. The transposed 90-degree-angled flap is smaller than the defect, but this deficiency is compensated by local tissue advancement.[26] A double rhombic flap can also be developed for the reconstruction of larger defects.[27]

Island Flap

Although many years ago Manchot (1889)[28] noted that the most important blood supply of skin derives from the subjacent tissue, flaps have traditionally been designed with an attachment to adjacent skin as though this were invariably essential to their survival. In the limited use of island flaps in the past, the pedicle was always designed to contain an identified major artery, the superficial temporal being commonly used in the eyelid area.[29,33] The use of island flaps only nourished by the random blood supply of the underlying subcutaneous pedicle has been advocated for the repair of small cutaneous defects in the facial area.[31–33] In 1977, I began to use a small temporally based musculocutaneous island flap, dependent on random blood supply, for the reconstruction of eyelid defects.[34] It has become an important part of my armamentarium. Most cases have been full-thickness defects involving the lid margin, but it can also be useful in reconstructing nonlid margin defects. In this context, it is most commonly used to enhance the mobility of a musculocutaneous advancement or rotation flap that does not readily span the defect being reconstructed (Fig. 40-5A). In these circumstances, the skin of the flap can be completely incised around the base of the flap to form an island of skin, (Fig. 40-5B) nourished by the underlying muscle that remains attached to its pedicle base (Fig. 40-5C). This permits the muscular component of the flap, with the overlying island of skin, to be further advanced into position. The skin at the base is then closed in a V–Y fashion (Fig. 40-5D).

Z-Plasty

The Z-plasty is a specialized transposition flap primarily used for scar revision. It is designed to accomplish one or more of the following functions: (1) lengthen a contracted scar, (2) interrupt a scar, (3) realign a scar toward natural skin lines, and (4) transpose tissue.[35]

* This has been traditionally labeled a rhomboid flap. Since the geometric pattern described, a parallelogram with equal sides, is a rhombus, it would seem that the adjectival form, rhombic is appropriate here. A rhomboid is a parallelogram with unequal sides.

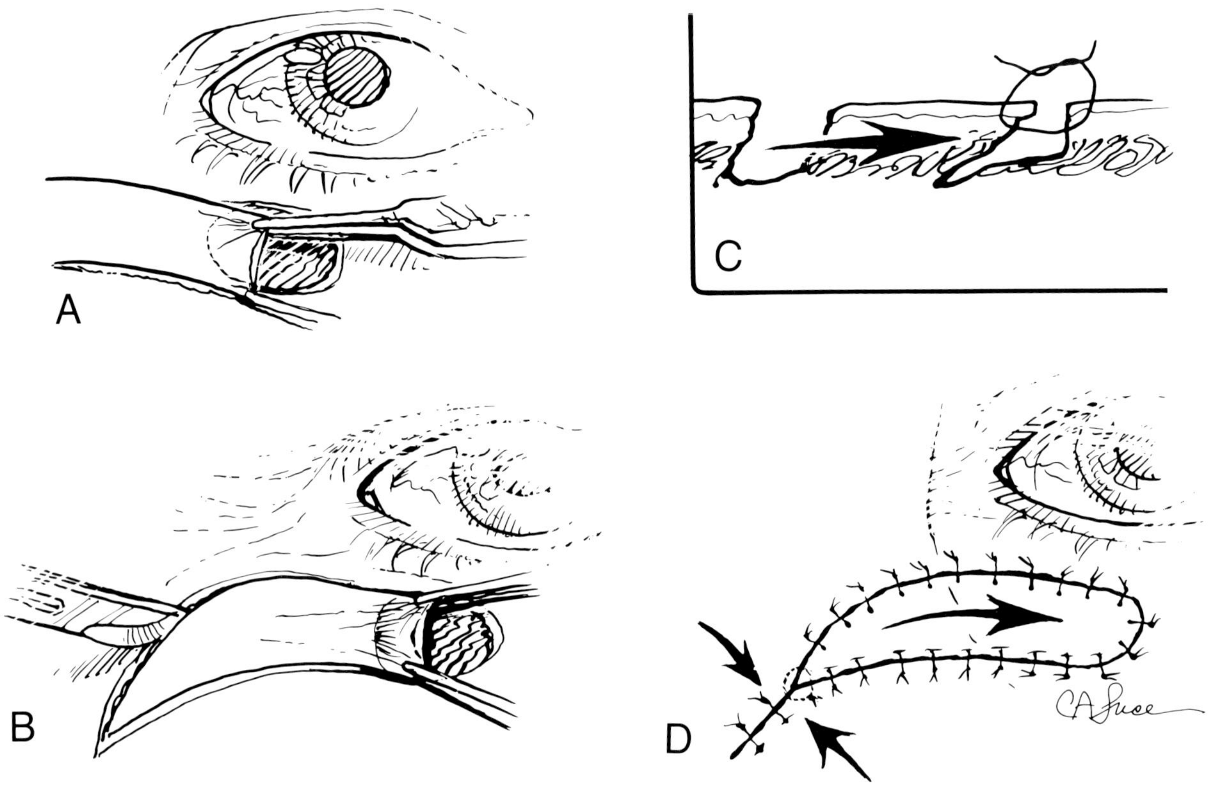

Fig. 40-5. Island flap combined with advancement or rotation flap. **(A)** Unable to cover defect fully. **(B)** Island flap formed of skin. **(C)** Skin nourished by underlying muscle pedicle. **(D)** V–Y closure.

As classically described, a Z-plasty is composed of two 60-degree triangular flaps of equal size. Each flap configuration, however, should be custom crafted to best resolve a specific problem. Scar relaxation occurs along the central limb of the Z (Fig. 40-6A,B). When the angles are 60 degrees, the central limb may lengthen as much as 75 percent. The longer this limb is in proportion to the other limbs, and correlatively the larger the angle, the more difficult the flap transposition. Multiple small Z-plasties are therefore preferred when extensive relaxation is required.[23] In oculoplastic surgery, the Z-plasty is commonly used to revise medial canthal scars or epicanthal folds and to elevate or lower a canthal angle. It can be used to revise vertically contracting scars in the eyelids. However, I usually prefer to excise such a scar and reconstruct with advancement flaps or skin graft.

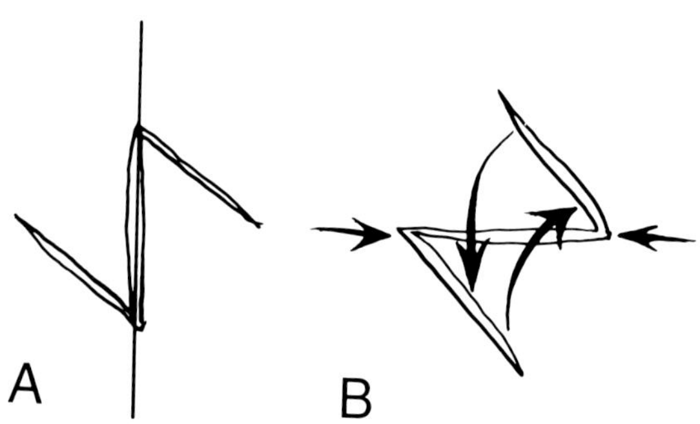

Fig. 40-6. Z-plasty transposition flap. **(A)** Relaxation occurs along central limb of Z. **(B)** Flaps transposed.

O–Z-Plasty

This flap can be used to close a small, circular skin defect. In order to obtain the best cosmetic result, it should be planned so that the final skin closure parallels the natural lines in the skin.

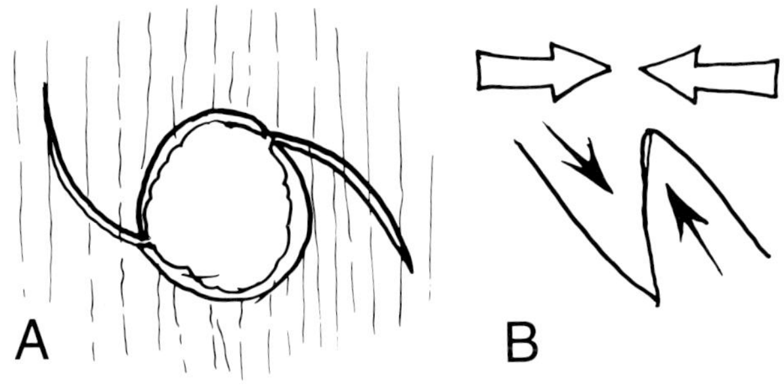

Fig. 40-7. O–Z flap. **(A)** Closure preferentially oriented with skin lines. **(B)** Flaps advanced and rotated into position.

Curved incisions are made on opposite sides of the circular defect, with the curvatures placed in opposite directions (Fig. 40-7A) and the flaps approximated in a Z-shaped pattern (Fig. 40-7B). This flap should only be used when a moderate amount of tissue elasticity is present.

V–Y and Y–V Flaps

The V–Y plasty is a simple, effective technique for releasing tissue in a linear fashion. While it has many uses, the oculoplastic surgeon finds a particular role for it in lengthening contracted scars in the medial canthus (Fig. 40-8). The Y–V-plasty has the reverse effect of contracting tissue. One of its uses is in the repair of telecanthus (Fig. 40-9A,B).

SKIN GRAFTS

A skin graft is customarily used when a surface defect cannot be readily reconstructed with a flap and when only the skin needs replacement. The full-thickness skin-grafting technique is not difficult to learn and greatly extends a surgeon's reconstructive options. A full-thickness graft is composed of epidermis and dermis and a split-thickness graft of epidermis and part of the dermis. Compared with a split graft, the full-thickness graft contracts less, usually provides better cosmesis, and is less fragile. A split-thickness graft survives better on a devitalized surface and can be obtained in large quantity. Principal indications in the eyelid area for a split graft are for resurfacing after an extensive burn. Some also use it after extensive Moh's fresh tissue tumor resection.

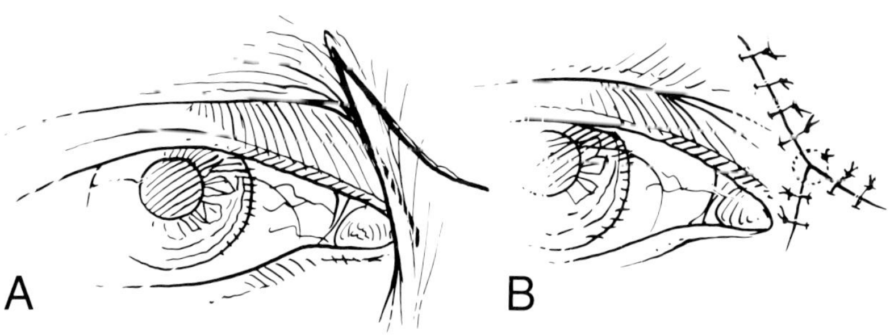

Fig. 40-8. V–Y flap in epicanthal–pseudoepicanthal fold repair. **(A)** Apex oriented superiorly in upper lid problem. **(B)** Flap advanced in Y.

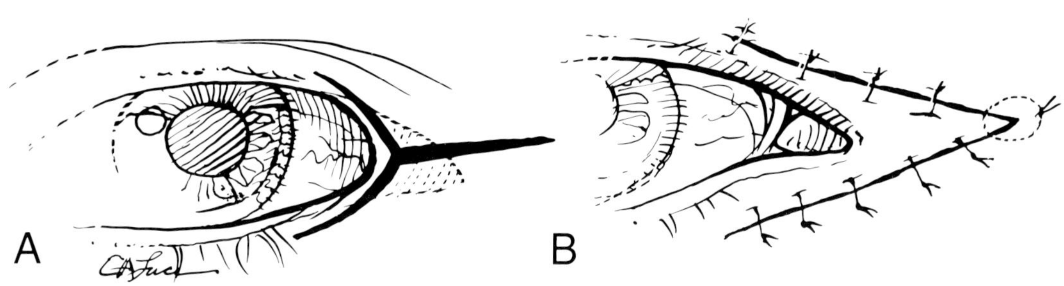

Fig. 40-9. Shortening medial canthus with Y–V flap. **(A)** Y incision. **(B)** V-flap closure.

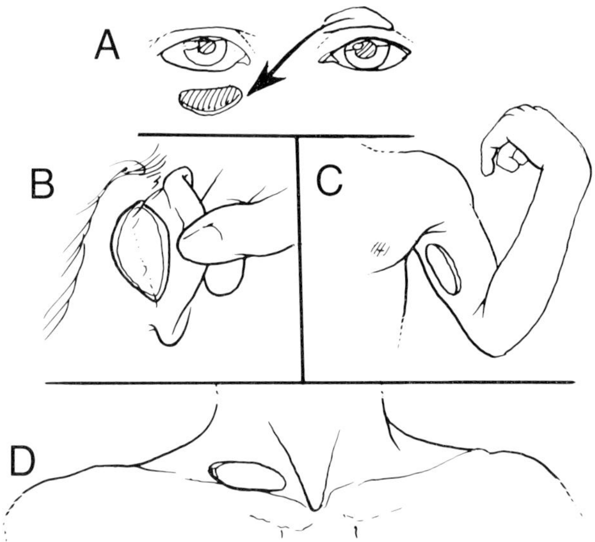

Fig. 40-10. Donor sites of eyelid–canthal grafts. **(A)** Upper eyelid. **(B)** Postauricular. **(C)** Inner upper arm. **(D)** Supraclavicular.

Donor Sites

The best site for replacement of eyelid skin is the opposite upper eyelid (Fig. 40-10A). Lower lid skin also provides an excellent match but is seldom available in adequate amount. When sufficient donor eyelid skin is not available, grafts are harvested from the postauricular, inner upper arm, and supraclavicular areas (Fig. 40-10B–D). For the best cosmetic result, a graft from these areas should be meticulously thinnned until part of the dermis has been removed. These same areas are also good donor sources for grafts to the canthi, paranasal, and temporal areas.

Graft Placement

A full-thickness skin graft contracts very little when maintained on some stretch during the healing period. A graft to an upper eyelid can usually be tailored to fit the size of the defect that is present when the eyelid is closed. A graft to the lower lid should have the same horizontal dimension as the

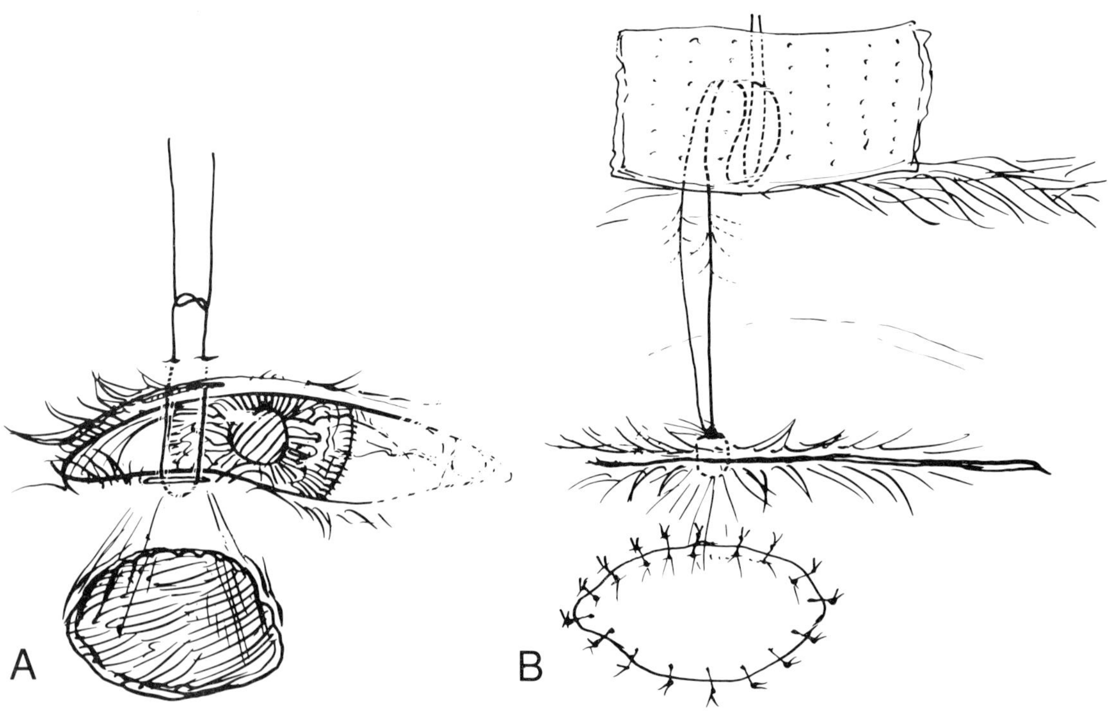

Fig. 40-11. Graft placement. **(A)** Defect vertically elongated with traction suture. **(B)** Intermarginal traction suture postoperatively.

defect. The appropriate vertical dimension is determined, to some extent, by the amount of tension in the tissue around the graft site. Usually, if the margin of the lower lid is elevated about 6 mm with a traction suture, the graft can be cut to the size of the resulting defect (Fig. 40-11 A). If a graft is too large, it will contract, and the surface will become wrinkled. In most cases, the eyelids should be immobilized and the grafts maintained on a gentle stretch for 7 to 10 days (Fig. 40-11B). Vertical traction sutures are particularly important to the success of a lower lid graft.

Contact between the graft and the recipient bed is obtained with a soft bolster. Many surgeons accomplish this by leaving long ends on every other suture used to secure the graft in place. These suture ends are then tied over the bolster. I do not use tieover sutures, but secure the bolster with tape. A Telfa pad or equivalent is first placed over the graft, and a segment of an eyepad is cut to the size of the graft and taped over the Telfa. Supplemental pressure is provided by two eyepads taped over the graft and eyelid area. This dressing is not changed for 5 days.

MEDIAL CANTHUS

The medial canthus is the second most common site of basal cell carcinoma in the eyelid area[36]; the recurrence rate after tumor resection is quite high. In most cases, this is probably because the excision of the original tumor was limited by the surgeon's fear of damaging the lacrimal drainage system. An inadequately treated medial canthal basal cell has a lethal potential, as it can readily invade the sinuses, nasopharynx, and cranial cavity.[37]

TREATMENT OF MEDIAL CANTHAL TUMORS

Irradiation is not recommended for treatment of medial canthal malignant epithelioma, especially when it is a morpheaform basal cell carcinoma.[38]

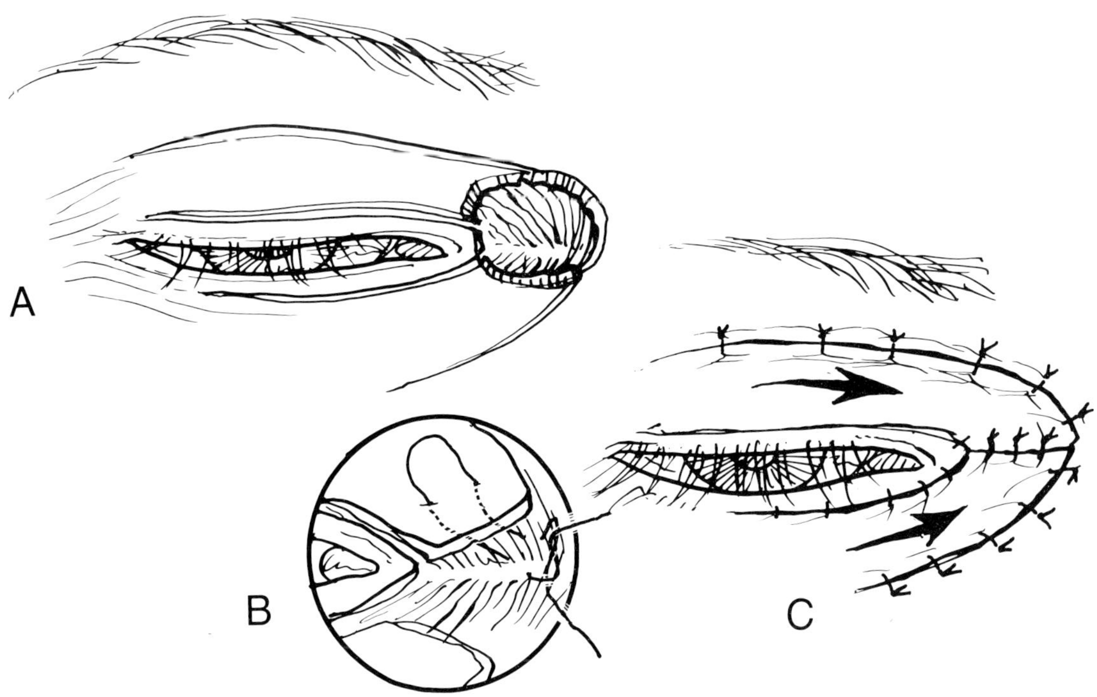

Fig. 40-12. Advancement flap reconstruction of medial canthus. **(A)** Flaps developed in upper and lower lids. **(B,C)** Flaps anchored into medial canthus.

Such tumors require thorough surgical excision. The extent of the tumor is determined by free strip-margin histologic frozen sections[39,40] or by Moh's fresh tissue-mapping technique.[43]

Laissez-Faire Treatment

A medial canthal defect may be permitted to heal by spontaneous granulation.[42,43] Depending on the defect size, this process requires 2 to 3 months and frequently produces a relatively normal-appearing skin surface. The advantages of this method are that it reduces the operative time and requires no reconstructive skills. The disadvantages are the tendency of the medial canthus to become displaced by the granulation process and the length of time required for healing.

Reconstruction with Flaps and Grafts

In a mature adult, there is frequently sufficient tissue laxity to permit reconstruction of a medial canthal defect with eyelid advancement flaps. At times, part of the defect may be closed with a flap and the remainder covered with a graft or by granulation. Advancement flaps can be developed from both upper and lower lids[44] (Fig. 40-12A–C). When the eyelid tissue is not lax, a skin graft tends to be a simpler method of reconstruction than flaps.

A forehead or glabellar flap can be used to reconstruct medial canthal defects.[45] On the basis of some problem cases seen in consultation, I believe that thick flaps of this type should be used with great caution following resection of a malignancy. The early signs of recurrence of the tumor are not detectable beneath these flaps, with potentially disastrous consequences. I have not found it difficult to reconstruct medial canthal defects satisfactorily without the use of forehead flaps.

MANAGEMENT OF EPICANTHAL AND PSEUDOEPICANTHAL FOLDS

Congenital epicanthal folds can be reconstructed, when necessary, by means of a V–Y-plasty or a V–W-plasty.[46] The medial canthal area is also predilected to the postoperative development of a pseudoepicanthal fold (bowstring). This vertical traction band commonly occurs following an upper lid blepharoplasty when excess skin has been excised or when the excision was more medial than is customary. It is especially common after correction of the patient with loose medial canthal skin. This can sometimes be prevented in the predilected patient by anchoring loose skin and muscle to the deep fascia of the medial canthus with 7-0 Vicryl suture or closing the medial area with a W-plasty. Another approach is to relieve epicanthal tension at the time of primary surgery by advancing the eyelid skin nasally and fixating it there with lid crease sutures. An established pseudoepicanthal fold should be intensively massaged and stretched for several months. Local steroid injections may also be indicated if hypertrophic scarring develops (see Chapter 41). If this does not resolve the problem, a V–Y-plasty can be done. In the upper lid, the apex of the V is placed at the superotemporal end of the elevated fold (Fig. 40-8A). After the skin incisions have been made, the skin is freed from the underlying tissue and repositioned into the medial canthus and a Y closure done (Fig. 40-8B). When the problem is severe, Z-plasties or a skin graft may be required.

LATERAL CANTHUS

When the tissues are lax, most lateral canthal defects can be rather easily reconstructed with advancement flaps from above and below the defect. The tissue should be closed in layers to prevent widening of the incision. When simple advancement flap closure is not possible, a rhombic flap or a skin graft may be used.

REFERENCES

1. von Graefe CF: Rhinoplastik. Reimer, Berlin, 1818
2. Fricke JCG: Die Bildung neuer Augenlider (Blepharoplastick). Perthes und Besser, Hamburg, 1829
3. Dieffenbach JF: Die operative Chirurgie. FA Brockhaus, Leipzig, 1845
4. Blasius E: Beitrage zur praktischen Chirurgie. A Forstner, Berlin, 1848

5. Horner WE: Clinical report on the surgical department of the Philadelphia Hospital. Am J Med Sci 21:99, 1837
6. Burow CA: Zur Blepharoplastik. Monatsschr Med Augenheilkd Chir 1:57, 1838
7. Tenzel RR: Treatment of lagophthalmos of the lower lid. Arch Ophthalmol 81:366, 1969
8. Borges AF: Relaxed skin tension lines (RSTL) versus other skin lines. Plastic Reconstr Surg 73:1, 1984
9. Burow, CA: Beschriebung einer neuen Transplantations Methode. Albert Nauck, Berlin, 1855
10. Harii K, Ohmori K, Ohmori S: Successful clinical transfer of ten free flaps by microvascular anastomoses. Plast Reconstr Surg 53:259, 1974
11. Harii K, Ohmori K, Sekiguchi J: The free musculocutoneous flap. Plast Reconstr Surg 57:259, 1976
12. McGregor IA: Fundamental Techniques of Plastic Surgery. Churchill Livingstone, Edinburgh, 1980
13. Converse JM: Reconstructive Plastic Surgery. Vol. I. WB Saunders, Philadelphia, 1977
14. Myers MB, Combs B, Cohen G: Wound tension and wound sloughs: A negative correlation. Am J Surg 100:711, 1965
15. Smith B, Cherubini TD: Oculoplastic Surgery. CV Mosby, St. Louis, 1970
16. Gibson T, Kenedi RM: The structural components of the dermis. p. 19. In Montagna W, Bentley JP, Dobson RL (eds): The Dermis. Appleton-Century-Crofts, East Norwalk, CT, 1970
17. Austad ED, Pasyk KA, McClatchey KD, Cherry GW: Histomorphologic evaluation of guinea pig skin and soft tissue after controlled tissue expansion. Plast Reconstr Surg 70:704, 1982
18. Cherry GW, Austad E, Pasyk K, et al: Increased survival and vascularity of random-pattern skin flaps elevated in controlled, expanded skin. Plast Reconstr Surg 72:680, 1984
19. Neumann CG: The expansion of an area of skin by progressive distension of a subcutaneous balloon. Plast Reconstr Surg 19:124, 1957
20. Radovan C: Development of adjacent flaps using a temporary expander. Plast Surg Forum 2:62, 1979
21. Radovan C: Tissue Expansion in soft-tissue reconstruction. Plast. Reconstr Surg 74:482, 1984
22. Tenzel RR: Reconstruction of the central one half of an eyelid. Arch Ophthalmol 93:125, 1975
23. Mustarde JC: Repair and Reconstruction in the Orbital Region. 2nd ed. Churchill Livingstone, Edinburgh, 1980
24. Bullock JD, Koss N, Flagg SV: Rhomboid flap in ophthalmic plastic surgery. Arch Ophthalmol 90:203, 1973
25. Limberg AA: Mathematical Principles of Local Plastic Procedures on the Surface of the Human Body. Megiz, Leningrad, 1946
26. Lister GD, Gibson T: Closure of rhomboid skin defects: The flaps of Limberg and Dufourmentel. Br J Plast Surg 25:300, 1972
27. Bullock JD, Hamdi B: Double rhomboid flap in ophthalmic plastic surgery. Ophthalmic Surg 11:431, 1980
28. Manchot C: Die Hautarterien des menschlichen Korpers. Vogel, Leipzig, 1889
29. Converse JM: Kazanjian and Converse's Surgical Treatment of Facial Injuries. Vol. 1. 3rd ed. Williams & Wilkins, Baltimore, 1974
30. Esser JF: Studies in plastic surgery of the face. I. Use of skin from the neck to replace face defects. II. Plastic operations about the mouth. III. The epidermic inlay. Ann Surg 65:297, 1917
31. Kubacek V: Transposition flaps on the face on a subcutaneous pedicle. Acta Chir Plast 2:108, 1960
32. Barron JN, Emmett AJJ: Subcutaneous pedicle flaps. Br J Plast Surg 18:51, 1965
33. Emmett AJJ: The closure of defects by using adjacent triangular flaps with subcutaneous pedicles. Plast Reconstr Surg 59:45, 1977
34. Stephenson CM: Reconstruction of the eyelid using a myocutaneous island flap. Ophthalmology 90:1060, 1983
35. Roggendorf E: The planimetric Z-plasty. Plast Reconstr Surg 71:834, 1983
36. Reese AB: Tumors of the Eye. 3rd ed. Harper & Row, New York, 1976
37. Collin JRO: Basal cell carcinoma in the eyelid region. Br J Ophthalmol 60:806, 1976
38. Wiggs EO: Morphea-form basal cell carcinoma of the canthi. Trans Am Acad Ophthalmol Otolaryngol 79:649, 1975
39. Older JJ, Quickert MH, Beard C: Surgical removal of basal cell carcinoma of the eyelids utilizing frozen section control. Trans Am Acad Ophthalmol Otolaryngol 79:658, 1975
40. Chalfin J, Putterman AM: Frozen section control in the surgery of basal cell carcinoma of the eyelid. Am J Ophthalmol 87:802, 1979
41. Mohs FE: Prevention and treatment of skin cancer. Wisc Med J 73:85, 1974
42. Fox SF, Beard C: Spontaneous lid repair. Am J Ophthalmol 58:947, 1964
43. Fier RH, Older JJ: Spontaneous repair of the medial canthus after removal of basal cell carcinoma. Ophthalmol Surg 13:737, 1982
44. Anderson RL, Edward JJ: Reconstruction by myocutaneous eyelid flaps. Arch Ophthalmol 97:2358, 1979
45. Mustarde JC: Repair and reconstruction in the orbital region. Churchill Livingstone, Edinburgh, 1966
46. Flowers RS: Surgical treatment of the epicanthal fold. Plast Reconstr Surg 73:571, 1984

Prevention and Management of Cutaneous Scarring

41

Charles M. Stephenson, Sr.

It is important to explain to the patient preoperatively that some scar formation is unavoidable and is an intrinsic part of the healing process of any wound. Many factors affect the final appearance of a scar, including the age of the patient, genetic predisposition to scar formation, location of scar, axial position of scar in relationship to natural skin patterns, precision of alignment of wound margins, tension on repaired wound, motion in wound, and presence or absence of infection, necrosis, and foreign body.[1] A consideration of these factors will aid in planning and performing the surgery. It will also assist in counseling the patient as to the expected final result.

AGE OF PATIENT

A healing skin wound in a young person usually has more visible scar formation at any given time after repair than does a comparable wound in an older person. There is greater skin elasticity in the young, and this creates higher wound tension.[2] In adults it is usually best to wait about 1 year before making a determination as to the necessity of scar revision. In a child, a scar may need to mature for 2 or 3 years before this decision can be made.

LOCATION

Repaired skin wounds in different areas about the eyes have varying propensities to visible scar formation. For example, a well-positioned and carefully closed defect in the thin skin of the eyelids tends to heal with less visibility than does a comparable one in the thicker skin of the forehead and cheek. In a young person, even a well-repaired wound in the lateral canthus tends to widen and remain conspicuous, whereas a well-repaired defect in an adult usually heals with minimum visibility. The closing of defects in the medial canthal area has a unique tendency to form an elevated scar called a pseudoepicanthal fold or bowstring (see Chapter 40).

ALIGNMENT OF SCAR IN RELATIONSHIP TO NATURAL SKIN PATTERNS

The axial position of a wound in relationship to the natural patterns in the skin is a most important factor in determining the final appearance of the wound. An incision or other wound lying parallel with these *lines of election* will form a much less conspicuous scar than one oriented at an angle to them.[3] Langer's early description (1861) of these natural skin patterns was based on cadaver studies.[4] It is now recognized that his representation is not entirely accurate when extrapolated to the living body. A more valid pattern is based on the relaxed skin tension lines (Fig. 41-1). These lines are coincident with the direction of the maximum tension in the skin when the musculature is relaxed and there is minimal skin distention by the underlying bony skeleton. In an adult, these preferred skin incision lines frequently, but not always, coincide with wrinkle lines. They can be determined by pinching the skin in different directions and observing the furrows that form. The furrows develop with greater ease and extend for a greater distance in the axis of the relaxed skin tension lines.[5] These lines lie in the horizontal axis in the eyelids and lateral canthus. They are oriented vertically in the medial canthus, gradually changing to the horizontal axis as the medial canthus merges with the eyelids (see Fig. 41-1). When a defect does not parallel these lines, it is desirable, when possible, to reorient the final closure so that it will be more consonant with them.

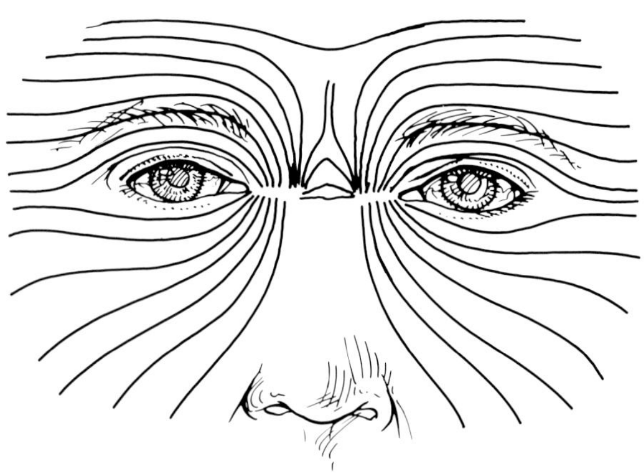

Fig. 41-1. Relaxed skin tension lines in the periocular skin.

CONDITION OF WOUND

Anything that delays the healing of a wound promotes an increase in scar formation. This includes the presence of foreign material, infection, tissue necrosis, and hematoma. A dirty wound should be thoroughly irrigated with saline solution and all possible foreign matter removed with meticulous care. Sharp dissection should be used to remove pigmented material that might otherwise permanently tattoo the skin. Eyelid tissue, even when severely traumatized, can usually be conserved and incorporated into the repair. The excellent blood supply to this area inhibits the development of infection and facilitates the survival of apparently devitalized tissue.

HEMATOMA

A persistent hematoma interferes with wound healing and increases scar formation. If not properly managed, this can induce ptosis, ectropion, or other eyelid malposition. Several precautions may be taken to reduce the incidence of hematoma formation. The patient should take no aspirin for 10 days prior to elective surgery. Ten or 15 minutes before an incision is made, the site should be injected with a solution containing epinephrine. Bleeding at surgery is carefully controlled with cautery and temporary local pressure. The patient should remain quiet after surgery, with the head elevated and an ice pack in place.

If a hematoma should develop immediately after

surgery, local pressure is applied for 5 to 10 minutes. If the hematoma continues to enlarge, the wound should be reopened and the bleeding controlled with cautery, if possible. After bleeding has stopped, firm pressure is briefly applied to the hematoma to express accumulated blood from the tissue. If some bleeding persists, a small drain is used for 1 or 2 days.

If the hematoma is first observed a day or more after surgery, I usually defer treatment for about 10 days. If the hematoma has not sufficiently absorbed in that time, it will have begun to liquefy and can be partially aspirated with an 18-gauge needle. If the aspiration does not adequately diminish the hematoma, the wound should be opened and the clots removed with small bayonet forceps.

WOUND CLOSURE

The technique used in repairing a wound obviously has a major effect on its final appearance. In order to secure the least visible scar, a wound must be approximated with precision, and there must be minimum tension and motion in the healing wound. The least scar reaction is caused by use of the finest suture materials that are strong enough to do the job. A synthetic absorbable suture, such as Vicryl (Ethicon) or Dexon (Davis & Geck), provides more strength and causes less reaction than does gut when used to close the deep layers of a wound. Sutures of 6-0, and occasionally 5-0, are appropriate for this purpose.

For skin closure, silk is the easiest material to work with. An extra-fast-absorbing 5-0 and 6-0 plain gut suture (Ethicon 1915G and 1916G) has recently been marketed. It falls out spontaneously within a few days and, reportedly causing minimal reaction. It is recommended for skin closures in infants, small children, and others in whom removal of sutures is not feasible. Nylon and prolene (polypropylene) cause less tissue reaction and probably have less tendency to cause suture tract cysts. They are generally preferable when a skin suture must be left in place for more than 3 or 4 days. Because of its ease of removal, prolene is especially suitable for use as a running subcuticular suture.

Interrupted 7-0 silk sutures are commonly used in careful skin closures in the eyelids (Fig. 41-2A). A running suture may be used, however, when the skin edges readily fall together in near-perfect alignment (Fig. 41-2B). Sutures should be placed equidistant from each skin margin to deter one margin from overriding the other. They should be tied with no more tension than required to approximate the tissues. Excessively tight sutures cause pressure necrosis and scarring. Sutures in eyelid skin should be removed within 3 or 4 days, if possible, to preclude the development of suture tract cysts and stitchmarks.

I frequently include 7-0 silk wipeoff sutures[6] in the skin closures in the periocular area (Fig. 41-2C). These sutures are placed very close to the skin margins and tied so tightly that they will either erode through and be wiped off or spontaneously fall off within 3 to 7 days. The special merits of these sutures are that they provide absolutely accurate skin approximation, need not be removed, and do not cause suture track cysts. To work properly, this stitch must be placed as close as possible to the wound margins.

In the forehead and cheek, a deep incision or other wound should always be repaired in layers to prevent development of a depressed or spreading scar. The subcutaneous layer is closed with interrupted 5-0 or 6-0 synthetic absorbable sutures, such as Vicryl or Dexon. A subcutaneous horizontal mattress stitch is effective for the deep closure of gaping forehead wounds (Fig. 41-2D). Subdermal and intradermal sutures may also be required to ensure that no tension is present in the skin closure line. Nylon, prolene, or silk suture (6-0) are used for skin closure in the cheek, lateral canthus, and eyebrow areas; nylon or prolene is preferred when the sutures must be left in place for more than 3 or 4 days. To prevent inversion of the skin edges and to close dead space, skin sutures in these areas should be passed outward from the perpendicular, so that the deep segment encompassed by the suture is wider than the superficial segment (Fig. 41-2E). When necessary to ensure eversion of the wound

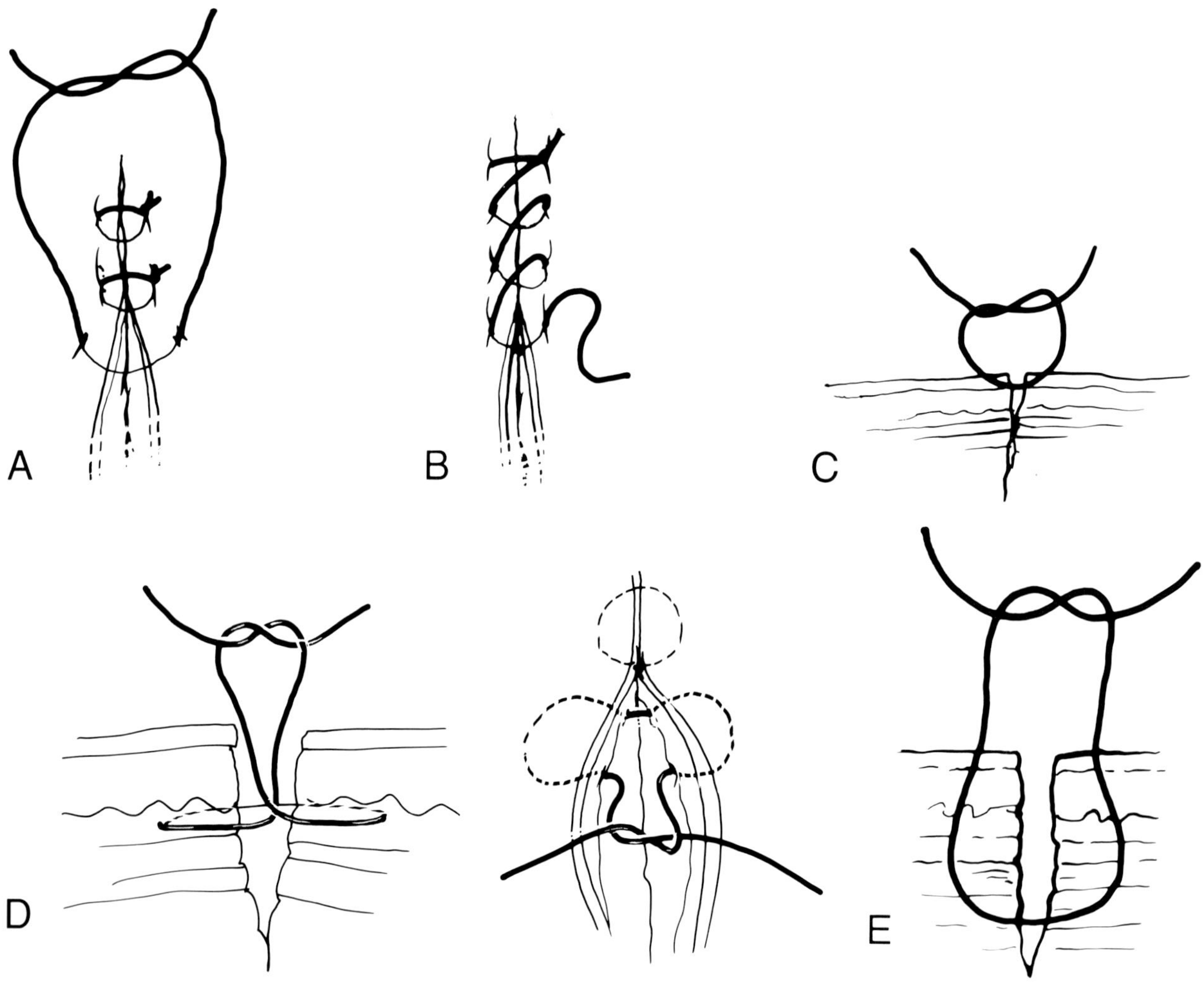

Fig. 41-2 (A–G). Methods of wound closure. **(A)** Interrupted sutures. **(B)** Running suture. **(C)** Wipeoff suture. **(D)** Horizontal mattress suture. **(E)** Deep suture to close dead space. *(Figure continues.)*

margins and relieve tension, vertical mattress sutures (Fig. 41-2F) can be alternated with simple skin-closure sutures. The near-far–far-near suture is also excellent for relieving tension on the wound margins.[7] (Fig. 41-2G).

An eyelid laceration that incises the orbicularis parallel with its muscle fibers does not usually require repair of the muscle and can usually be closed with skin sutures alone. For a laceration that divides the orbicularis transversely, the muscle should be repaired with 6-0 or 7-0 synthetic absorbable sutures.

TYPES OF SCARS: PHYSIOLOGIC AND PATHOLOGIC

Physiologic Scars

There are two types of healing processes. One is a normal physiologic development, the final scar product of which results from a combination of the factors previously discussed. The visible scar in

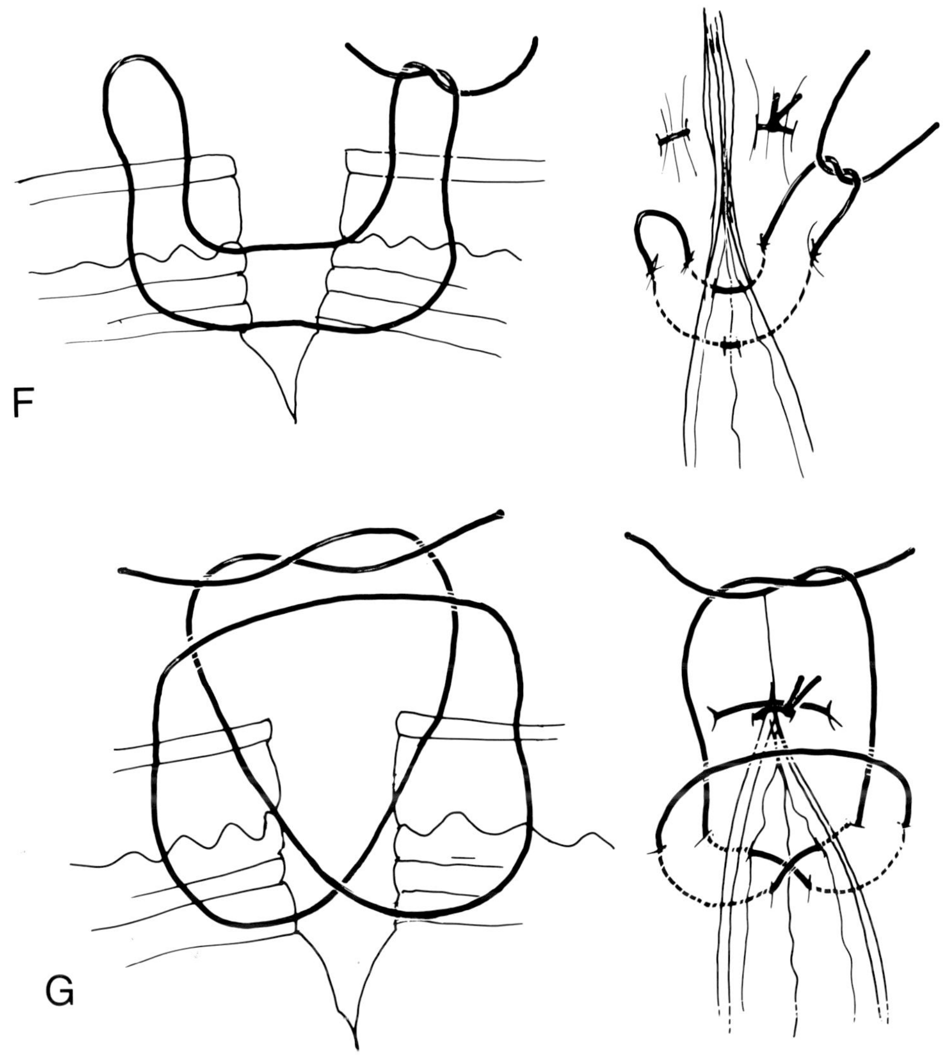

Fig. 41-2 *(Continued).* **(F)** Vertical mattress suture. **(G)** Near-far–far-near suture.

physiologic healing usually improves with time and massage. Massage may be commenced about 1 month after wound closure and can markedly improve the final appearance of the scar.

If a scar does not begin to improve satisfactorily within 6 to 8 weeks, one should consider intralesional injection of the corticosteroid, triamcinolone acetonide. Corticosteroids inhibit collagen synthesis,[8] and are more effective when used before extensive fibrosis has developed. It is my preference to inject lidocaine, 1 percent, beneath the scar after outlining the area to be treated with a marking pen. Triamcinolone, 40 mg/ml, is injected into the scar with a 30-gauge needle on a tuberculin syringe. A volume of 0.1 to 0.3 ml will usually suffice in small scars in the periocular area. Definite resistance should be felt during injection into the dense scar tissue. Undesirable atrophy and depigmentation may occur if corticosteroids are inadvertently injected into surrounding normal tissue.[9] Several injections may be required, at 3- to 4-week intervals.

Corticosteroids may also be instilled without a needle using a device that impregnates the medication under pressure (DermoJet, Robbins Instruments, Inc., Chatham, NJ). The advantage of this method is that the treatment is less painful and does not require a local anesthetic. A possible disadvantage is that the dose delivered and the distribution pattern vary somewhat with the density of the scar.[10]

It is usually best to wait about 1 year in an adult before making a determination as to the necessity of scar revision. In a normal physiologic scar, simple re-excision and skillful wound closure are frequently all that are required for a satisfactory result. If there are cicatrizing elements in the scar that are distorting the adjacent anatomy, it may be necessary to use special procedures, such as Z-plasty, V-Y plasty, or skin graft (see Chapter 40).

A rough irregularly elevated mature scar in the cheek or forehead may be improved by dermabrasion. This procedure can actually increase scarring, however, if used in the thin eyelid skin, where there are no pilosebaceous structures in the dermis.[11] Dermabrasion should also not be used on skin that has been devitalized by irradiation or infection.

Pathologic Scars

Hypertrophic scarring or keloid formation is a pathologic healing process that generally fails to improve with time and massage. It does not commonly occur in the eyelid area. The term *keloid* was coined by the French dermatologist Jean Alibert (1816)[12] and derives from the Greek word for claw (of a crustacean). Clinically, keloidal scars are elevated, hard, irregular, and frequently pruritic. Traditionally, they were considered to be distinct from hypertrophic scars. A keloid was defined as a scar that invaded beyond the margins of the original wound, showed more histologic disorganization, and had a greater tendency to recur.[13] As research in cell biology and immunology has demonstrated more about this phenomenon, it appears probable that keloids and hypertrophic scars are a continuum that represent different stages of the same abnormal healing process.[14]

Hypertrophic scars/keloids occur when there is an aberration in the normal wound healing of the dermis, and the process becomes arrested in the proliferative phase.[15] Recent immunofluorescent antibody studies[16] support previous findings[17] that the underlying pathogenesis in hypertrophic scarring involves a localized immune response. The histologic picture is that of an excess of hyalinized collagen bundles, fibroblasts, and blood vessels.[18] Each fibroblast in a hypertrophic scar has been shown to synthesize two to three times more collagen than does a normal fibroblast.[19] There are also increased numbers of mast cells and histamines. These cause abnormal vasodilation and protein release that enhance the hyperplasia.[20] Experimental attempts to inhibit this process with antihistamines have been inconclusive.[21]

There is evidence of a hereditary predisposition to hypertrophic scars/keloids. It is more likely to occur in some black family groups.[22,23] The tendency to hypertrophic scar formation is not constant throughout life[24] but has the highest incidence occurring during preadolescence and adolescence.[25] Keloids are predilected to the sternum, neck, upper limbs, and face.[26] An authentic keloid/hypertrophic scar probably does not develop in the very thin skin of the eyelids. It sometimes occurs in the transition area between eyelids and cheek, forehead, and nose. When a prominent scar develops in the eyelids, it is unlikely to be caused by a pathologic scar process. It is usually caused by interference with the normal healing process, such as an embedded foreign body, inversion of wound margin, tension in wound, or healing by granulation after wound separation.

The fundamental treatment of hypertrophic keloid/scars is the intralesional injection of triamcinolone acetonide. Steroids are less inhibitory of collagen synthesis in keloidal tissue, however, than in a scar in the normal dermis.[27] If several steroid instillations at 3- to 4-week intervals fail to involute a hypertrophic scar, surgical excision may be considered. It is especially important that a wound repair after hypertrophic scar excision be free of tension. It should also parallel the natural lines of election in the skin, if possible. Triamcinolone should be injected into the dermis of the wound edges immediately after a secondary scar resection, and at 3- to 4-week intervals thereafter, as the clinical course dictates.[28]

Because of concern over possible long-term adverse effects, the treatment of hypertrophic scars exclusively by irradiation is probably less common now than in the past. Low-dose radiation may be helpful, however, as an adjunct after surgical revision of such a scar.[29] Hypertrophic scars have also been treated by freezing,[30] constant controlled pressure,[31] topical application of retinoic acid,[32] and methotrexate.[33]

REFERENCES

1. McGregor IA: Fundamental Techniques of Plastic Surgery. 7th Ed. Churchill Livingstone, Edinburgh, 1980
2. Converse JM (ed): Reconstructive Plastic Surgery. Vol. 1. WB Saunders, Philadelphia, 1977
3. Cox HT: The cleavage lines of skin. Br J Surg 29:234, 1941
4. Gibson T: Karl Langer and his lines. Br J Plast Surg 31:3, 1978
5. Borges AF: Relaxed skin tension lines (RSTL) versus other skin lines. Plast Reconstruct Surg 73:1, 1984
6. Beard C: Ptosis. CV Mosby, St. Louis, 1976
7. Smith, B, Cherubini TD: Oculoplastic Surgery. CV Mosby, St. Louis, 1970
8. Cohen IK: The biology of keloid and hypertrophic scar and corticosteroid. Clin Plast Surg 4:297, 1977
9. Abdel-Fattah AM: Unusual complications of triamcinolone injected keloids: Tissue necrosis and systemic corticosteroid effect. Br J Plast Surg 29:283, 1976
10. Berry RB: A comparison of CO_2 powered needleless injectors in the treatment of keloids and triamcinolone. Br J Plast Surg 34:458, 1981
11. Rees TD: Aesthetic Plastic Surgery. Vol. II. WB Saunders, Philadelphia, 1980
12. Alibert JL: Note sur la kéloide. J Univ Sci Med 2:207, 1816
13. Blackburn WR, Cosman B: Histologic basis of keloid and hypertrophic scar differentiation. Arch Pathol Lab Med 82:65, 1966
14. Lee CP: Keloids—Their epidemiology and treatment. Int J Dermatol 21:504, 1982
15. Bornstern P, Sage H: Structurally distinct collagen types. Annu Rev Biochem 49:957, 1980
16. Kischer CW, Shetlar MR, Shetlar MS, Chvapil M: Immunoglobulins in hypertrophic scars and keloids. Plast Reconstr Surg 71:821, 1983
17. Cohen IK, McCoy BJ, Mohanakumar T, Diegelmann RF: Immunoglobulin, complement, and histocompatibility antigen studies in keloid patient. Plast Reconstr Surg 63:689, 1979
18. Soderberg T: Treatment of keloids and hypertrophic scars with adhesive zinc tape. Scand J Plast Reconstr Surg 16:261, 1982
19. Cohen IK, Diegelmann RF, McCoy B: Elevated collagen synthesis in cultural keloid fibroblasts. Surg Forum 28:526, 1977
20. Kischer CW, Bunce H III, Shetlar MR: Mast cell analyses in hypertrophic scars, hypertrophic scars treated with pressure and mature scars. J Invest Dermatol 70:355, 1978
21. Topol BM, Lewis VL Jr, Benveniste K: The use of antihistamine to retard the growth of fibroblasts derived from human skin scar, and keloid. Plast Reconstr Surg 68:231, 1981
22. Barrett JL: Keloids. P. 553. In Bergsma D (ed): Birth Defects: Atlas and Compendium. Williams & Wilkins, Baltimore, 1973
23. Bloom D: Heredity of keloids, review of the literature. NY State J Med 56:511, 1956
24. Lee CP: Keloids—Their epidemiology and treatment. Int J Dermatol 21:504, 1982
25. Cosman B, Crikelair GF, Gaulin JC, Lattes R: The surgical treatment of keloids. Plast Reconstr Surg 27:335, 1961
26. Tempest MN: Hypertrophic scarring and keloids. p. 80. In Tropical Surgery. Schwartz SI, et al. (eds): McGraw-Hill, New York, 1971
27. Russell JD, Shirley B, Trupiro KN: Fibroblast heterogeneity in glucocorticoid regulation of collagen metabolism: Genetic or epigenitic? In Vitro 18:557, 1982
28. Pollack S, Goslen JB: The surgical treatment of keloids. J Dermatol Surg Oncol 8:1045, 1982
29. Ollstein RN, Siegel H, Gillooley JF, Barsa JM: Treatment of keloids by combined surgical excision and immediate postoperative x-ray therapy. Ann Plast Surg 7: 181, 1981
30. Shepherd JP, Dawber RPR: The response of keloid scars to cryosurgery. Plast Reconstr Surg 70:677, 1982
31. Fujimori R, Hiramoto M, Ofuji S: Sponge fixation method for treatment of early scars. Plast Reconstr Surg 42:322, 1968
32. De Limpens J: The local treatment of hypertrophic scars and keloids with topical retinoic acid. Br J Dermatol 103:319, 1980
33. Onwukwe MF: Treating keloids by surgery and methotrexate. Arch Dermathol 116:158, 1980

42

Trichiasis and Distichiasis

John H. Sullivan

Any condition of the eyelids that causes cilia to contact the globe is generally referred to as trichiasis. In such circumstances, the eye displays conjunctival injection and the patient complains of the sensation of a foreign body. The inflammation resulting from chronic trichiasis may induce localized corneal vascularization and opacification. Aberrant eyelashes may create corneal epithelial defects and expose the patient to the risk of severe infection.

Specific categories of trichiasis can be identified. Entropion is easily distinguished by tarsal malposition and internal rotation of the lid margin. The pathogenesis and management of entropion is the subject of Chapter 35.

In epiblepharon the tarsus and lid margin are in normal alignment. Eyelashes are directed toward the cornea by an epicanthal skinfold in the medial aspect of the lower eyelid. It is most frequently observed in Oriental children. In these patients, spontaneous improvement usually occurs with maturation of the face at about 4 years of age. Management is further discussed in Chapter 37.

Distichiasis refers to a second row of eyelashes (*di:* "two"; *stichos:* "rows") posterior to the normal cilia. These accessory lashes are directed toward the cornea and often arise from the stomae of meibomian glands. In congenital distichiasis, the accessory cilia are often of normal size and form a single row. They usually occur in all four lids, although asymmetric involvement is frequent. The affliction is uncommon and may be transmitted as an autosomal dominant trait. It is sometimes associated with pitting edema of the lower extremities and mandibulofacial dysostosis.

Acquired distichiasis is much more common and is usually the result of chronic inflammatory lid disease. New cilia are usually generated from inflammatory metaplastic changes in the pilosebaceous units of the lid and conjunctiva. These cilia are irregularly spaced, short, of small caliber, and devoid of pigment. Occasionally in mucous membrane inflammatory disease, such as Stevens-Johnson syndrome and benign mucous membrane pemphigoid, the new cilia arise from a single row of meibomian glands, similar to congenital distichiasis.

Misdirected growth is the most common form of trichiasis. Most often found in a segment of the lower eyelids of elderly patients, it is sometimes accompanied by inflammatory metaplastic distichiasis. Chronic blepharitis, trauma, and previous lid surgery can be responsible. Scar formation within the lid misdirects the growth of the cilia toward the globe. The distinction between misdirected growth and entropion is blurred when cicatrization is sufficient to rotate the lid margin internally.

SURGICAL ANATOMY

The eyelashes are arranged in two or three irregular rows anterior to the intermarginal sulcus. The orifices of the meibomian glands lie posterior to this sulcus at the mucocutaneous junction. Eyelashes replace themselves every 100 to 150 days. Following epilation, a new shaft begins to grow within days, reaching full length in 70 days. The lash follicles are based 1.5 to 2.5 mm from their point of exit on the skin surface. The bulbs are often embedded on the outer surface of the tarsus immediately below the marginal arterial arcade.[1] The lash follicles of congenital distichiasis may sometimes be sufficiently posterior to the normal follicles to be separated surgically and selectively ablated. This is rarely possible in acquired distichiasis.

INDICATIONS FOR TREATMENT

Most patients with trichiasis are symptomatic and require treatment to provide comfort. Reduced corneal sensation from chronic trichiasis, especially in the elderly, may delay presentation of the patients for treatment until more serious complications arise. Caution is indicated in treating patients with active inflammatory mucous membrane disease, such as benign mucous membrane pemphigoid. In these cases, often an acute exacerbation develops following surgery or cryosurgery; marked conjunctival shrinkage and severe symblepharon with adhesion of the lids to the globe can result. When trichiasis is causing discomfort, however, cryosurgery is usually indicated. Pretreatment with systemic and topical corticosteroids or sulfones may be useful, but insufficient evidence exists to advocate this practice.

METHODS OF TREATMENT

Aberrant cilia are treated by either displacement or ablation. Eyelashes can be displaced from the cornea by soft contact lenses. Contact lenses are of limited use in the long-term management of trichiasis, however, because of mucus formation and lens dislocation. Ablation is most easily accomplished by epilation, but electrolysis offers a more permanent solution. The problem with electrolysis is frequent recurrence. Small-caliber cilia with long subcutaneous shafts are the most difficult to treat because of the technical difficulty of threading the hair shaft with an electrolysis needle. Scarring after electrolysis may deform the position of an adjacent lash. Galvanic current causes less scarring then does hyfercation and is therefore preferred when using electrolysis. Despite the high recurrence rate, electrolysis remains the best treatment when only a few lashes are involved and preservation of adjacent lashes is desirable.

Displacement of aberrant lashes by surgery has many variations (see Chapter 35). Tarsal fracture and wedge resection of the affected region are simple and useful operations. Interposition of mucous membrane, tarsoconjunctiva, or nasal septal cartilage can be very effective in displacing the lashes from the cornea.[2] These procedures are complex, however, and the functional and cosmetic results are often less than optimal. Recurrence of trichiasis is a common problem.

Cryosurgery is a simple, effective method of treatment suitable for most patients with trichiasis. It is easy to perform as an office procedure, and recurrence is rare.

RECOMMENDED TECHNIQUE

Cryosurgery is the preferred method of treating most cases of trichiasis. Liquid nitrogen or nitrous oxide can be used. The low boiling point (−196°C) of liquid nitrogen permits its use as a direct spray[3] or through a circulating probe, but with a higher risk of overtreatment.

Nitrous oxide can be stored in cylinders indefinitely but, because of its warmer boiling point (−95°C), must be used with a high-flow design cryoprobe.[4] Ophthalmic cryoprobes are inadequate. Cervical or rectal cryoprobes are satisfactory but cumbersome. Specially designed oculoplastic probes such as the Wallach LL-100 and MK 650 are both easy to use and effective.

Thermocouple monitoring of the freezing lesions is essential to avoid overtreatment and resultant cryonecrosis. Probe-tip geometry, surface-area contact, gas pressure, the blood supply to the lid, and other variables make propagation of the iceball somewhat unpredictable. However, errors in positioning or malfunction of the thermocouple require the ability to make a clinical judgment to determine the adequacy of the lesion. Lids with compromised vasculature may require and tolerate only 15 to 20 seconds of freezing. No treatment should be continued for more than 60 seconds.

Skin and conjunctiva are infiltrated with lidocaine; a microthermocouple is implanted beneath the skin close to the anterior surface of the tarsus, anterior to the lash follicles. The cryoprobe is positioned on the conjunctival surface and the iceball is generated through the follicles before being monitored (Fig. 42-1). In this way it is certain the follicles themselves have achieved the recorded temperature. The lid is frozen to −20°C, or a maximum of 60 seconds, and allowed to thaw spontaneously; the process is then repeated.

Antibiotic ointment and cold compresses are ap-

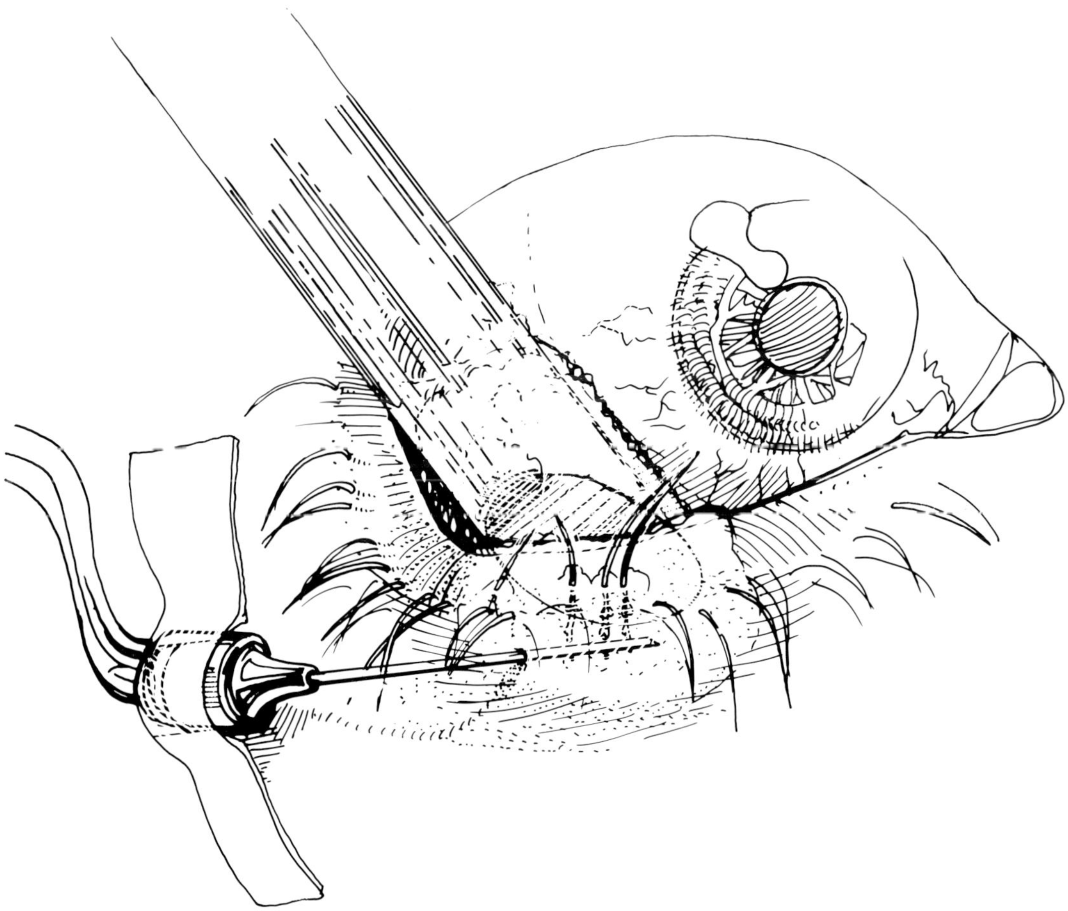

Fig. 42-1. Cryosurgery for trichiasis with thermocouple placed transcutaneously anterior to lash follicles and cryoprobe on conjunctival surface.

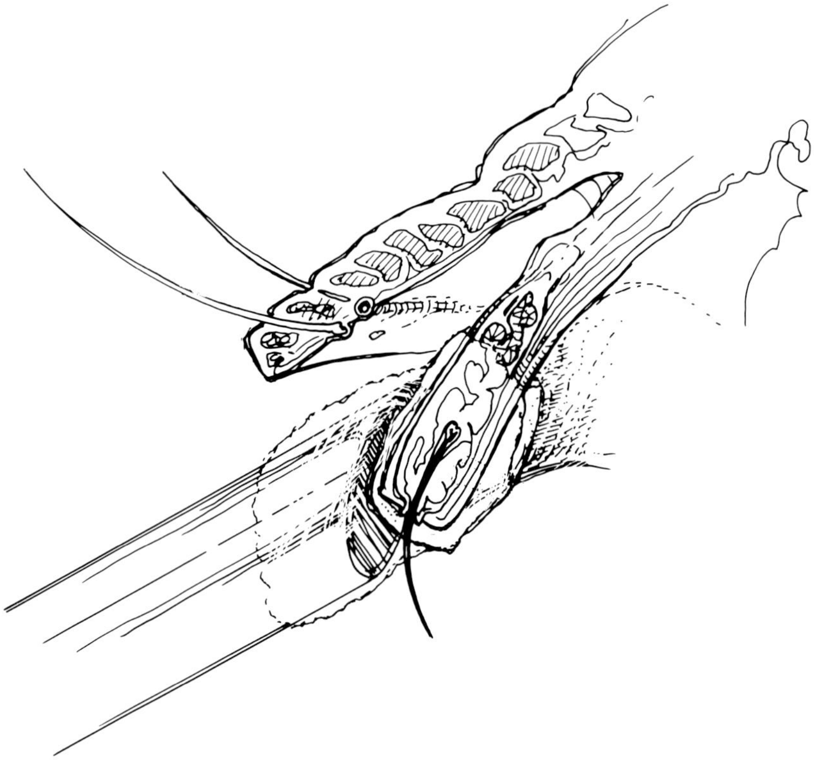

Fig. 42-2. Lid-splitting technique for treating congenital distichiasis with cryotherapy.

plied intermittently for several days until the swelling has subsided. In 3 to 4 days, if treatment has been successful, eyelashes can be epilated without resistance.

A technique in congenital distichiasis sometimes used to preserve the normal lashes involves surgically dividing the lid anterior to the distichiasis follicles (Fig. 42-2). The abnormal lashes are then selectively frozen with a double-cycle technique for 10 seconds, and the lid is closed with a running suture. Thermocouple monitoring is unnecessary because the thin layer of tissue freezes instantly to the temperature of the cryoprobe. The technique is usually effective in congenital distichiasis when the abnormal lashes arise from the meibomian gland. In acquired distichiasis, the follicles usually originate more anteriorly and cannot be surgically separated from the normal lashes (Fig. 42-2).

The thawing phase induces cellular necrosis.[5] The rapid-freeze technique leads to the formation of intracellular ice crystals that, when slowly thawed, undergo expansion through recrystalization. Cell destruction occurs as a result of this expansion and other complex biophysical factors. Certain tissues have a lower threshold for survival than do others. Hair follicles are relatively sensitive to the effects of freezing and thus can be ablated without major damage to surrounding tissue.

Because the cryogenic lesion spreads laterally and vertically with the same velocity, the minimum effective diameter of an adequate lesion, regardless of probe size, is about 4 mm. This limits the value of cryosurgery on individual lashes, especially in the upper lid, unless the patient is prepared to lose adjacent lashes as well.

PROGNOSIS AND COMPLICATIONS

Most patients exhibit significant swelling following cryosurgery of the eyelids. If multiple applications are required in a single sitting, the eyelids are likely to swell closed for 24 to 48 hours. Edema can extend into the cheek and lower face. Pain is common during the first few hours and uncommon after this period. The conjunctiva may exude discharge for several days. Periodic use of topical antibiotic ointment provides comfort and may prevent infection. Cold compresses help reduce swelling.

The swelling following cryosurgery may be mistaken for cellulitis, although such serious infection is rare. Lesser infections and overtreatment may result in segmental tissue destruction, with notching of the lid margin. This complication is more likely to occur when treating the elderly, who may have a poorer blood supply or diseased lids, such as those having been infected with trachoma.

Recurrence is the result of inadequate freezing. Normal cilia at the periphery of the cryosurgical lesion may become misdirected because of scarring. Retreatment of an area is possible but likely to cause further thinning of the lid. Overtreatment is characterized by permanent injection of the lid margin and pseudoepitheliomatous hypertrophy. Depigmentation of the skin can be anticipated and may be permanent even without overtreatment. This problem limits the clinical value of cryosurgery in darkly pigmented patients.

REFERENCES

1. Argyris TS: Wound healing and control of growth of skin. p. 231. In Montagna W, Billingham RE (eds): Advances in Biology of Skin. Vol 5: Wound Healing. Pergamon Press, New York, 1964
2. Fox SA: Ophthalmic Plastic Surgery. 4th ed. Grune & Stratton, Orlando, FL, 1970
3. Fraunfelder FT: Trichiasis. p. 375. In Fraunfelder FT, Roy HF (eds): Current Ocular Therapy. Vol. 2. WB Saunders, Philadelphia, 1985
4. Sullivan JH: The use of cryotherapy for trichiasis. Trans Am Acad Ophthalmol Otolaryngol 83:703, 1977
5. Farrant J: Cryobiology: The basis of cryosurgery. p. 15. In Von Leder H, Cahau WG (eds): Cryogenics in Surgery. Medical Examination Publishing Company, New Hyde Park, NY, 1971

Index

Page numbers followed by *f* refer to figures; those followed by *t* refer to tables.